ALLE ZEIT WACH
1842

Ciclosporin in Autoimmune Diseases

1st International Symposium, Basle, March 18–20, 1985

Editor: Rosemarie Schindler

With 149 Figures and 127 Tables

Springer-Verlag
Berlin Heidelberg New York Tokyo

Mrs. R. Schindler
Sandoz Ltd
Pharmaceutical Department
MPP/PAI, Journals and Monographs
CH-4002 Basle

ISBN-13:978-3-642-70609-7 e-ISBN-13:978-3-642-70607-3
DOI: 10.1007/978-3-642-70607-3

2329/3321.543210

Table of Contents

8. Hematology

9. Rheumatoid Arthritis

10. Glomerulonephritis and Systemic Lupus Erythematosus

Authors' addresses

Dr. Miriam Adhikari
Dept. of Paediatrics and Child Health
Faculty of Medicine, Univ. of Natal
P.O. Box 17039
Congella 4013 Durban
South Africa

Dr. Miles Allison
The Royal Free Hospital
Academic Dept. of Medicine
Pond Street
Hampstead
London NW3 2QG
England

Prof. Dr. Bernard Amor
Hôpital Cochin
7, rue du Faubourg Saint Jacques
F-75674 Paris Cedex 14

Prof. Dr. R. Assan
Service de Diabétologie
Hôpital Bichat
F-75018 Paris

Prof. Dr. J. F. Bach
Service d'Immunologie Clinique
INSERM U25 CNRS LA 122
Hôpital Necker
161, rue de Sèvres
F-75015 Paris

Prof. Dr. med. habil. B.-R. Balda
Dermatologische u. Allergologische Abteilung
Stenglinstrasse
D-8900 Augsburg

Dr. med. R. Bambauer
Abteilung für Nephrologie
der Medizinischen Universitätsklinik
D-6650 Homburg/Saar

Dr. H. Barthélémy
Clinique Dermatologique
Hôpital Edouard Herriot
F-69374 Lyon Cedex 08

Prof. J. R. Batchelor
University of London
Royal Postgraduate Medical School
Hammersmith Hospital
Ducane Road
London W12 OHS
England

Dr. K. Bendtzen
Department TA 7551
Rigshospitalet
Tasgensvej 20
DK-2200 Copenhagen N

David BenEzra, MD, PhD
Department of Ophthalmology
Hadassah University Hospital
P.O. Box 12000
91120 Jerusalem
Israel

Prof. Dr. U. Besinger
Neurologische Klinik und Poliklinik
der Technischen Universität München
Möhlstrasse 28
D-8000 München 80

Dr. R. Beukers
Academic Hospital
Dijkzigt Internal Medicine
Dr. Morleywaterplein 40
3002 Rotterdam
Netherlands

Dr. H. A. Bird
Clinical Pharmacology Unit
Royal Bath Hospital
Cornwall Road
Harrogate HG1 2PS
England

Dr. Claire Bombardier
420A Jones Building
Wellesley Hospital
160 Wellesley St. East
Toronto, Ontario M4Y 1J3
Canada

Prof. Dr. J.-F. Borel
Präklinische Forschung
Pharmazeutisches Department
SANDOZ AG
CH-4002 Basel

Cand. med. Michael Braida
Universitäts-Hautklinik Münster
von-Esmarch-Strasse 56
D-4400 Münster

Prof. Dr. J. Brodehl
Medizinische Hochschule
Kinderklinik
Abteilung Pädiatrische Nieren- u. Stoffwechselerkrankungen
Konstanty-Gutschow-Strasse
D-3000 Hannover

Dr. H. A. Capell
Centre for Rheumatic Diseases
Royal Infirmary
Glasgow G4 OSF
Scotland, GB

Dr. D. Cattran
Nephrology Service
Toronto General Hospital
Room 3/215 – College Wing
Toronto, Ontario M5G-JL7
Canada

Dr. Bertrand Coiffier
Service d'Hématologie, Pavillon H
Hôpital Edouard Herriot
5, place d'Arsonval
F-69374 Lyon Cedex 08

Dr. P. Deteix
Clinique de Néphrologie, Pavillon P
Hôpital Edouard Herriot
F-69374 Lyon Cedex 08

Dr. B. A. C. Dijkmans
Department of Rheumatology
University Hospital
Rijnsburgerweg 10
2333 AA Leiden
The Netherlands

Prof. Dr. D. Dommasch
Max Planck-Gesellschaft
Klinische Forschungsgruppe für multiple Sklerose
Postfach 6120
D-8700 Würzburg 1

Dr. J. Dupré
Dept. of Endocrinology
University Hospital
PB 5339, Postal Station A
London, Ontario N6A 5A5
Canada

Dr. G. Feutren
Service d'Immunologie clinique et
INSERM U25 CNRS LA 122
Hôpital Necker
161 rue de Sèvres
F-75015 Paris

Dr. Oystein Førre
Oslo Sanitets. Rheumatism Hosp.
University of Oslo
The National Hospital
Akersbakken 27
Oslo 1
Norway

Dr. B. von Graffenried
Klinische Forschung
Pharmazeutisches Departement
SANDOZ AG
CH-4002 Basel

Dr. E. Graham
St. Thomas Hospital
Dept. of Ophthalmology
Lambeth Palace Road
London SE1 7EH
England, GB

Dr. P. Halloran
Nephrology and Immunogenetics
Mount Sinai Hospital
6000 University Av., Suite 435
Toronto, Ontario M5G 1X5
Canada

Dr. med. Ch. R. Herzog
Klinik für Rheumatologie und Rehabilitation
Stadtspital Triemli
CH-8063 Zürich

PD Dr. P. Imbach
Universitätskinderklinik
Inselspital
CH-3010 Bern

Prof. P. Jacobs
Dept. of Haematology
University of Cape Town Medical School
Anzio Road
Observatory 7925
Cape Town
South Africa

Prof. J. R. Joubert
Dept. of Internal Medicine
University of Stellenbosch
P.O. Box 63
Tygerberg 7505
South Africa

Dr. A. Karlsson
Department of Internal Medicine
University Hospital
S-751 85 Uppsala

Dr. P. Keown
University Hospital
339 Windermere Road
London, Ontario N6A 5A5
Canada

Prof. Dr. med. J. Knop
Universitäts-Hautklinik
von-Esmarch-Str. 56
D-4400 Münster

Prof. Dr. P. Krupp
Klinische Forschung
Pharmazeutisches Departement
SANDOZ AG
CH-4002 Basel

Prof. Dr. R. Landgraf
Medizinische Klinik Innenstadt
der Universität München
Ziemssenstr. 1
D-8000 München 2

Dr. P. Le Hoang
Service d'Ophtalmologie
C.H.U. Pitié-Salpetrière
83, bd de l'hôpital
F-75013 Paris

Dr. M. R. Lucey
Liver Unit
King's College School of Medicine and Dentistry
Denmark Hill
London, SE5 8BX
England, GB

Dr. med. U. Marbet
Gastroenterologie
Dept. für Innere Medizin
Kantonsspital
CH-4031 Basel

Dr. Kanjiro Masuda
Dept. of Ophthalmology
Branch Hospital of Tokyo University
Mejirodai 3-86-6, Bunkyo-ku
Tokyo
Japan

Dr. A. M. McGregor
University of Wales
Welsh National School of Medicine
Dept. of Medicine
Heath Park
Cardiff CF4 4XN
Wales, GB

Prof. Dr. Alain Meyrier
Head, Nephrology and Hemodialysis Unit
Hôpital Avicenne
Route de Stalingrad
F-93000 Bobigny

Prof. Dr. P. A. Miescher
Hôpital Cantonal
Division d'Hématologie et
Centre de Transfusions
25, Rue Micheli-du-Crest
CH-1211 Genève 4

PD Dr. M. J. Mihatsch
Institut für Pathologie
Kantonsspital Basel
Schönbeinstrasse 40
CH-4003 Basel

Prof. Dr. Asuman Müftüoglu
Nisbetije Caddesi 2
Etiler
Istanbul
Turkey

Dr. J. Nerup
Steno Memorial Hospital
Niels Steensens Vej 2
DK-2820 Gentofte

Dr. J. Neuberger
King's College School
of Medicine and Dentistry
Liver Unit
Denmark Hill
London SE5 8RX
England, GB

Dr. R. B. Nussenblatt
Clinical Ophthalmic Immunology Section,
National Eye Institute, Clinical Branch, NIH,
9000 Rockville Pike
Building 10, Room 10D19
Bethesda, Maryland 20205
USA

Prof. Dr. R. Nyberg-Hansen
Department of Neurology
Rikshospitalet
The National Hospital
University of Oslo
Oslo 1
Norway

Prof. Dr. med. U. Patzold
Medizinische Hochschule
Neurologische Klinik
Karl-Wiechert-Allee 9
D-3000 Hannover 61

Prof. A. S. Rebuck
Toronto Western Hospital
Diversion of Respiratory Medicine
399 Bathurst Street
Suite 204, Edith Cavell Wing
Toronto, Ontario M5T 2S8
Canada

Prof. I. M. Roitt, F.R.S.
Department of Immunology
Arthur Stanley House
The Middlesex Hospital Medical School
40–50 Tottenham Street
London W1P 9PG
England

Dr. P. Rudge
Institute of Neurology
The National Hospital
Queen Square
London WC1 3BG
England

Prof. C. R. Stiller
University Hospital
339 Windermere Road
P.O. Box 5339, Station A
London, Ontario N6A 5A5
Canada

Prof. Dr. P. Stryckmans
Institut J. Bordet (ULB)
Rue Héger Bordet, 1
B-1000 Bruxelles

Dr. Karin Svenson
Section of Rheumatology
Department of Internal Medicine
University Hospital
S-751 85 Uppsala

Dozent Dr. med. G. Tappeiner
I. Universitäts-Hautklinik
Alserstrasse 4
A-1090 Wien

Dr. T. Tötterman
Clinical Immunology Section
Blood Center
University Hospitalet
S-751 85 Uppsala

Prof. Dr. Niels Tygstrup
Rigshospitalet
Medical Department A
9, Blegdamsvej
DK-2100 Copenhagen

Dr. Christa Utech
Deutsche Klinik für Diagnostik
Aukammallee 33
D-6200 Wiesbaden

Prof. R. Volpé, FRCP(C), FACP
The Wellesley Hospital
Department of Medicine
160 Wellesley Street East
Toronto, Ontario M4Y 1J3
Canada

Dr. J. de Vries
Oogzienkenhuis
Schiedamsevest 180
3001 Rotterdam
Netherlands

Prof. Dr. med. M. Wiederholt
Klinikum Steglitz, FU Berlin
Institut Klinische Physiologie
Hindenburgdamm 30
D-1000 Berlin 45

Dr. Roger Williams
Liver Unit
King's College School
of Medicine and Dentistry
Denmark Hill
London SE5 8RX
England

Preface to CyA Proceedings

Ciclosporin (Sandimmun®) has attained a predominant position and worldwide recognition in organ transplantation. In the light of its presumed mechanisms of action it was self-evident that the new substance should be tested also in the wide field of autoimmune diseases. With this volume an attempt has been made to provide full information to the scientific community about the status of ciclosporin as a possible treatment in these indications.

Needless to say, the necessary studies raise questions of an entirely different character, for the autoimmune diseases are themselves still imperfectly understood as regards their etiology, pathogenesis and the course of their pathophysiological processes. Moreover, in contrast to a severely impaired organ in need of replacement, prognosis as to the duration and course of the condition is difficult with many autoimmune diseases.

Clinicians and basic researchers are thus confronted with a large number of unsolved problems, and any drug capable of shedding explanatory light on the complexities of disturbed autoregulation and at the same time of raising hopes of genuine possibilities of treatment will meet with spontaneous interest. With all due reserve, ciclosporin may be regarded as such a substance. This also explains the great success of the first international symposium on ciclosporin and autoimmune diseases.

Access to this extensive and complex material is provided by basic papers presented by leading specialists dealing with established knowledge and theories about the processes of autoimmune disease, followed by detailed accounts of various scientific aspects of ciclosporin. If the reader then turns his attention to the clinical experience obtained to date with ciclosporin in certain autoimmune diseases, he must realise clearly that the results reported in many of the papers reproduced here are very much of a preliminary nature and make no claim to general validity. Needless to say, we can at present give no results for double-blind studies which have been instituted but are still uncompleted; all we can do is state the protocols adopted.

It will be noticed that, with the small groups of patients studied so far, the results are not always identical in terms of therapeutic effectiveness and side effects. Why, in the same disease, should ciclosporin help one patient but not another? Why can outcome in the same indication vary from study to study? Such cases show very clearly how imperfect our knowledge still is concerning the disease and the optimal therapeutic strategy.

It would also be interesting to know what part is played by genetic disposition to the disease or by acquired factors. What acute and chronic destructive processes are under way before the disease becomes clinically recognizable? It is in the light of these intricately inter-related pathophysiological processes that the discussion on the side effects of ciclosporin must be broached. To be able to differentiate their occurrence and degree exactly in relation to dosage and treatment, and thus to reduce them to the minimum, is one of the most important tasks of research.

In most indications, we shall not know whether the use of ciclosporin represents an acceptable risk/benefit ratio for the patient until the controlled studies now ongoing, and further investigations, have been evaluated.

The keen participation of speakers and audiences from the first to last day produced a crop of questions which are a stimulus to further thought and at the same time constitute a challenge to research and clinical medicine.

30. 05. 1985 *R. Schindler*

Nomenclature:
Sandimmun®
Sandimmune® (US regd)
Ciclosporin (INN prop.)
Cyclosporin (BAN)
Cyclosporine (USAN)
Cyclosporin-A (scientific name)

1. Autoimmunity and Ciclosporin (CyA)

Prevailing Theories in Autoimmune Disorders

I. M. Roitt[1]

The spectrum of autoimmune disease

It is helpful to regard the human diseases associated with autoimmunity as a spectrum with organ-specific disorders such as Hashimoto's thyroiditis at one pole, and non-organ-specific disorders like systemic lupus erythematosus (SLE) at the other (Table 1). The organ-specific disorders appear to involve immunological attack on a particular organ by virtue of an organ-specific immune response directed against target antigen within, and restricted to that particular organ. Non-organ-specific disorders involve lesions which are widespread throughout the body, to a large extent caused by immune complexes between auto-antibodies and antigens which are common to most cells in the body. An important feature is the overlap within diseases at each pole. For example, patients with autoimmune thyroid disease have a high incidence of gastric autoantibodies and, to a lesser extent, pernicious anaemia. On the other hand, patients with rheumatological disorders tend to have a combination of rheumatoid arthritis with features of systemic lupus, and so on. In the same way, there is familial aggregation at each pole of the disease spectrum with relatives of organ-specific diseases being specially prone to similar disorders, whereas probands with rheumatological disorders tend to have an unexpectedly high incidence of relatives with non-organ-specific disease. The genetic factors underlying such familial clustering are discussed further by Professor Batchelor in the following paper.

Autoantigens and self-reactivity

Most autoantigens are accessible to circulating immunocompetent lymphocytes. Even thyroglobulin, the iodine-containing protein of the thyroid gland which was once thought to be completely imprisoned within the colloid space of the thyroid follicle, is now known to circulate normally in concentrations of the order of 10 to 100 ng/ml. Thyroglobulin can be readily demonstrated by appropriate radioimmunoassay in the lymph draining the thyroid gland, and after a physiological stimulus to the gland with thyrotrophic stimulating hormone the concentration of thyroglobulin rises dramatically (Fig. 1), showing that the

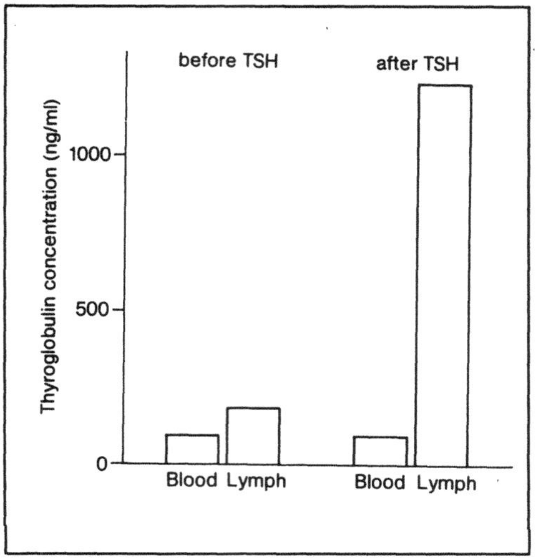

Fig. 1. Thyroglobulin in the cervical lymph draining the thyroid in the rat. The concentration of thyroglobulin is increased after injection of pituitary thyroid stimulating hormone (TSH) suggesting that the release from thyroid follicles is linked to the physiological activity of the acinar cells [8].
(From[8]; reproduced by kind permission of the publishers)

---

1 Department of Immunology, The Middlesex Hospital Medical School, London W1, UK

Table 1. Spectrum of autoimmune disease

Organ-specific ←——→ Non-organ-specific

Hashimoto's thyroiditis	Myasthenia gravis	Autoimmune haemolytic anaemia	Primary biliary cirrhosis	Systemic lupus erythematosus (SLE)
Primary myxoedema	Juvenile diabetes	Idiopathic thrombocytopenic purpura	Active chronic hepatitis HB_s-ve	Discoid LE
Thyrotoxicosis	Goodpasture's syndrome	Idiopathic leucopenia	Cryptogenic cirrhosis (some cases)	Dermatomyositis
Pernicious anaemia	Pemphigus vulgaris		Ulcerative colitis	Scleroderma
Autoimmune atrophic gastritis	Pemphigoid		Sjögren's syndrome	Rheumatoid arthritis
Addison's disease	Sympathetic ophthalmia			
Premature menopause (few cases)	Phacogenic uveitis			
Male infertility (few cases)	(?? Multiple sclerosis??)			

release from the gland is associated with a physiological reaction. Likewise, the hormone receptors on the surface of cells, which figure prominently in the many different autoimmune disorders, are accessible to contact with lymphocytes. The range of different nuclear components which provoke autoantibody formation so characteristically in SLE can also be recognized by circulating lymphocytes when they are released from effete cells in the body.

In addition, there is strong evidence for autoreactive lymphocytes which have not been eliminated by some type of clonal abortion related to self-tolerance. For example, we know that a small percentage of circulating B cells in normal individuals will bind either radioactive thyroglobulin [2] or DNA to their immunoglobulin surface receptors. There are reports of thyroglobulin autoantibody production by cell lines from normal individuals induced by Epstein-Barr (EB) virus, but particularly convincing is the general finding that in all vertebrate species so far studied, stimulation by autologous thyroglobulin in some fairly powerful adjuvant will provoke autoantibody formation with a time scale of response comparable to that which would be expected with any exogenous immunogen. Evidence for autoreactive T cells comes from studies in which experimental allergic encephalomyelitis could be transferred to a normal recipient with T cells from a sensitized animal, and especially from the isolation of T-cell clones from autoimmunized animals which react with the relevant autoantigen [4]. Thus it is we see that all the components required for self-reaction to produce an autoimmune response are present in the body and clearly, since the majority of individuals do not suffer the embarrassment of reacting to their own body constituents, there must be regulatory control mechanisms which inhibit the interaction of autoantigens with their respective self-reactive lymphocytes. In Figure 2 is set out one possible scheme to envisage the interactions involved, which lays stress on the recognition of autoantigens by T inducer (also known as T helper) cells as the point where the control mechanisms tend to focus. One of these

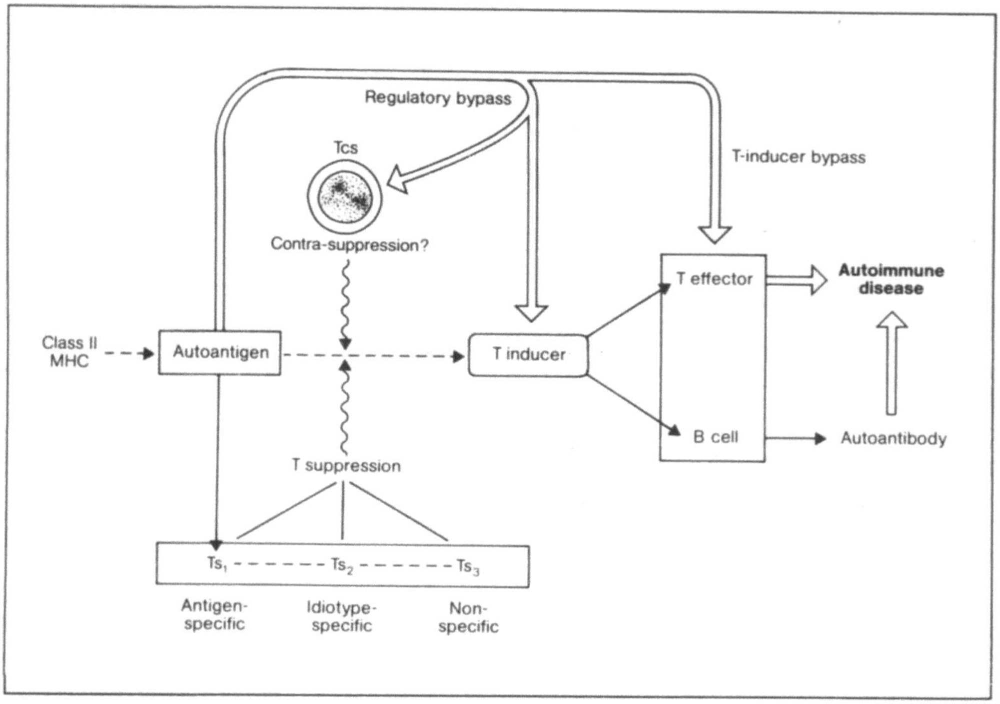

Fig. 2. The conrol of autoreactivity. The constraints on the stimulation of autoantigen with self-reactive inducer/helper T cell can be circumvented either through bypassing the inducer cell or by disturbance of the regulatory mechanisms

mechanisms depends upon the necessity for T-inducer cells to recognize autoantigen in association with a class II major histocompatibility complex molecule. In the absence of this association, for example a hormone receptor on the surface of a thyroid cell which does not express class II molecules, there will be what Mitchison has termed 'immunological silence' [22]. The interaction with T helper will also come under the control of a complicated network of suppressor T cells which includes antigen-specific, idiotype-specific and the final non-specific effector T suppressors. In addition I have included the rather controversial contra-suppressor cell whose function is said to be to render T inducer cells refractory to the influence of T suppressors [13]. In other words, if the contra-suppressor gets there first, the T helper is no longer capable of being suppressed.

Now these control mechanisms can be bypassed in essentially two different ways, either through a bypass of the T inducer, or through a bypass involving the regulatory mechanisms themselves. These possibilities will be considered in turn.

T inducer bypass

Provision of a new carrier

In essence, Allison [1] and Weigle [36] independently proposed that effector self-reactive cells would be rendered impotent if they were deprived of T inducer help through tolerization of the helper cells by mechanisms discussed in the last section. However, these effector cells would be stimulated if the autoantigen acquired a new carrier determinant which would then be recognized by T inducer cells which had not had the opportunity to be tolerized (Fig. 3). One way in which this might happen would be if an autoantigen were to become abnormal through some modification. We have looked at this possibility using the obese strain (OS) chicken as a

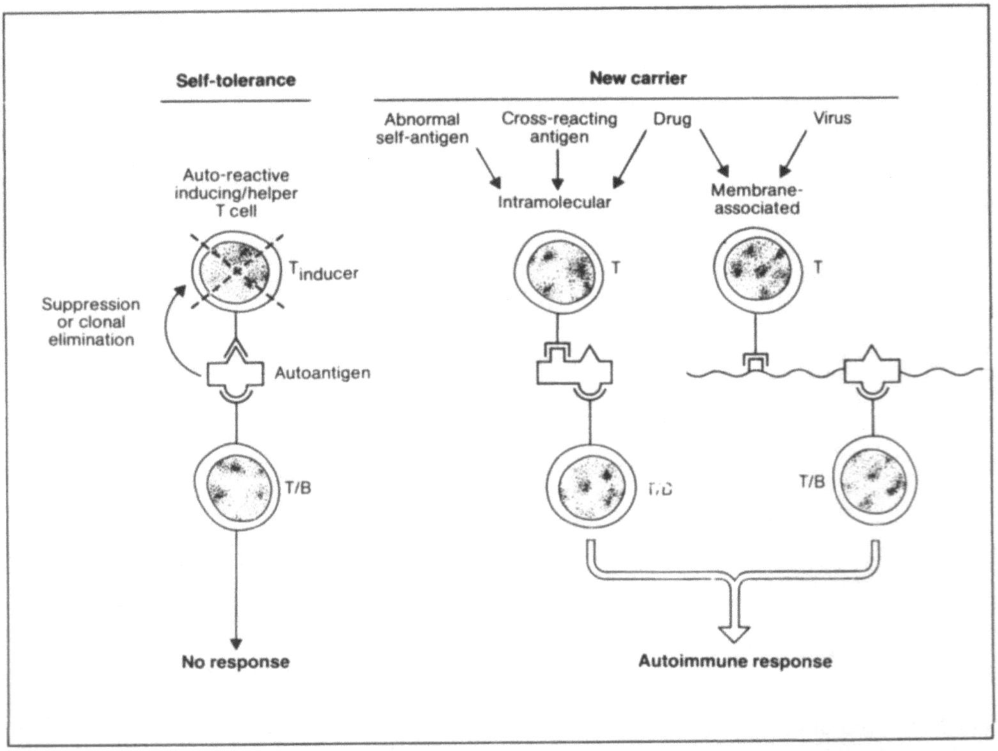

Fig. 3. T. inducer bypass through new carrier determinant generates autoimmunity

model. This bird is known to develop spontaneously an autoantibody response to thyroglobulin and eventually to destroy its own thyroid through the invasion of chronic inflammatory cells. Neonatally thyroidectomized OS chickens do not produce thyroglobulin autoantibodies, which incidentally shows that antigen is needed to drive the auto-immune response. When these birds are injected with thyroglobulin obtained from normal white leghorns, they make an autoantibody response, showing that it is not necessary for the thyroglobulin to be abnormal for the immunological system in the obese strain bird to be provoked into autoreactivity. Further evidence for a lack of abnormality in the obese strain thyroglobulin came from displacement studies with radioactive thyroglobulins from normal and OS chickens, in which no discrimination between the thyroid proteins could be discerned [27]. Nonetheless, there is some evidence that the thyroid gland itself may show abnormalities; thus, the iodine uptake by the newborn OS thyroid is considerably higher than that seen in normal strains, and was associated with an abnormally increased ratio of mono- to di-iodotyrosine in the thyroid and a low serum thyroxine [29]. Other evidence pointing to an organ-related component in autoimmune disease comes from a study of the relatives of patients with organ-specific autoimmunity, where it is seen that the first-degree relatives of patients with pernicious anaemia have a far higher incidence of gastric autoimmunity than do close relatives of patients presenting with Hashimoto's thyroiditis [10]. Another straw in the wind pointing to antigen is the observation by Bell and colleagues [3] of a relationship between a tendency to develop insulin-dependent diabetes and a particular sequence of DNA upstream of the gene encoding insulin as determined by restriction enzyme fragmentation.

Another way of acquiring a new carrier, and this is how Allison and Weigle first envisaged the operation of this mechanism, is through infection with a cross-reacting antigen which shares epitopes with an autoantigen but, in addition, has a new carrier determinant which can be recognized by T-helper cells which have not been tolerized. Examples are the cross-reaction between certain strains of *Streptococci* and heart muscle as seen in rheumatic fever and the postulated cross-reaction between *Trypanosoma cruzi* and heart which is said to be responsible for the immunopathological lesions observed late in Chagas' disease. Yet another example is post-rabies vaccination encephalomyelitis, involving cross-reaction between brain tissue from foreign species and self.

Theoretically, drugs could provide new carrier determinants either by substituting within the autoantigen itself, or by linking to a membrane close to an autoantigen where it may act to provide associative recognition. Although certain drugs like procainamide and alpha-methyl dopa are related to the development of SLE and autoimmune haemolytic anaemia respectively, as yet there is no hard evidence that this is a result of the drug acting as a new carrier determinant.

Viruses which encode new viral proteins in the surface membrane of cells may enable autoantigens to provoke an autoimmune response through associative recognition with the viral protein. That viruses may enhance the antigenicity of otherwise weak membrane proteins was demonstrated clearly by Lindenmann [19] when he showed that influenza-infected tumour plasma membranes effectively produced an immune response to the tumour-related antigen. Recently, Notkins and colleagues [24] showed that infection of mice with reovirus resulted in the production of autoantibodies to a variety of endocrine organs. No unequivocal relationships between viral infection and the development of autoimmunity have been established, although numerous attempts have been made to link Coxsackie virus infection with the onset of insulin-dependent diabetes.

Idiotype cross-reaction

Instead of a cross-reaction between a foreign antigen and self, one could also envisage cross-reactions involving idiotypes. Cooke and Lydyard [7] put forward the idea that if autoreactive T or B cells carried an idiotype which cross-reacted with the idiotype on an antibody to a microbe or even to a structure on the microbe itself, then infection by that particular micro-organism could generate T help directed to the idiotype, which could then stimulate the autoreactive T or B cell bearing the idiotype, possibly acting in conjunction with the autoantigen itself (Fig. 4). Indeed, preliminary reports have been made concerning cross-reactions between idiotypes on antibodies to *Klebsiella* polysaccharide K30 and on DNA autoantibodies [23] and between an epitope on *Streptococcus pyogenes* peptidoglycan and an idiotype on rheumatoid factor [17]. Yet another variation, the cross-reaction between idiotype on an antibody to an exogenous antigen and a corresponding determinant on an autoantigen, has been proposed by Plotz [26]. Figure 5 illustrates the different ways in which cross-reactions between idiotypes and antigens in general can contribute to the development of an autoimmune response.

Polyclonal activation

Autoimmunity could arise from the triggering of autoreactive lymphocytes, not through their antigen-specific receptor but through their receptor for the so-called polyclonal activators. Some examples of this are known. For instance, bacterial lipopolysaccharide can induce anti-DNA on injection into mice [15] while EB virus, which is a polyclonal B cell activator in the human, can persuade a relatively high proportion of the cells in certain B lymphocyte subsets to synthesize IgM rheumatoid factor [11]. Other evidence said to favour the action of polyclonal activators in the rheumatological disorders includes the observation that lymphocytes from patients with SLE, or from certain murine models of this disease [16], secrete relatively large amounts of immunoglobulin when placed in culture, even without further stimulation.

This view should be treated with some caution. Thus when one looks at the IgM-

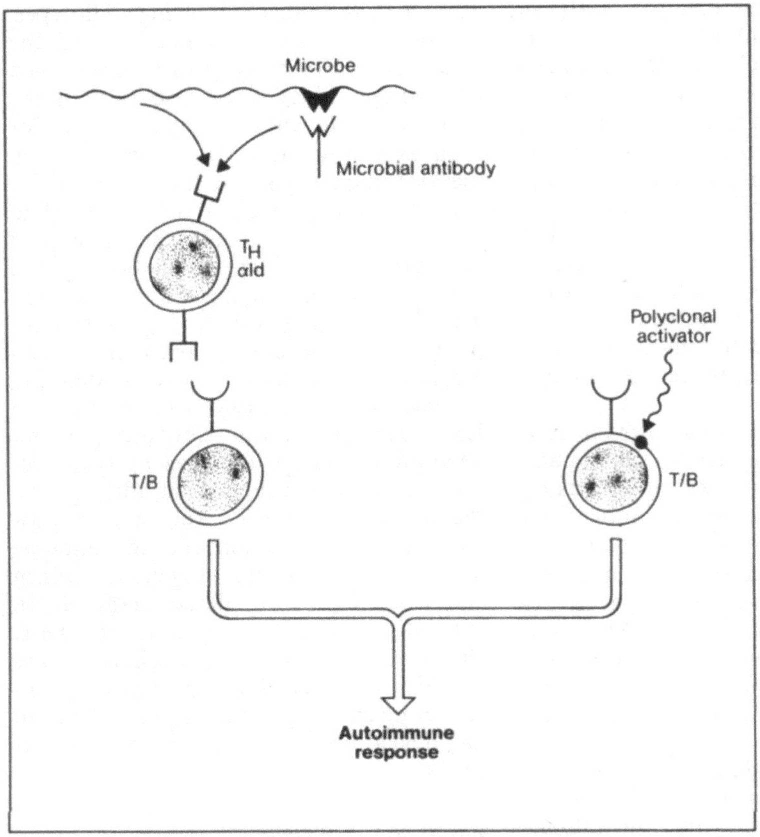

Fig. 4. T inducer bypass through idiotype cross-reactions or polyclonal activation can trigger an autoimmune response

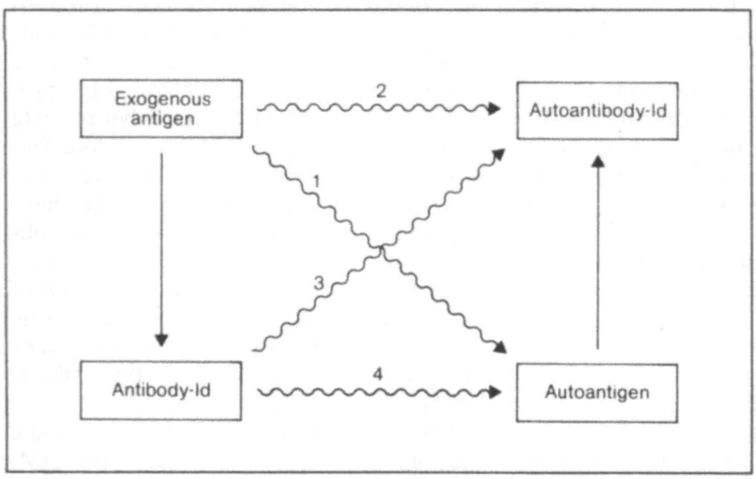

Fig. 5. Cross-reactions leading to autoimmunity:
1) Exogenous antigen and autoantigen [1, 36]
2) Exogenous antigen and autoantibody-Id [7]
3) Idiotypes on antibody to exogenous antigen and autoantibody [7]
4) Idiotype on antibody to exogenous antigen and autoantigen [26]

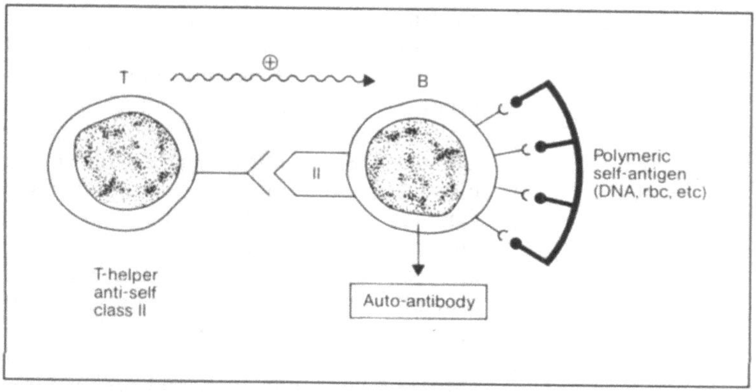

Fig. 6. Polyclonal T cell help for autoantibody production to polymeric antigens. Signal 1 for B cell activation arises from cross-linking of surface Ig receptors by polymeric autoantigen, while signal 2 is provided through recognition of class II major histocompatibility molecules by a self-reactive T helper cell specific for class II

producing plasma cells in the rheumatoid synovium, 90 to 95% are found to be synthesizing rheumatoid factors [38], a number which would seem to be rather high even in the light of the evidence produced above for the action of EB virus. Furthermore, in systemic lupus, the autoantibodies are directed against a wide variety of antigens, but these collectively have the feature of being components of the nucleus; there is not an indiscriminate production of autoantibodies against any other cellular components. Furthermore, in the obese strain chicken, the work cited showing that antigen is obligatory for the development of autoantibodies would be difficult to reconcile with a mechanism dependent only on polyclonal activation, although it must be said that it is difficult to exclude the possibility of antigen and polyclonal activators operating synergistically in genetically predisposed individuals.

It may be of interest to consider one way in which this situation could arise. Our own experience and that of others concerned with the establishment of T cell clones and hybridomas from immunized mice, is that T cells capable of reacting to self major histocompatibility class II molecules in the absence of exogenous antigen can be identified with surprising frequency. Since we know that chronic graft-vs-host reactions involving recognition of class II molecules by allogeneic T cells provide help for B cells reacting with polymeric but not univalent antigens [35], we could envisage that the emergence of T cells with specificity for autologous class II molecules would provide polyclonal help for B cells whose Ig receptors had been cross-linked by polymeric self-antigens such as DNA, erythrocytes or immune aggregates, with consequent production of autoantibodies (Fig. 6).

Regulatory bypass

Even if autoimmunity does arise by any of the mechanisms which have been described above, there do appear to be regulatory systems in normal individuals which attempt to correct this. For example, when rat red blood cells are injected into CBA mice, the cross-reactive antigen induces an autoantibody response to mouse erythrocytes which is expressed as a positive Coombs' test (Fig. 7). The Coombs' test reaches a peak of positivity at two weeks and then declines. Studies of this model by Cooke and her colleagues [5] indicate that the decline is associated with the generation of suppressor cells. The fall-off in Coombs' positivity is far slower in the NZB, a strain known to have a propensity to develop autoimmunity, while in the SJL, which is known to have prematurely ageing suppressor systems, treatment with rat red

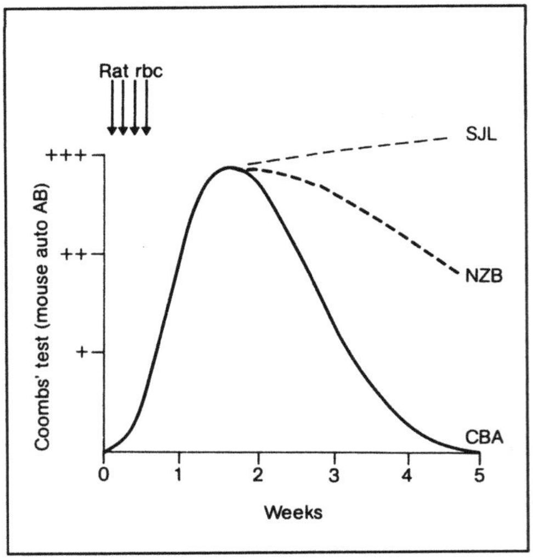

Fig. 7. Regulation of self-reactivity. When CBA mice are injected with rat red cells, autoantibodies are produced by this cross-reacting antigen which coat the host erythrocytes and are detected by the Coombs' test. The SJL strain, in which suppressor activity declines rapidly with age, is unable to regulate the autoimmune response and develops particularly severe disease. The response is also prolonged in the autoimmune NZB strain [5]

cells leads to death of the animal. In other words, the indications are that, to sustain a chronic autoimmune response, it may be necessary to have in addition some regulatory defect. We will now look at some possible ways by which these defects might arise.

Abnormalities in immunocompetent cells

Evidence for an intrinsic abnormality in the stem cells of NZB and other autoimmune strains comes from their ability to transfer autoimmunity to otherwise normal H-2-matched recipient strains. The defect may appear in both T and B cells. On the one hand, several authors have shown that the T cells in the NZB are difficult to tolerize [25], on the other, abnormalities in certain B cell subsets, particularly of the thymus-independent categories, have been demonstrated. For example, in the NZB it is difficult to tolerize the B cells responding to type I thymus-independent antigens by hapten on a human gammaglobulin carrier [12]. In addition, introduction of the Xid gene from the CBA/N mouse into the NZB produces congenic strains which do not make autoantibodies [33]. It is interesting also that CBA/N mice injected with rat red blood cells do not give rise to positive Coombs' tests even though they make good anti-rat red cell responses [6]. These experiments point to the CBA/N B cell subset, thought to be concerned in the response to type II thymus-independent antigens, as the subpopulation intimately bound with autoantibody production, and perhaps imply that the threshold for tolerance induction to self in this subset in strains prone to autoimmunity may be high. Curiously, abnormal numbers of Lyt 1-positive B cells have been found in NZB mice and the counterpart in the human, namely OKT1/surface Ig-positive cells, have been demonstrated in rheumatoid arthritis. Their relationship to the B cell subsets responding to thymus-independent antigens which we discussed above could be of interest.

Suppressor cell defects

We have already drawn attention to the diversity of suppressor T cells. Methods for demonstrating antigen-specific T suppressors in the human are not readily available although this is clearly likely to be an important area. Volpé and his colleagues have made a brave attempt to identify a defect in thyroid-specific suppressor cells in autoimmune thyroid disease and these results have been reported and discussed elsewhere. In patients with rheumatoid arthritis a defect in the T cell handling of EB virus transformation of B cells has been identified and the evidence suggests that EBV-specific suppressor T cells are not functioning as effectively as they do in normal individuals who have had prior infection with the virus [34]. The finding of major cross-reactive idiotypes associated with thyroglobulin autoantibodies in Hashimoto's disease [9, 20], with antibodies to acetyl choline receptors in myasthenia gravis [18], and with anti-DNA in SLE [31] could be interpreted as an indication that important suppressor T cells controlling the idiotype in question were defective. However, another interpretation would be that, as with normal immune responses, it is not unusual for a dominant cross-reactive idiotype to appear, probably owing to the recruiting action of T helper anti-idiotypes. The antigen- and idiotype-specific T suppressors appear to exert their effects through a population of non-specific suppressor T cells. In SLE, numerous studies have confirmed a defect in non-specific suppressor activity of peripheral blood lymphocytes activated by concanavalin A. That this depression of reactivity is intimately linked to the disease, rather than being a consequence of disease activity or even of therapy, seems likely from the studies of Miller and Schwartz [21] who showed that Con A-induced suppressor activity was low in the majority of first-degree relatives of SLE patients. The paradoxical exacerbation of thyroiditis which results from neonatal thymectomy of obese strain chickens is also considered indicative of an operative role for suppressor T cells in attempting to control an auto-immune response [37].

Contra-suppressors

I have already drawn attention to these somewhat controversial cells. The case for them is discussed by Green and his colleagues [13]. One experiment referred to is the production of soluble factors by lymphocytes from mice which have been thymectomized and injected with polyclonal activators which, when added to an antibody generating system, protected it from the action of soluble suppressor factors [32]. While suggesting that contra-suppressors had been activated in an animal lacking suppressors, it may be true to say that in general somewhat harder evidence is awaited. Nonetheless, the concept of the contra-suppressors might be quite important in autoimmunity. It is often said that T helper cells have a somewhat wider reactivity toward antigens than do B cells and there is some evidence that this wider reactivity may include a certain degree of self-recognition. If tolerance to self-T cells were very highly effective, it is argued that one might delete the majority of the cells from the T helper repertoire. This problem could be circumvented if there were another level of T cell at which tolerance to self could be effected but with a much narrower specificity, resembling more that of the B cell. Supposing that self-reacting contra-suppressors were exquisitely sensitive to tolerization by deletion or silencing by self-components, they would leave self-reactive T suppressors (which are presumed not to be tolerizable) to dominate the helper T cell population and prevent it reacting against self. This would not be so for exogenous antigens, so that the contrasuppressors to such antigens, when activated, would make the T helpers refractory to suppression, except under very special circumstances. Clearly, any circumstance which leads to an enhancement or precocious development of contra-suppressor cell activity directed to self would make an autoimmune reaction that much more likely.

Inappropriate expression of class II major histocompatibility complex molecules

If certain cell surface components are immunologically silent because T inducer cells cannot perceive them in the context of class II MHC (major histocompatibility complex) molecules, it could be argued that de-repression of the genes encoding such molecules would allow them to be expressed at the cell surface and possibly break silence. Bottazzo and his colleagues have shown that this can happen if, for example, human thyroid cells in tissue culture are activated either with phytohaemagglutinin or with gamma interferon [28]. That this is not an artefact of the culture system seems likely in view of their further observations that sections of frozen thyroid obtained from patients with thyrotoxicosis show intracytoplasmic fluorescence when stained with various antisera directed against the human class II molecule, HLA-D (human leucocyte antigen) [14]. These are indeed intriguing observations and it will be fascinating to see whether they are of primary consequence in terms of the initiation of an autoimmune response, or are concerned with the sequence of events which leads to autoimmune damage of the thyroid gland by a pre-established autoimmunity.

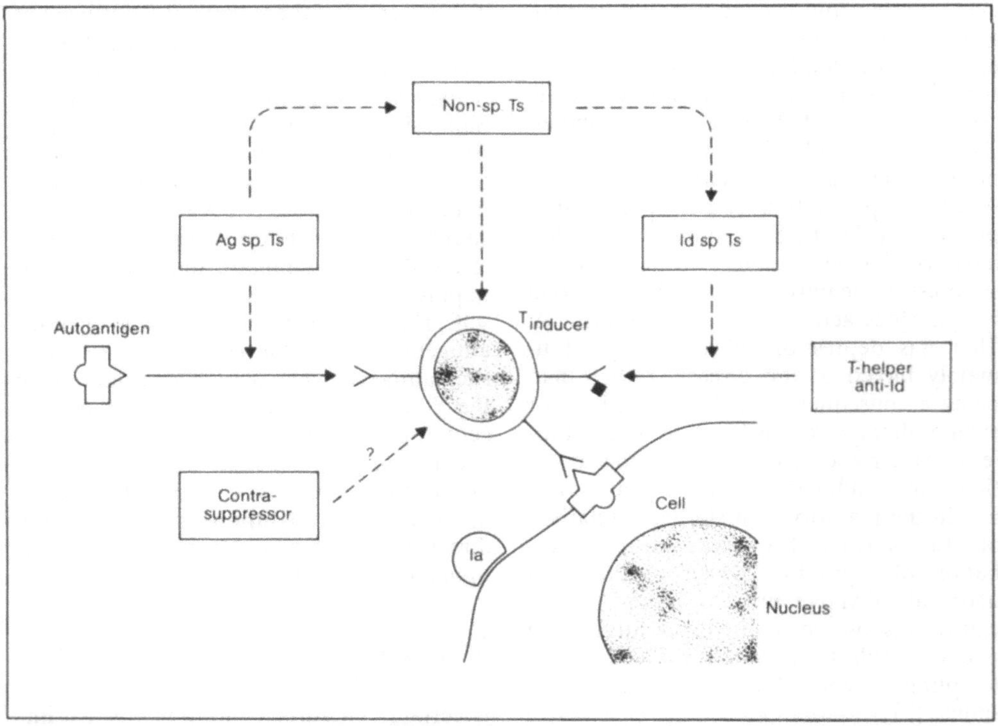

Fig. 8. Bypass of regulatory mechanisms leads to triggering of autoreactive T inducer cell through defects in (1) antigen-specific, (2) idiotype-specific or (3) non-specific suppressors, through (4) stimulation of contra-suppressors or (5) de-repression of class II genes with inappropriate cellular expression of Ia

The ways in which these different factors may influence the control of autoimmunity are indicated in Figure 8.

Conclusion

We cannot point to any one defect which is likely to be responsible for autoimmune diseases in general. The infrequency of overlap between organ-specific and non-organ-specific diseases as compared with the high frequency of overlap within each group strongly suggests that very different mechanisms underlie these two poles of the autoimmune spectrum. Almost certainly, most of these defects will prove to be involved in one disease or another and the evidence points strongly to the disorders having a multifactorial basis. It may well turn out that auto-immune diseases result from a combination of several different disorders, each in itself relatively common.

References

1. Allison AC (1971) Lancet ii: 1401
2. Bankhurst AD, Torrigiani G, Allison AC (1973) Lancet i: 226
3. Bell GI, Horita S, Karam JH (1984) Diabetes 33: 176
4. Ben-Nun A, Cohen IR (1981) Eur J Immunol 11: 949
5. Cooke A, Hutchings PR, Playfair JHL (1978) Nature 273: 154
6. Cooke A, Hutchings PR, Marshall-Clarke S (1980) Immunology 41: 815
7. Cooke A, Lydyard PM, Roitt IM (1983) Immunol Today 4: 170
8. Daniel PN, Pratt OE, Roitt IM, Torrigiani G (1967) Q J Exp Physiol 52: 184
9. Delves PJ, Roitt IM (1984) Clin Exp Immunol 57: 33
10. Doniach D, Roitt IM (1964) Semin Hematol 1: 313
11. Fong S, Vaughan JH, Carson DA (1983) J Immunol 130: 162
12. Goldings EA (1983) J Immunol 131: 2630

13. Green DR, Flood PM, Gershon RK (1983) Ann Rev Immunol 1:439
14. Hanafusa T, Pujol-Borrell R, Chiovato L, Russell RCG, Doniach D, Bottazzo GF (1983) Lancet ii:1111
15. Izui S, Lambert PH, Fournie PH, Turler H, Miescher PA (1977) J Exp Med 145:1115
16 Izui S, McConahey PJ, Dixon FJ (1978) J Immunol 121:2213
17. Johnson P, Phua K, personal communication
18. Lefvert A-K (1981) Scand J Immunol 13:493
19. Lindenmann J, Klein PA (1967) J Exp Med 126:93
20. Matsuyama T, Fukumori J, Tanaka H (1983) Clin Exp Immunol 51:381
21. Miller KB, Schwartz RS (1979) N Engl J Med 301:803
22. Mitchison NA (1982) In: Receptors, Antibodies and Disease. Ciba Foundation Symposium 90:p 57
23. Naparstek Y et al. (1984) Clin Res 32:507 A
24. Onodera T, Ray VR, Melez KA, Suzuki H, Toniolo A, Notkins AL (1982) Nature 297:66
25. Playfair JHL (1971) Immunology 21:1037
26. Plotz PM (1983) Lancet ii:824
27. Pontes de Carvalho LC, Templeman J, Wick G, Roitt IM (1982) J Exp Med 155:1255
28. Pujol-Borrell R, Hanafusa T, Chiovato L, Bottazzo GF (1983) Nature 304:71
29. Rose NR, Bacon LD, Sundick RS (1976) Transpl Rev 31:264
30. Rosenberg YJ, Steinberg AD, Santoro TJ (1984) Immunol Today 5:64
31. Schoenfeld Y, Isenberg DA, Rauch J, Madaio MP, Stollar BD, Schwartz RS (1983) J Exp Med 158:718
32. Smith HR, Green DR, Smathers PA, Gerson RK, Raveche ES, Steinberg AD (1983) Clin Exp Immunol 51:579
33. Smith HR, Steinberg AD (1983) Ann Rev Immunol 1:175
34. Tosato G, Steinberg AD, Blaese RM (1981) N Engl J Med 305:1238
35. Van Rappard-Van der Veen FM, Kiesel U, Poels L, Schuler W, Melief CJM, Landegent J, Gleichmann E (1984) J Immunol 132:1814
36. Weigle WO (1971) Clin Exp Immunol 9:437
37. Wick G, Kite JH, Witebsky E (1979) J Immunol 104:45
38. Youinou P, Morrow J, Lettin AWF, Lydyard PM, Roitt IM (1984) Scand J Immunol (in press)

Genetic Role in Autoimmunity

J. R. Batchelor [1]

It is perhaps not generally appreciated to what extent immune responses, including autoimmune ones, are under genetic control. Analysis of the mechanisms of this control at the cellular and molecular levels is one of the major challenges facing medicine today. One reason why considerable progress has already been made is that studies on human responses can be made against a theoretical and experimental background derived from work upon inbred strains of mice. For those unfamiliar with inbred strains, their usefulness rests on the fact that members of the same strain (and sex) are genetically identical, thus allowing responses of any sort, immunological or other, to be examined against a uniform genetic background [15]. Furthermore, several series of inbred strains have been developed, in which each strain of the series differs from sister strains only by a small part of the genome, the remainder of the genome being common to all the strains in the series. With such congenic strains, as they are called, it is possible to examine the effect of a defined cluster of genes and, in some instances, of a single gene.

Early studies with inbred mouse strains demonstrated that there was marked variation in susceptibility to bacterial infections [39]. Interest quickened when susceptibility of mice to a virus-induced leukaemia was found to be linked with inheritance of the major histocompatibility complex (MHC) genes [23]. Within a year there were reports of genetic control of immune responses to synthetic polypeptides [18, 24, 30], and in 1969 McDevitt and Chinitz [25] showed that the genes responsible for the control of antibody responses to three synthetic polypeptides were closely linked to the mouse MHC genes, the H-2 system.

1 Department of Immunology, Royal Postgraduate Medical School, London, UK

Naturally these exciting discoveries led many to ask whether human immune responses were similarly under genetic control, and if so whether the human MHC genes, ie the HLA (human leucocyte antigen) system genes, were responsible for control. The approach used was based on the argument that if the HLA genes have a controlling effect on immune responses, diseases of disordered immunity should be more prevalent in individuals with (a) particular HLA gene(s) than in others who lack that gene or genes. Therefore groups of patients with such diseases were HLA typed, and the frequencies of their HLA antigens were compared with those of healthy control populations of the same racial origin. This approach was dramatically vindicated by the discovery of the very close association between HLA-B27 and ankylosing spondylitis [9, 38].

As a result, a very large number of studies on a variety of other diseases have followed, and numerous significant associations have been observed [34]. A few examples are given in Table 1. The exam-

Table 1. Some examples of HLA-associated (human leucocyte antigen) diseases. (Data from [34, 42])

Condition	HLA antigen	Relative risk
Ankylosing spondylitis	B27	87.4
Reiter's disease	B27	37
Graves' disease	DR3	3.7
Hashimoto's thyroiditis	DR5	3.2
Insulin-dependent diabetes mellitus	DR3	3.3
	DR4	6.4
	DR2	0.2
Myasthenia gravis	DR3	2.5
Multiple sclerosis	DR2	4.1
Goodpasture's syndrome	DR2	15.9

ples include conditions in which there is strong evidence that autoimmunity is responsible for the pathological tissue damage, eg Hashimoto's thyroiditis or myasthenia gravis, and others where the evidence is much less clear, eg multiple sclerosis. Although many obscurities in aetiology and pathogenesis remain, all chronic autoimmune diseases studied have shown an association with one or other HLA antigen, and failure to find such an association can now be considered as evidence against an autoimmune pathogenesis. It is reasonable to conclude, on this evidence alone, that the HLA region genes do influence immune responsiveness.

Genetics, structure, and expression of HLA molecules

The HLA gene region consists of a series of closely linked genetic loci situated on the short arm of the 6th chromosome [7]. The genes and their protein products are normally classified as follows:

Class I: HLA-A, B, and C

Class II: HLA-DP, DQ, and DR

Class III: Genetic loci coding for polymorphisms of the 4 complement system proteins C2, Factor B, C4A, and C4B. In the strict sense these are not HLA genes.

The probable gene order is illustrated in Figure 1; the position of DQ and DR relative to one another remains uncertain, and although the order of the Class III genes relative to one another has been established [11] it has not been formally proven that C2 maps closer to the HLA-D region than C4B does.

One of the characteristics of the HLA system genes is their polymorphism. At the most recent International Histocompatibility Workshop [7] 23 HLA-A, 47 HLA-B, and 8 HLA-C series alleles were considered well enough defined to be assigned an identifying number. The polymorphism of the Class II genes may be slightly less but is still marked. Within Class III, polymorphism is also observed, particularly for C4A and C4B.

The HLA genes are inherited as codominants, so that an individual will express a pair of allelic variants for each locus, ie one transmitted from the mother, and one from the father.

Structurally, both Class I and II molecules are cell surface glycoproteins which span the plasma membrane and terminate within the cytoplasm [8, 19, 31]. Both classes are composed of 2 chains of unequal size (α and β chains) forming heterodimers. In the case of Class I molecules, only the α chain is encoded by the HLA genes, the β chain being B2 microglobulin encoded from chromosome 15. The gene products of the HLA-A, B, and C allelic series are found on virtually all nucleated cells and platelets, but there is quantitative variation in their expression

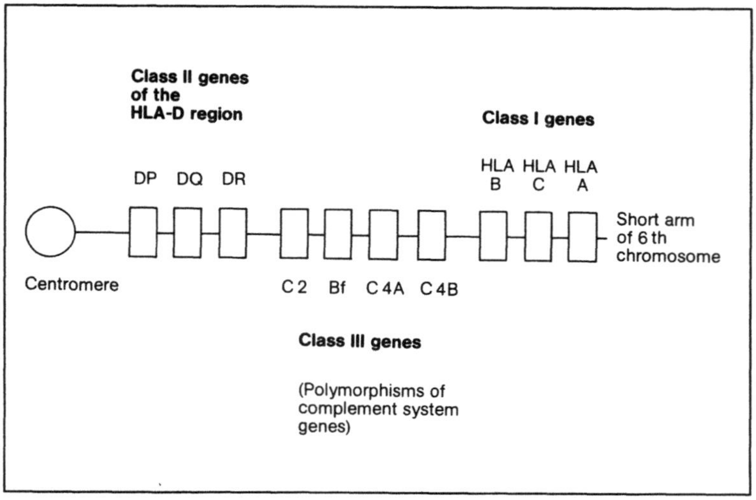

Fig. 1. HLA (human leucocyte antigen) region genes. Old terminologies for the Class II genes include: DQ = MB, DC or DS series; DP = SB

on cells of different tissues. Class II molecules differ significantly from those of Class I in a number of ways. One is that both the α and β chains are coded for by HLA region genes, and a second is that they are not present in detectable amounts on all nucleated cells. Until recently it was thought that Class II molecules were found only on accessory cells of the immune system such as monocytes, macrophages, and Langerhans cells, and on B lymphocytes and some vascular endothelia. However, interferon and possibly other lymphokines are now known to induce the expression of Class II molecules on cells in vitro [1, 32] and, similarly, immune reactions in vivo are associated with induced expression of Class II molecules by cells which otherwise do not express them [40]. Nevertheless the limited tissue expression of Class II molecules under non-pathological conditions is clearly important, since these molecules are obligatory partners in presenting antigens to certain subpopulations of T lymphocytes (see below). For example the paucity of Class II-bearing cells within the central nervous system is presumably one reason for its (relative) immunologically privileged status.

Function of HLA molecules

The cells of the immune system can be classified as effectors, regulatory, or accessory. For most protein antigens, T lymphocytes play an obligatory role and so the responses are said to be T-dependent. In any complex system of this sort, it is imperative that the interacting cells can recognize partner cells, and it has become evident that T cells use HLA as recognition molecules [28, 50]. The T cells using Class I HLA molecules for recognition are, in general, effectors belonging to the cytotoxic subpopulation, and can be identified with the monoclonal antibody OKT8. Those which use Class II HLA molecules usually belong to the helper subpopulation, and can be identified by the monoclonal antibody OKT4. Some exceptions to these generalizations do exist.

If an extrinsic antigen, eg tetanus toxoid, is introduced into the immune system diagrammatically illustrated in Figure 2, T helper cells with appropriate specificity for tetanus toxoid will not respond to the antigen alone – it is necessary for the antigen to be correctly presented by a specialized accessory cell. The antigen undergoes a preliminary processing, and is then presented to the T helper cell in association with Class II HLA molecules on the surface of the antigen-presenting accessory cell. Following correct presentation, the interacting T helper cell 'sees' the antigen in the context of the Class II HLA molecule and is thereby triggered to proliferate. The proliferation is accompanied by the synthesis of an array of soluble factors (lymphokines) which induce other cells of the immune system to differentiate and become activated by antigen [13, 17, 22, 48].

Like helper T cells, cytotoxic T cells require antigen, eg a virus-encoded molecule displayed on a infected cell, to become associated with an HLA molecule in order to provide both the correct stimulus for proliferation and the trigger for cytotoxicity. Thus, the cytotoxic T cell also 'sees' antigen in the context of an HLA molecule, usually of Class I. Much remains to be learned about the nature of the associations between antigens and Class I or II HLA molecules, and how this leads to T-cell activation but it is clear already that the effectiveness of T-cell activation depends on the precise MHC allele which associates with the antigen, some alleles being able to induce a vigorous activation while others lead to weaker or even no activation [36, 44].

Most of the analysis of function of MHC molecules has made use of mouse systems [50] but there is a growing body of data on HLA and human T-cell systems which leaves no doubt that the same principles hold for the function of human MHC molecules [6, 26, 44, 46].

In addition to the T-cell subpopulations already mentioned, there are also those with suppressor activity [21, 27, 43]. No general agreement has yet been reached as to the number of suppressor subpopulations but some authors have envisaged a cascade system, with a series of subpopulations being activated in sequence, the last one mediating the suppressive action

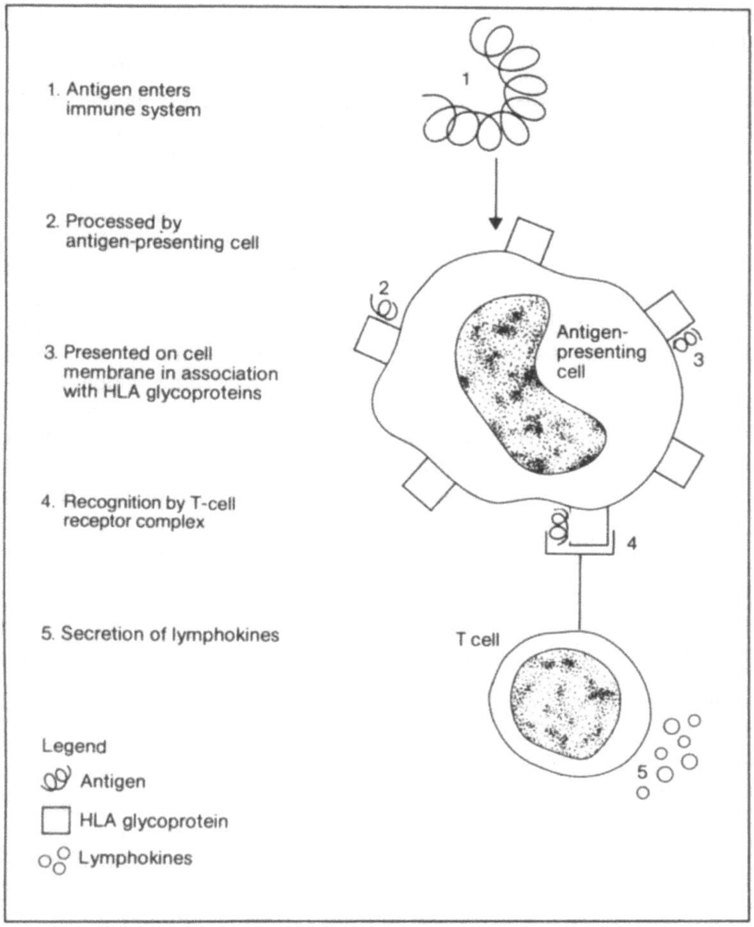

Fig. 2. HLA (human leucocyte antigen) molecules and antigen presentation to T cells

[41,49]. Within this sequence, MHC molecules also function as T-cell recognition structures.

HLA associations with autoimmune diseases

As yet, it is not possible to state in detailed cellular and molecular terms why susceptibility to auto-immune diseases is associated with the inheritance of specific HLA alleles. The most favoured explanation in the general sense is that susceptibility is directly governed by the configuration of the molecules encoded by any given HLA allele (usually Class II) which acts as a recognition unit for T-cell subpopulations responding to an autoantigen. According to such an hypothesis, the strength and duration of the response and the character of the T-cell subpopulation(s) activated (helper, suppressor, cytotoxic) could depend on the HLA allele providing the context against which the autoantigen was 'seen'. There are other possibilities, such as the idea that the repertoire of antigens against which a subject's T cells can respond is dictated by the MHC genotype [5].

Both of these concepts just described rest on the assumption that the HLA genes are themselves the ones responsible for susceptibility. However, one of the features of the HLA region is the tendency of specific alleles of different genetic loci to occur together in a subject more (or less) frequently than would be expected on the basis of their individual gene frequencies. A familiar example is provided by HLA-A1, HLA-B8, and HLA-DRW3 which in many Caucasoid populations would be expected mathematically to occur in the same individual in approximately 1% of the population, but actually are observed together in approximately 10 to 15% of the population. This tendency of certain alleles to occur in association (linkage disequilibrium) has relevance to genetic susceptibility to disease, including autoimmune diseases. The argument is that the HLA allele found in association with the disease may not itself be directly involved in the pathogenesis, but because of linkage disequilibrium with an allele of the 'true' disease susceptibility gene it appears to be associated with the disease under study.

An example of linkage disequilibrium between a disease susceptibility gene and HLA is found in idiopathic haemochromatosis [2, 14]. The (recessive) allele of the locus responsible for haemochromatosis is in linkage disequilibrium with HLA-A3; approximately 75% of patients with haemochromatosis have A3 (compared with a 21% frequency in control populations). Although this explanation is acceptable for a disease which is clearly not of autoimmune pathogenesis, postulating other linked disease susceptibility genes in addition to the HLA genes appears unnecessary in the case of the autoimmune diseases because of the evidence discussed earlier that MHC molecules are recognition structures used by T cells responding to an antigenic stimulus, and thus one of the factors influencing immune responses.

One objection raised to the assumption that the HLA molecules are themselves responsible for genetic variation in susceptibility to autoimmune diseases is that none of the diseases shows an absolute correlation with the presence of any given HLA allele. Several interesting possibilities may provide the explanation. First, analysis of the HLA genes, particularly those belonging to Class II, is far from complete, and alleles of an adjacent Class II locus in linkage disequilibrium may show a higher correlation. For example, coeliac disease originally appeared to be associated with HLA-DR3 and 7 [4]. Recent studies [45] have shown that the association is much stronger with DQW3, an allele of the DQ locus in linkage disequilibrium with DR3 and 7. Presumably, therefore, DQ3 is the allele conferring susceptibility to coeliac disease. Secondly, it may be that more than one HLA allele needs to be present to confer maximum susceptibility. In insulin-dependent diabetes mellitus, the highest relative risk is associated with the presence of *both* DR3 *and* DR4 [42]. Thirdly, other genetically determined traits may be of importance. An example here is the lupus erythematosus-like syndrome which sometimes occurs as a toxic complication of treatment with the antihypertensive drug hydralazine [29]. In hydralazine-induced lupus, one predisposing factor is a genetic difference in the activity of the liver N-acetyl transferase enzyme. Individuals are either slow or rapid acetylators, and hydralazine-induced lupus is observed almost exclusively in the slow acetylators. Another factor is the patient's sex, females being more commonly affected than males in a ratio of 4:1. A third genetic factor appears to be the HLA phenotype; in our experience 19 of 26 patients (73%) expressed HLA-DR4, a frequency significantly higher than that found in control groups [3]. It therefore seems that in hydralazine-induced lupus, at least 3 genetically determined traits govern susceptibility.

But perhaps the most important reason why an absolute correlation between HLA and autoimmune disease is not to be expected is that this would imply that non-genetic factors play an insignificant aetiological role; such an implication has only to be stated to be immediately rejected. There is strong evidence, which cannot be reviewed here, that environmental agents, eg infective agents, drugs and toxins, are important initiating factors of autoimmune responses. Obviously the extent and nature of the initial tissue-damaging event is an important parameter in this pathogenic scheme, and the outcome would not depend solely on an individual's genetically determined susceptibility. There presumably must be critical threshold levels of antigens necessary for induction of damaging autoimmunity even in susceptible individuals.

The possible role of Class III gene products

As mentioned earlier, linkage disequilibrium may be seen between HLA and adjacent genes, including those belonging to Class III [10]. The possibility that in some instances HLA-associated genetic susceptibility to a disease may be partly or wholly due to a Class III gene product needs, therefore, to be considered.

The most provocative case can be assembled for systemic lupus erythematosus (SLE). Firstly, inherited deficiencies of components of the complement system, although uncommon, have been observed, and subjects with these deficiencies are unusually prone to systemic lupus erythematosus [20, 35]. The inherited complement deficiencies associated with susceptibility to SLE include all the classical pathway components, some of which are encoded by genes not located in the HLA region of the 6th chromosome. However, these homozygous deficiencies of a complement component account for only a very small proportion of idiopathic SLE encountered in practice.

The second piece of evidence is that idiopathic SLE has been reported to be associated with several HLA antigens [47]. Working on the hypothesis that these associations might be secondary to linkage disequilibrium with a Class III gene allele, Fielder et al [16] showed in a family study that 83% of a group of 29 patients with SLE had one or more null or silent alleles for C4A, C4B, or C2. A null or silent allele results in failure to synthesize the corresponding protein gene product. The study suggested that partial (ie heterozygous) deficiencies of a complement component might confer susceptibility to SLE. Interpretation of the study was complicated by the high frequency of DR3 in the patient group, so that it remains uncertain at present whether susceptibility to SLE is most closely associated with the null alleles of C4 and C2 or with HLA-DR3, or whether both the Class II and III genes are involved. Further studies should resolve these questions.

It is tempting to speculate that the Class III genes are particularly likely to be involved in genetic susceptibility to diseases such as SLE in which much of the tissue damage is thought to be caused by antigen/antibody complexes. Inhibition of formation of insoluble complexes and, when formed, their resolubilization are critically influenced by the complement system [12, 37]. It is therefore plausible that polymorphic variation of the molecules of this highly reactive system should have functional consequences [33].

Concluding comments

It should not be assumed that HLA region genes are the only ones of significance in genetic susceptibility to autoimmune diseases. For reasons of space, justice has not been done to the associations between several autoimmune diseases and the Ig allotypes. There is clearly a fascinating problem to be resolved here. In addition, the old observations that most autoimmune diseases are heavily biased towards females indicates another genetically based cause of susceptibility which deserves further investigation.

Limitations of space have also prevented a proper discussion of autoimmune reactions arising from drug treatments or exposure to environmental toxins. Genetic susceptibility is a major factor here, which has been investigated in only a few instances. Table 2 lists some associations already reported. In the case of gold-induced

Table 2. Some examples of chemical- or drug-induced HLA-associated (human leucocyte antigen) toxicity syndromes

Condition	HLA antigens
1. Hydralazine-induced lupus	DR4
2. Gold-induced renal damage in rheumatoid arthritis patients	Haplotype: A1, B8, CW7, DR3
3. Susceptibility to vinyl chloride-induced scleroderma;	DR5
severity of syndrome	DR3
4. Penicillamine-induced myasthenia gravis in rheumatoid arthritis patients	DR1

renal damage arising in patients with rheumatoid arthritis, the association with the haplotype carrying HLA-B8, CW7, and DR3 is very strong; approximately 50% of patients with gold nephropathy have this haplotype, and more than 90% with this haplotype develop nephropathy if given a full course of gold therapy. Such figures argue that rheumatoid patients should be screened for this haplotype before embarking on gold treatment.

In conclusion, it seems inescapable to the author that, if we successfully identify the genes and their products which determine susceptibility to a wide variety of autoimmune reactions, this information will profoundly affect our strategies of both prevention and therapy of autoimmunity.

References

1. Basham TY, Merigan TC (1983) J Immunol 130:1492
2. Batchelor JR, Morris PJ, Dick H, Kennedy LJ (1978) In: Bodmer WF, Batchelor JR, Bodmer JG, Festenstein H, Morris PJ (eds) Histocompatibility Testing 1977. Munksgaard, Copenhagen, p 205
3. Batchelor JR, Welsh KI, Mansilla Tinoco R, Dollery CT, Hughes GRV, Ryan P, Bernstein R, Naish PF, Aber GM, Bing RF, Russell GI (1980) Lancet i:1107
4. Betuel H, Gebuhrer L, Descos L, Bertrand J, Freycon F, Lepetit JC (1980) In: Terasaki PI (ed) Histocompatibility Testing 1980. UCLA Tissue Typing Laboratory, Los Angeles, p 668
5. Bevan MJ (1981) In: Zaleski MB, Abeyounis CZ, Kano K (eds) Immunobiology of the Major Histocompatibility Complex
6. Biddison WE, Payne SM, Shearer GM, Shaw S (1980) J Exp Med 152:2045
7. Bodmer J, Bodmer W (1984) Immunol Today (in press)
8. Bodmer WF, Bodmer JG, Crumpton MJ, Lee J, Trowsdale J (1983) Transplant Proc 15:36
9. Brewerton DA, Caffrey M, Hart FD, James DCO, Nicholls A, Sturrock RD (1973) Lancet i:904
10. Brunn-Peterson G, Lamm LU, Sorensen IJ, Buskjaer L, Mortensen JP (1981) Hum Genet 58:260
11. Carroll MC, Campbell RD, Bentley DR, Porter RR (1984) Nature 307:237
12. Czop J, Nussenzweig V (1976) J Exp Med 143:615
13. Farrar WL, Mizel SB, Farrar JJ (1980) J Immunol 124:1371
14. Fauchet R, Simon M, Genetet B, Bourel M (1980) In: Terasaki PI (ed) Histocompatibility Testing. UCLA Tissue Typing Laboratory, Los Angeles, p 707
15. Festing MFW (1979) Inbred strains in biomedical research. Macmillan, London
16. Fielder AHL, Walport MJ, Batchelor JR, Rynes RI, Black CM, Dodi IA, Hughes GRV (1983) Br Med J 286:425
17. Gillis S, Smith KA (1977) Nature 268:154
18. Kantor FS, Ojeda A, Benacerraf B (1963) J Exp Med 117:55
19. Kaufman JF, Auffray C, Korman AJ, Shackelford DA, Strominger JL (1984) Cell 36:1
20. Lachmann PJ, Hobart MJ (1978) Br Med Bull 34:247
21. Lamb JR, Feldmann M (1982) Nature 300:456
22. Larsson EL, Iscove NN, Coutinho A (1980) Nature 283:664
23. Lilly F, Boyse EA, Old LJ (1964) Lancet ii:1207
24. McDevitt HO, Sela M (1965) J Exp Med 122:517
25. McDevitt HO, Chinitz A (1969) Science 163:1207
26. McMichael AJ (1978) J Exp Med 148:1458
27. Nishimura Y, Sasazuki T (1983) Nature 302:67
28. Parham P (1984) Immunol Today 5:89
29. Perry HM (1973) Am J Med 54:58
30. Pinchuck P, Maurer PH (1965) J Exp Med 122:673
31. Ploegh HL, Orr HT, Strominger JL (1981) Cell 24:287
32. Pober JS, Gimbrone MA, Cotran RS, Reiss CS, Burakoff SJ, Fiers W, Ault KA (1983) J Exp Med 157:1339
33. Porter RR (1983) Mol Biol Med 1:161
34. Ryder LP, Anderson A, Svejgaard A (1979) HLA and Disease Registry, Tissue Antigens [Suppl]
35. Rynes RI (1982) Clin Rheum Dis 8:29
36. Sasazuki T, Kohno Y, Iwanoto I, Tanimura M (1978) Nature 272:359
37. Schifferli JA, Bartolotti SR, Peters DK (1980) Clin Exp Immunol 42:387
38. Schlosstein L, Terasaki PI, Bluestone R, Pearson CM (1973) N Engl J Med 288:704
39. Schutze H, Gorer PA, Finlayson MH (1936) J Hyg 36:37
40. Suitters AJ, Lampert IA (1982) Br J Exp Pathol 63:207
41. Sunday ME, Benacerraf B, Dorf ME (1981) J Exp Med 153:811
42. Svejgaard A, Platz P, Ryder LP (1980) In: Terasaki PI (ed) Histocompatibility Testing

1980. UCLA Tissue Typing Laboratory, Los Angeles, p 638
43. Tada T, Taniguchi M, Okumura K, Hayawaka K, Hiramatsu K, Suzuki G (1981) In: Zaleski MB, Abeyounis CZ, Kano K (eds) Immunobiology of the Major Histocompatibility Complex. Karger, Basel, p 69
44. Thorsby E, Berle E, Braathen L (1983) Transplant Proc 15:282
45. Tosi R, Vismara D, Tanigaki N, Ferrara GB, Cicimarra F, Buffolano W, Follo D, Auricchio S (1984) Clin Immunol Immunopathol (in press)
46. Wallace LE, Rickinson AB, Rowe M, Epstein MA (1982) Nature 297:413
47. Walport MJ, Black CM, Batchelor JR (1982) Clin Rheum Dis 8:3
48. Williams N (1982) Nature 296:605
49. Zembala M, Asherson GL, Colizzi V (1982) Nature 297:411
50. Zinkernagel RM, Doherty PC (1974) Nature 248:701

The Mechanism of Action of Ciclosporin: A Continuing Puzzle

J. F. Borel, B. Ryffel

Ciclosporin (CyA) exerts a number of pharmacological effects (Fig. 1). Its most interesting action by far, however, consists of selectively modulating defined subpopulations of immunocompetent cells. CyA can therefore be considered as the first drug of a new generation of immunosuppressants which has substantially contributed to immunopharmacology.

activation is the recognition of a foreign antigen on the surface of an antigen-presenting cell (macrophage, dendritic cell) (Fig. 2). This antigen is recognised by means of the specific recognition structure only in association with the histocompatibility antigen of class II (D region in man; I region in the mouse) for T helper cells or class I for cytolytic T cells. This specific signal 1 activates the T cells from the G_0 phase of the cell cycle and leads these cells to express, 6 to 12 h later, receptors for IL-2 (interleukin 2 or T cell growth factor) [53]. This receptor expression, induced by antigen or mitogen, is called stage 1 of T cell activation (Fig. 3).

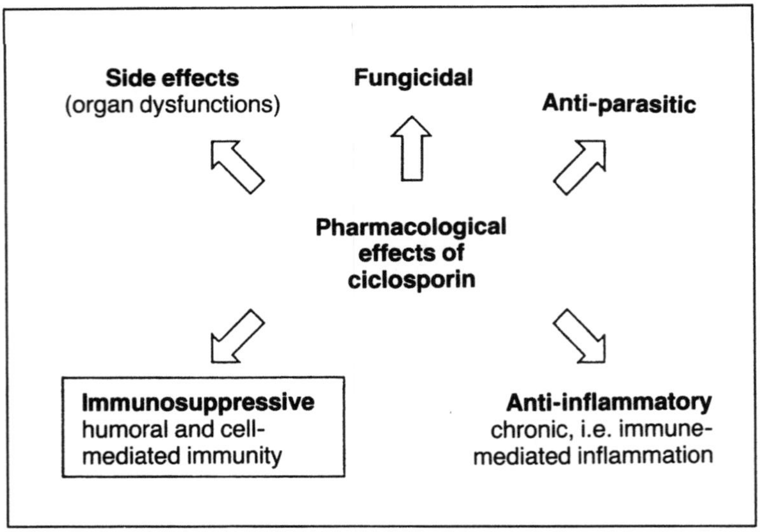

Fig. 1. The various pharmacological effects of ciclosporin

The basis of the immune response

It was realised in the last decade that the interaction between an antigen and its receptor on a lymphocyte is not a sufficient signal to stimulate the resting T or B cell to replicate and mature into an effector cell. The induction of the resting T cell into an activated T cell (T') requires two signals: first, the antigen specific signal 1; second, an unspecific costimulating factor (signal 2) [34]. Indeed, the specific step in lymphocyte

Concomitantly with the antigen recognition, the interaction with the histocompatibility class II antigen causes the antigen-presenting cell to release IL-1 (interleukin 1) (Figs. 2 and 3). This is the second signal required for the T cell to become activated and to be induced to produce IL-

Preclinical Research, Sandoz Ltd, 4002 Basle

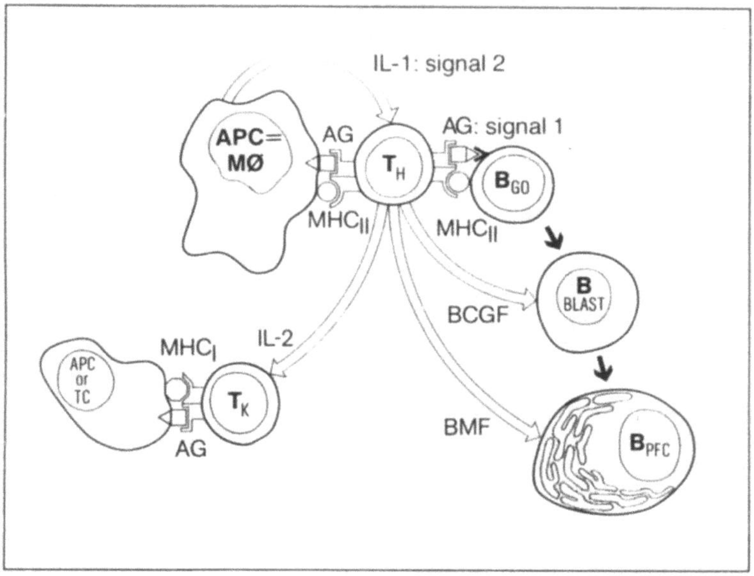

Fig. 2. Signal requirements for lymphocyte activation, proliferation and differentiation

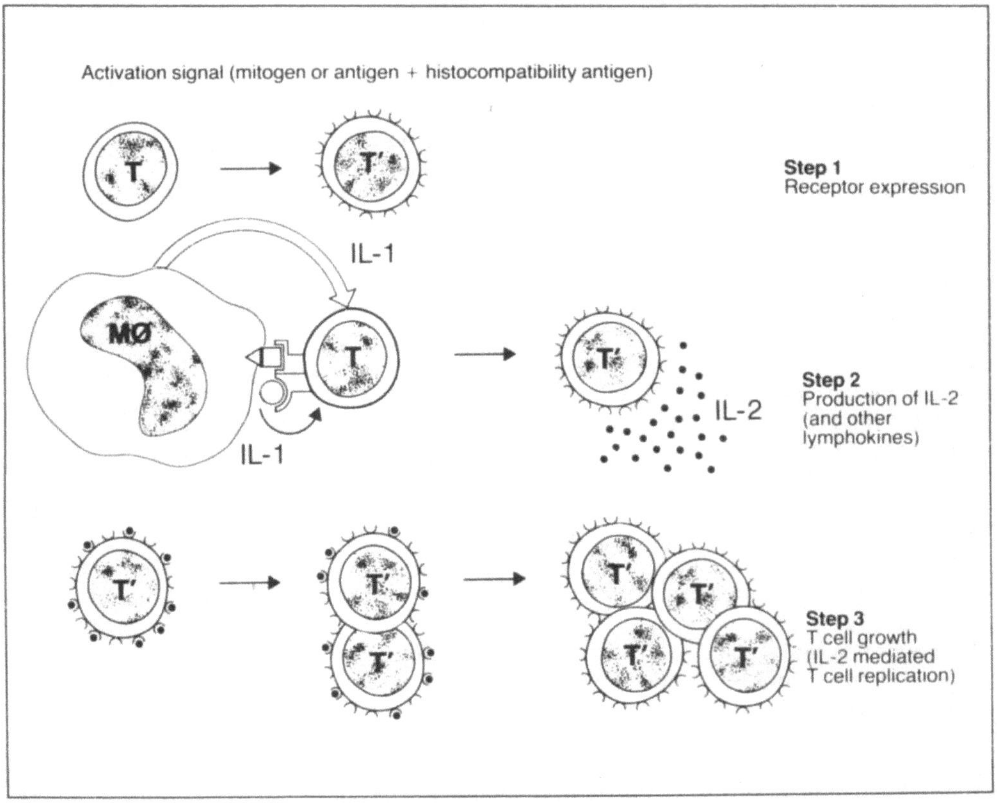

Fig. 3. Schematic representation of the interleukin-2 (IL-2) concept (Modified from M. Schreier [53])

2. It is generally agreed that IL-2 is released exclusively by T cell subpopulations, mainly by T helper cells, although cytolytic T cells, but not T suppressor cells, can also secrete IL-2. The promotion of IL-2 production is the second stage of the T cell response (Fig. 3) [53].

The third stage of the T cell activation, the actual T cell replication, is the result of the interaction of IL-2 with the IL-2 receptor, irrespective of the subpopulation to which the IL-2 receptor-expressing T cell belongs (Fig. 3). This step leads to further differentiation and maturation depending partly on the various lymphokines available and partly on the different effector potential of the T cell subsets involved in the ongoing immune reaction.

Table 1. Steps in the conversion of resting T cells (T) to activated T cells (T′)

Reactions	Ciclosporin sensitivity
Reaction A: Primary activation	
$T \xrightarrow[(2)]{(1)} T'$	+
Reaction B: Clonal expansion	
$T' \xrightarrow[(2)]{} nT'$	–
Reaction C: Triggering of lymphokine release	
$T' \xrightarrow{(1)} L$	+
Reaction D: Cytotoxic effector function	
T'_c = expression of cytotoxicity	–

Immunopharmaocology of CyA in vitro

Early studies have already emphasised the sparing effect of CyA on haemopoietic tissues and on leukocyte functions, except those of lymphocytes. The promt in vitro and in vivo reversibility of its immunosuppressive activity demonstrates that it is not due to a lymphocytotoxic action, such as an antimitotic effect [2, 60]. The compound is known mainly to inhibit the expression of helper function, i.e. the capacity of T cells to synthesise and release IL-2 [8, 13, 20]. Although it affects the production of several other lymphokines [26, 45, 47, 58], CyA does not interfere with their effects on target lymphocytes, such as IL-2 dependent T cell proliferation [21, 35], or on the phagocytic, migratory and monokine releasing activity of granulocytes or macrophages [9, 14, 27, 46, 54, 58].

The steps in the transformation of resting T cells (T) into activated T cells (T′) with receptors for IL-2, and the functions of these T′ cells such as the production of lymphokines, have different sensitivities to CyA (Table 1).

In these reactions, signal 1 is provided by antigen or mitogen binding to a receptor on the T cell surface, signal 2 by costimulator activity such as IL-1 or other postulated products of antigen-presenting cells. Reaction B is mediated by the T cell product IL-2 or T cell growth factor. CyA interferes with reaction C at concentrations of 5 to 100 ng/ml, but has no effect on reaction B at concentrations below 5 to 10 µg/ml. The cytolytic effector function of cytotoxic T cells (T'_c) is completely resistant to CyA [5].

Because it is multifactorial in nature, reaction A is more difficult to analyse. In fact, the involvement of multiple interactions in the conversion of T to T′ may account for the divergent results reported from different laboratories.

Current theories of T cell biology

While there is agreement concerning the regulation of activation, clonal proliferation and triggering of T cells expressing helper function, views diverge on the response of other T cells to CyA. These divergencies lead to two theories of T cell biology: The signalling model claims that all T cells are physiologically similar and have similar effector potential. Acccording to this hypothesis, CyA affects all T cells in essentially the same way, but the expression of different functions of the cells is regulated by differing receptor sensitivities to the compound.

The subset model postulates that CyA defines two T cell subsets, those that are sensitive to CyA (among which are helper and cytotoxic precursor cells) and those that are insensitive (including several suppressor and all cytotoxic cells).

The knowledge available to us at present does not permit the rejection of either of these models, and there is need of further experimental work designed to distinguish between them [6].

Finally, it has been suggested that CyA may affect B cell function in a manner similar to that in which it regulates T cells; that is, the signalling model, according to which CyA would define B cells at various stages of differentiation on the way to immunoglobulin synthesis, or the subset model, in which only B cells of one of several physiologically different subsets are CyA sensitive, would also be applicable [12, 30].

Effect of CyA at the level of molecular cell biology

It is deduced, from a vast number of both in vitro and in vivo results, that the compound reversibly affects the early steps immediately following antigen or mitogen recognition. As a result the T cells remain in the resting phase of the cell cycle, are unable to transform and to release lymphokines, and thus fail to induce and mount an immune response.

In addition, it has been conclusively shown that CyA may also effectively suppress an ongoing immune reaction such as (e.g.) a rejection crisis or an autoimmune relapse [2, 4, 11, 25, 51]. This therapeutic as opposed to preventive effect may be explained by CyA inhibiting the renewed antigen-triggered lymphokine release from activated cells [25] as well as interfering concomitantly with the activation and recruitment of further effector cells.

a) Interaction at the level of the lymphocyte membrane

CyA binds to cell membranes, but until now no specific receptor protein has been demonstrated. Saturable and reversible binding of labelled CyA occurs on the lymphocytic membrane, the binding sites having a K_D of about 10^{-7} M [37]. Inactive congeners do not displace bound CyA. However, the binding of CyA to membranes is not limited to lymphocytes. Similar binding characteristics are shown for macrophages, granulocytes, erythrocytes, hepatocytes and other cells [37, 50].

Flow cytometry using dansylated CyA reveals the existence of a dim and a bright staining T cell population. The weakly staining subset, which is CyA sensitive, responds to mitogen and alloantigen, whereas the bright staining population, which proves CyA resistant, proliferates only in response to IL-2 in vitro [22].

With regard to the specificity of binding, several ligands were tested, e.g. mitogens (including OKT3), HLA-DR, IL-1, IL-2, insulin and prolactin. There is no interference between CyA and OKT3 recognition sites, which are closely associated with T cell receptor, since binding of OKT 3 is not reduced by CyA and, conversely, labelled CyA is not displaced by OKT 3 [52]. In contrast, OKT 3 induced proliferation of human peripheral T cells is inhibited by CyA [56]. The attractive hypothesis of CyA blocking the receptors for HLA-DR antigens is dismissed [43] because there is much evidence that antigen recognition is not affected (see also Table 1; [3]). It has been claimed that CyA inhibits IL-1 binding [1, 44]. IL-2 and insulin receptors are not expressed on quiescent lymphocytes [19, 59], and therefore cannot be receptors for CyA. Prolactin has been shown to displace CyA and vice versa [24, 49]. Prolactin appears to modulate the immune reactivity of lymphocytes by rendering them susceptible to an antigenic stimulus [24]. Prolactin or a prolactin-like peptide might possibly behave as a lymphokine [39].

There is little information about CyA inducing any biochemical and physical changes in the membrane. However, it facilitates membrane immunoglogulin capping on murine B cells (Loor et al., unpublished results). Furthermore, the emergence of activation receptors such as IL-2, transferrin, insulin and Ia, was studied in the presence of CyA. IL-2 receptor expression seems not to be affected by CyA [33, 42], at least not during the first 24 h [38]. This observation is strongly supported by the fact that exogenous IL-2 reverses the inhibitory activity of CyA [8, 21]. However, the expression of transferrin and Ia receptors was significantly reduced [36, 42]. It has also been suggested that CyA inhibits T cell stimulation by interfering with the early activation of plasma membrane phospholipid metabolism [57].

However, currently available data do not support a direct effect of CyA at the membrane level, but argue in favour of this agent interfering with events distal to the calcium increase and proximal to gene translation [15, 17, 33, 41, 61].

b) Interaction within the cytoplasm

Among the earliest intracellular events following mitogen activation are changes in cytosolic calcium concentration. This calcium ion influx is either not influenced in the presence of CyA [41, 61] or it is even enhanced [23]. Similarly, the early uptake of nucleoside occurring simultaneously with the calcium influx in mitogen-stimulated lymphocytes remains unaffected by this drug [29]. Therefore, the CyA-sensitive step of the activation cascade lies after the calcium increase and seemingly before the ornithine decarboxylase activation, which is reported to be inhibited [16, 48].

Studies concerned with the subcellular localisation of radiolabelled CyA demonstrate that about 80% of the drug is recovered in the cytosol and that its intracellular concentration is markedly higher than in the medium [40]. It has been further shown that uptake of CyA is largely due to a cytosolic, drug-binding protein termed "cyclophilin". This high affinity-binding component consists of a single homogeneous polypeptide chain of about 117 amino acids [18]. No apparent sequence relationship between cyclophilin and any other protein could be detected.

The concentrative and biphasic uptake of CyA in the cytoplasm may be similar to that of steroids. CyA may diffuse passively through cell membranes and be retained by the high affinity cytosolic binding protein cyclophilin. However, the specific relationship of cyclophilin to the mechanism of CyA remains to be established [40].

Another ubiquitous cytosolic protein like cyclophilin is calmodulin. It was recently demonstrated that CyA binds to calmodulin and inhibits calmodulin-dependent enzymatic activation [10].

CyA causes the emergence of highly refringent globular bodies and the use of dansylated drug suggests that within a few hours CyA is contained in those globules. The latter are not identical with normal mitochondria or lysosomes, but are most likely lipid droplets [31]. The mitogen-induced increase of mitochondrial and lysosomal activity is strongly reduced by CyA [32].

There is no evidence for metabolic degradation of CyA taking place in cultured lymphocytes [40]. Moreover, no convincing data are available indicating that CyA might interfere with other metabolic events within the cytoplasm.

c) Interaction at the nuclear level

Nuclear localisation of CyA has been shown by means of labelled drug (Wiesinger and Weil, unpublished results; [40, 55]). This finding is of interest, since specific inhibition by CyA of mRNA synthesis encoding for some lymphokines has recently been demonstrated. The inhibition by CyA of RNA polymerase II specific for immunoglobulin gene transcription in HeLa cell lysates has been reported [7]. Whether this inhibition of RNA polymerase also occurs in lymphocytes has not been tested. However, three concordant papers confirm this assumption by showing that specific mRNA synthesis for lymphokines is inhibited by CyA [15, 17, 33]. Since transcription of these specific lymphokine mRNAs is known to appear within a few hours after stimulation of resting T lymphocytes [61] and reaches a high concentration during the transition from the G_0/G_1 to the S phase of T cell growth, this might well constitute the crucial step interfered with by CyA. This is further substantiated by the findings that the expression of other inducible genes, such as those for IL-2 receptor, HT 3 [33] and actin [61], are not inhibited; however, CyA suppresses synthesis of IL-2, gamma-interferon, B cell- and cytolytic T cell-stimulating factors by blocking the induction of active lymphokine mRNA. In contrast, the bulk protein

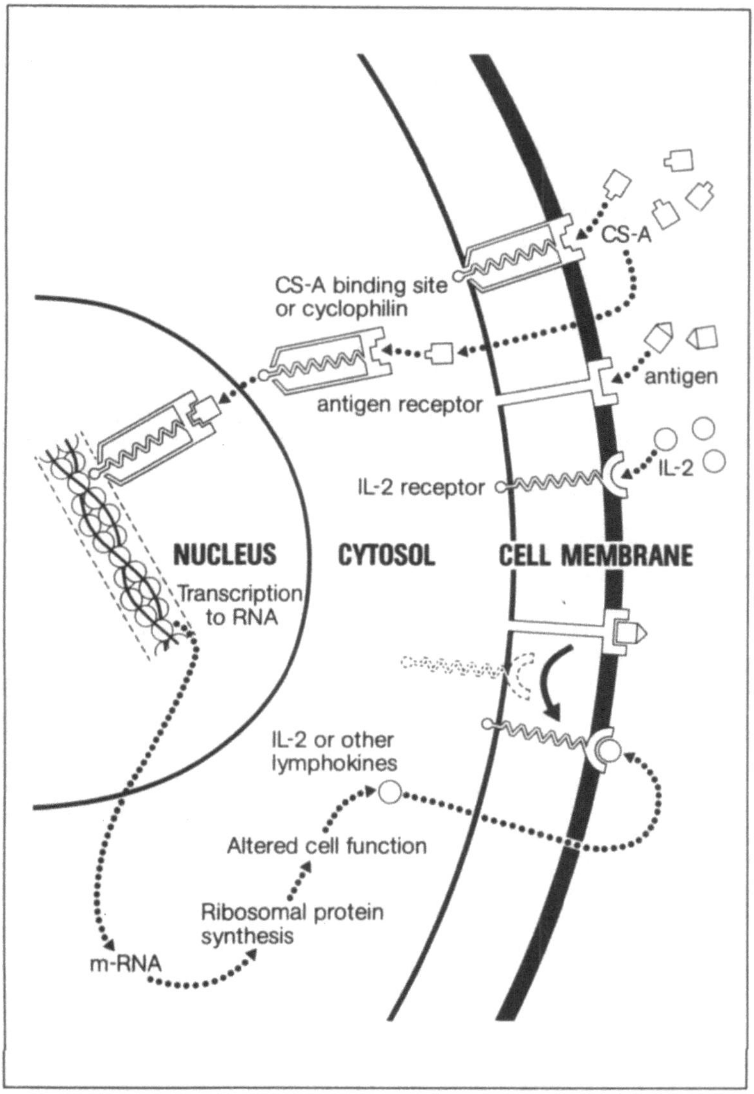

Fig. 4. Proposed mechanism of action of ciclosporin (CyA). CyA binds and is internalised into the cytoplasm. There the drug is bound to a protein termed cyclophilin. The CyA-receptor complex is transported into the cell nucleus, where it interacts with specific sites on the chromosome. This process interferes with the transcription of messenger ribonucleic acid (mRNA), i.e. specifically with the mRNAs encoding for lymphokines. As a consequence the translation of mRNA and subsequent synthesis and release of lymphokines, such as e.g. IL-2 , are inhibited

synthesis induced by ConA is not modified [17].

Conclusions

Although tempting, it seems risky to speculate on the mode of action of CyA, which still remains largely hypothetical despite important recent progress. Moreover, the molecular biology of lymphocyte activation, proliferation and maturation itself is far from being completely explored. Because of the undeniable selective activity of CyA on lymphocytes, the most promising approach for uncovering its mechanism of action would focus on the cellular functions which are peculiar to the lymphocyte and distinct from other more general events occurring during cell activation (see also Fig. 4). The most attractive explanation today would be that both CyA and prolactin bind to the same, still undefined binding protein, which definitely is not identical with the antigen recognition site or T cell receptor. CyA is then internalised and concentrated into the cytoplasm, where it is bound to cyclophilin. This process bears some similarity to that for steroid hormones. Both compounds appear to have receptors in the cytosol and to be able to penetrate into the nucleus [28] where CyA in particular inhibits specifically the transcription of mRNA coding for lymphokines, but not for the bulk of other proteins [17]. This might be the crucial CyA-sensitive step, because addition of the drug beyond this stage (i.e. 2–4 h after stimulation) remains ineffective; for instance the subsequent translation and protein (lymphokine) synthesis proceed normally [33]. The advantage of this hypothesis is its simplicity and its compatibility with the numerous in vivo results demonstrating that CyA not only prevents a primary immunisation, but that it may also terminate an ongoing immune reaction. This may be most likely to occur through inhibition of continued lymphokine release [25] as well as through suppression of further activation and recruitment of effector cells.

References

1. Bendtzen K, Dinarello CA (1984) Mechanism of Action of Cyclosporin A. Effect on T-Cell-Binding of Interleukin 1 and Antagonizing Effect of Insulin. Scand J Immunol 20:43–51
2. Borel JF, Feurer C, Gubler HU, Staehelin H (1976) Biological Effects of Cyclosporin A: A New Antilymphocytic Agent. Agents Actions 6/4:468–475
3. Borel JF (1976) Comparative study of in vitro and in vivo drug effects on cell-mediated cytotoxicity. Immunology 31:631–641
4. Borel JF (1981) Cyclosporin A – Present Experimental Status. Transplant Proc 13:344–348
5. Borel JF, Lafferty KJ (1983) Cyclosporine: Speculation about its mechanism of action. Transplant Proc 15:1881–1885
6. Borel JF, Lafferty KJ (1983) Basic Science Summation. Transplant Proc 15 [Suppl 1]:3097–3102
7. Brack C, Mattaj IW, Gautschi J, Cammisuli S (1984) Cyclosporin A is a Differential Inhibitor of Eukaryotic RNA Polymerases. Exp Cell Res 151:314–321
8. Bunjes D, Hardt C, Röllinghoff M, Wagner H (1981) Cyclosporin A mediates immunosuppression of primary cytotoxic T cell responses by impairing the release of interleukin 1 and interleukin 2. Eur J Immunol 11/8:657–661
9. Bunjes D, Hardt C, Solbach W, Deusch K, Röllinghoff M, Wagner H (1982) Studies on the mechanism of action of Cyclosporin A in the murine and human T-cell response in vitro. In: White DJG (ed) Cyclosporin A. Elsevier Biomedical Press, Amsterdam, pp 261–280
10. Colombani PM, Robb A, Hess AD (1985) Cyclosporine binding to calmodulin: a possible site of action on T lymphocytes. Science 228:337–339
11. Deeg HJ, Storb R, Gerhard-Miller L, Shulman HM, Weiden PL, Thomas ED (1980) Cyclosporin A, a powerful immunosuppressant in vivo and in vitro in the dog, fails to induce tolerance. Transplantation 29:230–235
12. Dongworth DW, Klaus GGB (1982) Effects of Cyclosporin A on the Immune System of the Mouse. I. Evidence for a Direct Selective Effect of Cyclsoporin A on B Cells Responding to Anti-Immunoglobulin Antibodies. Eur J Immunol 12/12:1018–1022
13. Dos Reis GA, Shevach EM (1982) Effect of Cyclosporin A on T Cell Function in Vitro: the Mechanism of Suppression of T Cell Proliferation Depends on the Naure of the T Cell Stimulus as well as the Differentiation State of the Responding T Cell. J Immunol 129/6:2360–2367
14. Drath DB, Kahan BD (1984) Phagocytic cell function in response to immunosuppressive therapy. Arch Surg 119:156–160
15. Elliottt JF, Lin Y, Mizel SB, Bleackley R, Harnish DG, Paetkau V (1984) Induction of Interleukin 2 Messenger RNA Inhibited by Cylosporin A. Science 226:1439–1441
16. Fidelus RK, Laughter AH, Twoney JJ, Taffet SM, Haddox MK (1984) The effect of cyclosporine on ornithine decarboxylase induction with mitogens, antigens, and lymphokines. Transplantation 37:383–387
17. Granelli-Piperno A, Inaba K, Steinman RM (1984) Stimulation of Lymphokine Release from T Lymphoblasts. J Exp Med 160:1792–1802

18. Handschumacher ER, Harding MW, Rice J, Drugge RJ (1984) Cyclophilin: A Specific Cytosolic Binding Protein for Cyclospoin A. Science 226:544–547
19. Helderman JH, Raskin P (1980) The T lymphocyte insulin receptor in diabetes and obesity. An intrinsic binding defect. Diabetes 29:551
20. Hess AD, Tutschka PJ, Santos GW, Pu Z (1982) Effect of Cyclosporin A on Human Lymphocyte Responses in Vitro. J Immunol 128/1:355–367
21. Hess AD (1985) Effect of Interleukin 2 on the Immunosuppressive Action of Cyclosporine. Transplantation 39:62–68
22. Hess AD, Colombani PM, Donnenberg AD, Fischer AC, Ryffel B (1985) Binding of dansylated Cyclosporine discriminates functional T lymphocyte subsets. Transplant Proc 17:1419–1427
23. Hiestand PC (1984) Cyclosporin A (Sandimmun®) modulates the Ca^+ uptake of mitogen-stimulated lymphocytes. Agents Actions 15:556–561
24. Hiestand PC, Mekler P, Nordmann R, Grieder A: Prolactin: an autocrine modulator of lymphocyte responsiveness. A possible mechanism of action of Ciclosporin. Proc Natl Acad Sci USA (in press)
25. Hodgkin PD, Agostino M, Sellins K, Prowse SJ, Bellgrau D, Lafferty KJ: T lymphocyte function **in vivo:** Ambivalence of the class I MHC antigen reactive subset. Transplantation (in press)
26. Horowitz M, Baron R, Mart J, Andreoli M, Vignery A (1984) Osteoclast Activating Factor Production by Murine Spleen Cells is Sensitive to Cyclosporin A and is Distinct from IL-2 and Interferon. Calcif Tissue Int 36:462
27. Janco RL, English D (1983) Cyclosporine and human neutrophil function. Transplantation 35:501–503
28. Karin M, Haslinger A, Holtgreve H, Richards RI, Krauter P, Westphal HM, Beato M (1984) Characterisation of DNA sequences through which cadmium and glucocorticoid hormones induce human metallothionein-II_A gene. Nature 308:513–519
29. Kay JE, Benzie CR, Borghetti AF (1983) Effect of cyclosporin A on lymphocyte activation by the calcium ionophore A23187. Immunology 50:441–446
30. Klaus GCB, Hawrylowicz CM (1984) Activation and proliferation signals in mouse B cells. II. Evidence for activation (G_0 to G_1) signals differing in sensitivity to cyclosorine. Eur J Immunol 14:250–254
31. Koponen M, Loor F (1983) Cytoplasmic Lipid Droplets as the Possible Eventual Cellular Fate of Active Forms of Cyclosporin. Exp Cell Res 149/2:499–512
32. Koponen M, Grieder A, Loor F (1984) Interference of Cyclosporin with Lymphocyte Activation: Blockage of the Mitogen-Induced Increases of Lysosomal and Mitochondrial Activities. Immunology 53/1:55–62
33. Kronke M, Leonard WJ, Depper JM, Arya SK, Wong Staal F, Gallo RC (1984) Cyclosporin A Inhibits T-Cell Growth Factor Gene Expression at the Level of mRNA Transcription. Proc Natl Acad Sci USA 81/16:5214–5218
34. Lafferty KJ, Woolrough J (1977) The origin and mechanism of the allograft rejection. Immunol Rev 35:231
35. Lafferty KJ, Borel JF, Hodgkin P (1983) Cyclosporine-A (CsA): Models for the Mechanism of Action. Transplant Proc 15 [Suppl 1]: 2242–2247
36. Leapman SB, Strong DM, Filo RS, Smith EF, Brandt GL (1982) Cyclosporin A Prevents the Appearance of Cell Surface "Activation" Antigens. Transplantation 34:94–95
37. LeGrue SJ, Friedman AW, Kahan BD (1983) Binding of Cyclosporine by Human Lymphocytes and Phospholipid Vesicles. J Immunol 131/2:712–718
38. Lillehoj HS, Malek TR, Shevach EM (1984) Differential Effect of Cyclosporin A on the Expression of T and B Lymphocyte Activation Antigens. J Immunol 133/1:244–250
39. Linzer DIH, Nathans D (1984) Nucleotide sequence of a growth-related mRNA encoding a member of the prolactin-growth hormone family. Proc Natl Acad Sci USA 81: 4255–4259
40. Merker MM, Handschumacher RE (1984) Uptake and Nature of the Intracellular Binding of Cyclosporin A in a Murine Thymoma Cell Line, BW5147. J Immunol 132: 3064–3070
41. Metcalfe S (1984) Cyclosporine does not prevent cytoplasmic calcium changes associated with lymphocyte activation. Transplantation 38:161–164
42. Miyawaki T, Yachie A, Ohzeki S, Nagaoki T, Taniguchi N (1983) Cyclosporin A Does Not Prevent Expression of Tac Antigen, A Probable TCGF Receptor Molecule, on Mitogen-Stimulated Human T Cells. J Immunol 130/6:2737–2742
43. Palacios R, Moller G (1981) Cyclosporin A Blocks Receptors for HLA-DR Antigens of T Cells. Nature 290/5809:792–794
44. Palacios R (1982) Mechanism of T cell activation: Role and functional relationship of HLA-DR antigens and interleukins. Immunol Rev 63:73–110

45. Palacios R (1985) Cyclosporin A inhibits antigen- and lectin-induced but not constitutive production of interleukin 3. Eur J Immunol 15:204–206
46. Pedersen C, Permin H, Stahl Skov P, Norn S, Svenson M, Mosbech M, Bendtzen K (1985) Inhibitory Effect of Cyclosporin A on Histamine Release from Human Leukocytes and Rat Mast Cells. Allergy 40:103–107
47. Reem GH, Cook LA (1983) Gamma Interferon Synthesis by Human Thymocytes and T Lymphocytes Inhibited by Cyclosporin A. Science 221/ 4605:63–65
48. Russell DH, Larson DF, Cardon SB, Copeland JG (1984) Cyclosporine inhibits prolactin induction of ornithine decarboxylase in rat tissues. Mol Cell Endocrinol 35:159–166
49. Russell DH, Matrisian L, Kibler R, Larson DF, Poulos B, Magun BE (1984) Prolactin receptors on human lymphocytes and their modulation by cyclosporine. Biochem Biophys Res Commun 121:899–906
50. Ryffel B, Gotz U, Heuberger B (1982) Cyclosporin Receptors on Human Lymphocytes. J Immunol 129/5:1978–1982
51. Ryffel B, Feurer C, Heuberger B, Borel JF (1982) Immunosuppressive Effect of Cyclosporin A in Two Lymphocyte Transfer Models in Rats: Comparison of in Vivo and in Vitro Treatment. Immunobiology 163:470–483
52. Ryffel B (1984) Cyclosporine: Effects on human T lymphocyte activation and clinical application. Clin Immunol Newsletter 5:164–168
53. Schreier MH (1984) Interleukin-2 and its role in the immune response. Triangle 23:141–152
54. Shennib A, Padilla-Longoria R, Chiu RCJ, Mulder DS (1982) Preservation of alveolar macrophage function during immunosuppression: Cyclosporin A versus Methylprednisolone. Surgical Forum 33:338–341
55. Simons JW, Noga SJ, Colombani PM, Coffey DS, Hess AD: Cyclosporin A induces alterations in the nuclear morphology of human mononuclear leukocytes. J Cell Biochem (in press)
56. Suthanthiran M, Evelyn M, Rubin AL, Stenzel KH (1984) A reappraisal of the effects of monoclonal antibodies directed at T cell differentiation antigens. Transplantation 38:720–726
57. Szamel M, Berger P, Resch K (1984) Cyclosporin A inhibits lymphocyte activation by interfering with the early activation of plasma membrane phospholipid metabolism. Immunobiology 167:208
58. Thomson AW, Moon DK, Geczy CL, Nelson DS (1983) Cyclosporine and Lymphokines Affecting Macrophage Behavior. Transplant Proc 15 [Suppl 1]:2390–2393
59. Uchiyama T, Broder S, Waldmann TA (1981) A monoclonal antibody (anti- Tac) reactive with activated and functionally mature human T cells. I. Production of anti-Tac monoclonal antibody and distribution of Tac(+) cells. J Immunol 126:1393
60. Wiesinger D, Borel JF (1979) Studies on the mechanism of action of cyclosporin A. Immunobiology 156:454–463
61. Wiskocil R, Weiss A, Imboden J, Kamin-Lewis R, Stobo J (1985) Activation of a human T cell line: A two- stimulus requirement in the pretranslational events involved in the coordinate expression of interleukin 2 and γ-interferon genes. J Immunol 134:1599–1603

Contrasting Effects of Ciclosporin on Humoral and Cell-mediated Immunity in Patients with Autoimmune Diseases

J. F. Bach and G. Feutren

Introduction

Experimental and clinical autoimmune responses usually demonstrate an association between autoantibodies and cell-mediated autoimmunity. It is reasonable to ask whether antibodies or effector T cells are responsible for the onset of disease (creation of lesions). Several arguments listed in Table 1 indicate a link between specific diseases and antibody- or cell-mediated immunity. One may thus speculate that a number of autoimmune diseases are due to the direct effect of antibodies whereas other diseases may be tentatively classified as dependent on cell-mediated immunity (Table 2). The problem is not simple, however, since even in the most typical cases (such as myasthenia gravis), the role of cell-mediated immunity has been demonstrated in the early phase of the experimental disease and antibody transfer from mother to newborn is not always associated with disease onset; it is as if in some cases the disease was due to T cells that do not cross the placenta.

Ciclosporin (CyA) has been shown to be a potent immunosuppressive agent in organ transplantation. It has been more recently used in a number of autoimmune diseases [4, 5]. With regard to our previous comments, it is important to determine whether in these autoimmune diseases the drug acts on antibody- or cell-mediated immunity. Data obtained in three disease states (autoimmune hemophilia, systemic lupus, Type I diabetes) indicate that ciclosporin preferentially affects cell-mediated autoimmune responses.

Service d'Immunologie Clinique, Inserm U 25, CNRS LA 122, Hôpital Necker, 161, rue de Sèvres, 75730 Paris Cedex 15, France

CyA and the production of an anticoagulant autoantibody

The occurrence of an autoantibody against Factor VIII_c that induces an acquired hemophilia is a rare but well-known event in the course of various autoimmune diseases [7]. We have treated with CyA a 41-year-old man suffering since 1977 from Cogan's syndrome (with polyarthritis, bilateral perceptive deafness, interstitial keratitis and aortic regurgitation) who spontaneously developed an autoantibody to Factor VIII_c responsible for acquired hemophilia (with spontaneous joint or muscle bleeding). In 1983, the patient was treated for a 6-month period with CyA: 3 months at 2.5 to 4.8 mg/kg/d and 3 months at 7.5 mg/kg/d reduced to 5.5 mg/kg/d after 50 days because of transient and minor nephrotoxicity. No significant modification of the anticoagulant titer was observed although ciclosporin whole blood trough levels were in the active range (Fig. 1). Three spontaneous haemorrhages requiring replacement treatment occurred in this period (left knee, right calf and right forearm).

In contrast to the complete inefficacy of CyA on the titer of anti VIII_c, the patient was successfully treated in 1978 with plasmapheresis plus high doses of corticosteroids and cyclophosphamide. This treatment had induced a ten-fold decrease in the anticoagulant titer.

CyA and anti-DNA antibody production in lupus

Similarly, CyA was observed to have no effect on anti-DNA titers in lupus treated with 5 mg/kg/d of CyA (blood trough level above 200 ng/ml) (Fig. 2a). In 8 patients, anti-DNA antibodies were above the normal level before CyA and remained so in

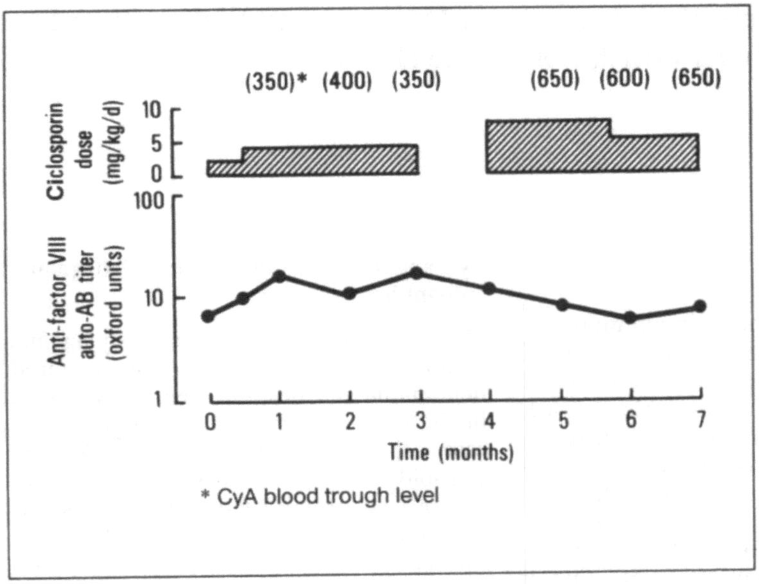

Fig. 1. Absence of change in titers of autoantibody to F. VIII_c (expressed as Oxford Units) during ciclosporin treatment

Table 1. Arguments for cellular or humoral pathogenic mechanisms in autoimmune diseases

Humoral immunity	Cell-mediated immunity
1. Disease transfer to animals by serum	1. Lymphocytic infiltration
2. Disease transfer from mother to newborn	2. Disease transfer by lymphoid cells in animal models
3. In vivo effect of monoclonal autoantibodies	3. Delayed type hypersensitivity skin reactions
4. Effects of bursectomy	4. Autoantigen-induced lymphocyte proliferation and inhibition leukocyte migration
	5. Suppression of the disease by T cell inactivation (neonatal thymectomy, ALS)
	6. In vitro lymphocytotoxicity

Table 2. Humoral versus cell-mediated immunity in autoimmune diseases

Antibody	Effector T cells
Myasthenia gravis	Uveitis
Autoimmune cytopenias	Type I diabetes
Pernicious anemia	Chronic active hepatitis

six cases after 6 months of treatment by CyA, and in four of those six patients at 9–15 months. Antinuclear factor activity (assessed by immunofluorescence tests) was not modified either. Parallel persistence of a decreased C4 level indicated the absence of an effect of CyA on the production of immune complexes that activate the classical pathway of the complement system (Fig. 2b). Contrasting with this inefficacy, clinical improvement was observed in seven of the eight patients [6].

Interestingly, we observed a clear-cut rise in IgG levels in most patients (Fig. 3). This was probably linked to the decrease of steroid dosage permitted by the clinical improvement.

CyA and anti-islet autoimmunity in diabetes

Analogous data were obtained in Type I diabetes. As shown in Table 3, islet cell

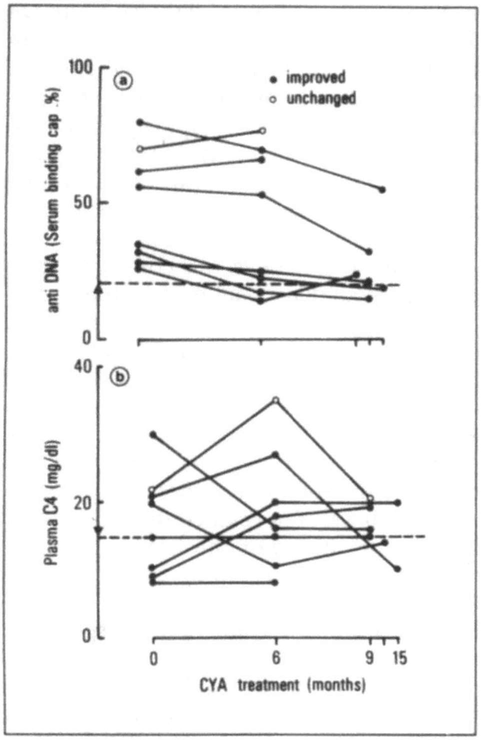

Fig. 2. Time-course of (a) anti-DNA antibodies (Farr test) and (b) plasma C4 level (nephelometry) during ciclosporin treatment in patients with severe systemic lupus. Dotted lines and arrows: normal values

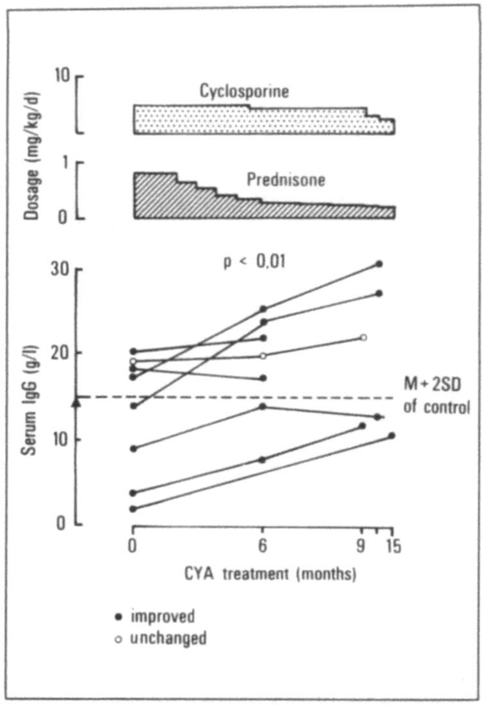

Fig. 3. Increase in serum IgG level (nephelometry) in patients with steroid-dependent or resistant systemic lupus treated with ciclosporin

Table 3. Islet cell antibodies (ICA) titer in recent Type I diabetics treated with ciclosporin

	Patient No.	CyA treatment (months)						
		0	0.5	1	2	3	4	5
Complete remission	1	–[a]	–	–	–	–	–	–
	2	–	–	–	–	–	–	–
	3	–	–	–	–	–	–	
	4	–	1	1	1	1	–	
Partial remission	5	8	8	8	–	–	–	
	6	20	10	10	10	10		
	7	1	2	2	1	1		
	8	–	–	–	–	–		
Failure	9	40	40	40	40	40		
	10	40	20	20	20	·[b]	20	
	11	20	20	·	20			
	12	·	·	·	·			

(a) – : Negative
(b) · : Not determined

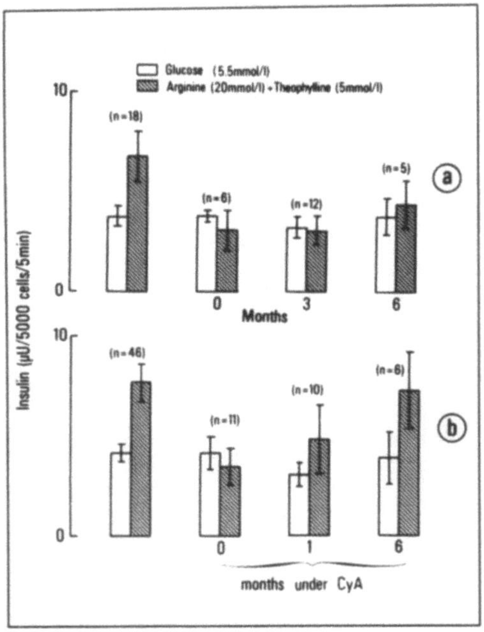

Fig. 4. Immunoreactive insulin secretion of in vitro cultured mouse islet cells in the presence of control or Type I diabetics' lymphocytes. (a): non CyA treated diabetics in the first 6 months after onset of diabetes. (b): ciclosporin-treated diabetics. Open columns: insulin secretion in basal state. Hatched columns: insulin secretion after a 5-min stimulation by arginine + theophylline. Results are expressed as mean ± SEM

antibody (ICA) titer was not substantially modified during the first months of ciclosporin treatment (mean dose: 8 mg/kg/d). Similar data were obtained with cytotoxic antibodies (assessed by a ^{51}Cr release assay), whose titers were not significantly reduced by CyA. In contrast with these results, CyA induced a decrease in cell-mediated immunity directed against islet cells. This effect was evidenced by using an in vitro assay described in our laboratory [2] where dispersed mouse islet cells are incubated for 18 hours in the presence of the patients' lymphocytes. The ability of these lymphocytes to block insulin secretion by islet cells after a 5-minute stimulation with glucose at high concentration or arginine is a strictly T cell dependent phenomenon, thought to be an in vitro correlate of anti-islet cell-mediated immunity [3]. As previously described [2], lymphocytes from the vast majority of Type I diabetics (but not from Type II diabetics) inhibit insulin secretion in vitro. The blocking effect is exerted by highly purified E^+ lymphocytes and $OKT3^+$, $OKT4^-$ lymphocytes, is not suppressed by aggregated immunoglobulins, and is specific to insulin-secreting cells since glucagon and somatostatin-secreting cells were not inhibited.

Figure 4a illustrates the course of lymphocyte-mediated insulin secretion inhibition in the first 6 months after the onset of diabetes in non CyA treated Type I diabetics. The blocking effect clearly persisted during this period. Contrasting with this evolution, CyA-treated diabetics' lymphocytes progressively lost their blocking capacity, the 6-month values being identical with those of normal controls (Fig. 4b). This disappearance of anti-islet cellular immunity paralleled the progressive onset of CyA-induced immunosuppression assessed by IL-2 production and PHA responsiveness [1].

Importantly, a favorable clinical effect was observed in 8 of the 12 treated patients with partial or complete remission, indicating that the clinical course paralleled that of cell-mediated rather than humoral immunity [1].

Discussion

These data indicate that in three different diseases, ciclosporin shows the same contrasting effect on humoral and cell-mediated immunity. It remains essentially without effect on autoantibody production (assessed in the three diseases studied) and shows a clear-cut action on cell-mediated immunity in the only model in which it could be studied with an appropriate in vitro assay.

The absence of effect on antibody production probably relates to the relative inefficacy of the drug on established antibody production [9]. Stiller et al. reported some effect of ciclosporin on ICA titer but this effect was only a minor one and appeared only after several months of treatment [10, 11]. Resistance to ciclosporin of autoantibody production probably explains the failure of ciclosporin to prevent spontaneous allergic thyroiditis in the chicken, where antibodies probably play the major role since bursectomy prevents occurrence of the disease [13].

The significant effect of ciclosporin on cell-mediated immunity is more difficult to assess because of the absence of suitable tests. In Type I diabetes however, an assay is available for detecting T cell-mediated autoreactivity. The value of this assay, which is based on blocking of insulin secretion by cultured islet cells, is still open to speculation and the method needs further investigation because of its apparent lack of HLA restriction (it uses xenogeneic mouse islet cells). The fact remains, however, that documented experiments have shown the assay to depend only on T cells without interference by K cells or antibody [3]. In any case, it is obvious that in contrast to the absence of effect on antibody production, ciclosporin significantly depressed the in vitro lymphocyte blocking assay, indicating that clinical remissions observed under ciclosporin are associated with depression of cell-mediated immunity, rather than of anti-islet autoantibodies producing B lymphocytes.

The situation is more complex in lupus, where no test of cell-mediated immunity is available. It is only on the indirect basis of the absence of an effect on antibody production that one can speculate about the preferential effect of ciclosporin on T cell mediated immunity. One should recognize, however, that there are few data in favor of such a direct effect of T cells in a disease generally thought to be due to immune complexes. Additionally, one cannot rule out that pathogenic antibodies are not detected by the tests used (so that the decrease in their production is missed) or that ciclosporin acts on immune complex induced inflammation in which T cells may participate, notably through lymphokine production.

The contrasting effect of ciclosporin on antibody and T cell mediated immunity is based on findings made in several independent series of patients. However, the absence of an effect of ciclosporin on autoantibody production is probably not an absolute phenomenon since we have ourselves shown that ciclosporin used at high doses (60 mg/kg/d) depresses anti-DNA antibody production in (NZB/NZW)F1 mice even when treatment is started late in the disease after the onset of the autoimmunity [8]. The same is observed for anti-skin autoantibodies in human pemphigus [12]. The reasons for these discrepancies are not clear (higher dosage, special nature of the autoimmune response?).

Acknowledgements

We are grateful to the clinicians and investigators who actively contributed towards the collection of the data presented in this article: R. Assan, M. Debray-Sachs, M. C. Quiniou-Debrie, G. F. Bottazzo for Type I diabetes; M. F. Kahn, P. Bourgeois, C. Gazengel for the anti Factor VII autoimmune patient; and S. Querin, Ph. Lesavre, L. Chatenoud, P. Godeau, J. Dormont for lupus.

References

1. Assan R, Feutren G, Debray-Sachs M, Quiniou-Debrie MC, Laborie C, Thomas G, Chatenoud L, Bach JF (1985) Metabolic and immunological effects of cyclosporin in recently diagnosed type 1 diabetes mellitus. Lancet I:67
2. Boitard C, Debray-Sachs M, Pouplard A, Assan R, Hamburger J (1981) Lymphocytes from diabetics suppress insulin release in vitro. Diabetologia 21:41
3. Boitard C, Chatenoud LM, Debray-Sachs M (1982) In vitro inhibition of pancreatic B cell function by lymphocytes from diabetics with associated autoimmune diseases: a T cell phenomenon. J Immunol 129:2529
4. Borel JF (1983) Cyclosporine: historical perspectives. Transplant Proc [Suppl 1] 15:2219
5. Borel JF, von Graffenried B (1984) Sandimmun® (Cyclosporin A) and autoimmunity. In: Lamber PH, Perrin L, Izui S (eds) Recent Advances in Systemic Lupus Erythematosus. Academic Press, New York, p 313
6. Feutren G, Querin S, Chatenoud LM, Noel LH, Beaurain G, Lesavre Ph, Bach JF (1985) The effects of cyclosporine in twelve patients with severe systemic lupus. In: Schindler R (ed) Ciclosporin in Autoimmune Diseases. 1st International Symposium, Basle, march 18–20, 1985. Springer, Berlin Heidelberg New York Tokyo, p 366

7. Green D, Lechner K (1981) A survey of 215 nonhaemophilic patients with inhibitors to F VIII. Thromb Haemost 45:200
8. Israel-Biet D, Noel LH, Bach MA, Dardenne M, Bach JF (1983) Marked reduction of DNA antibody production and glomerulopathy in thymulin (FTS-Zn) or cyclosporin A treated (NZB × NZW) F1 mice. Clin Exp Immunol 54:359
9. Kunkl A, Klaus GGB (1980) Selective effects of cyclosporin A on functional B cell subsets in the mouse. J Immunol 125:2526
10. Mandrup-Poulsen T, Nerup J, Stiller CR, Marner B, Bille G, Heinrichs D, Martell R, Dupre J, Keown PA, Jenner MR, Rodger NW. Wolfe B, v. Graffenried B, Binder C (1985) Disappearance and reappearance of islet cell cytoplasmic antibodies in cyclosporin-treated insulin-dependent diabetics. Lancet I:599
11. Stiller CR, Dupre J, Gent M, Jenner MR, Keown PA, Laupacis A, Martell R, Rodger NW, v. Graffenried B, Wolfe BMJ (1984) Effects of cyclosporine immunosuppression in insulin-dependent diabetes mellitus of recent onset. Science 223:1362
12. Thivolet J, Barthelemy H, Rigot-Muller G, Bendelac A (1985) Effects of cyclosporin on bullous pemphiloid and pemphigus. Lancet I:334
13. Wick G, Muller PU, Schwarz S (1982) Effect of cyclosporin A on spontaneous autoimmune thyroiditis of obese strain (OS) chickens. Eur J Immunol 12:877

Pharmacokinetics and Interactions of Ciclosporin

P. A. Keown, C. R. Stiller, M. Stawecki, J. McMichael and W. Howson

Ciclosporin (CyA) is a potent immunosuppressive agent which acts selectively upon the immune response by inhibition of the lymphokine cascade, thus inhibiting cell-cell communication [1]. In addition, augmentation of the inflammatory response is attenuated by blockade of macrophage migration inhibition factor (MIF) and macrophage arming factor (MAF), limiting the delayed-type hypersensitivity response and immunologically nonspecific tissue injury [2]. By virtue of its efficacy and immunologic specificity, CyA is employed extensively in organ transplantation, and also appears to be of major potential importance in the area of autoimmunity.

The clinical use of CyA is complicated, however, by its highly lipophilic nature, its limited bioavailability, and the complexity of its metabolism, interactions, and elimination. In this article we will review these features, and examine the therapeutic levels which have been established for optimal clinical use of this agent.

Pharmacokinetics of CyA

CyA is absorbed from the small bowel with a bioavailability of approximately 30%. The absorption half-life is approximately 1 hour, and maximum concentration (C_{max}) is achieved between 2 and 6 hours post administration with a mean of 4 hours. CyA is absorbed into the lymphatic system and delivered to blood via the thoracic duct. Elimination is ensured almost exclusively by the liver, with a biphasic half life. The α phase of elimination is approximately 1 hour, reflecting tissue distribution, and the β phase is between 4 and 10 hours. A longer terminal elimination half life of up to 27 hours has also been reported [3].

Following intravenous administration, high concentrations may be achieved rapidly in the central blood compartment. Absorption from intramuscular administration is unreliable, and this route is seldom employed now in man [4].

Within the blood compartment, approximately 10% is bound to white cells, 50% to red cells, and the remainder is in the serum. Enterohepatic recycling may be observed in approximately 25% of patients, with a second peak observed approximately 8 hours post administration. CyA is distributed through the body tissues with a volume of distribution of approximately 8.7 litres/kg body weight. At equilibrium, about 12 hours following administration, there is approximately 8 times as much CyA in the peripheral as in the central compartment.

Measurement of CyA

CyA concentrations may be measured by radioimmunoassay (RIA) or high performance liquid chromatography (HPLC). The former measures both parent drug and immunoreactive metabolites, of which 18 have so far been described. In contrast, HPLC measures the parent compound alone. CyA has been most extensively measured in the serum compartment. Distribution between serum and red cell compartments is temperature-dependent, so

---

Department of Medicine, University Hospital, London, Ontario, and University of Western Ontario, Canada

Supported in part by grants from the Medical Research Council of Canada, the Ivey Foundation, and the Kidney Foundation of Canada

P. A. Keown is a Career Scientist of the Ontario Ministry of Health that at 4 °C or 22 °C a 20% reduction in measurable CyA occurs within the serum compartment after approximately 20 minutes, after which time equilibration is complete. Attempts to correct for this by incubation of the blood sample at 37 °C produce an error, owing to further partitioning of CyA into the serum compartment accompanying progressive erythrocyte lysis.

In an attempt to compensate for the variability induced by redistribution, some centers, predominantly in Europe, have increasingly adopted whole-blood measurements of CyA. The whole-blood concentration is also subject to bias, however, being intrinsically dependent upon the hematocrit, and may vary dramatically with this parameter [5].

Measurement of CyA by RIA is simple, rapid and reliable, and for clinical monitoring is superior in most instances to HPLC, which is employed predominantly for research purposes. The ratio of parent compound to total immunoreactive compound is approximately 70% at C_{max} and 30–40% at trough levels. In liver transplantation, however, the relationship between the parent molecule and the metabolites is distorted, perhaps by injury to the liver following hypothermic storage. The ratio of parent compound to immunoreactive metabolite falls to less than 10% by two weeks post transplant, secondary to an apparent block in elimination of metabolite [6]. This latter is less immunosuppressive, and in these circumstances measurement of parent CyA levels by HPLC is mandatory.

Factors influencing CyA metabolism

The absorption of CyA, which is approximately 30–40% under optimal conditions, is markedly depressed by gastrointestinal disorders. Vomiting and diarrhea of any cause markedly diminish uptake, and a similar effect is observed following renal transplantation, owing to uremic enteropathy. The kinetics of drug absorption are not affected by the presence of food in the gastrointestinal tract, but absorption is diminished by approximately 25%. Continued therapy appears to lead to progressive saturation of the peripheral compartment, necessitating a reduction in dosage to avoid excessive concentrations within the central or blood compartment.

Elimination of the drug is naturally influenced by liver disease and biliary tract obstruction, as this is the principle mode of excretion. CyA metabolism occurs within the liver and is predominantly dependent upon the mixed function oxidase enzyme system. Induction of cytochrome P450 by agents such as phenytoin, rifampin or phenobarbitone rapidly decreases the levels of CyA in the blood by hastening elimination [7]. The effect of enzyme induction is evident after approximately 48 hours, and is characterized by a rapid fall in serum CyA levels with a marked decrease in the concentration/dose ratio. Following withdrawal of the inducing agent, a period of approximately 2–3 weeks is required to establish normal function oxidase activity, during which time the dose of CyA must be carefully regulated [7]. An opposite effect, which may be related to cytochrome P450 inhibition, is observed with certain drugs, particularly ketoconazole [8]; this results in a dramatic increase in CyA concentrations in the blood compartment without a change in dose. A similar interaction has recently been observed with erythromycin, although the mechanism of this is not yet clearly established.

A further pharmacokinetic interaction has been described with corticosteroids; this is of importance because of the frequent association with these drugs. High dose intravenous methylprednisolone has been shown to cause a rise in blood CyA concentrations, and CyA may decrease the rate of elimination of corticosteroids.

In addition to the pharmacokinetic interactions described above, pharmacodynamic effects have also been described. The relation between CyA concentrations in the central compartment and its toxic effects may be considered to describe a sinusoidal curve, with progressive toxicity accompanying increasing CyA levels [9]. The threshold of renal toxicity is diminished by simultaneous administration of a number of compounds, including aminoglycosides, amphoteracin-B, sulfamethoxazole or co-trimoxazole and nonsteroidal anti-inflammatory agents, which all accentuate the renal adverse effects of CyA either by further compromising renal blood flow or by a direct toxic effect on the proximal tubule. Certain physical injuries may also exert a synergistic deleterious effect on renal function; these include prolonged warm ischemia, and perfusion damage to the transplanted kidney, which serves to shift the toxicity/concentration curve to the left and promote the development of acute and chronic nephrotoxicity.

Blood levels and clinical events

The relationship between CyA concentrations in the blood compartment and immunosuppressive or adverse effects has been studied most extensively in the renal allograft recipient. In this setting, a relationship between these parameters can be clearly defined. Within the first months following transplantation, allograft rejection occurs most frequently with mean trough serum levels of approximately 170 ng/ml, while clinical and immunological quiescence is maintained with trough levels of 200 ng/ml [10]. The relationship between CyA concentration and effect in the renal allograft recipient is clearly time-dependent, however, and immunological adaptation between graft and host post transplant may reduce progressively the degree of immunosuppression required. Beyond 90 days, adequate immunosuppression may be maintained with trough levels of 50–100 ng/ml, in which range both graft rejection and progressive nephrotoxicity may normally be avoided [10].

A relationship between these parameters may also be seen in autoimmune disease, although the therapeutic range may differ. Complete remission in newly diagnosed patients with Type 1 diabetes mellitus, resulting in reduction and cessation of exogenous insulin requirement [11], was observed most commonly in those who attained a trough serum level of 100 ng/ml CyA within the first 15 days of therapy (69% complete remission). In contrast, those who did not achieve this level within the first 30 days of therapy had a clearly deficient response as measured by insulin requirement (22% complete remission). Further, maintenance therapy in this disease appeared to necessitate continued trough levels of at least 100 ng/ml, below which immunological breakthrough and clinical relapse was observed.

The clinical studies described above are paralleled by pharmacodynamic measurements of the immunosuppressive ability of serum from patients receiving this drug, using a third-party mixed lymphocyte culture bioassay. In these studies, immunosuppression is maintained with serum CyA concentrations in excess of 100 or 150 ng/ml, while levels below this threshold do not reproducibly inhibit the immune response.

Renal effects of CyA

Of the adverse effects of CyA which have been described, its effect upon the kidney is of greatest clinical concern. Studies in the experimental animal have suggested that CyA exerts a dual effect on the kidney, decreasing renal blood flow and causing direct structural changes to the proximal tubule [12]. In man, the renal adverse effects of CyA appear in most uncomplicated situations to be dose-related. An acute, reversible deterioration in renal function accompanied by hyperkalemia and occasionally hypertension normally follows an acute elevation in serum CyA levels, with a lag time of up to 14 days. Following a decrease in CyA dose and restoration of normal levels, renal function returns to normal with a corresponding lag period of up to 21 days.

A reproducible fall in glomerular filtration rate is observed in all patients commencing CyA therapy, and can be limited to approximately 20% in the vast majority of patients by careful monitoring of CyA levels.

Following renal transplantation, the use of therapeutic drug monitoring and the maintenance of CyA concentrations within strict limits minimizes the adverse renal effects of this drug. Allograft function reaches a nadir at approximately 4 months, and plateaus by 6 months post transplant, showing no progressive change in studies pursued between 3 and 5 years post transplant. However, in cases where the concentrations of CyA in the central compartment are inappropriately maintained, particularly, it now appears, within the early treatment period, long-term renal function is jeopardized. Optimal therapeutic ranges can thus now be defined with reasonable confidence, within which the majority of patients treated will maintain satisfactory immunological quiescence with minimal toxicity. For the renal allograft recipient, initial trough serum concentrations of 150–250 ng/ml are required to achieve this effect, but this may be reduced rapidly so that by 3 months post transplant the target therapeutic trough serum range is from 50–100 ng/ml. In part, the reduction in therapeutic range is due to host-graft immunological adaptation which occurs following transplantation. In the patient with autoimmune disease, however, such adaptation may not occur to a similar extent, and the target range for adequate immunosuppression appears to be higher, extending from 100–150 ng/ml.

References

1. Bunjes, Hardic D, Rollinghoff M, Wagner H (1981) Cyclosporin A Mediates Immunosuppression of Primary Cytotoxic T-Cell Responses by Impairing the Release of Interleukin 1 and Interleukin 2. Eur J Immunol 11:657–661
2. Thompson AW, Moon DK, Geczy CL, Nelson DS (1983) Cyclosporin A Inhibits Lymphokine Production but not the Responses of Macrophages to Lymphokines. Immunology 48:291–299
3. Beveridge T, Gratwohl A, Michot F et al. (1981) Cyclosporin A: Pharmacokinetics after a Single Dose in Man and Serum Levels after Multiple Dosing in Recipients of Allogeneic Bone-Marrow Grafts. Current Therapeutic Research 30:5–18
4. Keown PA, Stiller CR, Ulan RA et al. (1981) Immunological and Pharmacological Monitoring in the Clinical Use of Cyclosporin A. Lancet 1:686–689
5. Lemaire M, Tillement JP (1982) Role of Lipoproteins and Erythrocytes in the In Vitro Binding and Distribution of Cyclosporin A in the Blood. J Pharm Pharmacol 34:715–718
6. Wall WJ, Keown PA, Stiller CR, McKenzie N, Devinini R, Stawecki M, McMichael J, Howson W, Muirhead N, Hollomby D (1984) Efficacy and Safety of Low Dose Continuous Intravenous Cyclosporine (CyA). Abstracts: 10th International Congress of The Transplantation Society, Minneapolis S 3.6, 61–62
7. Keown PA, Laupacis A, Carruthers G, Stawecki M, Koegler J, McKenzie FN, Wall W, Stiller CR (1984) Interaction between Phenytoin and Cyclosporine following Organ Transplantation. Transplantation, Vol 38, No 3, 304–306
8. Ferguson RM, Sutherland DE, Simmons RL, Najarian JS (1982) Ketoconazole, Cyclosporin Metabolism, and Renal Transplantation (Letter). Lancet 2:882–3
9. Keown PA (1984) Cyclosporine Blood Level Monitoring. Transplantation Immunology Letter Supplement, Vol 1, No 2, November
10. Keown PA, Stiller CR, Laupacis AL et al. (1982) The Effects and Side-effects of Cyclosporine: Relationship to Drug Pharmacokinetics. Transplantation Proceedings 14:659–661
11. Stiller CR, Dupre J, Gent M, Jenner MR, Keown PA, Laupacis A, Martell R, Rodger NW, Graffenried B, Wolfe BMJ (1984) Effects of Cyclosporine Immunosuppression in Insulin-Dependent Diabetes Mellitus of Recent Onset. Science 223:1362–1367
12. Petric R, Keown PA, Stiller CR, Wallace AC, McDonald JWD (1985) Affect of Cyclosporine (CyA) on Renal Function, Blood Flow, and Prostacyclin A and Thromboxane Generation in Experimental Animal Model. 1st International Meeting on Experimental Cyclosporine Nephrotoxicity, Basel, April (Abstract)

Side Effects and Safety of Sandimmun® in Long-term Treatment of Transplant Patients

P. Krupp, P. Timonen and A. Gülich *

The introduction of Sandimmun® (ciclosporin) into immunosuppressive therapy has improved the results of organ transplantation with respect to patient survival, graft survival and the main post-transplant complications [5, 6, 16, 26], and the adverse reaction profile of this potent immunosuppressive agent has been established [7]. However, long-term safety experience is still limited. To broaden knowledge in this respect, a long-term safety follow-up, primarily of bone marrow and renal transplant recipients treated with Sandimmun, has been initiated. Preliminary data of this ongoing investigation from renal transplant recipients, who provide the bulk of the information, are presented here.

Methods

67 transplantation centers around the world are actively participating in this prospective, open, non-randomized, non-comparative investigation which is primarily aimed at assessing the adverse reactions of Sandimmun in bone marrow and kidney transplant recipients. At each center every patient treated for at least 2 weeks with the drug is registered and follow-up examinations are done after 3, 6, 12 and 24 months. Some centers follow their patients over a 5-year period. The survey started 2 years ago and the recruitment period terminated at the end of 1984.

The register encompasses data on 3,038 renal transplant recipients. For this cohort follow-up information on the first 6 postoperative months is available for 2,188 patients, and after 1 and 2 years the available information relates to 1,591 and 728 patients respectively. As the survey is still ongoing, the data have not yet been analyzed in depth. The results are based on an interim evaluation.

Results

In the surveyed cohort of renal transplant recipients male patients predominate. 4% of the patients were less than 17 years of age and 12% were over 55 years at the time of transplantation.

The disease leading to transplantation was glomerulonephritis in over 40% of the patients and in about 20% the reasons were congenital anomalies and diabetic nephropathy.

The dosages of Sandimmun used in the surveyed cohort for the first post-transplant year are given in Table 1. It is evident that the highest doses were administered at the beginning; almost 25% of the patients received more than 15 mg/kg/day. According to present recommendations the initial dose of Sandimmun should not exceed 10–15 mg/kg/day in this patient population. However, this survey includes patients from an early period of the use of this drug when higher dose regimens were common. Over the first post-transplant year the daily doses administered were reduced and after 12 months one fourth of the patients were on 5 mg/kg/day or less, 78% of them still receiving the drug.

In Table 2 the principal concomitant medication is listed. Over 18% of the patients were receiving azathioprine either as an additional immunosuppressive agent – most often in combination with corticosteroids – or as a replacement after discontinuation of Sandimmun medication. In only a

---

Clinical Research, Pharmaceutical Division, Sandoz Ltd, Basle, Switzerland

* We are indebted to all investigators who are participating in this ongoing long-term safety survey, and to Miss Götz for processing the data

Table 1. Dosage of Sandimmun in the cohort surveyed

Post-Tx (months)	1	3	6	12
mg/kg/day (mean)	13	8	7.3	7.2
mg/kg/day	Number of patients in %*			
≦ 5	3.1	10.8	16.7	24.2
5.1 – 10	17.3	53.9	56.1	49.8
10.1 – 15	51.4	14.9	5.6	2.9
> 15	24.5	0.8	0.5	0.5
Number of patients not on Sandimmun (%)	3.4	19.3	20.5	22.1
Total number of patients	3,038	2,100	2,188	1,591

* Patients with missing data excluded

Table 2. Concomitant medication in the cohort surveyed*

	%
Immunosuppressants	
Azathioprine	18.4
ALG/ATG	2.2
Corticosteroids	
Methylprednisolone	32.7
Prednisolone	48.7
Prednisone	21.6
Hydrocortisone	5.2
Antimicrobial agents	
Antibacterials	
Antibiotics	15.6
Sulfonamides	12.1
Tuberculostatics	1.9
Antivirals	1.5
Antifungals	17.7
Antihypertensives	
Beta-blocking agents	48.0
Captopril	7.1
Clonidine	10.7
Hydralazine	19.8
Anticonvulsants	2.0

* 100% = 3,038 patients

small percentage were antilymphocyte or antithymocyte globulins used as a further immunosuppressive therapy. However, a quite considerable number of patients were treated with corticosteroids which were administered either for acute rejection episodes or for continued immunosuppression. The other drugs listed were given either to overcome the complications which can occur with any immunosuppressive therapy, e.g. antimicrobials for various infections, or agents for the treatment of possible adverse reactions directly associated with the use of the various immunosuppressive agents.

Taking into consideration these and other drugs not listed, it is obvious that the adverse events reported were not only induced by Sandimmun medication, but were also to some extent caused by the concomitant therapy.

Figure 1 shows the graft survival probability of the monitored cohort of patients. The probability amounted to over 80% at the end of the first year and did not change to a relevant extent during the second year.

In Table 3 the adverse events reported are reviewed. With one exception, namely the occurrence of lymphoma, only those events are listed which were observed in at least 10 of the 3,038 patients surveyed. For a particular patient a given adverse event is indicated only once even though it may have been reported at several examinations. However, more than one adverse event may have occurred in the same patient. The reported adverse events were grouped according to the organ system affected in order to allow a functional classification.

Skin reactions were reported in about one third of the patients, mainly consisting of hypertrichosis, an established side effect of Sandimmun whose cause is unknown. Acne developed in 2% of the patients and was in most cases caused by concomitant corticosteroids. The rashes were either due to GvH reactions or could have resulted from antimicrobial treatment, particularly from aminopenicillins.

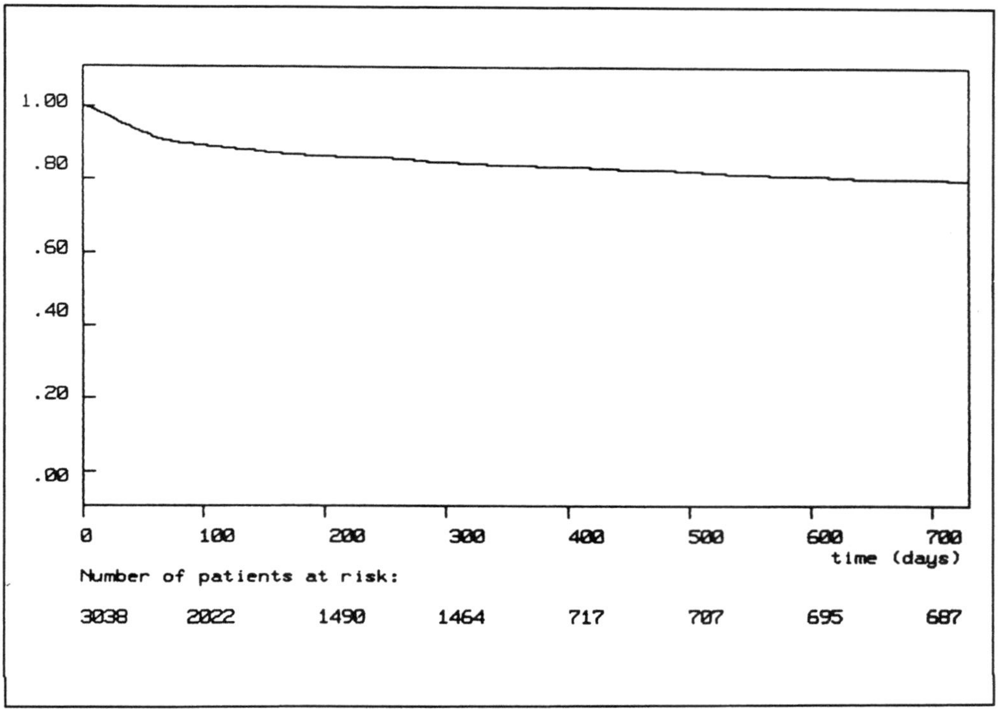

Fig. 1. Graft survival probability in the surveyed renal transplant recipients

Joint and muscle pain were experienced by some patients; the etiology of these symptoms remains unexplained, whereas bone disorders, which include bone pain, could be caused by disturbances of calcium metabolism.

It is known that tremor and hyper- and paresthesia can be experienced by patients on Sandimmun. In 1.6% of the patients convulsions occurred. There is some evidence that the following factors could play a contributory role in the pathogenesis: high plasma concentrations of ciclosporin, high-dose corticosteroids, hypertension, especially in young patients, and perhaps hypomagnesemia.

Psychic disorders developed in a few patients. These effects have to be seen in relation to the basic disease and the postoperative situation of the kidney transplant recipients.

The 25 cataracts reported were in all probability associated with the concomitant corticosteroid treatment.

Gum hyperplasia, nausea and vomiting are frequently reported side effects of Sandimmun. A multifactorial etiology, however, has to be considered for the occurrence of gastrointestinal ulcers and hemorrhages. In addition to stress factors, concomitant corticosteroid medication could have played a contributory role, although it is still debated whether steroids cause an increased risk of peptic ulcer. However, pancreatic disorders, including pancreatitis, have been shown to occur any time during long-term corticosteroid treatment. Moreover, an increased incidence of pancreatitis is reported to occur after renal transplantation.

Liver dysfunction was reported in 18% of the patients and included cases with elevated transaminases as well as with bilirubin. It has been shown that the alkaline phosphatase contributing to the increased levels of this enzyme is primarily derived from bone [21].

Regarding metabolic changes, it is now recognized that hyperuricemia can occur during Sandimmun medication owing to impaired renal function, but only exceptionally have actual attacks of gout been re-

Table 3. Adverse events reported for the cohort surveyed

	n	%
Skin		
Hypertrichosis	1000	32.9
Acne*	62	2.0
Rash	19	0.6
Musculoskeletal system		
Joint/muscle pain	32	1.1
Bone disorder	22	0.7
Nervous system		
Tremor	629	20.7
Hyper-/paresthesia, neuropathy	160	5.2
Convulsions	50	1.6
Headache	25	0.8
Spinal cord disorder	25	0.8
Psychic functions		
Weakness, fatigue	22	0.8
Depressive reaction	18	0.6
Eye		
Cataract*	25	0.8
Vision impairment	19	0.6
Gastrointestinal system		
Gum hyperplasia	449	14.8
Nausea/vomiting/loss of appetite	289	9.4
G.I. ulcer/hemorrhage*	91	3.1
Pancreatic disorder	17	0.6
Liver		
Liver dysfunction	558	18.4
Metabolism		
Hyperuricemia	122	4.0
Increase of triglycerides and cholesterol	108	3.6
Diabetes/hyperglycemia	62	2.1
Endocrine system		
Cushing-like symptoms*	157	5.1
Parathyroid disorder	16	0.5
Hypercalcemia	16	0.5
Heart		
Myocardial infarction	37	1.2
Cardiac failure	27	0.9
Cardiac arrest	17	0.6
Angina pectoris	14	0.5
Vascular system/blood clotting		
Hypertension	1170	38.5
Thromboembolism	19	0.6
Coagulation disorder	10	0.3
Respiratory system		
Pulmonary edema	13	0.4
Blood cells		
Anemia	29	0.9
Leukopenia	31	1.0
Thrombocytopenia	29	0.9

Table 3. (Continued)

	n	%
Urinary system		
Renal dysfunction	1571	51.7
Urinary tract infection	319	10.5
Reproduction		
Breast disorder (gynecomastia)	21	0.7
Contraceptive failure	10	0.3
Infections		
Bacterial (including pneumonia)	559	18.3
Viral	383	12.6
Fungal	97	3.2
Tumors		
Lymphoma	5	0.2
Malignant tumor	18	0.6

* Adverse reactions which are in all probability associated with corticosteroid medication

ported. Disturbances of fat and carbohydrate metabolism are well known adverse effects of long-term corticosteroids; however, the influence of Sandimmun on these parameters has not been fully elucidated.

Cushing-like symptoms were obviously related to concomitant administration of corticosteroids, whereas the parathyroid disorders were mostly complications of impaired renal function.

The occurrence of myocardial infarction and other cardiac disorders had to be expected in this patient group. There is no evidence of adverse effects of Sandimmun on cardiac function.

Hypertension is known to occur in certain patients on Sandimmun medication; the pathogenesis is unknown. However, hypertension has also been described in renal transplant recipients on conventional immunosuppressive therapy, and long-term corticosteroids can induce such an effect. A clustering of thromboembolic complications in Sandimmun-treated transplant recipients has recently been reported [27]. Attempts are being made to elucidate whether Sandimmun medication may influence hemostatic function to any relevant extent.

Anemia, of a mild degree, occurred in 1% of the patients. In about the same percentage leukopenia, probably due to the con-

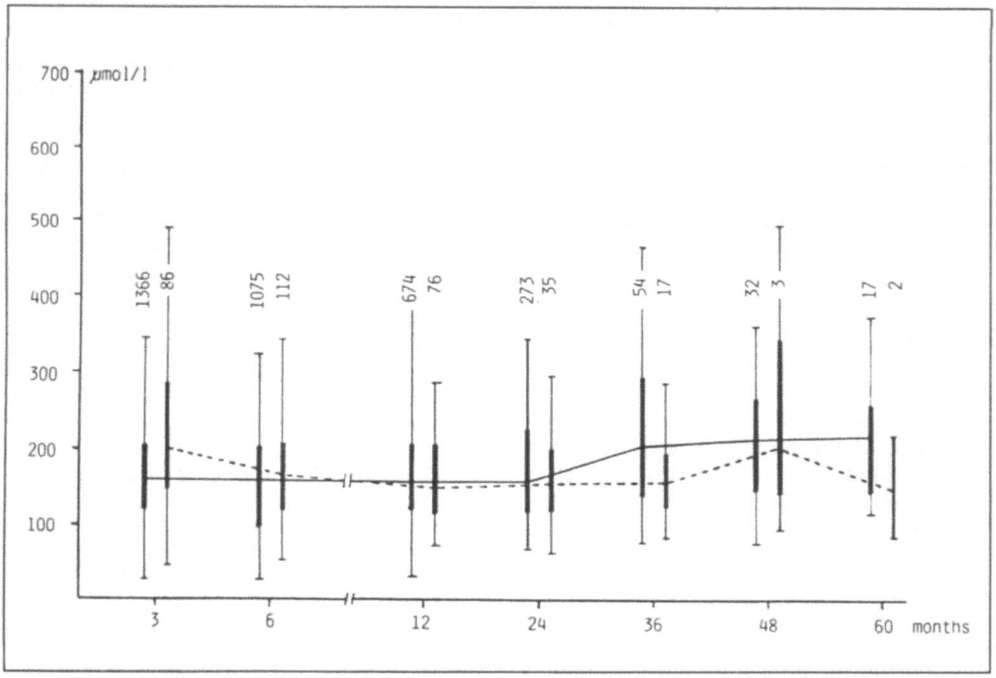

Fig. 2. Serum creatinine concentrations in kidney transplant recipients. The points connected by the continuous line (Sandimmun treated patients) and the dotted line (patients not on Sandimmun) are median values; the wider bars include 50% and the smaller bars 95% of all values (box and whisker plot). The numbers give the patients whose creatinine concentrations are available

comitant azathioprine medication, was noted. The same incidence of thrombocytopenia was reported. It has been speculated that anemia could be due to red cell antibodies produced by donor B-cells which are transferred along with the kidney and which would tend to proliferate because of the specific action of Sandimmun on T-cells [15].

Renal dysfunction is the most frequent side effect of Sandimmun medication, being reported in over 50% of the patients now surveyed. The renal histopathological findings have been thoroughly investigated [17]. In this cohort the functional aspects of this adverse effect have been analyzed with respect to serum creatinine concentrations. Figure 2 shows that this parameter, although limited in its predictive value, did not change to a relevant extent during the monitoring period. In addition, no marked difference exists between the patients on long-term Sandimmun medication and those who were converted to conventional therapy.

In 0.7% of the patients gynecomastia developed. No influence of Sandimmun on endocrinological functions has been found [8, 9].

It is well established that the incidence of different types of infection is increased in immunosuppressed patients. There is, however, ample evidence that opportunistic infections do not occur more frequently with Sandimmun than with conventional immunosuppressive therapy [18].

Finally, 5 cases of lymphoma and lymphoproliferative disorders and 18 malignant tumors located in various organs were reported, the total incidence of malignancies being 0.8%. This figure compares favorably with the published incidence of cancer in transplant recipients, which varies from 1.6 to 24% in different geographical areas [2, 11, 20, 23]. Four of the 5 patients presenting with lymphoproliferative disorders were on concomitant ALG. The incidence of lymphoproliferative disorders in this survey is of the same order as a recent estimate which took into consideration the worldwide clinical experience with Sandimmun [1] as well as the figure published for renal transplant recipients on conventional immunosuppressive therapy [14].

Conclusion

Sandimmun exhibits a characteristic profile of adverse reactions, the most prominent side effect being nephrotoxicity. However, there is good evidence that this as well as most other side effects can be diminished by carefully monitoring the blood concentration of ciclosporin and by individually adjusting the dosage [12, 13, 25].

The serious complications of any immunosuppressant, such as the occurrence of opportunistic infections and malignancy, are also observed with Sandimmun. In patients on Sandimmun, however, the infections are less resistant to therapy and the overall incidence of malignancies appears to be lower in Sandimmun-treated patients [19, 22, 24]. This may be related to the fact that standard immunosuppressive medication relies on antimetabolite activity to produce immunosuppression whereas Sandimmun acts in a different manner primarily by inhibiting the secretion of lymphokines necessary to initiate a new immune response and leaving established immune reactions largely unaffected [3, 4, 10]. In any case, in contrast to conventional immunosuppressive therapy, bone marrow depression does not result from Sandimmun medication.

The preliminary analysis of the data collected so far with this ongoing long-term safety follow-up of Sandimmun-treated renal transplant patients confirms the knowledge gained in clinical trials and based on published case reports. No serious risks not already recognized have become apparent. Further evaluation of the data will show whether particular factors can be determined whose circumvention or elimination may further increase the safety of this drug.

References

1. Beveridge T, Krupp P, McKibbin C (1984) Lymphomas and lymphoproliferative lesions developing under cyclosporin therapy. Lancet 1:788
2. Birkeland SA (1983) Malignant tumors in renal transplant patients. The Scandia transplant material. Cancer 51:1571–1575
3. Borel JF, Bauer C, Gubler HU et al. (1976) Biological effects of cyclosporin A: a new antilymphocytic agent. Agents Actions 6:468–475
4. Borel JF (1984) Animal experiments with ciclosporin. Triangle 23: 3/4, 153
5. Calne RY, White DJG, Evans DB et al. (1981) Cyclosporin A in cadaveric organ transplantation. Br Med J 282:934
6. Canadian Multicentre Transplant Study Group (1983) A randomized clinical trial of cyclosporine in cadaveric renal transplantation. N Engl J Med 309:809–815
7. Cohen DJ, Loertscher R, Rubin MF et al. (1984) Cyclosporine: A new immunosuppressive agent for organ transplantation. Ann Intern Med 101:667–682
8. Handelsman DJ, McDowell IFW, Caterson ID (1984) Ovarian function after renal transplantation: comparison on cyclosporin A with azathioprine and prednisone combination regimens. Br J Obstet Gynaecol 91:802–807
9. Handelsman DJ, McDowell IFW, McDowell W et al. (1984) Testicular function after renal transplantation: comparison of Cyclosporin A with azathioprine and prednisone combination regimes. Clin Nephrol 22: No. 3, 144–148
10. Hess AD (1985) Effect of interleukin 2 on the immunosuppressive action of cyclosporine. Transplantation 39:62–68
11. Jacobs C, Brunner FP, Brynger H et al. (1981) Malignant diseases in patients treated by dialysis and transplantation in Europe. Transplant Proc 13:729–732
12. Kahan BD, Ried M, Newburger J (1983) Pharmacokinetics of cyclosporine in human renal transplantation. Transplant Proc 15:446–453
13. Keown PA, Stiller CR, Ulan RA et al. (1981) Immunological and pharmacological monitoring in the clinical use of cyplosporin A. Lancet 1:686–689
14. Kinlen LJ, Sheil AGR, Peto J, Doll R (1979) Collaborative United Kingdom-Australasian study of cancer in patients treated with immunosuppressive drugs. Br Med J 2:1461–1466
15. Mangal AK, Growe GH, Sinclair M et al. (1984) Acquired hemolytic anemia due to

"auto"-anti-A or "auto"-anti-B induced by group 0 homograft in renal transplant recipients. Transfusion 24:201–205

16. Merion RM, David MD, White DJG et al. (1984) Cyclosporine: Five years' experience in cadaveric renal transplantation. N Engl J Med 310:148–154
17. Mihatsch JM, Thiel G, Ryffel B (1985) Ciclosporin-associated Nephropathy. In: Schindler R (ed) Ciclosporin in Autoimmune Diseases. 1st International Symposium, Basle, March 18–20, 1985. Springer, Berlin Heidelberg New York Tokyo, p 50
18. Najarian JS, Ferguson RM, Sutherland DER et al. (1983) A prospective trial of the efficacy of cyclosporine in renal transplantation at the University of Minnesota. Transplant Proc 15: No. 1, 438–441
19. Oyer PE, Stinson EB, Jamieson SW et al. (1984) Cyclosporine in cardiac transplantation: A 2½ year follow-up. In: B. D. Kahan, Cyclosporine, Vol. 1, Biological Activity and Clinical Applications. Grune and Stratton, Orlando, p 330–336
20. Penn I (1970) Malignant tumors in organ transplant recipients. Springer, Berlin
21. Price CP, Deam SM, Calvin J (1983) Serum alkaline phosphatase isoenzyme in patients on cyclosporin A following renal transplantation. Clin Biochem 16, No. 5, Abstr. C314, A25
22. Reece IJ, Okereke OUJ, Painvin GA et al. (1984) Infection in cyclosporine-immunosuppressed cardiac allograft recipients. Heart Transplant 3:239–242
23. Sheil AGR, Mahony JF, Horvath JS et al. (1981) Cancer following successful cadaveric donor renal transplantation. Transplant Proc 13:733–735
24. Sheil AGR (1984) Cancer in organ transplant recipients: part of an induced immune deficiency syndrome. Br Med J 288:659–661
25. Thiel G, Harder F, Loertscher R, et al. (1983) Cyclosporin A used alone or in combination with low-dose steroids in cadaveric renal transplantation. Klin Wochenschr 61:991–1000
26. van Buren CT, Flechner SM, Kerman RH et al. (1984) Cyclosporine improves outcome in high-risk cadaveric renal allograft recipients. Transplant Proc 16:1162–1166
27. Vanrenterghem Y, Gresele P, Roels L et al. (1985) Thromboembolic complications and haemostatic changes in cyclosporin-treated cadaveric kidney allograft recipients. Lancet 1: 999–1002

Ciclosporin-associated Nephropathy

M. J. Mihatsch [1], G. Thiel [2], B. Ryffel [3]

Introduction

The topic of this review is the question of whether morphological changes in the kidneys are associated with ciclosporin (CyA) treatment. At the international conference on CyA held in Cambridge in 1981, it was concluded that CyA did not induce significant morphologic renal lesions in man [6], in contrast to animal experimental data [14]. Two years later, at the first international congress on CyA in Houston, several seemingly contradictory morphologic patterns of CyA nephrotoxicity were reported [5, 8, 12, 16, 19].

Because of this confused situation an international workshop of pathologists was held in Basel early in 1984, which resulted in a preliminary classification of morphologic changes seen in CyA-treated patients [1].

On the basis of the results of the Basel workshop and extensive re-evaluation of our own transplant biopsies [13] the different morphologic patterns of CyA nephrotoxicity will be described. The description will, however, be limited to forms which are most likely to occur in patients with autoimmune disease. The following classification is already widely accepted.

Classification of CyA nephropathy

According to time of presentation and pathogenesis, three major groups of lesions can be differentiated (Table 1).

Table 1. Classification of CyA nephropathy

1. Primary non- or poorly functioning transplant
   - Diffuse interstitial fibrosis
2. Acute toxicity
   - Toxic tubulopathy
   - Peritubular capillary congestion
   - Combination of both
   - No light microscopic lesions (associated with impaired renal function)
3. Chronic toxicity
   - CyA-associated arteriolopathy
   - Interstitial fibrosis, striped form with tubular atrophy
   - Combination of both

The first reaction pattern – diffuse interstitial fibrosis – does not play a role in autoimmune disease because it occurs only in patients with prolonged oligo-anuria or primary poor renal function [5, 13].

In the following the morphologic lesions associated with acute and chronic toxicity will be described separately.

Acute toxicity

By light microscopy three different types of lesions may be found: Toxic tubulopathy, peritubular capillary congestion, or essentially normal renal tissue and a combination of toxic tubulopathy and peritubular capillary congestion.

Toxic tubulopathy (TT) [10, 12]

The morphologic changes seen in toxic tubulopathy comprise inclusion bodies in tubular epithelial cells (corresponding to giant mitochondria) isometric tubular vacuolization and microcalcification. Vascular lesions are absent. Interstitial lesions are minimal (edema) or absent.

Giant mitochondria occur predominantly in the convoluted part of the proximal tubule, usually one per cell (Fig. 1a, b). Mul-

1 Department of Pathology, University of Basel
2 Department of Internal Medicine, Cantonal Hospital, Basel
3 Department of Preclinical Research, Sandoz Ltd, Basel

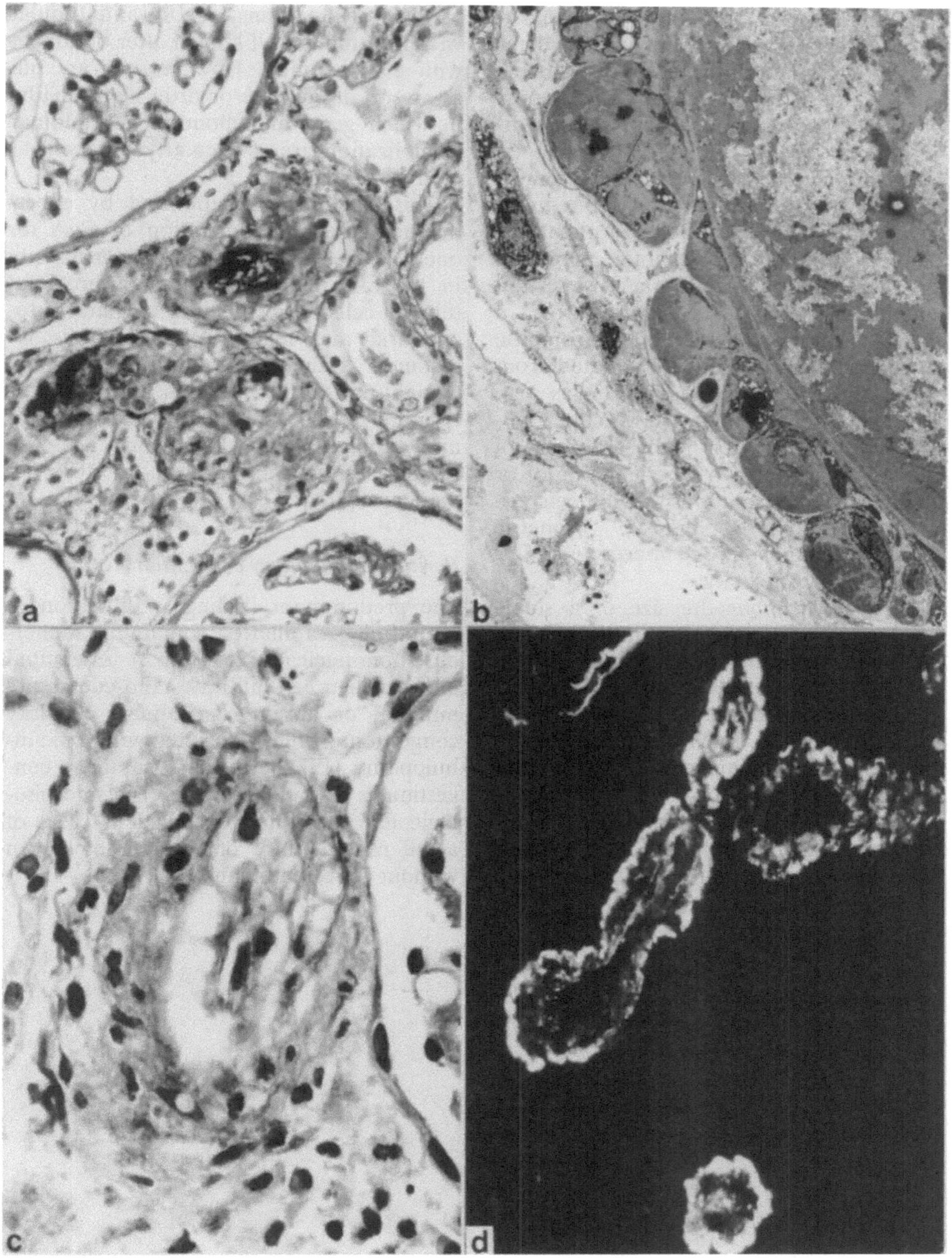

Fig. 1. Morphologic features of toxic tubulopathy
a) Giant mitochondria seen by light microscopy as tubular inclusion bodies ( ), CAB × 1240
b) Giant mitochondrion, EM × 22 000
c) Isometric tubular vacuolization, EM × 812
d) Tubular microcalcification, Kossa × 620

tiple tubular inclusion bodies can be classified as phagolysosomes. Unequivocal demonstration of giant mitochondria is possible only by use of electron microscopy, although this is impractical in routine diagnosis.

Isometric vacuolization is found almost exclusively in the straight part of the proximal tubule. The morphologic picture is identical to that of osmotic nephrosis (Fig. 1c). All tubular cells in a cross section contain densely packed, empty (free of lipids) vacuoles of equal size. Isometric vacuolization must be differentiated from coarse and irregular vacuolization as seen in ischemic renal damage (e.g. acute tubular necrosis (ATN)) or in the periphery of infarcts. In patients to whom mannitol or similar infusion solutions have been administered before biopsy, isometric vacuolization must not be interpreted as indicative of CyA toxicity.

Microcalcifications the size of a single tubular cell or of a small number of them are found in various parts of the nephron (Fig. 1d). They are the result of dystrophic calcification of necrotic tubular cells.

There has been much debate about the specificity of tubular giant mitochondria and/or vacuolization [5, 7, 11, 21]. There is no doubt that these morphologic lesions are unspecific, though highly characteristic. Giant mitochondria may be found under a variety of conditions [4, 18], and tubular vacuolization is well known after treatment with e.g. mannitol. However, we are not aware of any disease or drug nephropathy in which giant mitochondria and tubular vacuolization are as regularly observed as after CyA treatment.

This statement is supported by experimental data. Administration of CyA for one week results in similar tubular toxicity in the rat: inclusion bodies in proximal tubular cells corresponding to giant mitochondria and mainly polymorphous lysosomes, tubular vacuolization in the straight part of the proximal tubule (slightly more irregular in the rat than in man) and tubular microcalcification [12]. The tubular lesions show a clear-cut dose dependence [2].

Peritubular capillary congestion [16, 17]

The predominant finding is dilatation of peritubular capillaries containing numerous mononuclear cells (Fig. 2). Interstitial mononuclear cell infiltrates and edema are minimal or absent. Peritubular capillary congestion is often associated with toxic tubulopathy [13]. Peritubular capillary congestion is also not specific. This morphologic lesion is often observed in cases of acute renal failure of any etiology even without CyA treatment [13].

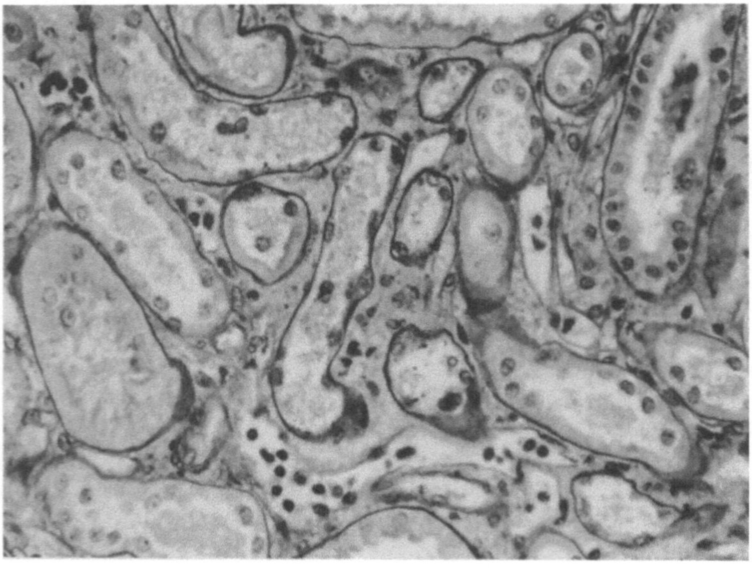

Fig. 2. Peritubular capillary congestion with dilated capillaries containing many mononuclear cells. HE × 387

Essentially normal renal tissue [1, 12]

Peritubular capillary congestion and essentially normal renal tissue probably differ in only one respect, namely the presence of mononuclear cells in peritubular capillaries. The lack of mononuclear cells may be due to concomitant therapy with steroids [1].

Whether toxic tubulopathy or peritubular capillary congestion or essentially normal renal tissue are found depends primarily on the quality of histologic technique (fixation of tissue, section thickness, stains etc.), the number of sections evaluated and the accuracy of histologic evaluation [1, 12]. Even under optimal conditions, the typical features of toxic tubulopathy may be absent in light microscopic sections. By electron microscopy, however, in some of these cases minor lesions of toxic tubulopathy may be found. It is still unclear, however, why only some patients with toxic CyA trough levels (see below) develop tubular alterations visible by light microscopy. The duration of overdosing as well as individual differences in sensitivity may play a significant role [12].

Peritubular capillary congestion and essentially normal renal tissue by light microscopy associated with impaired renal function are not, in our experience, found in animal experiments.

Acute toxicity and CyA trough levels

The morphologic lesions summarized under acute toxicity are found in renal transplants in patients with toxic whole blood trough levels of more than 1500 ng/ml [12, 13].

Patients with pre-existing renal disease or concomitant renal damage are more susceptible to acute toxicity [12, 13]. In renal transplants signs of acute toxicity may already be found at whole blood trough levels exceeding 500 ng/ml if additional damage, e.g. rejection, ATN, arteriolopathy, fibrosis etc., is present [13].

The last statement is supported by animal experimental data. Administration of CyA in a dose of 50 mg/kg for three days does not result in significant renal damage nor does the administration of mannitol alone. The combined use of CyA plus mannitol, furosemide, amphotericin B, aminoglycosides and non-steroidal anti-inflammatory drugs, however, results in severe acute tubular toxicity [3]. The same holds true for the combination of CyA and ischemia [19].

Chronic toxicity

Two different types of lesions may be found by light microscopy: CyA-associated arteriolopathy and interstitial fibrosis, striped form with tubular atrophy, or a combination of both.

CyA-associated arteriolopathy (CAA) [12]

The CyA vascular lesion begins and is predominantly located in the arterioles. It rarely extends to the vascular pole of the glomerulus or the peripheral glomerular capillaries, and may with time progress into small arteries.

Two types of CyA arteriolopathy, which may co-exist, can be identified:

a) Circular lumpy protein deposits permeate the arteriolar wall and narrow the vascular lumen, in a way rather similar to the lesions of arteriolar necrosis or arteriolosclerosis (Fig. 3 a).
   The protein deposits are sometimes arranged in a pearl-necklace-like pattern. Electron microscopy reveals that the protein deposits may replace areas of necrotic myocytes (Fig. 3 b).
b) Mucoid, paucicellular thickening of the intima resulting in narrowing of the vascular lumen predominates (Fig. 3 c). The thickened intima is rich in acid proteoglycans.
   Vacuolization of myocytes and endothelial cells may be found in both types of CAA. Circular lumpy deposits of IgM and/or complement (C3) are demonstrated in both types by means of immunofluorescence (Fig. 3 d). Fibrin is seen only in early biopsies.

The glomerular involvement is always slight and focal. Segmental obsolescence of glomerular loops or a cobweb-like neo-

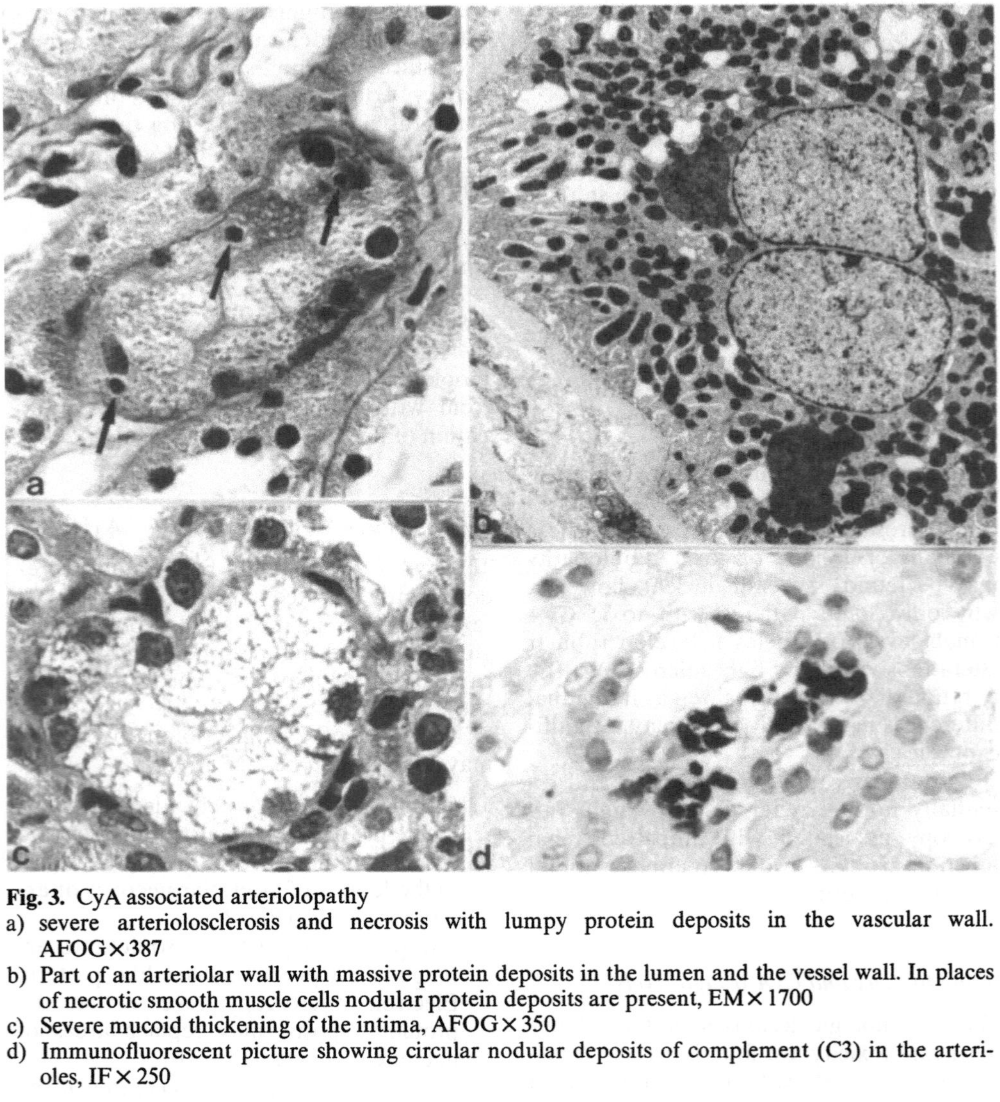

Fig. 3. CyA associated arteriolopathy

a) severe arteriolosclerosis and necrosis with lumpy protein deposits in the vascular wall. AFOG × 387
b) Part of an arteriolar wall with massive protein deposits in the lumen and the vessel wall. In places of necrotic smooth muscle cells nodular protein deposits are present, EM × 1700
c) Severe mucoid thickening of the intima, AFOG × 350
d) Immunofluorescent picture showing circular nodular deposits of complement (C3) in the arterioles, IF × 250

formation of basement membrane-like material may be present.

The long-term consequences as seen in repeat biopsies are:

a) progressive scarring of arterioles with marked narrowing or complete occlusion of the lumen,
b) progressive global or segmental glomerular obsolescence,
c) interstitial fibrosis, striped form, accompanied by tubular atrophy, and
d) concentric intimal fibrosis in arteries.

The pathogenesis of CyA-associated arteriolopathy is unknown, but a mechanism similar to thrombotic microangiopathy is most likely [12].

Not every arteriolar lesion in CyA treated patients is CAA. Differentiation from hypertensive or diabetic arteriolopathy (arteriolosclerosis, arteriolar hyalinosis) is usually simple, due to excentric nodular subendothelial protein deposits, whereas in CAA circular deposits are present, mainly occupying the sites of necrotic myocytes. In advanced cases of hypertensive or diabetic arteriolopathy, differentiation may be difficult or even impossible. Detailed clinical information and meticulous morphologic analysis is necessary.

In animal experiments, this arteriolopathy could not be induced in normotensive rats. In spontaneous hypertensive rats, however, hypertensive vasculopathy developed earlier and was more pronounced in CyA-treated animals than in control animals [15].

Interstitial fibrosis, striped form, with tubular atrophy (SF) [9, 12, 20]

Irregularly distributed areas or stripes of interstitial fibrosis and atrophic tubules are observed in the renal cortex (Fig. 4). Tubules in other areas appear essentially normal. Slight mononuclear cell infiltration is nearly always seen in the fibrotic areas or around blood vessels. Vascular or glomerular changes are not prominent.

Interstitial fibrosis, striped form with tubular atrophy, is also morphologically an unspecific lesion. Numerous pathogenic factors result in this form of interstitial fibrosis, and may include glomerulonephritis, segmental focal glomerulosclerosis, pyelonephritis, obstruction of the urinary tract etc. Interstitial fibrosis due to CyA therapy must not be diagnosed unless all these pathogenic factors are excluded or are at least highly unlikely to be present.

Interstitial fibrosis in the restricted sense was first described by Thiru et al. [20] as a CyA-associated lesion, whereas others [12] considered this form of interstitial fibrosis as the consequence of CAA. In fact, SF cases with and without CAA have been found. Furthermore, CAA precedes the development of SF, which also indicates a pathogenic relationship [13]. Finally, we have previously demonstrated that there is a correlation between the severity of CAA and the extent of SF in repeat biopsies [12].

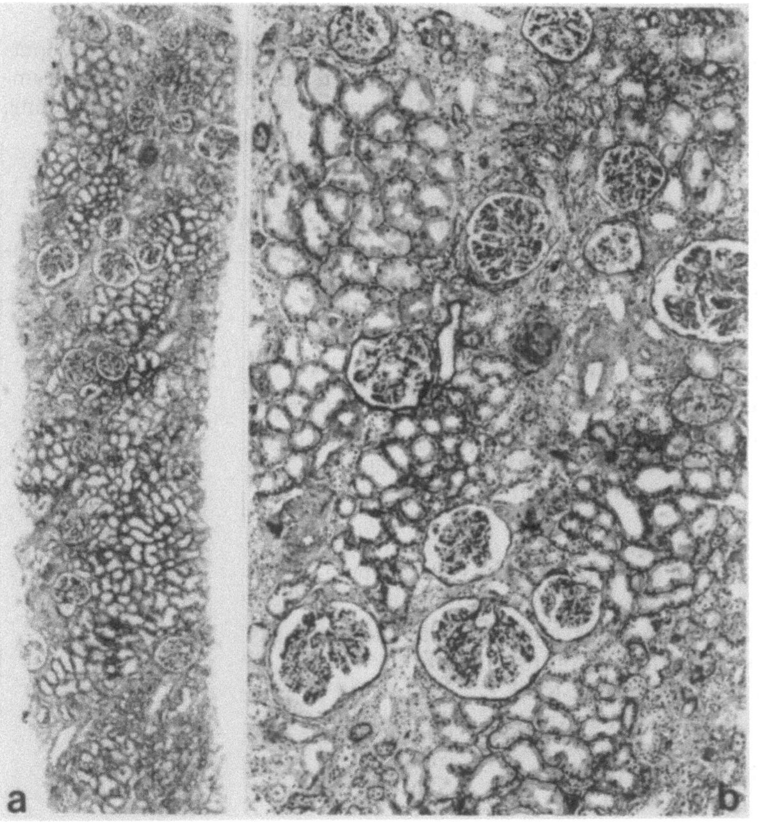

Fig. 4. Striped form of interstitial fibrosis with tubular atrophy, a) AFOG, ×70 b) AFOG, ×190

Nevertheless, CAA is not found in all cases of SF. This may be because:

1. SF may be due to progressive tubular damage,
2. CAA is difficult to identify in advanced cases.

The first possibility can be neither proven nor excluded on the basis of present knowledge. Several observations from our own files favor the second hypothesis: first biopsy – severe CAA, no significant fibrosis; second biopsy – severe CAA, moderately severe SF; third biopsy – no CAA, severe SF. The reason for the absence of CAA in the third biopsy was probably that the completely occluded and destroyed arterioles had merged with interstitial fibrosis. In our opinion CAA is the most important pathogenic factor in the development of SF.

If SF is not accompanied or preceded by CAA, or if SF is not clearly progressive (in repeat biopsies) or associated with signs of other defined nephropathy, one should be very cautious about interpreting SF as a CyA associated lesion.

Chronic toxicity and CyA trough levels

What is known about the relation of CyA trough level and chronic nephrotoxicity? Klintmalm et al. [9] demonstrated that patients with interstitial fibrosis experienced episodes of acute nephrotoxicity within the first 6 months after transplantation more frequently than patients without. Furthermore, the cumulative doses of CyA within the first 6 months were higher in this group. On the basis of these findings we calculated the average CyA trough levels at different time intervals after transplantation [13]. It could be demonstrated that patients with signs of chronic nephrotoxicity have significantly higher CyA trough levels within the first three months after transplatation than patients in the control group. The mean whole blood trough level within the first three months after transplantation in the control group was 1160 ng/ml whereas in the chronic nephrotoxicity groups it was 1520 ng/ml [13].

Summary and outlook on autoimmune disease

It should be remembered that CyA is a nephrotoxic drug. But its nephrotoxicity is dose-dependent and may not be inevitable if minimal therapeutic doses are used. However, various risk factors that should be treated are recognized, such as heart failure, hypertension and renal disease. Concomitant nephrotoxic drug administration should be avoided. Since in autoimmune disorders the renal parenchyma may also be involved in the disease process, special caution is indicated with the therapeutic use of CyA. The long-term effect of CyA therapy on kidney function and morphology is uncertain. However, there is currently no evidence that CyA nephrotoxicity is progressive if risk factors are optimally controlled and minimal therapeutic CyA blood levels are respected.

What can we learn from the experience obtained mainly with renal and other transplants for the treatment of patients with autoimmune disease?

1. Before starting with CyA therapy perform careful studies of renal function under control conditions (s-creatinine, creatinine clearance, urinalysis, etc.).

Table 2. Ciclosporin: Drug interaction

Decreased elimination
ketoconazole
erythromycin
steroids (?)
cimetidine (?)
thiazide diuretics (?)
Increased elimination
phenytoin
rifampicin
isoniazid
sulphadimidine
trimethoprim (i.v.)
sulfinpyrazone (?)
Additive nephrotoxicity
amphotericin B
aminoglycoside
melphalan
trimethoprim
cotrimoxazole
NSAID

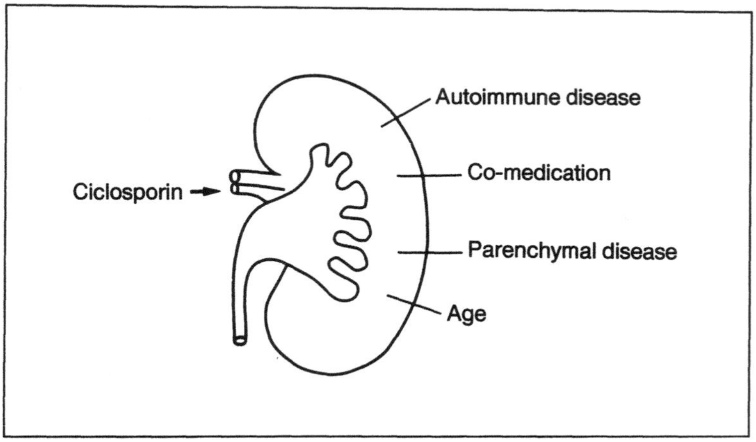

Fig. 5. Schematic presentation of different factors damaging to the kidney

2. Treat rigorously all co-existing diseases with possible renal side effects: hypertension, heart failure, diabetes mellitus, urinary tract infection, etc (Fig. 5).
3. Avoid co-medication with potentially nephrotoxic drugs (see Table 2). Also consider self-medication with analgesics by the patient.
4. Be very cautious in elderly patients in view of possible age-dependent attrition of renal tissue, co-existing arteriosclerosis etc.
5. Start with low doses of CyA, so that the trough levels within the first two weeks do not exceed 50–100 ng/ml (serum) or 300–500 ng/ml (whole blood) trough levels. Avoid extreme fluctuation of peak levels.
6. Increase CyA dose slowly. Whole blood trough levels should not exceed – if possible – 800 ng/ml serum. Repeated controls of renal function and blood pressure are necessary.

References

1. Bergstrand A, Bohman SO, Farnsworth A, Gokel JM, Krause PH, Lang W, Mihatsch MJ, Oppedal B, Sell S, Sibley RK, Thiru S, Verani R, Wallace AC, Zollinger HU, Ryffel B, Thiel G, Wonigeit K (1985) Renal histopathology in kidney transplant recipients immunosuppressed with cyclosporin A. Clin Nephrol, submitted for publication
2. Brunner FP, unpublished observation
3. Brunner FP, Mihatsch MJ, Thiel G (1984) Mannitol potentiates cyclosporin nephrotoxicity. 12th Int. Congress of Nephrology. Book of abstracts
4. Chedid A, Jao W, Port J (1980) Megamitochondria in hepatic and renal disease. Am J Gastroenterol 73:319–324
5. Farnsworth A, Hall BM, Ng ABP, Duggin GG, Horvath JS, Ross-Sheil AG, Tiller DJ (1984) Renal biopsy morphology in renal transplantation. A comparative study of the light microscopic appearances of biopsies from patients treated with cyclosporin A or azathioprine, prednisone and antilymphocyte globulin. Am J Surg Pathol 8:243–252
6. Hamilton DV, Evans DV, Thiru S (1982) Toxicity of cyclosporin A in organ grafting. In: White DJG (ed) Cyclosporin A. Elsevier Biomedical Press, Amsterdam New York Oxford pp 393–411
7. Kirwan PD (1982) Giant mitochondria and multiple cilia in proximal convoluted tubules of renal transplant patients receiving cyclosporin A immunosuppression. Micron 13: 353–354
8. Klintmalm G, Ringden O, Groth CG (1983) Clinical and laboratory signs in nephrotoxicity and rejection in cyclosporine-treated renal allograft recipients. Transplant Proc 15:2815–2820
9. Klintmalm G, Bohman SO, Sundelin B, Wilczek H (1984) Interstitial fibrosis in renal allografts after 12 to 46 months of cyclosporine treatment. Beneficial effects of lower doses early after transplantation. Lancet II:950–954
10. Marbet UA, Graf U, Mihatsch MJ, Gratwohl A, Müller W, Thiel G (1980) Renale Nebenwirkungen der Therapie mit Cyclosporin A bei der chronischen Polyarthritis und nach Knochenmarktransplantation. Schweiz Med Wochenschr 110:2017–2020

11. Mihatsch MJ, Olivieri V, Marbet U, Thiel G, Harder F (1982) Giant mitochondria in renal tubular cells and cyclosporin A. Lancet I:1162
12. Mihatsch MJ, Thiel G, Spichtin HP, Oberholzer M, Brunner FP, Harder F, Olivieri V, Bremer R, Ryffel B, Stöcklin E, Torhorst J, Gudat F, Zollinger HU, Loertscher R (1983) Morphological findings in kidney transplants after treatment with cyclosporine. Transplant Proc 15:2821–2835
13. Mihatsch MJ, Thiel G, Basler V, Ryffel B, Landmann J, Overbeck J von, Zollinger HU (1985) Morphologic patterns in cyclosporin A treated renal transplant recipients. Transplant Proc (in press)
14. Ryffel B (1982) Experimental toxicological studies with cyclosporin A. In: White DJG (ed) Cyclosporin A. Elsevier Biomedical Press, Amsterdam New York Oxford, pp 45–75
15. Ryffel B, Siegl H, Thiel G, Mihatsch MJ (to be published) Experimental nephrotoxicity of cyclosporine
16. Sibley RK, Ferguson RM, Sutherland DER, Simmons RL, Najarian JS (1983) Morphology of cyclosporine nephrotoxicity and of acute rejection in cyclosporine nephrotoxicity and of acute rejection in cyclosporine-prednisone immunosuppressed renal allograft recipients. Transplant Proc 15:2836–2841
17. Sibley RK, Rynasiewicz J, Ferguson MR, Fryd D, Sutherland DER, Simmons RL, Najarian JS (1983) Morphology of cyclosporine nephrotoxicity and acute rejection in patients immunosuppressed with cyclosporine and prednisone. Surgery 94:225–234
18. Suzuki T, Furusato M, Takasaki S, Ishikava E (1975) Giant mitochondria in the epithelial cells of the proximal convoluted tubules of diseased human kidneys. Lab Invest 33:578–590
19. Thiel G, Torhorst J, Brunner FP (1982) Renal toxicity of cyclosporin A in the rat. Proc Clin Dial Transplant Forum 10:62–65
20. Thiru S, Maher ER, Hamilton DV, Evans DB, Calne RY (1983) Tubular changes in renal transplant recipients on cyclosporine. Transplant Proc 15:2846–2851
21. Verani RR, Flechner SM, Buren ChT van, Kahan BD (1984) Acute cellular rejection or cyclosporine A nephrotoxicity? A review of renal biopsies. Am J Kidney Dis 4:185–191

Ciclosporin in Autoimmune Diseases – Side Effects (with Emphasis on Renal Dysfunction) and Recommendations for Use

B. von Graffenried and W. B. Harrison

Based on theoretical considerations, results of animal studies in various autoimmune disease models and anecdotal experience in patients [3], a systematic clinical research programme of ciclosporin (CyA) treatment in various autoimmune diseases was undertaken in 1982. About 1000 patients have since been treated with CyA, and the side-effect profile is emerging.

Frequent side effects (Table 1)

The most commonly reported adverse effect is nephrotoxicity, which will be discussed in more detail below. Reversible hypertension of unknown pathogenesis develops in 5–15% of patients, mostly after 2–3 months of therapy. It is mainly of mild to moderate severity, is associated with low renin levels and usually responds to conventional therapy. The elderly and those treated with non-steroidal anti-inflammatory drugs seem to exhibit a higher risk of developing hypertension. Uncontrolled hypertension may enhance nephrotoxicity. Increases of serum potassium and uric acid are frequent and have previously been described [1, 13]. Hepatotoxicity has only rarely been of clinical relevance and usually reverts on lowering of the dose of CyA. A reversible decrease of hemoglobin of about 1 g/dl has occurred in various studies [13, 15]. The anemia is normochromic and normocytic. There is no evidence for iron deficiency or hemolysis, and since white blood cells and platelets remain unchanged it is not the expression of general bone marrow toxicity. Hypertrichosis is common. Gingival hyperplasia can be avoided to a large extent if patients with poor dentition have their teeth put into order and placques removed. Gastrointestinal intolerance (loss of appetite, nausea, vomiting) is quite frequent, as is fine tremor of the hands and a peculiar feeling of warmth, which usually disappear without discontinuation of CyA therapy. Infections have not so far been a problem, and when they have occurred, their course has not shown unusual features.

Table 1. CyA in autoimmune disease, frequent side effects

Nephrotoxicity
Hypertension
Hyperkalemia
Hyperuricemia
Hepatotoxicity
Anaemia
Hypertrichosis
Gingival hyperplasia
GI intolerance
Tremor
Paresthesia

Overall, these side effects have been the cause for discontinuation of CyA in about 5–20% of patients in the various studies.

Rare adverse events

It is not possible to make firm statements on the relationship to CyA of the events listed in Table 2. Benign mammary hyperplasia and epileptic seizures have also been reported in transplant patients treated with CyA and are probably drug-related. A lymphoma occurred in a patient who was treated for 2 years with cytostatic agents for a thymoma and then developped aplastic anemia which was treated successfully with CyA. After 5 months of CyA therapy a

Clinical Research Department, Sandoz Ltd., Basle, Switzerland

Published with kind permission of Grune and Stratton, Orlando, Florida

Table 2. CyA in autoimmune diseases, rare side effects (n patients out of about 1000)

Facial edema (9)
Benign mammary hyperplasia (6)
Skin rash (3)
Hemolytic-uremic syndrome (?1)
Thrombocytopenia (1)
Legionaire's disease (1)
Aseptic meningitis (3)
Benign papillary adenoma of thyroid (1)
T-cell lymphoma (1)
Squamous cell carcinoma of skin (1)
Myocardial infarction (2)
Epileptic seizures (3)

lymphoma was detected. It is important to note that this was a T-cell lymphoma, whereas lymphomas in immunosuppressed transplant patients are nearly always of B-cell origin. The aplastic anemia may have been the first symptom of the lymphoma.

Nephrotoxicity

Renal dysfunction is the most frequent side effect associated with effective CyA therapy and has been extensively described in transplant patients [2]. Acute CyA nephrotoxicity is dose-dependent, correlated with CyA levels in blood or plasma [8] and reversible after dose reduction [16] or stopping CyA therapy [4]. The morphological correlations of acute CyA nephrotoxicity appear to be tubular lesions characterized by inclusion bodies, isometric vacuolization and microcalcification [10]. Stimulation of the tubuloglomerular feedback mechanism [7] as well as disturbance of the microcirculation through interaction of CyA on local prostacyclin synthesis [12] have been postulated in order to explain the decline in glomerular filtration rate, as evidenced by the rapid increase of serum creatinine in CyA treated patients.

In the following, the currently available experience is reported with regard to renal function in patients with autoimmune diseases treated with CyA. In such patients the study of CyA nephrotoxicity is uncomplicated by certain factors which obscure interpretation of renal function data in renal transplant patients. In addition, lower initial dosage and differing concomitant medications further distinguish these patients from transplant patients. The data presented relate to renal function in patients on continuous therapy up to 24 months and to reversibility of nephrotoxicity in patients discontinuing treatment.

Methods

The data presented were extracted from case report forms of ongoing clinical studies in the following indications: multiple sclerosis, rheumatoid arthritis, diabetes mellitus Type I, uveitis posterior, primary biliary cirrhosis, endocrine ophthalmopathy and systemic lupus erythematosus. Additionally, data on some single patients in 7 further indications are included in this analysis.

In all study protocols, an initial CyA dosage is established (in most studies either 5 or 10 mg/kg/d in the form of a drink solution given once or twice daily). The dose is thereafter modified according to serum creatinine, side effects, blood or plasma trough levels of CyA and therapeutic response.

For the analysis of the effect of continuous CyA therapy, data was considered only from patients who had had at least 6 months of therapy. The following parameters were extracted: serum creatinine, trough CyA levels and CyA dose in mg/kg/d. These data were collected at baseline and at 1, 3, 6 months (all patients) and, if available, after 12 and 24 months of continuous therapy. As an indirect parameter of glomerular filtration rate, creatinine clearance (crcl) in ml/min was computed using the Cockcroft-Gault formula [5] which takes into consideration the reciprocal of serum creatinine, age, body weight and sex. The percentage change of serum creatinine and crcl from baseline was calculated at each time point for each patient.

For the analysis of reversibility of CyA-induced nephrotoxicity, data were obtained only from those patients who had undergone at least 4 weeks of treatment with CyA and in whom serum creatinine values were available after stopping CyA therapy. Data similar to those described above were extracted and calculated at baseline, at time of highest serum creatinine value recorded on CyA (with time in weeks from start of therapy) and at time of last measurement under CyA. All creatinine values recorded after stopping CyA were extracted with the respective time (weeks) after stopping CyA. If more than one such value was available, all data were used till baseline values were reached again. Treatment duration was also recorded. Percentage change of creatinine and crcl from baseline was calculated at time of highest and last value under CyA and at time of first and last recorded value after stopping CyA.

All data from patients meeting the above mentioned criteria which were accessible to Sandoz Ltd., Basle up to February 6, 1985 are presented.

Results

Demographic data from patients on continuous CyA therapy, CyA dosages used and CyA trough levels achieved are given in Table 3.

Data on renal function from patients on continuous CyA therapy up to at least 6 months (n = 349) and 12 months (n = 180) and 24 months (n = 12) are shown in Tables 4 and 5 and Figures 1 and 2. Renal function declines rapidly within the first month, then levels off between months 3 and 6 with only a slight further decline up to month 12 and thereafter constant values up to 24 months. The mean reduction of crcl at month 6 compared to baseline is 14%. Mean values are well within the normal range at all time points. The proportion of patients with serum creatinine above 130 μmol/l is 2.0% at baseline, 7.7% at month 1, 10.4% at month 3, 15.4% at month 6 and 20.6% at month 12.

Table 3. Characteristics of patients on continuous therapy

Disease	n patients treated during			age (years)	CyA dosage (mg/kg/day) $\bar{X} \pm SD$		
	6 mo	12 mo	24 mo	$\bar{X}$	0 mo	6 mo	12 mo
Multiple sclerosis (MS)	116	79	6	35	5.8±1.9	5.8±1.4	5.9±1.4
Uveitis posterior	63	32	3	35	9.2±1.9	8.7±3.4	7.7±3.5
Diabetes mellitus Type I	78	50	–	16	9.9±2.6	11.5±4.0	9.3±3.5
Primary biliary cirrhosis (PBC)	31	8	–	53	3.2±1.3	3.1±1.0	2.7±0.9
Rheumatoid arthritis (RA)	25	2	1	54	8.9±2.0	5.9±2.1	5.7±3.3
Endocrine ophthalmopathy	14	–	–	51	9.2±1.7	4.9±3.2	–
Systemic lupus erythematosus	8	3	–	30	5.8±1.2	5.6±1.0	3.9±1.2
Others	14	6	2	32	–	–	–
Total	349	180	12	34	7.5±3.0	7.6±4.7	7.0±3.1

CyA trough levels (ng/ml, RIA), $\bar{X} \pm SD$

	n	Month 1	n	Month 3	n	Month 6	n	Month 12
Whole blood								
All patients	142	385±296	136	345±266	128	322±199	59	298±148
MS	87	265±152	81	269±179	77	288±185	57	303±147
PBC	13	604±440	11	543±299	12	377±175		
RA	15	608±320	16	567±460	15	425±260		
Plasma								
All patients	81	153±132	81	118± 63	80	125± 79	47	116± 78
Diabetes mel. Type I	70	140± 91	69	116± 53	68	118± 50	44	116± 79

Table 4. Renal function of patients on continuous CyA therapy for 6 months

	n	0		Month 1			Month 3			Month 6		
		$\bar{X} \pm SD$	95% CL[1]	$\bar{X} \pm SD$	95% CL	%[2]	$\bar{X} \pm SD$	95% CL	%	$\bar{X} \pm SD$	95% CL	%
All patients												
Cr[3], µmol/l	349	78±20	75 – 80	89±28	86 – 92	+14	93±32	90 – 97	+21	98±34	94 – 101	+27
crcl[4], ml/min.	301	92±26	90 – 95	85±24	82 – 88	–7	80±23	77 – 83	–12	78±25	75 – 80	–14
Multiple sclerosis												
Cr, µmol/l	116	81±14	78 – 83	89±17	86 – 92	+11	93±27	88 – 98	+16	92±20	88 – 96	+15
crcl, ml/min.	112	97±26	92 – 102	89±22	84 – 93	–8	86±21	82 – 90	–10	86±22	81 – 90	–10
Uveitis posterior												
Cr, µmol/l	63	86±21	81 – 91	100±34	91 – 109	+17	106±31	98 – 114	+24	114±32	106 – 122	+35
crcl, ml/min.	24	92±24	82 – 103	88±25	77 – 98	–3	77±22	68 – 86	–15	75±23	65 – 84	–16
Diabetes mellitus Type I												
Cr, µmol/l	78	68±18	64 – 72	76±26	71 – 82	+13	81±22	76 – 86	+21	92±35	84 – 100	+37
crcl, ml/min.	78	95±29	89 – 102	89±26	83 – 95	–4	83±24	78 – 88	–11	76±26	70 – 81	–17
Primary biliary cirrhosis												
Cr, µmol/l	31	66±11	62 – 70	84±17	74 – 95	+25	86±39	70 – 101	+30	81±28	71 – 92	+23
crcl, ml/min.	31	84±18	77 – 90	70±18	59 – 81	–17	71±20	63 – 80	–16	72±24	63 – 81	–13
Rheumatoid arthritis												
Cr, µmol/l	25	79±22	70 – 88	101±31	88 – 115	+27	112±37	96 – 127	+41	112±47	93 – 131	+42
crcl, ml/min.	20	83±24	71 – 94	66±21	55 – 77	–19	59±20	49 – 68	–28	60±23	50 – 71	–28

[1] Confidence limits
[2] Mean % change from baseline
[3] Serum creatinine
[4] Creatinine clearance calculated using the Cockcroft-Gault formula (see text)
n lower than for Cr because for some patients data on age and sex not available

Table 5. Renal function of patients on continuous CyA therapy for 12 months

	n	0		Month 1			Month 3			Month 6			Month 12		
		$\bar{X}\pm SD$	95% CL[1]	$\bar{X}\pm SD$	95% CL	%[2]	$\bar{X}\pm SD$	95% CL	%	$\bar{X}\pm SD$	95% CL	%	$\bar{X}\pm SD$	95% CL	%
All patients															
Cr[3], μmol/l	180	76±19	76 – 81	88±28	84 – 93	+11	94±32	89 – 99	+20	100±35	95 – 106	+29	103±33	99 – 108	+34
crcl[4], ml/min.	155	95±26	91 – 100	89±24	85 – 93	–5	83±21	80 – 87	–11	79±24	76 – 83	–15	77±25	73 – 81	–18
Multiple sclerosis															
Cr, μmol/l	79	81±14	78 – 84	88±16	84 – 91	+9	95±31	88 – 102	+17	93±21	88 – 98	+15	96±24	90 – 101	+19
crcl, ml/min.	76	98±27	92 – 104	91±21	86 – 95	–6	86±20	81 – 91	–10	87±22	82 – 92	–9	84±21	79 – 89	–12
Uveitis posterior[5]															
Cr, μmol/l	32	88±19	81 – 95	100±35	87 – 113	+12	107±27	97 – 117	+22	118±33	106 – 130	+37	127±30	116 – 138	+49
1/Cr × 10	32	118±23	110 – 127	110±31	99 – 121	–7	98±23	90 – 107	–17	92±29	81 – 102	–21	84±22	76 – 92	–27
Diabetes mellitus Type I															
Cr, μmol/l	50	68±19	63 – 73	78±27	70 – 86	+15	82±23	75 – 89	+22	94±37	83 – 105	+40	98±36	88 – 108	+46
crcl, ml/min.	50	97±28	89 – 105	89±27	81 – 97	–6	83±22	77 – 90	–13	75±25	68 – 82	–21	73±27	66 – 81	–24

[1] Confidence limits
[2] Mean % change from baseline
[3] Serum creatinine
[4] Creatinine clearance calculated using the Cockcroft-Gault formula (see text)
n lower than for Cr because for some patients data on age and sex not available
[5] crcl not given, since age, which is required for the application of the Cockcroft-Gault formula, not available for most patients.

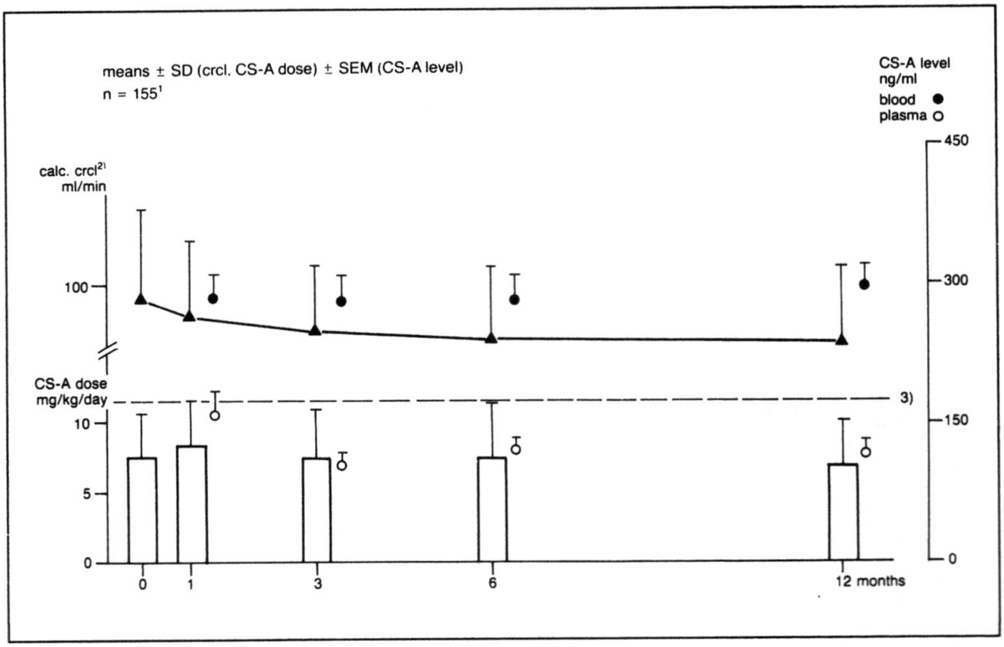

Fig. 1. 1) n for CyA levels in blood = 68 (months 1, 3), 64 (month 6), 59 (month 12); in plasma 47 (month 1), 48 (month 3), 49 (month 6), 47 (month 12); blood and plasma figures relate to different patients; 2) Creatinine clearance calculated using the Cockcroft-Gault formula (see text); 3) This line represents the calculated crcl for a serum creatinine of 130 μmol/l (= 1.47 mg/dl) and the data of the study population (mean age 31 years, mean body weight 61 kg, ratio male : female = 1 : 1.35) and indicates lower limit of normal range (= 57.4 ml/min)

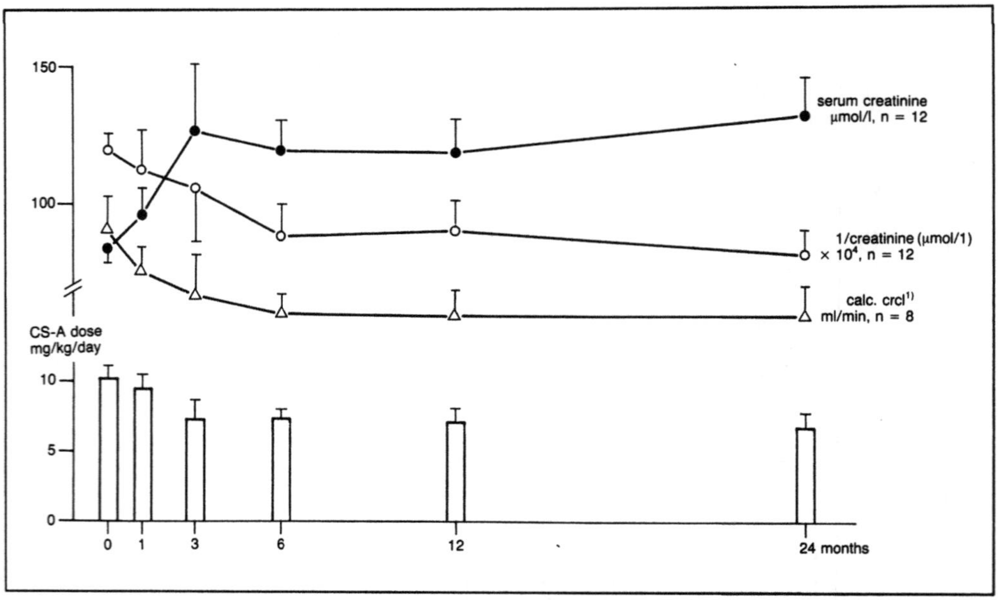

Fig. 2. 1) Creatinine clearance calculated by Cockcroft-Gault formula (see text)

Table 6. Subgroups of patients with continuous therapy ($\bar{X} \pm SD$)

	Baseline crcl	Month 6 crcl			Month 12 crcl			Age	Initial CyA dosage	CyA blood levels at month 1	
	ml/min	ml/min[1]	(n)	%[2]	ml/min	(n)	%	(years)	mg/kg/day	ng/ml	(n)
Age											
≦15 years	89±29	73±26	(54)	−12	71±25	(30)	−24	10±3	10.4±2.7	–	
16–50 years	97±26	82±24	(200)	−14	80±24	(110)	−16	34±9	6.7±2.5	338±239	(121)
>50 years	79±18	65±22	(47)	−17	60±22	(15)	−25	59±6	6.6±3.7	653±434	(21)
Initial CyA dosage											
≦7.5 mg/kg/day	94±27	83±25	(158)	−11	82±24	(89)	−14	37±13	4.7±1.1	342±275	(115)
>7.5 mg/kg/day	90±25	72±23	(143)	−17	69±23	(66)	−24	30±18	10.2±1.5	569±318	(27)
Baseline crcl											
>90 ml/min	111±21	89±22	(156)	−20	85±24	(91)	−22	30±13	7.2±2.8	370±323	(73)
≦90 ml/min	72±13	66±21	(145)	−8	64±20	(64)	−13	38±18	7.5±3.4	403±269	(68)
CyA blood level at month 1											
≦300 ng/ml	94±20	85±20	(77)	−8	86±21	(48)	−8	37±10	5.2±1.5	194±70	(77)
>300 ng/ml	95±32	80±27	(65)	−15	88±28	(20)	−17	41±13	6.6±2.4	610±304	(65)

[1] Calculated creatinine clearance using the Cockcroft-Gault formula (see text)
[2] Mean % change from baseline

The general pattern of renal function over time is very similar for a series of subgroups of patients subdivided by diagnosis (Tables 4, 5), age, initial CyA dosage, baseline crcl and CyA trough blood levels at month 1 (Table 6). For all these subgroups there is no evidence of relevant progressive deterioration over time.

Differences emerge, however, concerning the extent of reduction of renal function. Patients with multiple sclerosis, endocrine ophthalmopathy and SLE have a less than average reduction of crcl which may be related to the below average CyA dosage from month 3 onwards. On the other hand, patients with rheumatoid arthritis show an above average decline in crcl which remains stable from month 3 to month 6. This subgroup also exhibited higher mean age and above average CyA blood levels at month 3. Patients older than 50 years of age show a slightly higher mean percentage decrease of crcl at month 6 when compared to younger patients and also exhibit higher CyA levels. Patients treated with more than 7.5 mg/kg/d who had high CyA blood levels also show a more pronounced reduction in crcl than those with lower dosage and lower CyA levels. On the other hand, patients with low baseline crcl show less reduction in crcl over time than patients with high baseline values despite similar doses of CyA, similar CyA levels and similar age. A more pronounced mean reduction in crcl occurred in patients with trough CyA blood levels above 300 ng/ml at month 1 as compared to those with lower levels.

Data on reversibility of CyA-induced impairment of renal function were obtained in 144 patients in whom creatinine values were available before, during and after CyA therapy (Table 7, Fig. 3). Reasons for cessation of CyA therapy were: completion

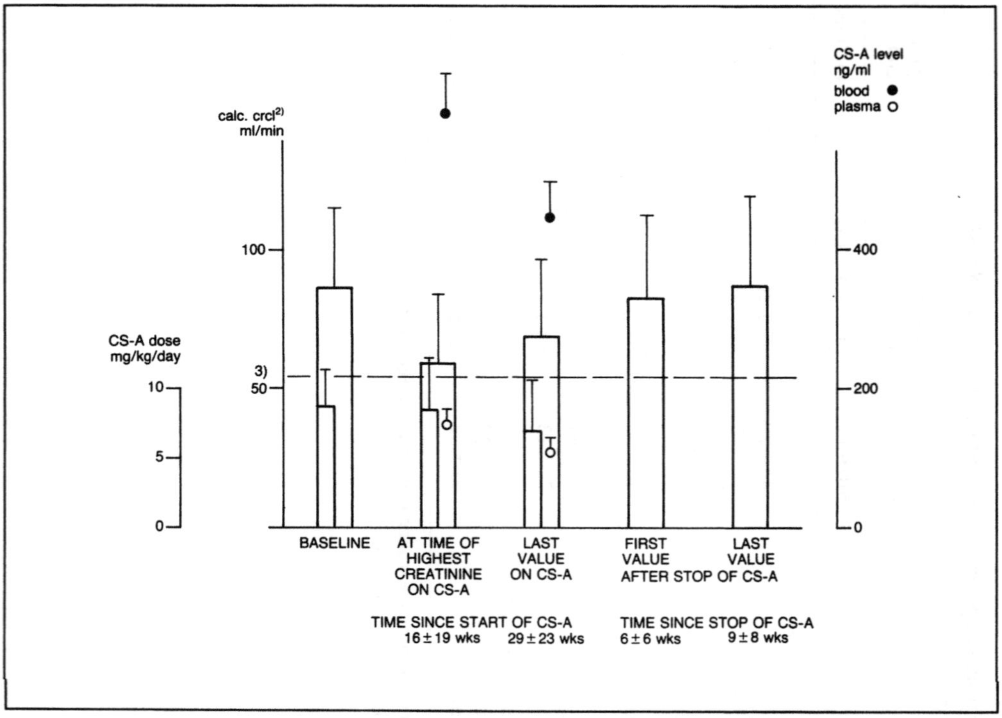

Fig. 3. 1) n for CyA levels in blood = 44, in plasma = 46 (different patients); 2) Creatinine clearance calculated by Cockcroft-Gault formula (see text); 3) This line represents the calculated crcl for a serum creatinine of 130 μmol/l (= 1.47 mg/dl) and the data of the study population (mean age 39 years, mean body weight 62 kg, ratio male : female = 1 : 1.8) and indicates lower limit of normal range (= 54.3 ml/min)

Table 7. Reversibility of CyA nephrotoxicity

	n	Baseline	Highest creatinine on CyA		At end of CyA therapy		First creatinine after stopping CyA		Last creatinine after stopping CyA	
		$\bar{X}\pm SD$	$\bar{X}\pm SD$	% [1]	$\bar{X}\pm SD$	%	$\bar{X}\pm SD$	%	$\bar{X}\pm SD$	%
Cr [2], μmol/l	144	86 ±49	136 ± 65	+64.1	115 ± 59	+37.9	95±51	+12.4	90±51	+5.5
1/Cr×10⁴	144	133 ±42	87 ± 32	−33.1	104 ± 44	−20.0	123±43	−6.4	130±44	−1.1
crcl [3], ml/min.	137	87 ±29	59 ± 25	−32.1	69 ± 28	−18.5	83±30	−4.4	87±33	+0.9
t since start CyA, weeks	144	–	16 ± 19		29 ± 23		–		–	
t since stop CyA, weeks	144	–	–		–		6± 6		9± 8	
CyA dose, mg/kg/day	144	8.9± 2.4	8.4± 3.8		6.9± 3.7		–			
CyA levels, ng/ml										
Whole blood	44	–	604 ±339		450 ±316		–		–	
Plasma	46	–	148 ±101		107 ± 90		–		–	

[1] Mean % change from baseline
[2] Serum creatinine
[3] Creatinine clearance calculated using the Cockcroft-Gault formula (see text)
n lower than for Cr because for some patients data on age not available

of study (56%), nephrotoxicity (10%), other side effects (16%) and inefficacy (18%). The maximum recorded reduction of crcl from baseline (mean −32%) was measured at 16 weeks (± 19) after start of therapy. At that particular time, 42.4% of patients had creatinine values above 130 µmol/ml. With reduction of CyA dose and correspondingly lower CyA levels an improvement of renal function occurred while patients continued CyA treatment up to a mean total duration of 29±23 weeks. At the time of the last value on CyA the mean percentage reduction of crcl from baseline had improved to −18.5%. 28.5% of the patients had creatinine values above 130 µmol/ml at end of therapy. Only one creatinine value after stopping CyA was available in the majority of patients (64%) and this was measured only relatively soon after stopping CyA (mean 6±6 weeks, median 4 weeks). At that time crcl had improved substantially but not yet quite reached baseline values (mean change from baseline −4%). When taking the last recorded value for all patients (which for 64% of patients was in fact the only value measured), mean crcl further improved and reached baseline values again at a mean interval of 9±8 (median 6) weeks after cessation of therapy. 15 patients (10.4%) still had creatinine values above 130 µmol/l at that time. In 8 of these patients baseline creatinine was already above the respective limits (patients with chronic glomerulonephritis).

For a more detailed analysis of the time course of reversibility, only those patients were considered for whom creatinine values were available within 12 weeks of stopping therapy (n=131). Mean creatinine values were computed for data collected within the first, second and third month after CyA (per time period only one value per patient). As shown in Figure 4, full reversibility of CyA nephrotoxicity is reached 2 months after stopping therapy.

Data on subgroups of patients are shown in Table 8. As already seen in the analysis of patients on continuous therapy, maximum impairment of renal function is greater in older patients, in those with longer duration of therapy, in those with a high initial dosage of CyA and in patients with rheumatoid arthritis. Improvement of renal function occurred in all subgroups until the end of CyA therapy and only small differences in the extent of reversibility after stopping CyA are apparent be-

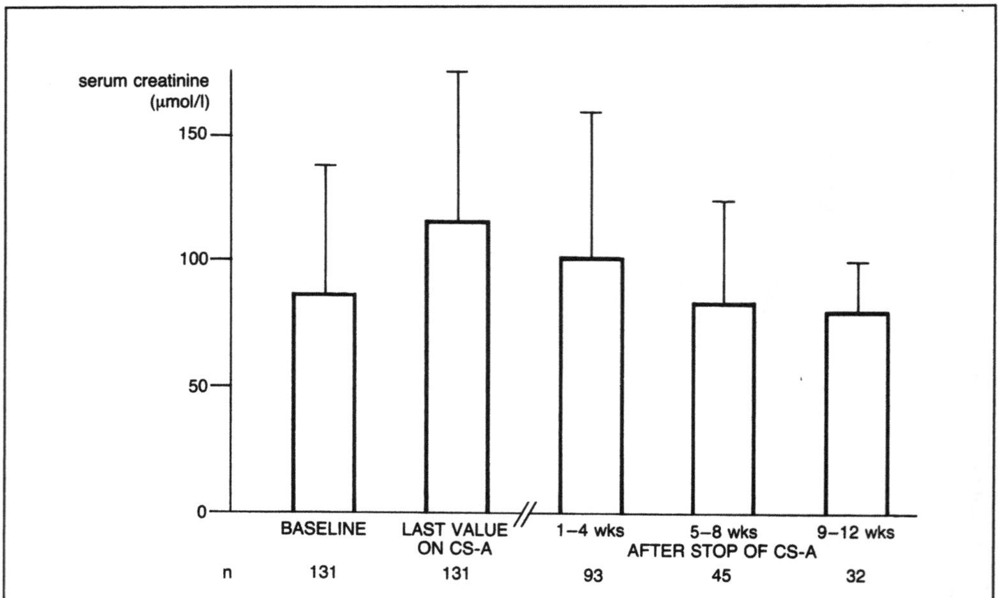

Fig. 4. Reversibility of nephrotoxicity; time course (means ± SD)

Table 8. Reversibility of CyA nephrotoxicity for subgroups of patients ($\bar{X} \pm SD$)

	n	Calculated creatinine clearance[1] ml/min.							Age (y)	Length of CyA therapy	Initial CyA dose	CyA blood levels at highest Cr	
		Baseline	At time of highest creatinine	%[2]	At end of CyA therapy	%	Last value after stopping CyA[3]	%			(mg/kg/d)	ng/ml	(n)
Age													
≦15 years	21	85±30	57±21	−29	70±22	−7	100±40	+23	10± 3	40±17	10.8±2.2	–	
16−50 years	71	95±32	65±29	−30	77±30	−17	92±33	−2	35±10	31±25	8.3±2.3	554±294	(24)
>50 years	45	77±19	46±16	−38	56±22	−27	72±22	−6	58± 6	22±21	9.2±2.2	664±386	(20)
Length of CyA therapy													
≦24 weeks	76	88±33	62±29	−28	72±31	−14	87±34	0	44±16	15± 6	8.7±2.3	552±344	(25)
>24 weeks	61	87±23	54±20	−37	66±23	−23	88±32	+1	32±18	45±26	9.3±2.6	672±330	(19)
Baseline crcl													
>84 ml/min.	68	109±22	71±27	−36	83±27	−24	107±31	−2	35±16	29±23	9.0±1.9	642±361	(24)
≦84 ml/min.	69	66±16	47±16	−29	57±21	−13	68±22	+4	42±19	29±24	8.9±3.0	559±314	(20)
Decrease of lowest 1/Cr from baseline													
≦30%	72	85±29	72±27	−16	80±27	−2	93±37	+10	36±17	23±16	8.4±2.7	512±360	(22)
>30%	65	90±29	46±16	−48	59±24	−34	82±28	−7	42±19	34±27	9.4±2.0	696±298	(22)
Initial CyA dosage													
≦7.5 mg/kg/day	31	80±28	59±26	−25	67±27	−13	75±28	−33	40±13	24±14	5.0±0.9	587±396	(15)
>7.5 mg/kg/day	106	90±29	58±25	−34	70±28	−20	91±33	+2	39±19	30±25	10.1±1.1	613±314	(29)
Diagnosis[4]													
IDDM	40	93±30	64±26	−30	76±25	−13	99±30	+10	19±12	38±20	9.7±2.5	–	
RA	31	83±24	49±22	−42	58±26	−32	77±28	−9	55±11	19± 8	9.4±1.7	691±347	(19)
EO	29	83±15	60±15	−27	72±20	−13	83±16	+1	50± 8	18± 7	9.3±1.5	490±207	(10)
Others	37	88±38	57±32	−32	68±34	−20	81±39	−5	38±12	35±34	7.6±2.9	690±414	(10)

[1] Calculated using the Cockcroft-Gault formula (see text)
[2] Mean % change from baseline
[3] Mean time after stopping for all patients 9±8 (median 6) weeks. Very similar times for all subgroups with the exception of age and dosage. Age >50 years=7±5 (median 4) weeks, 16−50 years=9±7 (median 7) weeks; dosage ≦7.5 mg/kg/day=8±6 (median 4) weeks, >7.5 mg/kg/day=9±8 (median 7) weeks.
Mean time after stopping for IDDM 8±4 (median 7) weeks, for RA 7±4 (median 6) weeks, for EO 7±5 (median 4) weeks and for others 13±12 (median 12) weeks.
[4] IDDM=Diabetes mellitus Type I; RA=Rheumatoid arthritis; EO=Endocrine opthalmopathy

tween the subgroups. Full reversibility is obtained in the subgroups with more than 6 months of therapy (45±26 weeks), with more than 7.5 mg/kg/d initial CyA dose (10.1±1.1 mg/kg/d) and in the group of patients with low baseline crcl (66±16 ml/min). Mean crcl after stopping CyA was lower than at baseline in the group of patients over 50 years of age and in patients with rheumatoid arthritis. In these groups, the median time at which the last measurement of creatinine (after stopping CyA) was performed was only 4 and 6 weeks respectively.

Discussion

Despite the relatively high numbers of patients analysed in this preliminary report (349 patients treated up to 6 months; 180 patients up to 12 months; 12 patients up to 24 months; 144 patients with data before, during and after stopping therapy), the interpretation of the data must remain cautious, mainly because of the heterogeneity of the data. They stem from a large number of still ongoing studies in very different diseases using varying research protocols. Major differences relate to age, baseline renal function, dosage of CyA and, for considerations of reversibility, duration of therapy. Age- and disease-dependent differences in pharmacokinetics of CyA may confound analysis of certain factors, e.g. in the young population with diabetes Type I or in primary biliary cirrhosis. An important factor complicating the analysis is that CyA dosage is not only variable between indications but also between studies within the same indication and is frequently adjusted individually on the basis of efficacy, serum creatinine, other side effects and CyA levels. Important factors such as concomitant medication (e.g. non-steroidal anti-inflammatory drugs, diuretics, antihypertensives), pre-existing hypertension or hypertension developing under CyA have not been taken into account for this analysis. A definite conclusion on reversibility of CyA-induced nephrotoxicity is hampered by the fact that in the majority of patients only one value of serum creatinine was taken after cessation of CyA therapy, at a time which may have been too short to allow full recovery. Finally, this report must be seen as an intermediate analysis of an ongoing process of safety monitoring and further statistical analyses will be performed in order to attempt to formulate definite conclusions.

CyA induces an increase in serum creatinine within the first 2 weeks of therapy. The period of steepest decline in renal function takes place within the first 3 months. At month 6 the mean reduction in creatinine clearance (crcl) calculated by the Cockcroft-Gault method [5] is 14%. After month 6 there is only a slight further impairment, and the limited data show no relevant further deterioration up to 2 years of CyA therapy. The extent of nephrotoxicity is related to CyA dosage and CyA levels, and may also be age-related. It is likely that these factors interact in patients with rheumatoid arthritis, who also show above-average nephrotoxicity. Concomitant therapy with NSAID's may be an additional contributing element in these patients [6]. It is important to note that patients with below-average baseline renal function have shown only little and stable renal dysfunction despite average doses of CyA. Despite differences in magnitude of renal toxicity between the subgroups mentioned, the pattern of nearly stable renal function from month 6 to month 12 applies for all of them and no risk factor studied has emerged for predicting progressive deterioration. It will be important, in future retrospective analyses, to include blood pressure in the list of parameters studied.

CyA-induced renal dysfunction markedly improves after reduction of CyA dose with subsequent lower CyA levels and is, for mean values of the total population studied, completely reversible within 2 months after stopping therapy. It is reassuring that this is true also for patients whose duration of therapy approaches 1 year, those with above average initial CyA dosage and those with below average baseline crcl. In patients older than 50 years and in those with rheumatoid arthritis mean crcl rose substantially after stopping CyA but did not quite reach baseline values. More data are needed at later time points after withdrawal of CyA in order to decide whether this is due to too short an interval after stopping therapy or if these groups are indeed those at potential risk. Reversibility of CyA-induced nephrotoxicity has previously been reported in patients with diabetes Type I [15] and ocular inflammatory disorders of autoimmune origin [13].

The previously reported increase in serum uric acid in patients with uveitis [13] is confirmed in this analysis (data not shown), as well as the increase in serum potassium described in transplant patients [1]. The increases are small, but are nevertheless more pronounced than would be expected from serum creatinine values if they were due only to decreased glomerular filtration, and therefore point to an effect of CyA on tubular function. Urinary excretion of beta-2-microglobulin, a marker of proximal tubular function, has been described as being increased in patients with rheumatoid arthritis under CyA treatment [9].

Recently, progressive and possibly irreversible CyA-induced deterioration of renal function has been described in heart-transplant patients [11]. This pattern has not emerged from the data so far available in patients with autoimmune diseases. There are, however, important differences between the two series of patients. Mean baseline serum creatinine was in the upper range of normal (115 µmol/l) in the heart patients, possibly indicating pre-existing nephropathy, and rose by over 60% to a mean value of 186 µmol/l at month 12. In the patients with autoimmune diseases presented in this report, mean serum creatinine at baseline was much lower (79 µmol/l) and remained well within the normal range (103 µmol/l at month 12). The much higher initial doses of CyA (17.5 mg/kg/d) and the resulting much higher mean CyA levels (300–350 ng/ml in plasma, which correspond to blood levels over 1000 ng/ml) in the heart transplant patients when compared with data from patients with autoimmune diseases (7.5 mg/kg/d; blood CyA levels 298–385 ng/ml) may be responsible for the different pattern of nephrotoxicity.

Although the data seem to demonstrate full reversibility of CyA-induced acute nephrotoxicity, a very slowly progressive chronic nephropathy cannot be excluded since the parameter used to assess renal function (serum creatinine) is not sensitive enough to detect early loss of nephrons. In addition, patient numbers beyond one year of treatment are small.

Possible irreversible histological findings in kidneys of transplant patients on CyA have been published [10, 11]. Renal biopsies have not been performed systematically in patients with autoimmune diseases treated with CyA. The only published result of a renal biopsy concerns a 58-year-old patient with progressive therapy-resistant Sézary-syndrome [14]. This patient was treated initially with 17 mg/kg/d of oral CyA. The dose was adjusted downwards because of distinct nephrotoxicity, but serum creatinine remained abnormal (130–160 µmol/l). After 10 months of CyA therapy, a renal biopsy was performed which showed "patchy tubular atrophy and quite extensive interstitial fibrosis". In a 52-year-old patient with therapy-resistant, life-threatening polychondritis who has been successfully treated with CyA for more than 3 years (initial dose 15.7 mg/kg/d; maintenance dose about 6 mg/kg/d), a recently performed renal biopsy has shown features similar to what has been described in biopsies of CyA-treated transplant patients (data on file, Sandoz Ltd.). The biopsy was performed because of the suspicion of chronic nephrotoxicity after rising creatinine, falling creatinine clearance and hypertension had been noted after some 15 months of therapy. More biopsies in well-documented patients in whom a suspicion of nephrotoxicity exists are needed to clarify the situation.

Recommendations for use of CyA in autoimmune diseases

In the interim, the data presented in this report seem to justify the continuation of a cautious and systematic programme of clinical trials whose aim is to assess the benefits and risks of CyA treatment in conditions with progressive deterioration for which either no accepted therapy exists or for which the available therapy is unsatisfactory in terms of both efficacy and toxicity. At present the following procedures are recommended to avoid excessive acute nephrotoxicity and thus possibly the development of chronic renal damage:

1. Patients should be treated with CyA only within formal clinical studies with established research protocols and systematic documentation, and Sandoz must receive data on a continuous basis with minimal time lag. Only in this way can continuous safety monitoring with rapid spread of new information regarding safety issues be established.
2. Patients with pre-existing impaired renal function should be excluded from studies unless amelioration of renal disease is the aim of therapy (e.g. SLE) or in the case of life-threatening and therapy-resistant situations.
3. Elderly patients, and those with pre-existing hypertension or hypertension developing on CyA should be regarded as high-risk patients and must be observed carefully.
4. Concomitant therapy with nephrotoxic drugs, potassium-sparing diuretics and drugs known to interact with the pharmacokinetics of CyA should be avoided.
5. Initial dosage of CyA should not exceed 3–5 mg/kg/d, with the possibility of increasing dosage after about 1 month in the event of insufficient effect and absence of relevant side effects or toxicity. In situations with severe inflammatory symptoms and/or threat of rapid and irreversible loss of organ function, 7.5 –10 mg/kg/d is recommended as the starting dose.
6. Depending on the clinical situation, CyA should be reduced by 25–50% in the case of increase of serum creatinine of more than 50–75% over baseline or above 130–150 µmol/l. If this does not correct this range of abnormality within 2–4 weeks, a further dose reduction is indicated. In patients with slowly progressing creatinine, even if within the normal range, dosage should also be reduced.
7. Regular measurements of CyA levels are recommended. Trough (=predose) blood levels over 600–800 ng/ml or plasma levels above 150–200 ng/ml should be avoided. Because of the large difference in sensitivity of patients to CyA nephrotoxicity, the indicated levels do not separate toxic from non-toxic levels for all patients. The likelihood of nephrotoxicity, and perhaps of other side effects like hypertension, increases with higher levels and furthermore it appears from initial experience that levels higher than those stated are not necessary for immunosuppression.
8. If long-term therapy is indicated (for maintenance of remission or prevention of chronic progression of disease), the lowest effective dose should be determined individually if parameters of disease activity are available. If this is not the case, the highest dose which does not induce relevant nephrotoxicity (see point 6) should be sought.
9. After stopping CyA, serum creatinine as well as any other CyA induced abnormality should be measured at least at monthly intervals until full normalization has occurred. If this does not occur, patients should be followed up long-term and data should be reported.

Acknowledgements

We would like to thank Miss S. Huggenberger for secretarial assistance and typing of the manuscript and Miss J. Fischer and Miss A. Barnes for data processing.

References

1. Adu D, Turney J, Michael J, et al. (1983) Hyperkalaemia in cyclosporin-treated renal allograft recipients. Lancet II:370
2. Bennet WM, Pulliam JP (1983) Cyclosporine nephrotoxicity. Ann Intern Med 99:851
3. Borel JF, von Graffenried B (1984) Sandimmun (cyclosporin A) and autoimmunity. In: Lambert PH, Perrin L, Izui S (eds) Recent Advances in SLE. Academic Press, London, p 313
4. Chapman JF, Griffiths D, Harding NGL, et al. (1985) Reversibility of cyclosporin nephrotoxicity after three months' treatment. Lancet I:128
5. Cockcroft DW, Gault MH (1976) Prediction of creatinine clearance from serum creatinine. Nephron 16:31
6. Dunn MJ (1984) Nonsteroidal anti-inflammatory drugs and renal function. Annu Rev Med 35:411

7. Gutsche HU, Delz E, Lüneburg M, et al. (1984) Effect of cyclosporine on the proximal tubular function of the rat kidney. IXth Int. Congress of Nephrology, Los Angeles, June 1984, Abstract, 475A
8. Kahan BD, van Buren CT, Lin S, et al. (1982) Immunopharmacologic monitoring of cyclosporin A-treated recipients of cadaveric kidney allografts. Transplantation 34:36
9. Marbet UA, Graf U, Mihatsch MJ (1980) Renale Nebenwirkungen der Therapie mit Cyclosporin A bei chronischer Polyarthritis und nach Knochenmarkstransplantation. Schweiz Med Wochenschr 110:2017
10. Mihatsch MJ, Thiel G, Spichtin HP, et al. (1983) Morphological findings in kidney transplants after treatment with cyclosporine. Transplant Proc 15:2821
11. Myers BD, Ross J, Newton L, et al. (1984) Cyclosporine-associated chronic nephropathy. N Engl J Med 311:699
12. Neild GH, Rocchi G, Imbert L, et al. (1984) Effect of cyclosporine on prostacyclin synthesis by vascular tissue in rabbits. In: Kahan BD (ed) Cyclosporine. Grune and Stratton, Orlando, p 182
13. Palestine AG, Nussenblatt RB, Chan CC (1984) Side effects of systemic cyclosporine in patients not undergoing transplantation. Am J Med 77:652
14. Puttick L, Pollock A, Fairburn E (1983) Treatment of Sézary syndrome with Cyclosporin A. J Soc Med 76:1063
15. Stiller CR, Dupré J, Gent M, et al. (1984) Effects of cyclosporine immunosuppression in insulin-dependent diabetes mellitus of recent onset. Science 223:1362
16. Verani RR, Flechner SM, van Buren CT, et al. (1984) Acute cellular rejection or cyclosporine nephrotoxicity? A review of transplant renal biopsies. Am J Kidney Dis 4:185

Clinical Effects and Renal Side Effects in Patients with Autoimmune Diseases Treated with Ciclosporin (CyA)

Karin Svenson[1], Sven-Olof Bohman[2] and Roger Hällgren[1]

We have used ciclosporin (CyA) since 1981 in the treatment of selected cases with severe autoimmune diseases. Our first patient suffered from life-threatening relapsing polychondritis. She had been treated with conventional immunosuppressive therapy without success, but after institution of CyA, a remarkable remission was seen [1]. Attempts to switch her over to chlorambucil met with failure. In four cases with inflammatory active rheumatoid arthritis we have observed remission of vasculitic ulcers and skin lesions during treatment with CyA but only modest effects on inflammatory synovial reactions. In accordance with others [2, 3] we have achieved excellent clinical effects of CyA in patients with Behçet's disease (n = 3) and patients with chronic uveitis (n = 3).

Our patients have suffered from various well-known side effects of CyA such as gingivitis, hirsutism, tremor, hypertension and liver toxicity. However, the renal side effects are our main concern. It is a well-known fact that CyA is a nephrotoxic substance. Earlier reports have described acute tubular damage [4] accompanied by an interstitial inflammatory reaction [5]. Until recently, this acute nephrotoxicity was considered completely reversible upon dose reduction or withdrawal of the drug [6]. However, studies of renal biopsies in recipients of heart and renal allografts suggest that CyA may cause chronic renal damage on long term administration [7, 8]. The relative contribution of CyA to the renal damage observed in these settings has been difficult to assess, since the patients may suffer from renal impairment due to longstanding cardiovascular disease or renal allograft rejection. Until now we have performed renal biopsies in six of our patients treated with CyA. A detailed report of the clinical data of these patients, their CyA dosages and plasma concentrations and renal glomerular and tubular function is given elsewhere [9] and the histopathological renal biopsy findings in these patients are briefly summarized in Table 1 with additional data where relevant. The CyA dosage, the CyA plasma concentrations and the serum creatinine levels and serum creatinine clearance in one of the patients (pat. 3) is illustrated in Figure 1.

The histological lesions varied considerably in degree between patients (Table 1) and consisted mainly of focal interstitial fibrosis (Figs. 2, 5, 6) with tubular atrophy and a slight degree of interstitial inflammation (Figs. 2, 5, 6), and arteriolar hyalinisation (Figs. 3, 4). In some cases there was also glomerular sclerosis (Fig. 2) and vacuolisation of tubular epithelium (Fig. 4). The lesions were thus largely unspecific with respect to pathogenesis but the consistency of the pattern of changes was remarkable. In addition, as observed in a previous report [7], there was a rough correspondance between the degree of histological changes and the cumulated CyA dose (Table 1). Together with the fact that these renal lesions are similar to those reported in kidney and heart transplant recipients treated with CyA [7, 8], our results support the view that CyA is a causative agent of chronic nephropathy in certain circumstances.

1 Section of Rheumatology, Department of Internal Medicine, University Hospital, Uppsala, Sweden
2 Karolinska Institute, Department of Pathology, Huddinge Hospital, Huddinge, Sweden

Karin Svenson, MD
Department of Internal Medicine
University Hospital
S-751 85 Uppsala
Sweden

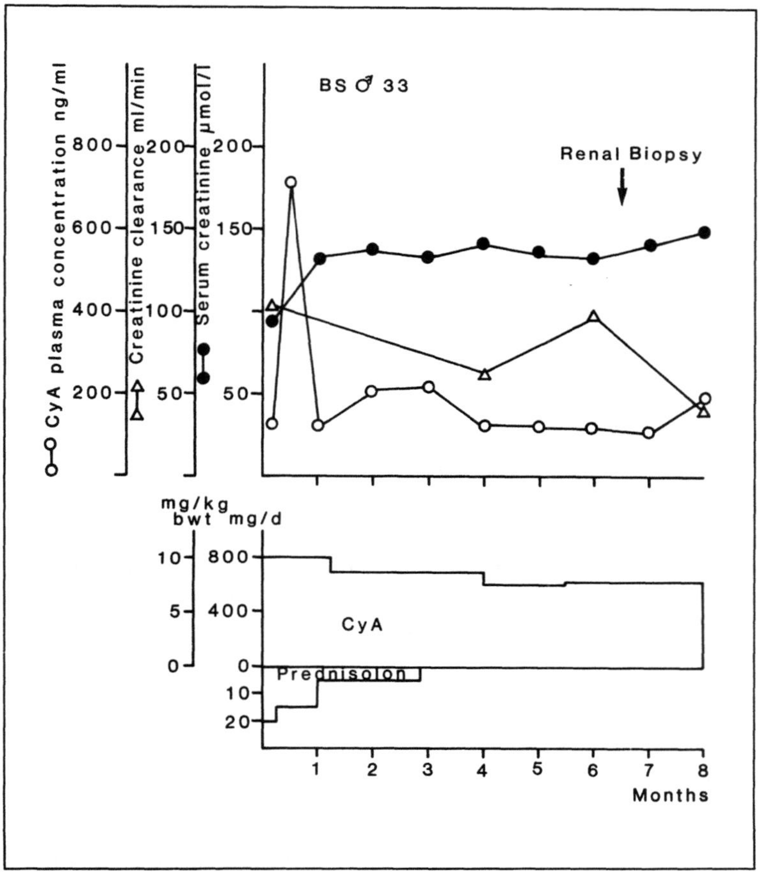

Fig. 1. A 33-year-old patient (pat. 3) with Behçet's disease of 6 years' duration, who despite treatment with immunosuppressive agents and high-dose corticosteroids developed progressive visual impairment, was successfully treated with CyA. After 6 months of CyA therapy a renal biopsy was performed showing slight focal interstitial fibrosis with tubular atrophy (Fig. 6) slight arteriolar hyalinisation and slight arterial intimal thickening. The blood pressure war normal. An elevation of serum creatinine was noted already after one month of CyA therapy

Table 1. Summary of histopathological renal changes* in patients treated with CyA for autoimmune diseases

Patient (Sex/age)	Diagnosis	Accumulated dosage of CyA (g)	Arteriolar hyalinisation	Focal interstitial fibrosis	Glomerular sclerosis
1 (f/51)	Relapsing polychondritis	500	+++	+++	++
2 (m/31)	Behçet's disease	150	○	++	○
3 (m/33)	Behçet's disease	120	+	+	○
4 (m/52)	Chronic uveitis	65	○	+	○
5 (f/53)	Chronic uveitis	55	++	+	+
6 (f/30)	Behçet's disease	65	+	○	○

* ++++ very severe lesions; +++ severe lesions; ++ moderately severe lesions; + slight lesions; ○ no pathological lesions

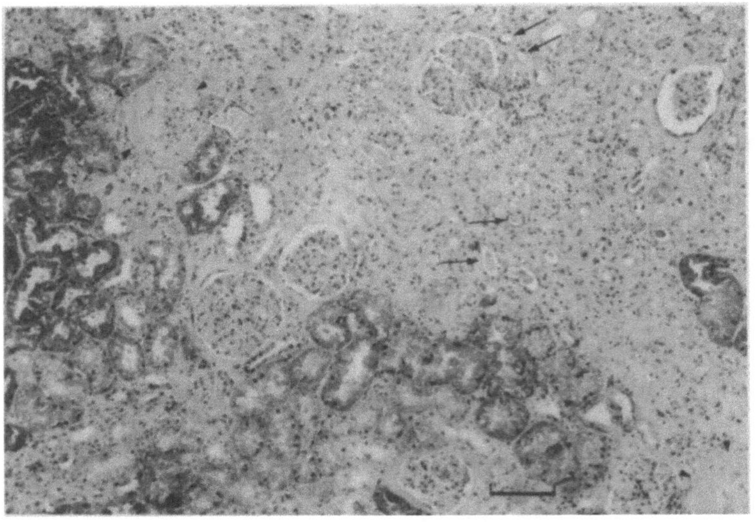

Fig. 2. Area with severe interstitial fibrosis in renal biopsy from a patient with relapsing polychondritis (pat. 1) treated with CyA for 3 years. Tubules in the fibrotic area are atrophic (arrows) and some glomeruli are sclerosed (arrowheads). Interstitial inflammation is minimal. Bar indicates 100 μm. The glomerular filtration rate at the time of biopsy was 55 ml/min · 1.73 m^2 (measured by ^{51}Cr EDTA clearance)

Original biopsy report:
Five out of 15 glomeruli are more or less completely sclerosed. The other glomeruli show slight capillary wall thickening. The dominating finding is a more-or-less moderately severe, irregularly distributed interstitial fibrosis with atrophy of tubules and a slight lymphocytic infiltration. The majority of tubules within non-fibrosed areas appear normal but some nephrons show vacuolisation of the epithelial cells. Close to the cortico-medullary junction there is part of an approximately 1.5 mm large cyst limited by a cuboidal to flat epithelium. Arteries show slight intimal thickening as in atherosclerosis. Arterioles show moderate to severe hyaline arteriolosclerosis, in some vessels with near occlusion of the lumen. Immunofluorescence microscopy has not been performed because of the somewhat sparse biopsy material. The pronounced interstitial fibrosis and glomerular sclerosis are, as such, unspecific findings, yet in agreement with what has been previously described as long-term effects of ciclosporin. The other glomerular lesions are slight and difficult to interpret. Glomerular changes other than sclerosis have so far not been described in connection with ciclosporin treatment. Relapsing polychondritis can, in some cases, be associated with a progressing glomerulonephritis but this does not agree well with the present biopsy findings. A hyalinosis of arterioles is most commonly seen in diabetes or hypertension.

Comment: Upon serial sectioning of the biopsy specimen interstitial fibrosis was found to be more extensive than was thought from the original slides. It was present in both the superficial and the deep part of the cortex.

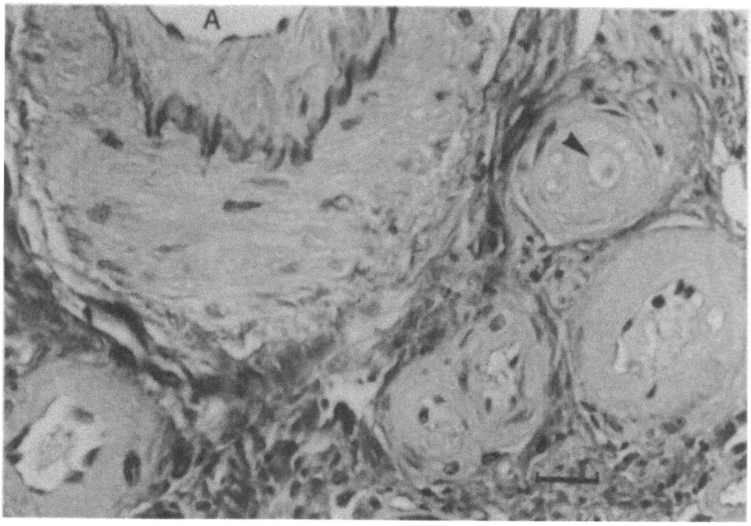

Fig. 3. Severe arteriolar hyalinosis in same biopsy as in Fig. 2. In some vessels the lumen appears nearly obliterated (arrowhead). An artery (A) shows slight intimal thickening. Bar indicates 20 µm

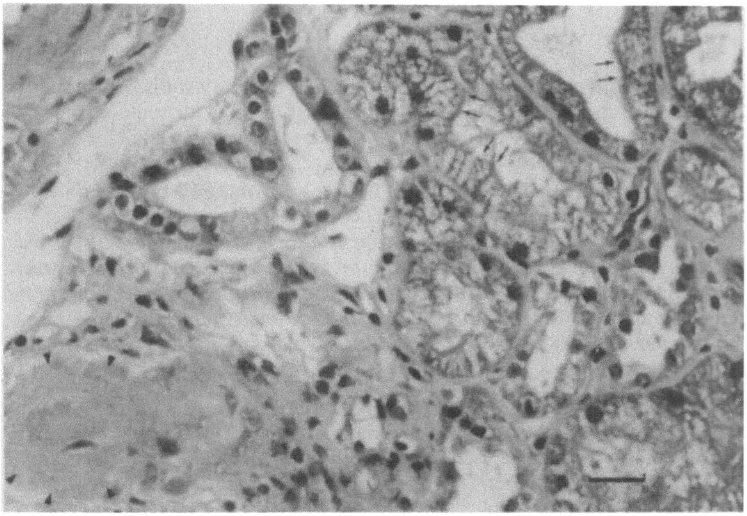

Fig. 4. Vacuolisation of proximal tubules (small arrows) in same biopsy as in Fig. 2. A hyalinised arteriole is also seen (arrowheads). Bar indicates 20 µm. Tubular vacuolisation was present in only one of our patients. This patient was the only one with tubular proteinuria

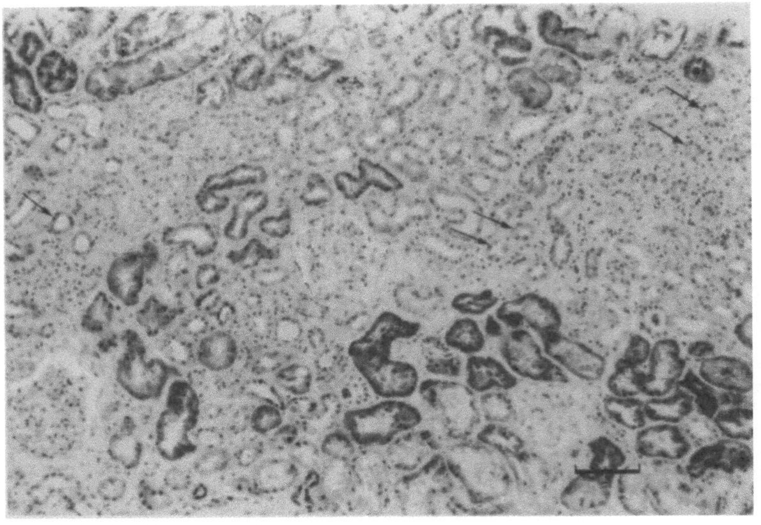

Fig. 5. Moderately severe interstitial fibrosis in renal biopsy from a patient with Behçet's disease (pat. 2) treated with CyA for 7 months. Atrophic tubules are seen in fibrotic areas (small arrows). Interstitial inflammation is very slight. Bar indicates 100 μm. The glomerular filtration rate at the time of biopsy was 62 ml/min · 1.73 m^2

Original biopsy report:
About 20 glomeruli are seen, some of which show slight thickening of the capillary walls. No glomerular sclerosis. In the interstitium there is a slight, irregularly distributed fibrosis with some atrophy of tubules and a very sparse lymphocytic infiltrate. The majority of tubules are unremarkable, as are the blood vessels. There is a focal change consisting of one or two nephrons with dilated tubules which contain large granulocyte cylinders. The tubular epithelium is partly destroyed and there is focal interstitial inflammation surrounding these tubules. This change could be interpreted as a sign of infection but it is remarkably focal. The completely normal appearance of the majority of tubules speaks against tubular damage as the primary cause. Immunofluorescence microscopy shows a weak linear staining with anti-IgG along the glomerular capillary walls. The interstitial fibrosis is, in principle, the same type of change as has been described from Stanford and recently also in renal transplants from our laboratory. However, the lesions appear to be less severe both in the present biopsy case and in the majority of the renal transplants; this is probably related to the dosage of ciclosporin.

Comment: Serial sectioning of the biopsy specimen showed stripes of fibrosis in nearly all parts, a situation clearly intermediate between that in patient 1 and in the majority of the other patients. In order to express this variability we therefore chose to present the semiquantitative data on a five-degree scale (0 to 4+) in the present communication (Table 1) instead of the four degree scale (0 to 3+) that we usually use in routine work. No clinical or bacteriological signs of urinary tract infection were found in this patient. Some patients with Behçet's disease may have renal involvement in the form of a focal proliferative or necrotising glomerulonephritis, but neither the clinical nor the biopsy findings in this case are compatible with this form of renal disease.

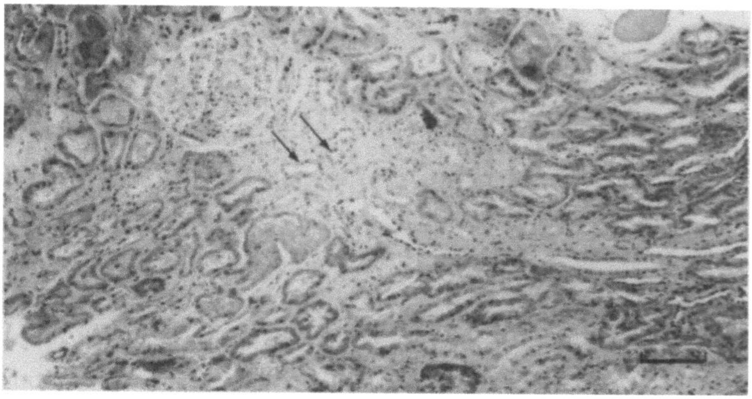

Fig. 6. Slight focal interstitial fibrosis with tubular atrophy (arrows) in renal biopsy from a patient with Behçet's disease treated with CyA for 6 months (pat. 3). Bar indicates 100 μm. The glomerular filtration rate at the time of biopsy was 79 ml/min · 1.73 m²

Original biopsy report:
Fifteen glomeruli are seen showing no light-microscopic changes. In the interstitium there are only occasional small stripes of fibrosis associated with a partly atrophic nephron. No interstitial inflammation. Immunofluorescence microscopy shows sparse deposits of IgM and occasional deposits of C3 in the glomeruli, which in this connection are difficult to interpret and probably without diagnostic significance. To my knowledge, ciclosporin does not cause such a fluorescence pattern and probably neither does Mb Behçet.

Comment: Review of the specimens for this study showed in this case also slight hyaline thickening of the walls of arterioles.

Acknowledgement

Supported by the Swedish Medical Research Council (grant no. B85-12x-05937-05B).

References

1. Svenson KLG, Boström H, Holmdahl R, Klareskog L, Klintmalm GBG, Sjöberg O, Wibell L (1984) Cyclosporin A treatment in a case of relapsing polychondritis. Scand J Rheumatol 13:329
2. Sanders MD, Geraint James D, Graham E (1983) Cyclosporin in Behçet's disease. Lancet 11:454
3. Nussenblatt RB, Palestine AG, Chan CC (1983) Cyclosporine therapy in the treatment of intraocular inflammatory disease resistant to systemic corticosteroids and cytotoxic agents. Am J Ophthalmol 96:275
4. Mihatsch MJ, Thiel G, Spichtin HP, Oberholzer M, Brunner FP, Harder F, Olivieri V, Bremer R, Ryffel B, Stöcklin E, Torhorst J, Gudat F, Zollinger HU, Loertscher R (1983) Morphological findings in kidney transplants after treatment with cyclosporine. Transplant Proc 15:2821
5. Sibley RK, Rynasiewics J, Ferguson RM, Fryd DF, Sutherland DER, Simmons RL, Najarian JS (1983) Morphology of cyclosporine nephrotoxicity and acute rejection in patients immunosuppressed with cyclosporine and prednisone. Surgery 94:225
6. Merion RM, White DFG, Thiru S, Evans DB, Calne RY (1984) Cyclosporine: five years experience in cadaveric renal transplantation. N Engl J Med 310:148
7. Klintmalm G, Bohman S-O, Sundelin B, Wilczek H (1984) Interstitial fibrosis in renal allografts after 12 to 46 months of cyclosporin treatment: Beneficial effect of low doses in early post-transplantation period. Lancet 2:950
8. Myers BD, Ross J, Newton L, Luetscher J, Perlroth M (1984) Cyclosporine-associated chronic nephropathy. N Engl J Med 311:699
9. Svenson K, Bohman S-O, Hällgren R: Renal interstitial fibrosis and vascular changes in patients with autoimmune diseases treated with cyclosporin. Submitted for publication

2. Multiple Sclerosis – Myasthenia Gravis – Polymyositis

The Use of Ciclosporin (CyA) in Multiple Sclerosis – Trial Design and Tolerance

P. Rudge[1]

Introduction

Although the aetiology of multiple sclerosis is unknown, there is a considerable body of evidence suggesting that immunological function is abnormal. For example, the cerebrospinal fluid contains abnormal immunoglobulins with evidence that they are produced within the central nervous system compartment, raised titres of various viral antibodies, especially measles, are found in the serum and there is evidence that T cell subsets are abnormal particularly in relation to relapses of the condition. While there is no adequate animal model of multiple sclerosis, experimental allergic encephalomyelitis (EAE) does to some extent mimic multiple sclerosis particularly in those models that have a relapsing and remitting course. There is no doubt that EAE is an immunological disease and certain of the abnormalities seen in it parallel those found in multiple sclerosis. As immunosuppression is an effective prophylactic therapy for EAE and the use of ciclosporin has been shown to be of value even if given after the first clinical signs have developed [1], it was logical to try giving CyA to patients with multiple sclerosis. In 1979 a pilot study in which 5 patients were given CyA at a dose of 10 mg/per kg/day for a short period showed that there were no adverse effects upon the course of the disease and certainly none of the patients deteriorated. For this reason it was decided to set up a small double-blind controlled study of CyA in multiple sclerosis.

Protocol

1. Patients

It was decided that only patients with definite multiple sclerosis who were aged 15 to 50 years and of either sex should be admitted to the trial. They were to be ambulant but to have significant disability. Patients with concomitant diseases limiting mobility, such as ankylosing spondylitis, and patients with malignancy or renal failure or who were pregnant were excluded from the trial. No patient was to be admitted who had had an immunosuppressant regimen in the previous three months.

It was initially planned to admit between 40 and 60 patients to the trial over a period of two years in London. These would be randomly assigned to a control and a treated group. The trial commenced in March 1982 but when it was clear that larger numbers would be required, and there was some difficulty in recruitment, collaboration with Dr. van Welbeck in Amsterdam was sought and an additional 40 patients were recruited there. These patients were stratified separately into treated and control subjects.

2. Assessment

The patients were assessed clinically by a "blind" neurologist at three-month intervals from 0–2 years and by a "blind" occupational therapist at six-month intervals from 0–2 years. An "unblind" neurologist also saw the patients at three-monthly intervals to monitor their clinical status. Two scoring systems were used by the "blind" observers, namely the Kurtzke scoring system for function and disability [2] and an occupational therapy scoring system concerned with activities of daily living.

In addition to clinical assessments, laboratory assessment was undertaken. Initially the spinal fluid was going to be examined at entry into the trial and at 1 and 2 years, and visual evoked potentials using whole field stimulation were also going to

---

1 The National Hospital, London, W.C.1.

be assessed at the same time. In fact both studies were done only at entry and at 24 months. At each assessment blood urea, uric acid and creatinine were determined and urine examination was carried out together with liver function tests and a full blood count. A variety of serum viral titres was also assessed. In addition T cell subsets were studied at six month intervals.

3. Drug administration

The patients received, after their initial assessment, CyA or placebo oil at a dose of 10 mg/kg per day in divided dosage. After two months the dose was reduced to 8 mg/kg per day and continued for two years. The drug was then stopped. Blood levels, although measured, were not used to monitor therapy. Alteration of the CyA dosage was controlled by the "unblind" observer on clinical criteria and the dosage was reduced if the creatinine exceeded 200 μmol/l.

Tolerance

The following data primarily concern the London group of patients in whom 21 took CyA and 22 were in the placebo group. Some of the data also include the Dutch patients, of whom 18 received CyA and 19 the placebo.

The majority of patients kept approximately to the protocol of drug administration. In a few there was difficulty in the first two months in getting the patient started on the drug and on occasion it was stopped for a week or two. After two months there was some variation in the dose taken over the next two years but on average 7 mg/kg was administered.

The well-recognised side effects of hirsuitism, gingivitis, nausea, pruritus, skin rash and paraesthesias were found in a number of patients (Table 1). Nausea was not confined to the CyA group in the London part of the study. The pruritus was associated with a skin rash in some of the patients and in one in Britain the rash was so severe the drug had to be stopped. The pruritus in this patient took nearly six months to disappear although the maculo-papular skin rash disappeared much more quickly. In addition to obvious rashes, some patients seemed to have telangiectases under the skin. Paraesthesias occurred in a proportion of patients taking CyA. These paraesthesias were usually in the extremities and were specifically related to the time of giving the drug. Usually they occurred within an hour or two of taking the drug and lasted only about 60 minutes. This side effect was more common in Holland and one patient who was taking the placebo preparation was withdrawn be-

Table 1. Side effects

	Britain		Holland	
	CyA (21)	Placebo (22)	CyA (18)	Placebo (19)
Hirsutism	9	0	15	1
Gingivitis	10 (2)*	0	10	0
Nausea	7 (2)	3	9	0
Pruritus/rash	5 (1)	0	2	0
Paraesthesias	3 (1)	0	14	0

* Figures in parentheses indicate severe symptoms.

Table 2. Neurological symptoms

	Britain		Holland	
	CyA (21)	Placebo (22)	CyA (18)	Placebo (19)
Vertigo	2	0	0	0
Tremor	0	0	6	0
Fits	3	0	0	0

cause of it. It is not clear why Dutch patients are more susceptible to the paraesthesias than the British ones.

A number of other side effects occurred. Headache was found in both Dutch and British patients in about 20% of the people taking CyA. Sometimes the headache had characteristics of migraine and in fact all the British patients who had headache of this type had had migraine before. Tiredness and depression occurred in about 10–20% of the patients taking CyA but was not confined to this group. In the British group, the side effect seemed to be a real one in that the tiredness undoubtedly improved shortly after the patient stopped the drug at the end of the trial. Arthralgia occurred in 30% of the British group of patients but not in the Dutch. It involved both small and large joints but not the axial skeleton. The cause was never ascertained. Routine X-rays and immunological studies were normal. The arthralgia was dose-dependent and in three patients the dose had to be reduced to control the symptoms.

A number of neurological symptoms occurred apart from headache and depression. It is difficult to ascertain their significance in a group of patients with multiple sclerosis but it is noteworthy that these side effects were confined to the CyA group (Table 2). Of particular interest is the tremor which occurred only in the Dutch patients; it was found in a third of the patients taking CyA. Unfortunately this symptom is a common one of multiple sclerosis and is difficult to interpret. Fits occurred in three patients in Britain but in none in Holland. One of the patients had previously had fits but the other two had not. One patient had focal motor seizures. This is interesting in that the amount of CyA crossing the blood brain barrier is small and perhaps suggests that the drug enters the nervous system more easily in areas of damage to the blood brain barrier in multiple sclerosis. None of the patients had to be withdrawn from the trial because of the fits.

In the London group of patients a number of laboratory data are available including blood pressure measurements. It is clear that, overall, the diastolic and systolic blood pressures rise with CyA administration (Fig. 1). Although there is great variation and there may be doubt about one or two of the patients actually taking the drug regularly because of wide swings of blood pressure, it is clear that the diastolic pressure does rise on average by 10–20 mm of mercury, this rise reaching its maximum at about 12 months. A similar rise also occurs in systolic blood pressure. The apparent fall of diastolic blood pressure at 24 months may well be an artefact of small numbers and the systolic blood pressure shows no tendency to fall. When the drug was stopped, the blood pressure returned to normal within three months. Renal function is well recognised to be abnormal with

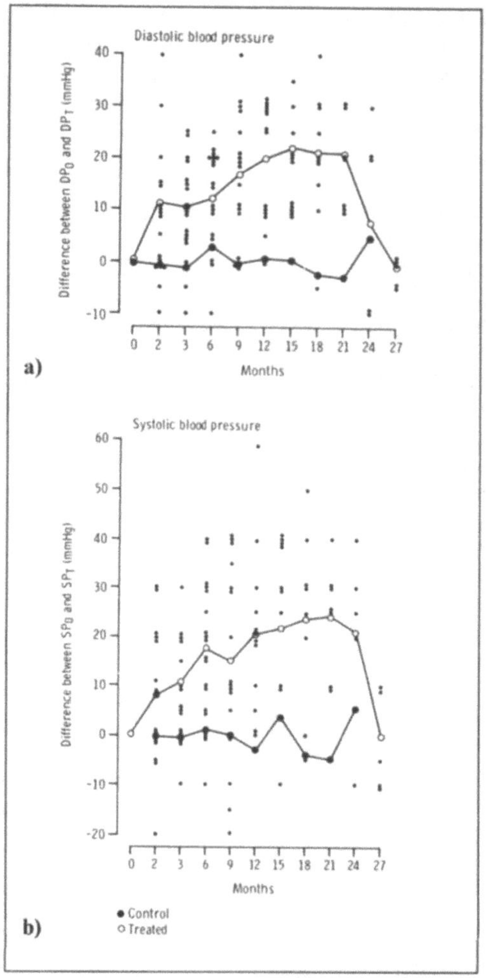

Fig. 1. Blood pressure measurements

CyA administration [3]. The creatinine level is extremely variable and in two patients greatly exceeded 200 μmol/l. requiring a gradual reduction of the dosage. With regard to the remainder, however, it is clear that the blood creatinine is elevated in the treated patients (Fig. 2). A plateau is reached at about six months and all measurements after one month are significantly deviated at the 1% level. The creatinine returned to normal in patients who had not had a level exceeding 200 μmol/l, within three months of cessation of the therapy. However, in two patients where this level was exceeded, the creatinine has not returned to the pre-treatment level although it is in the normal range six months after cessation of treatment. Urea also rose, and this rather more quickly than the creatinine. The level returned to normal

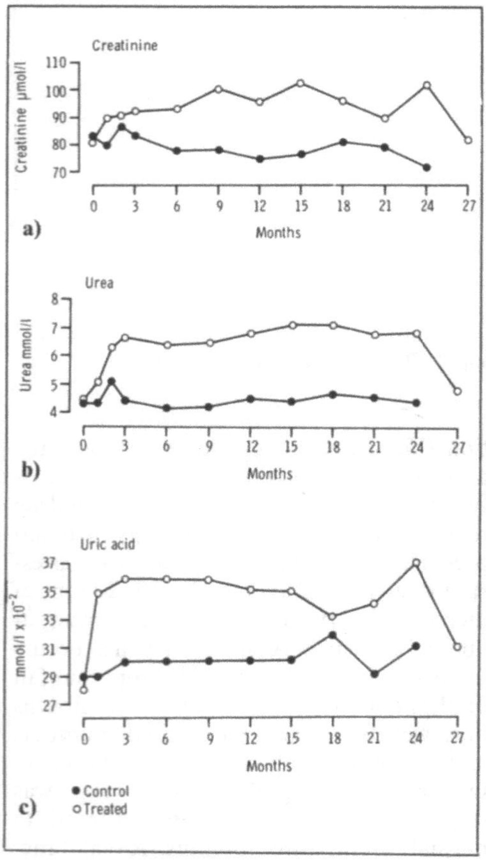

Fig. 2. Laboratory data

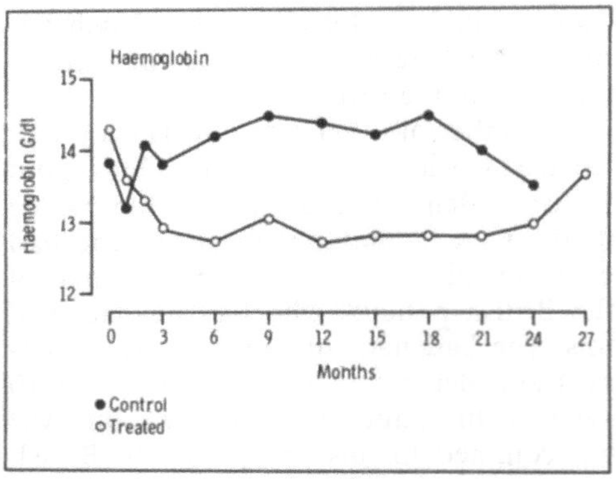

Fig. 3. Haemoglobin values

within three months of cessation of therapy. All the blood urea concentrations measured from one month through 24 months were significantly elevated in the whole group of patients at the 1% level. Uric acid rose even more sharply than urea throughout the period of the trial and returned to normal on cessation of therapy, but interestingly these levels were not significant at the 5% level at any time. A minor degree of anaemia occurred during the trial (Fig. 3). The haemoglobin slowly fell over the first three months by an average of 1.5 g/100 ml and returned to the pre-treatment value within three months of cessation of the drug. The white cell count and platelet count were not significantly altered throughout the trial. Bilirubin was elevated to a minor extent but no other liver function test showed any significant impairment. No viral titre altered significantly and there was no evidence of an increased incidence of bacterial infection in those patients receiving CyA.

Conclusion

This ongoing study has shown that ciclosporin is tolerated with some difficulty by patients with multiple sclerosis. A maintenance dose of 7 mg/kg/day is the average that they can tolerate and some patients require less. There is, however, great variability in the tolerance. Five patients have had to discontinue the trial in the British group, of whom three were in the CyA treated section. One had a severe skin rash, one had severe depression and one refused to comply. In the Dutch group, two patients have withdrawn in the CyA section; one because of hypertension and one because of psychosis. Three other patients in the placebo group have withdrawn, one of them having had paraesthesias and two depression and anxiety. The significance of these side effects will have to be considered in relation to the ultimate therapeutic efficiency of this drug in multiple sclerosis.

The results of this trial will be analysed in September 1986 when all the patients have completed two years of therapy.

References

1. Bolton C, Allsopp G, Cuzner ML (1982) Clin Exp Immunol 47: 127–132
2. Kurtzke J (1965) Neurology 15:654–661
3. Myers BD, Ross J, Newton L, Luetscher J, Perlroth M (1984) N Engl J Med 311:699–705

The Effect of Ciclosporin versus Azathioprine on the Course of Multiple Sclerosis; Design of a Long-term Follow-up Study and Side Effects

U. Patzold[1], D. Dommasch[2], Sigrid Poser[3], L. Kappos[2], J. Haas[1], J. P. Malin[1], P. Krauseneck[4]

Introduction

The investigation which we are conducting in Hanover and Würzburg is a double-blind randomised stratified parallel group study comparing the effect of continuous CyA treatment with that of azathioprine treatment in patients with multiple sclerosis (ms). The primary object of this study is the progression of the disease, defined as the increase of clinical pathoneurological findings over a 2-year period.

Criteria for inclusion and exclusion

We attempted to include in this study all out-patients between 18 and 50 years of age with defined MS. Included were patients with:

1. relapsing-remitting course, i.e. a course with relapses and "complete" remissions without functional deficit,
2. intermittent course with incomplete remissions of the relapses, i.e. a stepwise progression of the disease,
3. intermittent-progressive course, i.e. a course with relapses, and a steady progression between the relapses,
4. chronic progressive course without clear relapses from the beginning of the disease or in the last 2 years before entrance into the study.

Patients with a relapsing-remitting disease have been included not earlier than after the 2nd relapse, that is, 10 weeks after onset of the last attack. In patients with chronic progressive disease, treatment was not begun earlier than 6 months after onset of the disease. It was our goal to include a total of 200 patients within 1½ years, with new patients being added at 3-month intervals.

The study does not include patients whose MS had so far followed a benign course, i.e. patients who had had no relapse during the preceding 2 years or had shown no progression of the disease during that period. At the other extreme patients with far advanced disease were also excluded. It was obligatory for all patients to be able to walk.

Patients previously treated with cyclophosphamide were also excluded. Patients being treated with azathioprine have been included without discontinuing the medication. For these patients the previously prescribed medication was replaced at the beginning of the study by the preparation under evaluation.

General description of the experiment

Laboratory parameters necessary for the supervision of the therapy and for monitoring CyA levels and possible side effects of the administered medications could have impaired the double-blind character of the study. To prevent this the following measures have been taken:

1. Determination of the necessary laboratory values by a not otherwise involved

---

1 Neurologische Klinik und Poliklinik, Medizinische Hochschule Hannover

2 Klinische Forschungsgruppe für Multiple Sklerose der Max-Planck-Gesellschaft an der Neurologischen Klinik der Universität Würzburg

3 Abteilung Neurologie der Universität Göttingen

4 Neurologische Klinik der Universität Würzburg

We thank Dr. K. Wonigkeit, Abdominal- und Transplantations-Chirurgie, Medizinische Hochschule Hannover, for the determination of CyA blood levels in half of our patients.

background physician at each center who is also responsible for any necessary changes in dosage, discontinuation of medication and further investigations.
2. Each patient receives capsules of identical appearance containing either azathioprine or placebo as well as oral solutions of identical appearance and taste containing either CyA or placebo. Patients take the oral solution as well as the capsules without knowing whether the solution or capsule contains the active substance. The physicians carrying out the treatment are likewise uninformed.
3. For evaluation of the therapy, necessary clinical examinations of the patients are performed in each case by the physicians carrying out treatment at the other center. Each patient is always examined by the same physician.

Dosage of CyA and azathioprine

The administered dose of CyA is equal to 5 mg/kg bodyweight per day. Azathioprine is given in a dose of 2.5 mg/kg bodyweight per day. The dose is modified on the onset of side effects. It is further adjusted according to CyA whole-blood trough levels and the blood count. In the case of whole-blood trough levels above 750 ng/ml or under 150 ng/ml the dosage is modified by the above-mentioned background physician. The azathioprine dose is reduced if the leucocyte count falls below 3000/mm^3 and increased if after 6 months of treatment the MCV is not greater than 91 fl.

During an acute severe attack all patients receive prednisone in the same manner for several weeks in a dosage beginning with 100 mg/day, together with the coded medication.

Evaluation of success of therapy

The success of the therapy is measured as a change in clinical pathoneurological findings during the 2 years. The neurological examinations are performed in each case by the "blind" physician from the other center at 3-month intervals without knowledge of previous findings. All objective neurological findings are scored and quantified using a specially developed score, which is a modification of our previously used scoring system [1, 2]. With this score it is possible to record cranial nerve symptoms, impairments of coordination, paralyses, disturbances of muscle tone, sensation, urinary bladder function and vision, and mental disturbances.

Secondary study objects are:

1. Progression of the disease using Kurtzke's disability scale, which permits scoring of neurological disturbances from 1–10 [3].
2. Progression of the disease using functional parameters from the Kurtzke incapacity scale, Hauser's ambulation index and self-estimation scales [4].
3. Number of relapses during 2 years.
4. Changes in the latency of visually evoked potentials during the 2 years of treatment.
5. Changes in spinal fluid findings after 2 years of treatment.
6. Changes in immunological parameters during treatment. In particular B- and T-cell function as well as the ratio of lymphocyte subpopulations is examined during the progression of the disease.

Lists of patients included

Within the first year we were able to include 194 patients, 90 from Hanover, 106 from Würzburg. 98 received CyA, 96 azathioprine. There are no differences between the 2 groups with regard to the progression of the disease before inclusion in the study, the duration of the disease, age and sex of patients, severity of the disease, frequency of pretreatment with azathioprine and initial pathological findings in the spinal fluid.

The study has now been running for nearly 2 years. All patients have been treated for at least 1 year. So far 13 patients have dropped out. The most common reasons for drop-outs have been gastrointestinal (GI) symptoms. Among the remaining patients the compliance is remarkably good. We know from laboratory controls that the patients have taken their medication regularly and in the correct manner.

Side effects

The summary of the main side effects is based on the first 15 months of the therapy (Table 1). Data are complete only up to the 9th month. The data on 1 year's treatment in slightly more than 40 patients have so far been processed.

As expected the main side effects of CyA besides nausea and GI disturbances are hypertrichosis, paraesthesias and gingival hyperplasia. Upper respiratory infections are more common among patients treated with azathioprine. It is remarkable that as many as 7% of patients treated with azathioprine also complain of hypertrichosis. So far all patients have tolerated this symptom and on no occasion has it forced us to stop treatment. Gingival hyperplasia is also mild. Only in a few of the patients has a regular dental consultation been required, and one gingivectomy has been necessary.

Figure 1 shows the alterations of the blood count. One can see a clear increase in erythrocyte MCV during treatment with azathioprine whereas no change occurs with CyA. The initial decrease is only a reflection of the fact that patients pretreated with azathioprine have been included in this group. In both groups we have observed a slight decrease of hemoglobin. With the employed dose of azathioprine we note only a slight decrease in leucocytes and no change in the thrombocyte count.

Figure 2 shows the change in liver function. With CyA there is a slight increase of alkaline phosphatase and bilirubin. No pathological figures have been observed. GPT and GGT have shown only slight changes. At the beginning of treatment with azathioprine we saw an initial increase of GPT and GGT which then normalized. This is a known effect of azathioprine. In additon, in Hannover, we have determined the CHE during therapy. Neither with azathioprine nor with CyA has a change of CHE been noted.

As expected even with the low dose of CyA used there was an initial significant increase of serum creatinine which was still rising after half a year (Fig. 3). In some cases levels have increased up to more than 270 μmol/l. In all patients the creatinine level has so far fallen to normal after a reduction in dosage or a short-term discontinuation of therapy.

In comparison mean CyA whole-blood trough levels are shown to vary around

Table 1. Main side effects during therapy with CyA and azathioprine

Adverse events observed						
Event	CyA group (n=93)			AZA group (n=93)		
	No. of pts.	Severe events	Incidence	No. of pts.	Severe events	Incidence
Nausea, vomiting, loss of appetite, weight decrease, gastric pain	36	2	(39%)	47	7	(51%)
Hypertrichosis	36		(39%)	8		(7%)
Hyper-/Paraesthesia	20		(22%)	5		(5%)
Gingival hyperplasia	19	1	(20%)	6		(6%)
Loss of hair	8	1	(9%)	7	1	(8%)
Upper resp. tract infection	8		(9%)	13		(14%)
Joint/limb/skeletal pains	6		(6%)	4		(4%)
Tremor	5		(5%)	–		
Pruritus, skin rash	3	1	(3%)	2		(2%)
Weight/appetite increase	4		(4%)	6		(6%)
Angina pectoris	3		(3%)	–		
Muscle contractions	3	1	(3%)	1		(1%)
Headache	2		(2%)			

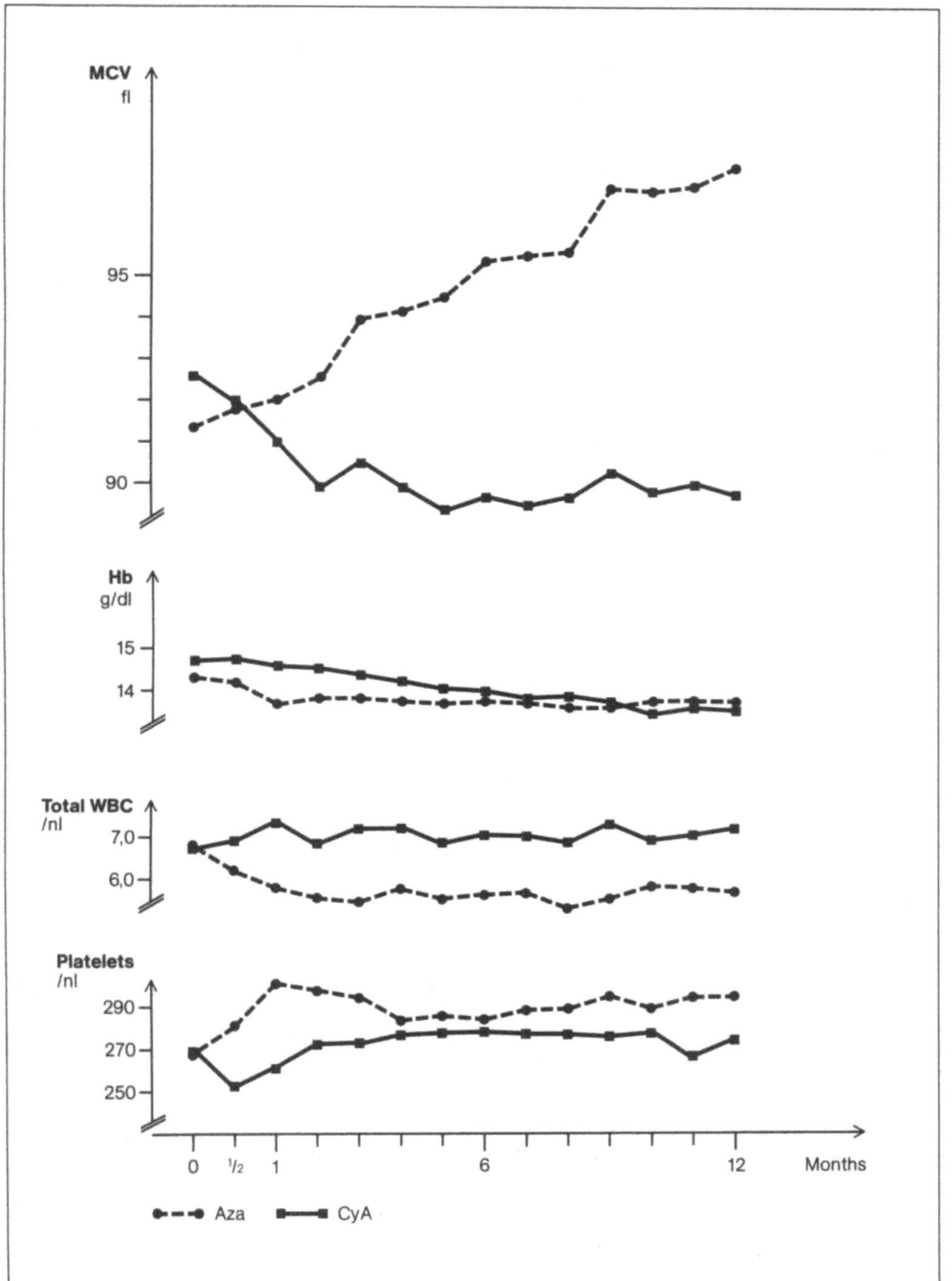

Fig. 1. MCV, Hb, leucocyte and thrombocyte counts during therapy with CyA and azathioprine

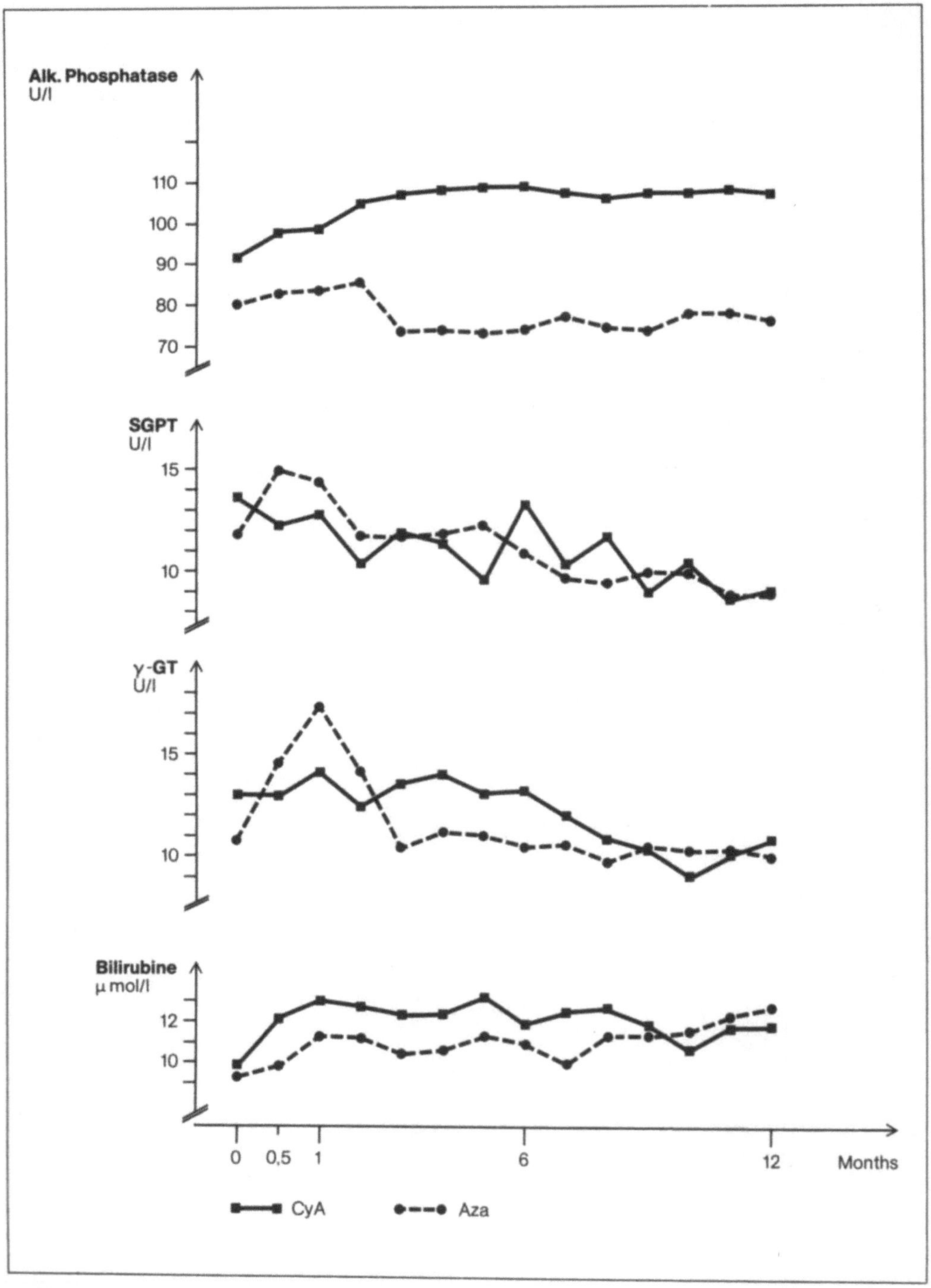

Fig. 2. Liver function during therapy with azathioprine and CyA

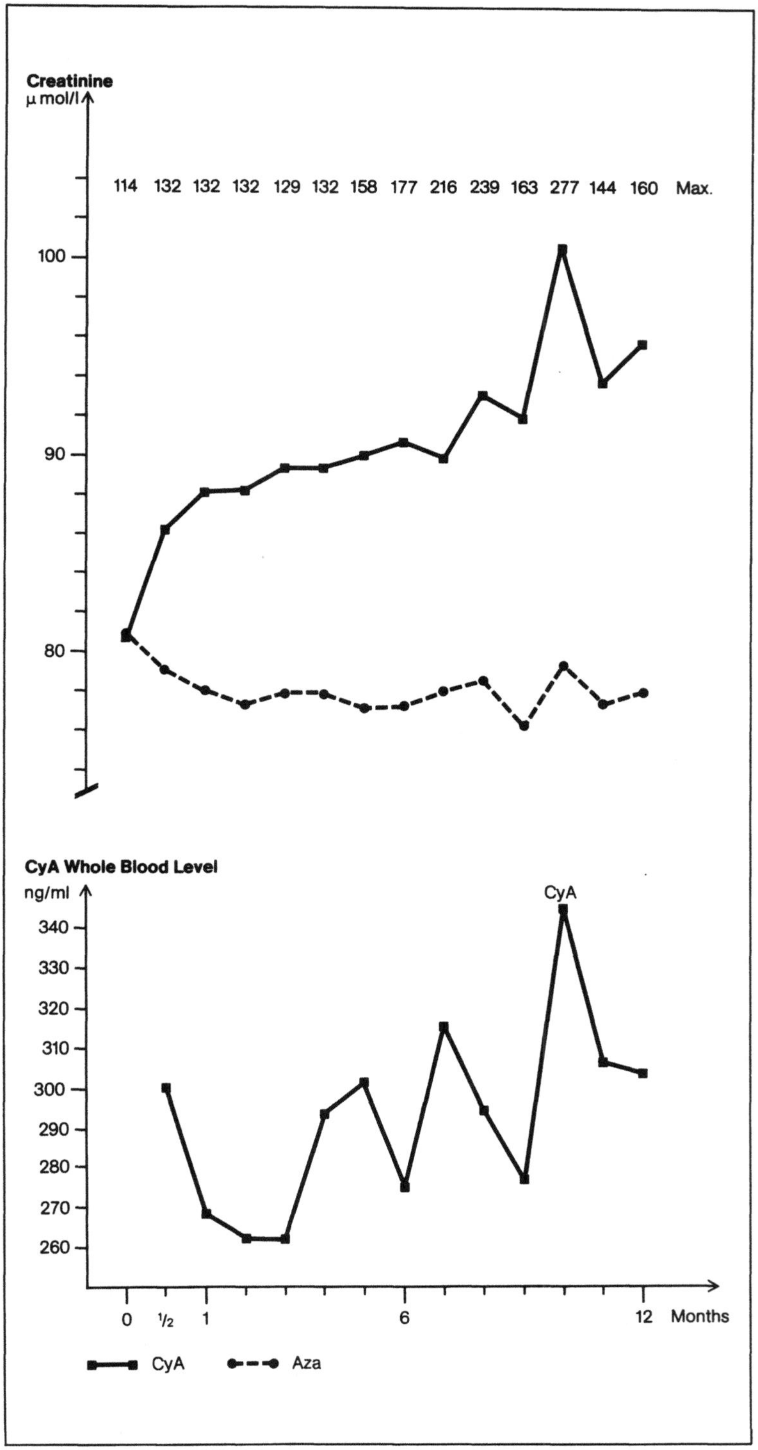

Fig. 3. Serum creatinine level during therapy with azathioprine and CyA. In addition the mean trough whole-blood levels of CyA are shown

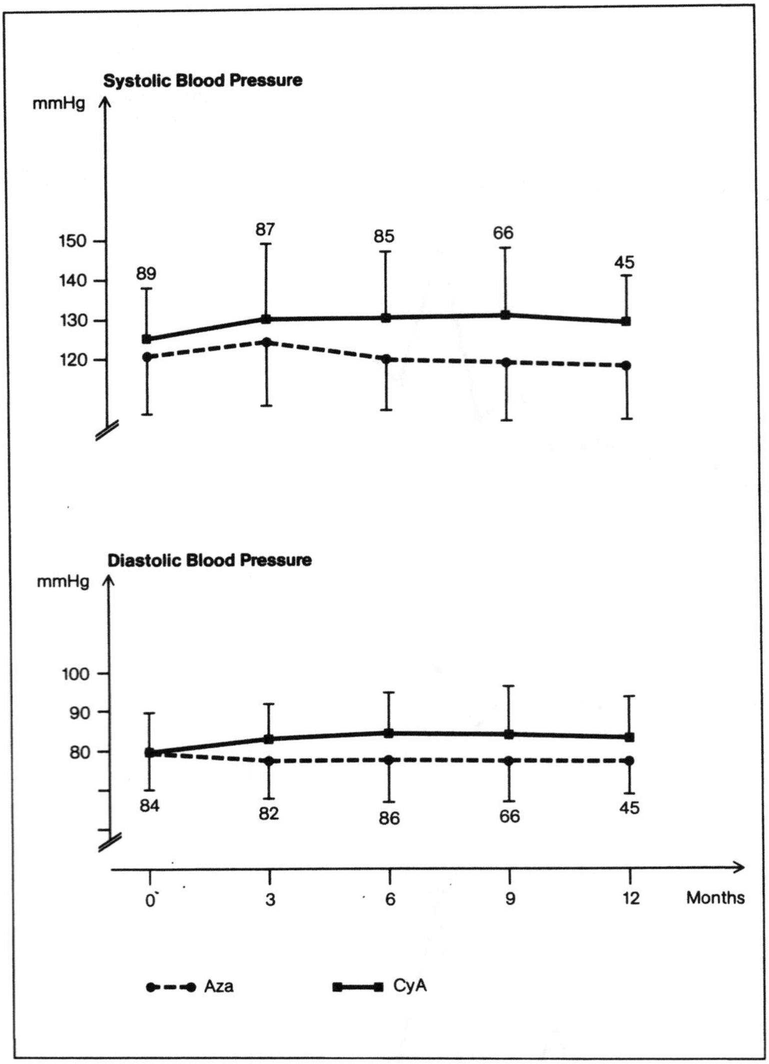

Fig. 4. Mean blood pressure during treatment with CyA and azathioprine. The number of patients evaluated is also given

300 ng/ml. There is no universal correlation between whole-blood levels of CyA and serum creatinine levels. In some cases this question needs further investigation.

The main side effect is hypertension, which develops surprisingly often among our patients (Fig. 4). Nearly 50% of our patients treated in Hannover with CyA for 1 year or longer have blood pressure values greater than 150/95 mm Hg. With azathioprine this is the case in only 2 patients.

Severe hypertension with systolic blood pressures of greater than 170 mm Hg and diastolic pressures greater than 110 mm Hg has not so far occurred very often. This has been easily controlled with beta blockers. So far we have not discontinued medication because of hypertension, but rather have tried to treat these patients with a reduced dose of CyA. The hypertension does not correlate with serum creatinine levels. We do not yet know whether long-term continuous treatment of MS with CyA will become impossible because of the occurrence of hypertension.

References

1. Patzold U, Hecker H, Pocklington P (1982) Azathioprine in treatment of Multiple Sclerosis – Final results of a 4½-year controlled study of its effectiveness covering 115 patients. J Neurol Sci 54:377–394
2. Patzold U, Haller P, Haas J, Pocklington P, Deicher H (1978) Therapie der multiplen Sklerose mit Levamisol und Azathioprin – Vergleich der Wirksamkeit einer „immunstimulierenden" und „immunsuppressiven" Behandlung. Nervenarzt 49:285–294
3. Kurtzke JF (1983) Rating neurologic impairment in Multiple Sclerosis: An expanded disability status scale (EDSS). Neurology 33:1444–1452
4. Hauser SL, Dawson DM, Lehrich JR, Flint Beal M, Kevy SV, Propper RD, Mills JA, Weiner HL (1983) Intensive Immunosuppression in Progressive Multiople Sclerosis – A randomized, three-arm study of high-dose intravenous cyclophosphamide, plasma exchange, and ACTH. N Engl J Med 308:173–180

Ciclosporin in the Treatment of Myasthenia Gravis: Preliminary Results from a Pilot Study

R. Nyberg-Hansen, L. Gjerstad[1]

Introduction

Aquired myasthenia gravis (MG) is an autoimmune disorder of neuromuscular transmission. It is characterized by variable weakness and fatigability of skeletal muscle due to interference with neuromuscular transmission by antibodies to acetylcholine receptors (AChR). Circulating polyclonal anti-AChR antibodies can be demonstrated in nearly 90% of patients with generalized MG [5].

The basic abnormality in MG is a decrease of AChR at neuromuscular junctions. Most anti-AChR antibodies are directed against the main immunogenic region of AChR [3]. They appear to impair neuromuscular transmission mainly by causing complement-mediated destruction of the postsynaptic membrane of neuromuscular junctions, and by accelerating the internalization and degradation (modulation) of AChR [2]. Blocking antibodies constitute only a minor fraction of anti-AChR.

In view of the immunopathogenesis of MG, the efficacy of prednisolone and other immunosuppressants is now well recognized. The purpose of the present study was to investigate the efficacy, safety and tolerance of ciclosporin (CyA) therapy in patients with MG in whom immunosuppressants other than prednisolone are indicated.

Patients and methods

The study is an open uncontrolled pilot study which is not yet completed. It includes six patients with generalized MG in whom CyA is being used for 28 weeks either alone or in combination with prednisolone. Informed consent has been obtained from all patients.

So far data are available from four patients, three females and one male aged 16–61 years, all of them severely affected. Two patients have been treated with CyA for 28 and two for 20 weeks. None of the patients had thymoma. Three patients had been thymectomized. All patients used an anticholinesterase drug (pyridostigmine) in unchanged dosage during the study.

Patient 1 had used prednisolone for two years without satisfactory effect. *Patient 2* used prednisolone with good effect for five years. This medication was stopped one year before the present study owing to osteoporosis. *Patient 3* had used prednisolone for five years with clinical improvement, and had received azathioprine for three years without satisfactory effect. Azathioprine was stopped one month before CyA therapy was started. *Patient 4* had used prednisolone for three years and azathioprine for seven months without satisfactory effect. The latter drug was stopped four months before the present study. Some other relevant clinical details are given in Table 1.

CyA was added to prednisolone in three patients, while one (No 2) received CyA alone. The dose of prednisolone was kept unchanged with alternate-day treatment in patients 3 and 4, while it was reduced from 20 mg daily to 20 and 15 mg every other day in patient 1 after 20 weeks of CyA treatment.

The starting dose of CyA was 5 mg/kg/day given in one daily dose as a drink solution. The dose was increased to 7.5 mg and 10 mg/kg/day in two divided doses after 8 and 16 weeks respectively, provided that no serious side effects occurred, that

1 Department of Neurology, Rikshospitalet, The National Hospital, University of Oslo, Oslo 1, Norway

Table 1. Some clinical data of the four patients treated with CyA for more than 20 weeks. For further details, see text

No.	Sex	Age	Duration	Thymectomy	HLA antigen	Prednisolone (mg)
1	F	16	5 yrs.	Yes	A1, B8 DR3	20/20
2	F	58	30 yrs.	No	A2, B8 DR3	0/0
3	M	61	21 yrs.	Yes	A1, A2, B8 DR3	40/0*
4	F	46	10 yrs.	Yes	A1, B8 DR3	35/0*

* Previously used azathioprine

the serum creatinine did not rise into the abnormal range, and that trough levels of CyA (blood sample taken immediately before next dose is due) did not exceed 750 μg/l whole blood. Owing to side effects (see below), the dose was not increased above 7.5 mg/kg/day in patients 2 and 4.

The efficacy of CyA therapy was evaluated by detailed clinical examination carried out before starting the CyA therapy and at regular intervals during the study. It included clinical neurological examination with special emphasis on muscle weakness, global assessment by the patients and by the investigators, and measurement of anti-AChR antibodies in the serum.

The presence of weakness on clinical examination was graded (0–3) and the sum of the scores for all muscle functions tested was used as an objective estimate for the degree of weakness. Similarily, the patients' own feeling of muscle strength was graded (1–4) and the sum of the scores was used to estimate their subjective evaluation of strength. The laboratory tests included full haematological examination, liver and renal tests, urinalysis, blood chemistry and the concentration of CyA in whole blood.

The patients were asked about particular sensations or symptoms occurring during the study. They were not directly asked about specific side effects of CyA.

Results

A definite clinical improvement in muscle strength and fatigability occurred during

Table 2. Anti-AChR antibody titre of the patients before and after treatment with CyA for 28 (x) and 20 (y) weeks, respectively. The analyses were carried out in the Department of Neurology, Haukeland Hospital, Bergen, Norway

Patient	Control	Ciclosporin
1	0.3	0.3 (x)
2	10.5	5.2 (x)
3	0.8	0.3 (y)
4	3.2	1.7 (y)

Normal value < 0.2 arbitrary units/L

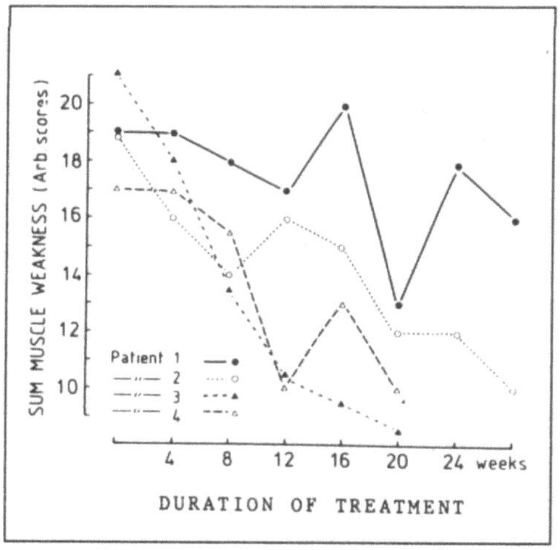

Fig. 1. The muscle weakness disclosed by clinical examination in relation to the duration of CyA treatment. The sum of muscle weakness represents the sum of scores for various muscle functions (eyelid, face, tongue, neck, respiration, proximal and distal upper and lower limbs, chewing and eye motility).

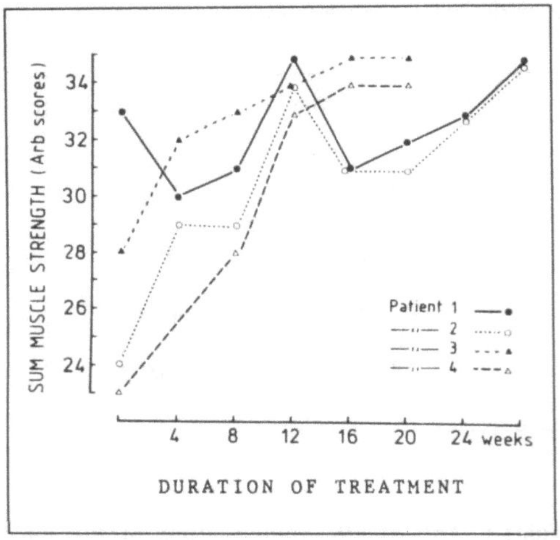

Fig. 2. The muscle strength according to the patient's own statement in relation to the duration of CyA treatment. The sum of muscle strength represents the sum of scores given by the patients for various muscle functions, expressing their subjective evaluation of muscle strength.

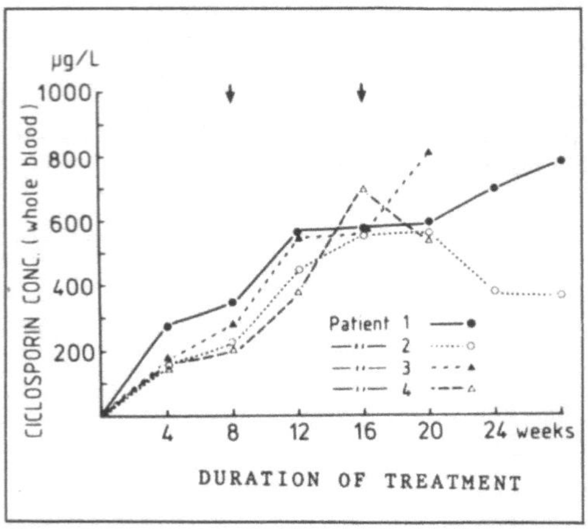

Fig. 3. The CyA concentration (whole blood) in relation to the duration of CyA treatment. The arrow to the left indicates the increase in the CyA dose from 5 to 7.5 mg/kg/day, and the arrow to the right the further increase to 10 mg/kg/day. In patients 2 and 4 the dose was not increased above 7.5 mg/kg/day. Note the decrease of CyA level in patient 2 after 16 weeks, which is probably related to gastritis.

CyA therapy in all patients. The scores for muscle weakness decreased (Fig. 1) and the patients' evaluation of muscle strength increased (Fig. 2) throughout the study. The effect was observed after four weeks treatment and a major improvement was achieved within twelve weeks. The effect was moderate to marked in patients 2, 3 and 4 and slight to moderate in patient 1.

There was a marked decrease (47–63%) in the anti-AChR antibody titre during CyA treatment in patients 2, 3 and 4, while patient 1, the subject with the least clinical improvement, showed no change in antibody titre (Table 2).

The concentration of CyA increased gradually and after 8 weeks all patients had reached a whole-blood level above 200 µg/l (Fig. 3). Owing to levels exceeding 750 µg/l the CyA dose was reduced after 20 and 28 weeks in patients 3 and 1, respectively. The blood level of CyA in patient 2 decreased after 16 weeks when she developed gastritis.

Side effects known to occur on CyA therapy were noticed (paraesthesias, hirsutism, tremor, nausea, diarrhoea, headache), but they were slight and tolerable in all patients. No serious side effects requiring withdrawal of CyA were seen. Patient 2, however, who was not using prednisolone, developed gastritis with multiple ulcers demonstrated both on x-ray and by gastroscopy. It responded well to treatment with histamine H2 antagonists and the dose of CyA was not increased above 7.5 mg/kg/day. Patient 4 with low serum albumin developed oedema probably owing to water retention. She was treated with furosemide and the dose of CyA was not increased above 7.5 mg/kg/day.

A gradual increase in serum creatinine and a reduction in creatinine clearance were seen in all patients. However, abnormal ranges were not reached. Otherwise no significant changes were disclosed by the laboratory tests.

Discussion

The beneficial effect of immunosuppressive therapy in the treatment of MG is well recognized. However, to the best of our knowledge no report on the effect of CyA has been published before. In the present study, a definite clinical improvement occurred in all four patients receiving CyA. The whole-blood CyA level was kept below

750 μg/l. All patients were severely affected and had suffered from MG for several years. Two had previously used azathioprine combined with prednisolone for several months without satisfactory clinical effect. It should be emphasized that the present study is an open uncontrolled pilot study with obvious limitations.

The degree of improvement was similar in the one patient who received CyA alone and in those in whom the drug was combined with prednisolone. Although this may indicate that CyA allows more sparing use of steroids in MG, prednisolone in combination with CyA probably has an additive effect in MG as in other immunological disorders [1].

Except for gastritis with ulcer in one patient and water retention in another, both requiring specific treatment, only slight side effects were noticed.

In three of our four patients CyA caused a decline in anti-AChR antibodies which correlated fairly well with the clinical improvement. A fall in antibody titre has previously been shown to correlate with long-term clinical improvement following treatment with prednisolone, azathioprine or thymectomy [4, 8–11]. In MG patients on azathioprine there is usually a delay of three to six months before improvement [6]. In the present study, the effect of CyA occurred a relatively short time after the start of CyA therapy, with a definite clinical improvement being noticed after four weeks.

The therapeutic effect of CyA in MG may possibly be explained by suppression of T-helper cell activiation of B-cells producing anti-AChR antibodies [1, 7].

Although the results of this limited pilot study seem promising, further properly controlled studies are needed to define the role of CyA in the treatment of MG patients. Furthermore, such studies should probably also include patients at an earlier stage of the disease than those of the present study.

Summary

Six patients with generalized myasthenia gravis are being treated with ciclosporin in a not yet completed open pilot study. Data from our patients treated for more than 20 weeks show a definite clinical improvement in muscle strength. Anti-AChR antibody titer had decreased in three of the four patients. Except for one case with ulcerating gastritis the side effects have been slight.

References

1. Borel JF, von Graffenried B (in press) Sandimmun (Cyclosporin A) and autoimmunity. In: Proceedings of the Workshop on recent advances in systemic lupus erythematosus, Geneva, Switzerland, 1–3 September 1983, Academic Press, London
2. Drachman DB (1981) The biology of myasthenia gravis. Annu Rev Neurosci 4:195–225
3. Engel AG (1984) Myasthenia gravis and myasthenic syndromes. Ann Neurol 16:519–534
4. Lefvert AK, Bergström K, Matell G, Osterman PO, Pirskanen R (1978) Determination of acetylcholine receptor antibody in myasthenia gravis: clinical usefulness and pathogenic implications. J Neurol Neurosurg Psychiatry 41:394–403
5. Lindström J, Seybold ME, Lennon VA et al. (1976) Antibody to acetylcholine receptor in myasthenia gravis. Neurology (Minneap.) 26:1054–1059
6. Mertens HG, Hertel G, Reuther P et al. (1981) Effect of immunosuppressive drugs (azathioprine). Ann NY Acad Sci 377:691–699
7. Muraguchi A, Butler JL, Kehrl JH, Falkoff RJM, Fauci AS (1983) Selective suppression of an early step in human B cell activation by cyclosporin A. J Exp Med 158:690–702
8. Olanow CW, Lane RJ, Roses AD (1981) Relationship between the acetylcholine receptor antibody titer and the clinical status in myasthenia gravis. Ann NY Acad Sci 377:856–857
9. Oosterhuis HJGH, Limburg PC, Hummel-Tappel E et al. (1983) Anti-acetylcholine receptors in myasthenia gravis. II. Clinical and serological follow-up of individual patients. J Neurol Sci 58:371–385
10. Tindall RSA (1981) Humoral immunity in myasthenia gravis: biochemical characterization of acquired antireceptor antibodies and clinical correlations. Ann Neurol 10:437–447
11. Vincent A, Newsom-Davis J (1980) Anti-acetylcholine receptor antibodies. J Neurol Neurosurg Psychiatry 43:590–600

Ciclosporin (CyA) in Myasthenia Gravis

U. A. Besinger[1], W. Mraz[2], A. Fateh-Moghadam[2]

Myasthenia gravis (MG) is a humorally mediated autoimmune disease. Circulating autoantibodies (ab) against the postsynaptic acetylcholine receptor (ACHR) are responsible for the postsynaptic transmission failure which is the cause of the abnormal weakness and fatigability of the skeletal muscles in myasthenics [16].

During the last decade, immunosuppression with azathioprine, sometimes in combination with prednisone, and given together with the cholinesterase inhibitor pyridostigmine has become a standard therapy for MG [12]. In addition, plasma exchange (PE) therapy has proven to be a very rapid and effective method of preventing myasthenic crises which are very rare in immunosuppressed patients [8]. In some cases azathioprine has to be withdrawn because of bone marrow depression and severe infections. For such patients CyA might have some therapeutic benefit as an alternative to azathioprine. As an immunomodulating drug, CyA inhibits peripheral lymphocyte interactions without bone marrow depression. It seems to be able to decrease antibody production by suppression of T-helper lymphocytes and to inhibit the B-cell activation at an early stage [6]. To evaluate this effect we treated patients with generalized myasthenia gravis with CyA in a pilot study after obtaining their informed consent.

1 Neurologische Klinik der Technischen Universität München, Möhlstraße 28, D-8000 München 80

2 Abteilung Klinische Chemie am Klinikum Großhadern, Ludwig-Maximilians-Universität München, Marchioninistraße 15, D-8000 München 70

Methods

Up to now 7 patients with generalized myasthenia gravis, confirmed by clinical and EMG findings and by the presence of ACHR-ab, have been included in this running pilot study (Table 1). The data of 4 patients, 1 woman and 3 men, are available at this time (Table 2), while the other 3 patients need further investigation.

Only patients with severe generalized myasthenic symptoms despite optimal pyridostigmine treatment were selected for this study (Table 3). Patients under immunosuppressive therapy with azathioprine were accepted for the alternative CyA treatment only if they previously had developed bone marrow depression or had needed plasma exchange (Table 4).

CyA therapy was discontinued in the case of severe adverse reactions and marked clinical progression of myasthenic symptoms during treatment (Table 5).

All patients with malignancy, chronic infections and symptoms of liver or renal dysfunction were excluded in conformity with the "Guidelines for the use of CyA in patients with autoimmune disease" (Sandoz, Basle).

CyA administration

Patients were admitted to hospital for 2 weeks at the beginning of the treatment. CyA therapy was started with a dose of 5 mg per kilogram of body weight, divided into 2 doses. every 12 hours. The dose was adjusted to trough plasma levels between 150 and 200 ng/ml in the early phase, and later to between 100 and 150 ng/ml, in order to avoid side-effects. After discharge the patients were seen every second week for 2 months and at monthly intervals thereafter (Table 6).

Table 1. Confirmation of MG

- Standardized neurological examination
- Classification by MG score
- EMG, repetitive nerve stimulation test (Harvey-Masland)
- Determination of specific ACHR-ab

Table 2. Selection of patients with confirmed generalized myasthenia gravis for CyA therapy

Pat.	Sex	Age	Duration of MG (y)	Previous immuno-suppression	Bone marrow depression	Pyrido-stigmine mg/day	Prednisone mg/day
Sch. W.	♂	71	12	azathioprine	+	600	0
St. T.	♂	59	8	azathioprine	+	720	20
Hi. O.	♀	72	15	azathioprine	+	720	0
R. G.	♂	53	1	0	0	450	0

Table 3. Patient selection criteria

- Patients with generalized, severe myasthenic symptoms
- No therapeutic effect from cholinesterase inhibitors
- MG score > 0.5
- Progressive life threatening symptoms

Table 4. Therapeutic groups

long-standing myasthenia gravis ↗ in/after plasma exchange ↘ bone marrow depression

previous immunosuppression changed to CyA

recently diagnosed myasthenia gravis ↗ before/without thymectomy ↘ after thymectomy

no previous immunosuppression without plasma exchange

Table 5. Criteria for the cessation of CyA therapy

- Clinical deterioration during therapy (life threatening symptoms, Δ MG score + 0.5)
- Increase in ACHR-ab titres (> 50%)
- Severe side effects from CyA therapy

Table 6. Therapy monitoring

Period of treatment		inpatient															outpatient			
		CyA																		
		1st week							2nd week								3rd week	4th week	5th week	6th week
		Mon	Tue	Wed	Thu	Fri	Sat	Sun	Mon	Tue	Wed	Thu	Fri	Sat	Sun					
MG Score	▲	▲	▲	▲	▲	▲	▲	▲	▲	▲	▲	▲	▲	▲	▲			▲		▲
Lab. invest.*		▲		▲		▲			▲		▲		▲					▲		▲
CyA	▲	▲		▲		▲			▲		▲		▲					▲		▲
ACHR-ab	▲	▲		▲		▲			▲		▲		▲					▲		▲
β_2-m, Alb. (S/U)	▲	▲		▲		▲			▲		▲		▲					▲		▲
C_3/C_4, Ig, LpX	▲	▲				▲			▲				▲					▲		▲
RBP	▲	▲		▲		▲			▲		▲		▲					▲		▲
Transferr.	▲	▲		▲		▲			▲		▲		▲					▲		▲
Urine	▲	▲		▲		▲			▲		▲		▲					▲		▲

* so, pot, bili, creatinine, urea, cholesterol, triglyceride, CHE, γGT, GOT, GPT, AP, Quick, PTT, BCC

Table 7. Listing of clinical score for patients with myasthenia gravis. For calculation, grades of each item are added and divided by the number of items tested. All patients were tested under optimal anticholinesterase treatment. The upper test limit was taken from patients and healthy controls without neuromuscular weakness

Generalized signs

A. Muscles of limbs and trunk

Test items	None 0	Mild 1	Moderate 2	Severe 3	Weakness grades
Arm outstretched (90°, standing) sec	>240	90 –240	10 –90	<10	
Leg outstretched (45°, supine) sec	>100	30 –100	0 –30	0	
Head lifted (45°, supine) sec	>120	30 –120	0 –30	0	
Grip strength (Vigorimeter®) (Decrement after 10 maximal closures), %	<15	15 –30	30 –75	>75	
Vital capacity, L	3.5	2.5– 3.5	1.5– 2.5	< 1.5	Male
	2.5	1.2– 2.5	1.2– 1.8	< 1.2	Female
B. Oropharyngeal muscles					
Facial muscles	Normal	Mild weakness on lid closure	Incomplete lid closure	No mimic expression	
Chewing	Normal	Fatigue on chewing solid foods	Only soft foods	Gastric tube	
Swallowing	Normal	Fatigue on normal foods	Incomplete palatal closure nasal speech	Gastric tube	

Clinical muscle testing (MG score)

Clinical muscle testing was done every day during the clinical treatment period and thereafter at each clinical visit. All examinations were carried out according to a standardized program (Table 7) within the first 2 hours after pyridostigmine treatment and at the same time of the day. The normal range was based on the data of 112 patients and volunteers without neuromuscular disease. The lower range of this group was used as the upper test limit in the MG patients. The four grades of muscle strength were chosen arbitrarily. The clinical score was calculated on the sum of the grades of each item and divided by the number of items tested [1, 2]. A good correlation of the score value and serially determined ACHR-ab levels was found in a long-term follow-up study in individual myasthenia gravis patients [3].

Laboratory investigations

Baseline laboratory tests were performed including β_2-microglobulin (β_2-m), creatinine, electrolytes, liver enzymes, immunoglobulins, transferrin, albumin, retinol-binding protein (RBP), and hematological status. Immunoglobulins were determined by laser nephelometry (Behring-Werke, Marburg), enzyme immunoassay was used for β_2-m, and radial immunodiffusion for RBP. All other tests were performed by standard methods of clinical chemistry.

During clinical treatment blood samples were taken every second day and later at each clinical visit, in order to monitor CyA levels, ACHR-ab titres and the panel of tests mentioned above (Table 6).

ACHR-ab assay

To determine the ACHR-ab concentration an immuno precipitation assay was used as described previously [17]. A Triton X-100 muscle ACHR extract from amputated human limbs was labelled with ^{125}I alpha-Bungarotoxin (New England Nuclear) and precipitated with serum from MG patients. All serial determinations were made in the same assay in each patient.

CyA assay

CyA determinations in the plasma [10] were performed by radioimmunoassay as described by Donatsch et al. [9]. Blood samples were taken in the morning, immediately before CyA intake. Before centrifugation the samples were incubated at 37 °C for 1 h by the method described by Wenk et al. [19] with minor modifications [11].

Results

Therapeutic effects:

1 of our 4 patients improved clinically (Fig. 1). His MG score decreased from 0.75 to 0.375, which correlated well with reduction of the ACHR-ab titres. Unexpectedly, serum IgG levels did not decrease. This patient has been under CyA treatment for 9 months and is now in an excellent clinical condition, so that we have been able to taper the pyridostigmine to half of the dose he was receiving before CyA treatment. A slow increase of creatinine and β_2-m was observed after CyA trough plasma levels had reached the therapeutic range. β_2-m showed a marked increase from 1.8 mg/l to 4 mg/l 90 days after the beginning of CyA therapy. In the same time creatinine increased only from 0.9 mg/dl to 1.4 mg/dl. The mild side effects, such as hirsutism, nausea, loss of appetite and slight tremor of the upper extremities were tolerated. In the second patient (Fig. 2) we could not observe any clinical response to the CyA therapy. The ACHR-ab titres showed a slight increase during CyA therapy. This patient refused to continue CyA treatment because she developed severe side effects coinciding with a progressive increase of CyA trough plasma levels. The creatinine and β_2-m levels, which were elevated before CyA treatment was started, suggest that this patient had a preexisting renal dysfunction. After the CyA treatment had been stopped, immunosuppressive therapy with azathioprine was started. Four weeks later she developed bone marrow depression with leucopenia of approximately 2000/mm^3 so that azathioprine treatment had to be discontinued.

In the third patient (Fig. 3) we found no significant changes in myasthenic symptoms, but a marked reduction in ACHR-ab titres. In this case we had to break off CyA therapy after 3 months because of gastric pain, nausea, vomiting and gingival hyperplasia. Interestingly, 1 week after CyA withdrawal MG deteriorated rapidly with progressive ocular and pharyngeal symptoms, while the side-effects from CyA treatment disappeared simultaneously. 4 weeks later the MG score was increased from 1.0 to 1.5, and we had to start plasma exchange therapy to prevent myasthenic crisis. During plasma exchange we introduced immunosuppression with a combined azathioprine/prednisone treatment. His clinical condition is now quite good with an MG score of 0.35 and markedly decreased ACHR antibody titres. In this patient, too, we observed a slight increase in creatinine and β_2-m levels in the serum, whereas no changes in liver functions or in the hematological status could be seen.

In the fourth patient, CyA treatment had to be discontinued because he developed myasthenic crisis during therapy and showed signs of cerebral infarction. The latter, however, was not thought to be CyA-related because this patient had a history of vascular disease and had undergone surgery for a thrombus of the right carotid artery before CyA therapy.

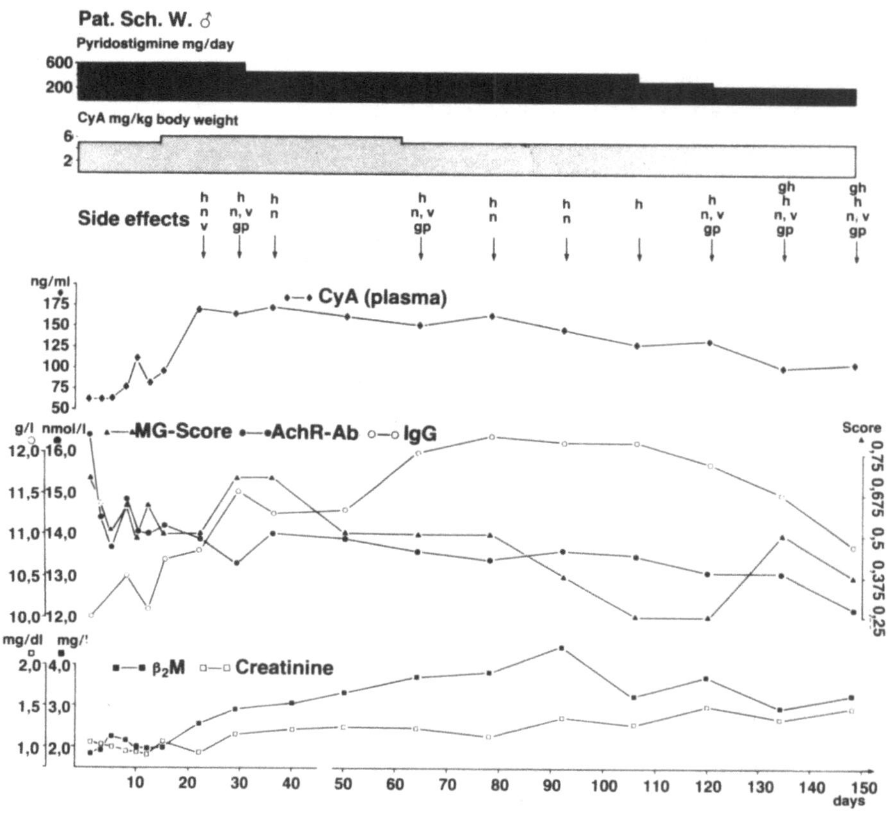

Fig. 1. Patient with generalized myasthenia gravis during CyA therapy. Note the correlation between the decrease in ACHR antibodies and MG score. In contrast to ACHR-ab, the IgG level is slightly increased. β_2-m and creatinine values are simultaneously elevated. CyA was given orally, divided into two doses, every 12 hours

Side effects

All patients complained of subjective side effects such as nausea, sometimes combined with vomiting, 1–2 h after CyA ingestion, and gastric pain which seemed to be related to the trough plasma levels (Fig. 2). After we had stopped CyA therapy we observed a rapid improvement of these complaints (Fig. 3). Gingival hyperplasia was prominent in 2 patients and improved after CyA treatment had been stopped (Fig. 3). One patient developed a tremor syndrome of the upper extremities and a mild elevation of blood pressure. In this case transient edemas of the lower extremities occurred about 2 weeks after the beginning of CyA treatment.

These side effects seemed to be more pronounced at higher CyA trough plasma levels (about 200 ng/ml), and to improve after adjusting the CyA dose to trough plasma levels between 100 and 150 ng/ml.

Toxic effects

In all patients creatinine and β_2-m in serum were elevated during CyA treatment (Figs. 1, 3). After CyA therapy had been withdrawn, the values decreased. In the patient who is still under CyA treatment,

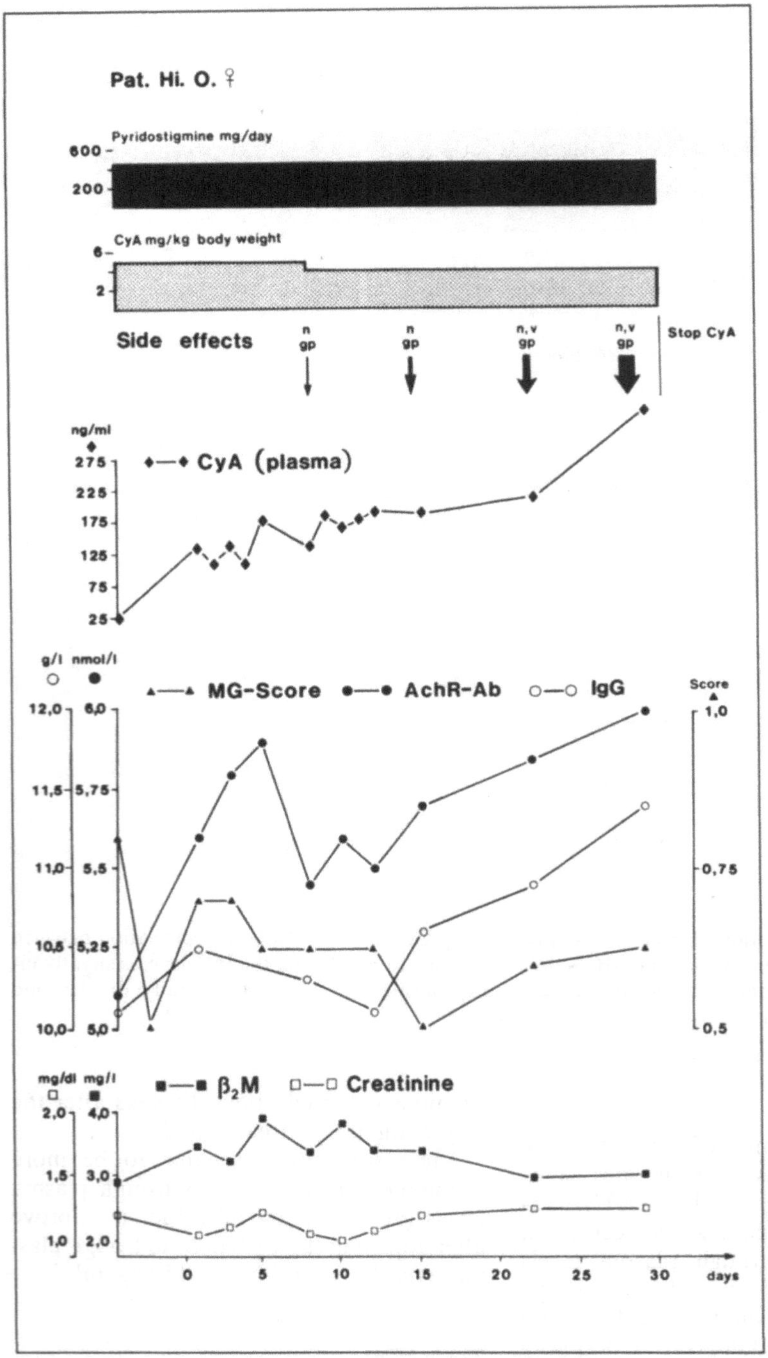

Fig. 2. Serial determination of ACHR-ab titres, MG score, β_2-m, creatinine and CyA trough plasma levels in a patient with generalized myasthenia gravis during CyA treatment. Note the accumulation of CyA with increasing side effects and the slight elevation of β_2-m and creatinine, indicating renal insufficiency before CyA treatment

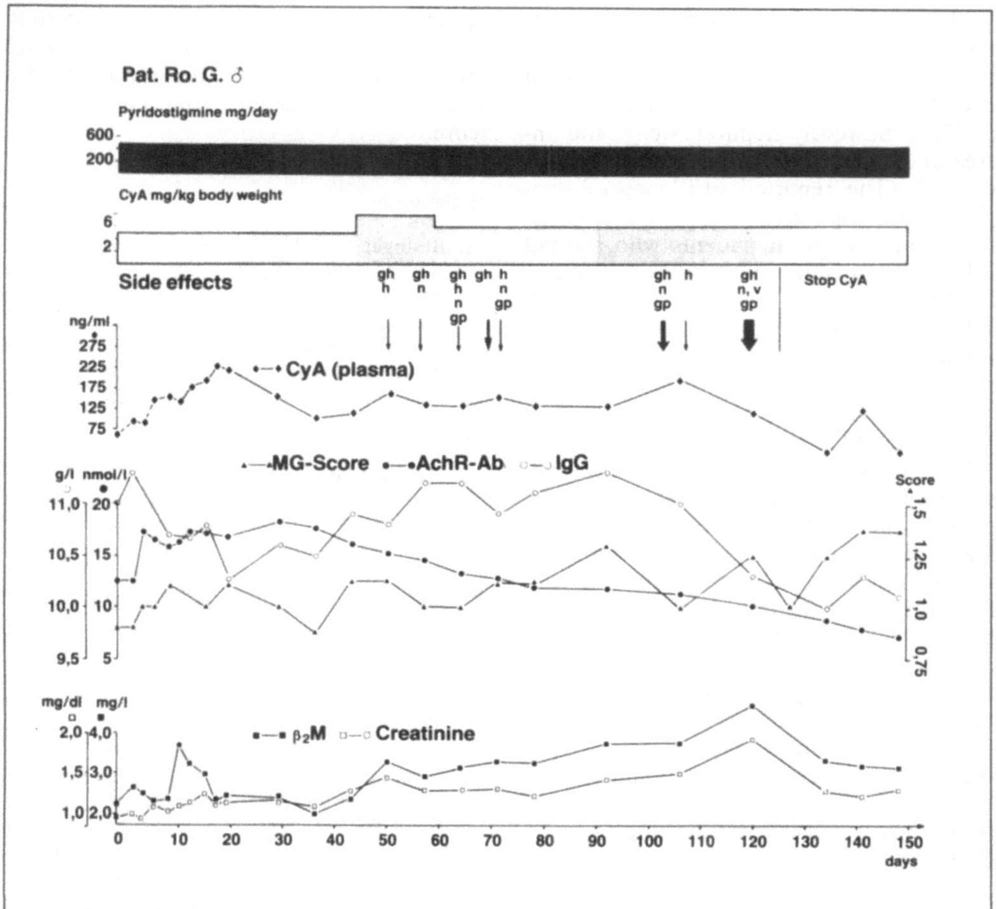

Fig. 3. Patient with generalized myasthenia gravis, without clinical response to CyA therapy but with decrease in antibody titres. Slight simultaneous elevation of β_2-m and creatinine during treatment, with reduction after break-off of CyA therapy

β_2-m and creatinine show elevated levels without signs of progressing nephrotoxicity.

There were no signs of hepatotoxicity, anemia, lymphopenia or other changes in the hemopoietic system.

Discussion

The results of the running pilot study reported here need a very cautious interpretation. CyA treatment seemed to be effective in two of our patients, who showed clinical improvement, or a decrease in ACHR-ab titres, or both. These observations are in agreement with the postulated immuno-suppressive mechanism of CyA, which primarily inhibits T-helper cell activity [5, 7], and interferes with other B-lymphocyte activating mechanisms [6, 4].

In myasthenia gravis the anti ACHR-ab production is induced by specific thymic anti-ACHR-T-helper lymphocytes [18]. CyA might inhibit these specific helper T-cell subsets, resulting in reduced ACHR-ab production. This effect was observed in 2 patients (Figs. 1, 3). The early onset about 10 days after the initiation of CyA treatment, might be due to the CyA-induced suppression of the peripheral lymphocyte interactions [5]. To confirm these first positive results of CyA as an immunosuppressive drug in MG, further study is necessary.

Most patients have been immunosuppressed successfully with long-term azathioprine without any adverse reactions or complications. In long-term administration of CyA, however, nephrotoxicity and increased incidence of lymphoma was reported [15]. (The reported incidence of lymphoma has since been shown to be within the normal range in patients who are not subjected to immunsuppression with a combination of several drugs [3a]). Although this was not observed in patients treated for autoimmune diabetes with lower doses [14], CyA cannot be considered as an alternative immunosuppressive drug in MG treatment.

Side effects as well as the immunosuppressive activity of CyA seem to be dependent on plasma level (Figs. 2 and 3). At lower plasma levels, side effects improved without reducing the immunsuppressive effect. This indicates that serial CyA trough plasma level determination is necessary in order to monitor patients during CyA therapy and to determine the optimal therapeutic plasma CyA levels.

This might help to avoid the side effects which have been the limiting factors for CyA therapy in two of our patients. Nephrotoxicity was not a limiting factor of CyA therapy as has been described for cardiac allograft recipients [13].

To monitor renal functions, β_2-m in serum and urine seems to be more sensitive than creatinine.

From these preliminary results we conclude that 1. CyA is effective in the treatment of some patients with myasthenia gravis, but cannot replace standard therapy with azathioprine. 2. Only in patients with bone marrow depression from immunosuppressive therapy might CyA be suggested as an alternative drug. The risks of long-term CyA treatment are not well established. 3. Further investigation is necessary to evaluate the minimal plasma levels of CyA needed to maintain immunosuppressive activity and to minimize the side effects. 4. Serial determination of plasma levels is necessary for monitoring the CyA therapy and for the determination of optimal plasma levels in the therapy of autoimmune diseases. 5. Myasthenia gravis may serve as a model to study the immunosuppressive activity of CyA in autoimmune disease, because it is possible to measure the specific ACHR-ab titres quantitatively and to correlate them to the clinical MG score.

References

1. Besinger UA, Toyka KV, Fateh-Moghadam A, et al. (1980) Die Bedeutung eines quantitativen klinischen Bewertungssystems für die Verlaufsbeobachtung der Myasthenia gravis: eine prospektive Studie. In: Mertens HG, Przuntek H (eds) Pathologische Erregbarkeit des Nervensystems. Springer, Berlin, pp 568–572
2. Besinger UA, Toyka KV, Heininger K, et al. (1981) Long term correlation of clinical course and acetylcholine receptor antibody in patients with myasthenia gravis. Ann NY Acad Sci 377:812–815
3. Besinger UA, Toyka KV, Hömberg M, Heininger K, Hohlfeld R, Fateh-Moghadam A (1983) Myasthenia gravis: long-term correlation of binding and bungarotoxin blocking antibodies against acetylcholine-receptors with changes in disease severity. Neurology 33:1316–1321

3a. Beveridge T, Krupp P, McKibbiu C (1984) Lymphomas and lymphoproliferative lesions developing and cyclosporin therapy. Lancet No. 8380, Vol I:788

4. Borel JF, Wiesinger D (1977) Effects of cyclosporin A on murine lymphoid cells. In: Lucas DO (ed) Regulatory mechanisms in lymphocyte activation. Academic Press, New York, p 716
5. Borel JF, Lafferty KJ (1983) Cyclosporine: Speculation about its mechanisms. Transplant Proc 15:1881–1885
6. Bouwer HGA, Hinrichs DJ (1983) Cyclosporine effects on mitogen induced T- and B-cell proliferation. Transplant Proc XVII, Suppl 1:2306–2310
7. van Buren CT, Kerman R, Flechner S, Kahan BD (1983) Cyclosporine effects on immunoregulatory cells in men. Transplant Proc 15:2293–2297
8. Dau PC (1981) Plasmapheresis and immunosuppressive drug therapy in sixty myasthenia gravis patients. Ann NY Acad Sci:700–708
9. Donatsch P, Abisch E, Homberger M, et al. (1981) A radioimmunoassay to measure cyclosporin A in plasma and serum samples. J Immunoassay 2:19–32
10. Mraz W, Zink RA, Graf A, Preis D, Illner WD, Land W, Siebert W, Zöttlein H (1983) Distribution and transfer of cyclosporine

among the various human lipoprotein classes. Transplant Prov 15:2426–2429
11. Mraz W, unpublished
12. Mertens HG, Hertel G, Reuther P, Ricker K (1981) Effect of immunosuppressive drugs (Azathioprine). Ann NY Acad Sci:691–699
13. Myers BD, Ross J, Newton L, Luetscher J, Perlroth M (1984) Cyclosporine-associated chronic nephrotoxicity. N Engl J Med 311:699–705
14. Stiller CR, Dupré J, Gent M, Jenner MR, Klown PA, Lampacis A, Martell R, Rodger NW, v. Graffenried B, Wolfe BMI (1984) Effects of cyclosporine immunosuppression in insulin-dependent diabetes mellitus of recent onset. Science 223:1362–1366
15. Thiru S, Calne RY, Nagington J (1981) Lymphoma in renal allograft patients treated with cyclosporin as one of the immunosuppressive agents. Transplant Proc 13:359
16. Toyka KV, Drachman DB, Griffin DE, et al. (1977) Myasthenia gravis: study of humoral immune mechanisms by passive transfer to mice. N Engl J Med 296:125–131
17. Toyka KV, Becker T, Fateh-Moghadam A, Besinger UA (1979) Die Bedeutung der Bestimmung von Antikörpern gegen Acetylcholinrezeptoren in der Diagnostik der Myasthenia gravis. Klin Wochenschr 57:937–942
18. Wekerle A, Hohlfeld R, Ketelsen UP, Kalden JR, Kalies J (1981) Thymic myogenesis, T-lymphocytes and the pathogenesis of myasthenia gravis. Ann NY Acad Sci:455–476
19. Wenk E, Follath F, Abisch E (1983) Temperatur dependency of apparent cyclosporin A concentration in plasma. Clin Chem 29:1865

Ciclosporin (CyA) in the Management of Polymyositis/Idiopathic Cardiomyopathy

K. Bendtzen, N. Tvede, V. Andersen and S. A. Mortensen [1]

Polymyositis comprises a group of relatively rare diseases characterized by inflammatory myopathy of unknown cause. The term dermatomyositis is applied in the presence of a characteristic skin rash. Cardiac involvement may occur, and certain cases of idiopathic cardiomyopathy without skeletal muscle disease may constitute a separate entity within the group of immunologically mediated myopathies.

Four major diagnostic criteria are used to define polymyositis [2]: 1) progressive, symmetrical weakness of the limb-girdle muscles and anterior neck flexors; 2) histological evidence of muscle necrosis with inflammation; 3) elevation in serum levels of skeletal muscle enzymes; and 4) characteristic electromyographic changes distinguishing polymyositis from primary neurogenic disorders. Characteristic dermatological features serve as a fifth criterion for dermatomyositis.

Corticosteroids are generally considered beneficial in the treatment of polymyositis, but some reports and our own experience show little evidence that corticosteroids are efficaceous in the longer term, while steroid-induced myopathy always threatens to worsen the condition. Similarly, cytostatic drugs often fail to control the disease, and the mortality rates in groups treated with cytostatic drugs are often similar to corticosteroid-treated or even untreated groups [3, 5]. Consequently, there is a need to offer alternative therapy to these unfortunate patients.

Case No. 1: Polymyositis

This patient is the subject of a recent report [1]: A 40-year-old man, he experienced sudden symmetrical weakness of the neck flexors and the limb-girdle muscles. Rapid progression was noted, and within 2 months almost all striated muscles were clinically affected. Polymyositis group I was diagnosed on the basis of the clinical findings, characteristic muscle biopsy and electromyography, and severe elevation of serum muscle enzymes (Fig. 1). Prednisolone and cyclophosphamide were administered with a favourable effect on the enzyme abnormalities, but the patient's muscle strength deteriorated and respiratory muscle involvement was noted. Biochemical signs of progressive disease were not pronounced, although slight elevations in serum aldolase levels were seen when reductions in corticosteroid dosage were attempted. Within a week of starting CyA therapy (7.5 to 10 mg/kg/day), the urinary creatine index (CI) and the serum aldolase levels decreased. More importantly, however, the patient gained 25% in measured muscle strength and his general feeling of illness disappeared. His functional disability grade [4] improved from 6 to 5. He has now been on CyA for more than 12 months. The glucocorticoid dose has been reduced to 10 mg/day, and the patient, who was bedridden before CyA therapy, can now walk around supported by sticks.

To evaluate the effect of CyA, the drug was withheld for a week. As shown in Figure 1, the patient's condition deteriorated markedly within a week with reappearance of the characteristic feeling of illness, progressive fatigue and loss of muscle strength. Only slight serum enzyme abnormalities were noted. Within a week after reintroduction of CyA the patient went into clinical remission.

Apart from transient gynaecomastia and gingivitis, there have been no signs of drug-induced side effects.

1 Medical Departments, Rigshospitalet University Hospital, Copenhagen, Denmark

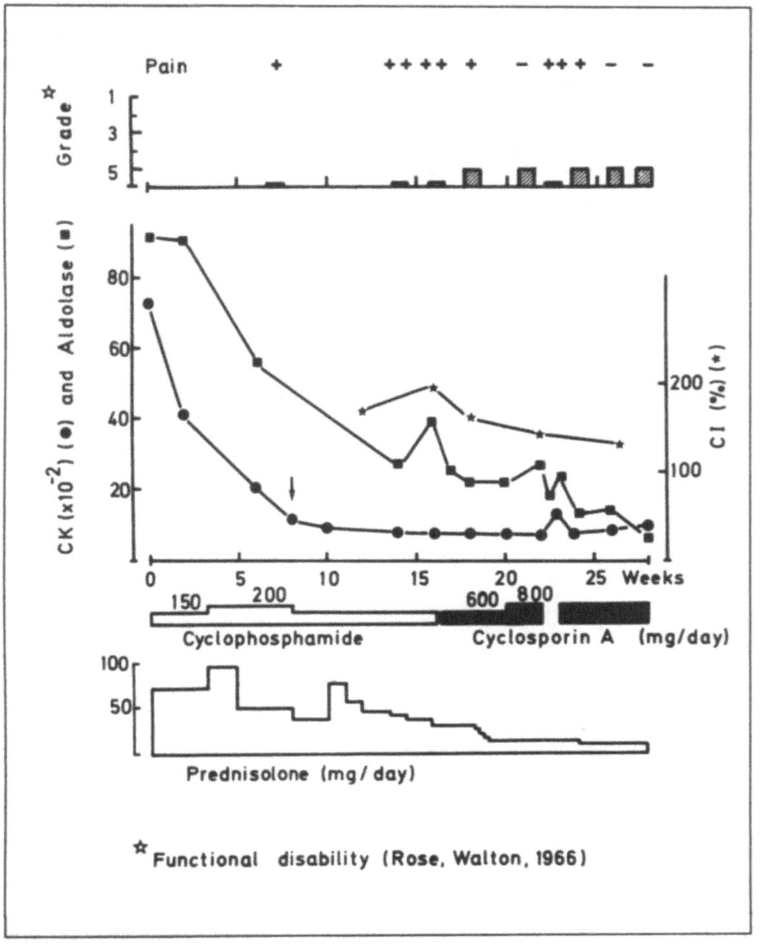

Fig. 1. Clinical course of case No. 1 (polymyositis)
CK: creatine kinase
CI: creatine index (24 h urine excretion of creatine plus creatinine/24 h urine excretion of creatinine × 100)

Case No. 2: Polymyositis

This patient has also been the subject of a previous report (1): A 41-year-old man, he abruptly developed symmetrical weakness and pain in the limb-girdle muscles, rapidly progressing to involve almost all striated muscles, possibly including the myocardium (right-bundle-branch block). The diagnosis of group I polymyositis was confirmed by characteristic electromyographic and muscle biopsy abnormalities. As shown in Figure 2, there was a good but brief clinical and paraclinical response to corticosteroid treatment. Suddenly, and despite therapy, his symptoms reappeared with concomitant increases in the serum muscle enzyme levels. Azathioprine was administered, but because of marked clinical progression the drug was replaced with CyA (7.5 mg/kg/day). At this point, the patient had severe Cushing's syndrome and the serum enzyme levels suggested severe myolysis. As shown in Figure 2, the enzyme abnormalities improved considerably after only 5 days of treatment. More importantly, the severe muscle pain, which had to be treated with morphine analogues, almost disappeared and the patient's muscle strength improved considerably.

The patient has been treated with CyA for 12 months (8.6 to 10 mg/kg/day). Apart from hypertrophic gingivitis, no side effects have been observed.

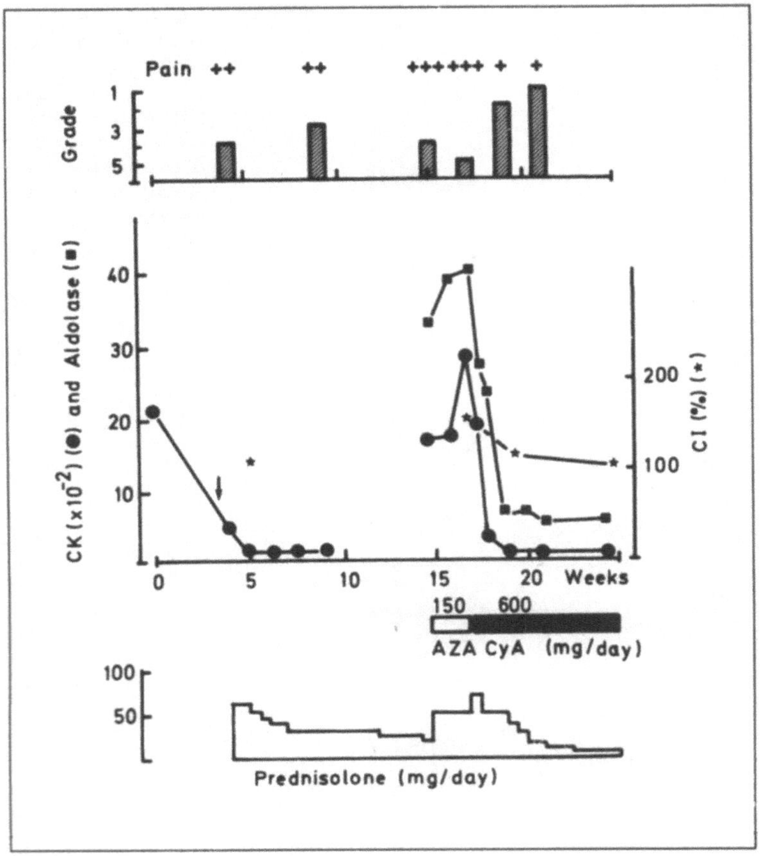

Fig. 2. Clinical course of case No. 2 (polymyositis)
AZA: azathioprine
CyA: ciclosporin
Also see legend to Fig. 1

Case No. 3: Cardiomyopathy

This patient is a 33-year-old man with insulin-dependent diabetes mellitus and a four-year history with enlarged liver and dyspnoea on exertion. Echocardiography, angiography and hemodynamic measurements revealed cardiomyopathy of restrictive type with pulmonary hypertension and grade I mitral valve incompetence. Endomyocardial biopsy from the right ventricle showed necrosis of muscle cells with lympho-histiocytic infiltration (Table 1). There was moderate, patchy round-cell infiltration along the small vessels. No signs of underlying illness, except diabetes, were found, and skeletal muscle involvement was absent. Physically, the patient was graded as class III (New York Heart Association (NYHA)) (Table 2). After one month on CyA (8.6 to 5.7 mg/kg/day), the patient improved to NYHA class II with markedly reduced fatigue, reduced palpitations and diminished dyspnoea and chest pain on exertion. His walking distance improved and he was able to walk to the fourth floor. Echocardiography showed improved myocardial contraction, and hemodynamic measurements revealed a 25% increase in the ejection fraction along with a slight increase in cardiac index. A repeat biopsy, however, showed unchanged, chronic active inflammation.

After 11 months on ciclosporin his condition remained stable, and a third endomyocardial biopsy at this time showed healing with fibrosis and muscle hypertrophy without signs of inflammation.

Because of renal toxicity (serum creatinine 0.17 mmol/l) the dose of CyA was reduced to 4.3 mg/kg/day. Other side effects were slight and included hypertrichosis, gingi-

Tab. 1. 33-year-old male with myocarditis treated with ciclosporin. Haemodynamic and endomyocardial biopsy data

	RA mm Hg	RV mm Hg	PA mm Hg	LVEDP/ wedge mm Hg	Cardiac index L/min m²	Biopsy findings light microscopy
Initial study	5	59/7	59/29	25/24	1.59	Severe mononuclear Cell infiltration
Control 2½ months	8	62/9	60/30	–/39	1.74	Cell infiltration unchanged
Control 11½ months	2	65/2	63/28	25/25	1.71	Cell infiltration absent; slight interstitial fibrosis

RA: Right atrium; RV: Right ventricle; PA: Pulmonary artery; LVEDP: Left ventricular end diastolic pressure; wedge: Pulmonary capillary wedge pressure.
Microscopy: Performed by U. Baandrup, University Institute of Pathology, Aarhus Municipal Hospital, Denmark

Tab. 2. 33-year-old male with myocarditis treated with ciclosporin. Clinical and non-invasive data

	NYHA class	Chest X-ray heart volume ml/m² BSA	MSS echo mm	FS echo %	RV echo mm	LA echo mm	MUGA LVEF% rest	CyA treatment mg/day
Initial study	III	610	18	13	29	46	20	–
Control 2½ months	II	610	10	22	22	44	25	600 mg initial 400 mg after 2 weeks
Control 11½ months	I	415	13	23	25	38	31	300 mg

MSS: Mitral septal separation; FS: Fractional shortening; RV: Right ventricle; LA: Left atrium; MUGA: Radionuclide Angiocardiography; LVEF%: Left ventricular ejection fraction; CyA: Ciclosporin

vitis, dysaesthesia of hands and feet, and tremor.

Conclusion

We feel that cautious optimism is justified concerning ciclosporin treatment of severe myositis. The beneficial effect may be seen within a week, and irreversible muscle damage may be prevented by prompt administration of CyA if conventional therapy fails. We do not know whether ciclosporin improves survival rates, nor whether the effect is long-lasting in these otherwise therapy-resistant disorders.

References

1. Bendtzen K, Tvede N, Andersen V, Bendixen G (1984) Cyclosporin for polymyositis. Lancet i:792
2. Bohan A, Peter JB (1975) Polymyositis and dermatomyositis I. N Engl J Med 292:344
3. Bohan A, Peter JB (1975) Polymyositis and dermatomyositis II. N Engl J Med 292:403
4. Rose AL, Walton JN (1966) Polymyositis: a survey of 89 cases with particular reference to treatment and prognosis. Brain 89:747
5. Winkelmann RK, Mulder DW, Lambert EH et al. (1968) Course of dermatomyositis-polymyositis: comparison of untreated and cortisone-treated patients. Mayo Clin Proc 43:545

3. Diabetes Mellitus Type 1

Type I Diabetes Mellitus: Rationale for Immune Intervention

H. Kolb[1] and J. Nerup[2]

Introduction

Pilot trials of immune intervention in recent onset Type I diabetes mellitus have been performed since 1978 and include a variety of immunosuppressive or immunomodulatory substances [1, 4, 6, 8, 9, 11, 12, 14, 15]. The decision in favour of such trials in general is based on two reasons. Firstly, insulin therapy of Type I diabetes mellitus is not satisfactory: a considerable proportion of patients face late complications and reduced life expectancy. Secondly, data are accumulating in favour of the immune nature of beta-cell destruction in Type I diabetics. Thus the disease process may be amenable to immunotherapy.

Late complications and survival in insulin-dependent (Type I) diabetic patients

The continuing Steno Studies [2, 5, 7] on the prognosis of insulin-dependent (Type I) diabetes mellitus (IDDM), comprise a large unselected segment of the Danish diabetic population. Table 1 lists the types of complication seen in patients surviving 30–40 years of insulin-dependent diabetes. The average survival time, with insulin-dependent diabetes diagnosed before the age of 31, is 37–40 years. Thus Table 1 gives data for the surviving population.

The predominant causes of death are diabetic nephropathy and cardiovascular catastrophies. It should be noted that some 25–30% of the patients do not develop late diabetic complications.

Expressed as relative mortality, insulin-dependent (Type I) diabetics are burdened with quite shocking excess mortality. When compared with age- and sex-matched control populations, relative mortality is increased 30–35, 20–25 and about 10 times for patients diagnosed at age 5, 15 and 25 years respectively. Diabetic nephropathy with or without myocardial infarction is responsible for almost all the increased relative mortality, reaching peak values after 20–25 years of diabetes.

It is noteworthy that even during the first 5–10 years of insulin-dependent diabetes mellitus, relative mortality is increased by a factor of 2–3.

The prognosis of insulin-dependent (Type I) diabetes mellitus has improved over recent years. Relative mortality has been reduced by about 40%, for example, for a patient aged 15 years at time of diagnosis in 1955 compared with a similar patient diagnosed ten years earlier.

What is the prognosis of patients who succumb to IDDM in 1985? Some improvement since 1955 is to be expected, since favourable changes have occurred in both insulin treatment and the monitoring of metabolism. Insulin therapy now centres

Table 1. Complications

After 30–40 years of IDDM. Data are compiled from 264 patients who developed diabetes between 1923 and 1953. The range given is due to different rates of late complications in patients with good and bad metabolic control respectively

Blindness	10–30%
Proteinuria	30–45%
Uremia	10–30%
Amputation/gangrene	10–20%
Cerebral vascular insult	5–15%
Myocardial infarction	15–25%

1 Diabetes Research Institute, University of Düsseldorf, Düsseldorf, Fed. Rep. Germany
2 Steno Memorial Hospital, Gentofte, Denmark
Correspondence: Prof. Dr. Hubert Kolb, Diabetes-Forschungsinstitut, Auf'm Hennekamp 65, 4000 Düsseldorf, Fed. Rep. Germany, Tel.: FRG 02 11/3 38 22 79

on better stimulation of the physiologic beta-cell response by reduced use of long-acting insulin preparations plus peaks of short-acting insulins with meals. Monitoring of metabolism has improved through the availability of more appropriate and intensive patient education, and repeated self-monitoring through urine and blood glucose determinations. Possibly the most important development has been the introduction of the analysis of non-enzymatic hemoglobin glycation as a measure of average blood glucose levels during the preceding months. The data obtained have very much facilitated the optimization of insulin therapy.

Still, the prognosis of Type I diabetics in 1985 must be regarded as unsatisfactory. At present, it still has not been possible to mimic endogenous insulin secretion fully with continuous and/or bolus injections, or to adjust to the variation in insulin needs due to differences in physical activity, food intake, stress situations and infectious complications. A second point is that compliance, especially in children and adolescent patients, is not easy to obtain; these subgroups, however, carry the highest risk for developing late complications.

Is Type I diabetes mellitus an immune-mediated disease?

Insulin deficiency in Type I diabetics is the result of chronic inflammation of pancreatic islets with specific loss of beta cells (Fig. 1). The disease develops only in genetically susceptible persons, with an environmental factor possibly as the initiating agent [3, 10, 13]. The basic assumption for

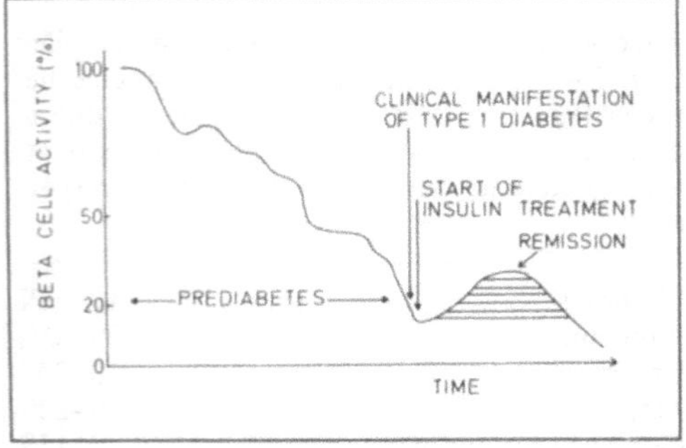

Fig. 1. Loss of beta-cell activity during the course of diabetes mellitus Type I

Table 2. Type 1 diabetes, an immune-mediated disease?

1. HLA immune response genes involved
2. Chronic organ inflammation
3. Organ-specific humoral autoimmunity
4. Organ-specific cellular autoimmunity

Table 3. Prevalence of islet-cell cytoplasmic antibodies (ICA) in Type 1 diabetics. Data are from a prospective study on children between 1 and 15 years of age at diagnosis of IDDM (Kolb et al., to be published).

Time	ICA-prevalence (No/total)
At diagnosis	593/692 (85.7%)
After 1 year	261/348 (83.0%)
After 2 years	138/234 (59.0%)
After 3 years	89/142 (62.7%)

immunotherapy protocols is that the progressive loss of beta cells is an immune-mediated process. Since at clinical manifestation of insulin deficiency some 10–20% of beta cells have not yet been destroyed, immunosuppression at this point may rescue residual beta-cell activity and allow uninhibited islet-cell regeneration to take place.

Several characteristics of Type I diabetes suggest that islet inflammation may be immune in nature (Table 2). Firstly, genes controlling diabetes susceptibility have been found within the HLA gene complex, near and/or at the DR locus. This locus contains putative immune response genes. Secondly, islet inflammation in pre-diabetic patients appears as a chronic progressive destructive process rather than an acute infectious inflammation. Thirdly, humoral autoimmunity to islet cells is present in the majority of Type I diabetics. Antibodies against cytoplasmic constituents of all islet cell types are seen with high prevalence around manifestation time and disappear within a few years in the majority of patients (Table 3). In addition, between 50 and 80% of patients show antibodies specific for surface determinants of beta cells. In general these antibodies display cytotoxicity in vitro. Early demonstrations of cellular immunity in islet inflammation were the observation of lymphocyte infiltrations in islets and of a positive leukocyte migration inhibition test when peripheral blood leukocytes from Type I diabetics were exposed to islet antigens. More recently cytotoxicity of lymphocytes towards islet cells has been shown in vitro.

It is essential to realize that none of the immune phenomena described so far permits any decision on whether immune reactions to islets are causative of or an epiphenomenon of beta-cell loss. However, recent experience with pancreas grafting to Type I diabetics furnishes almost certain proof that beta-cell destruction is immune mediated. This conclusion is derived from segmental pancreas transplants from living normal donors to diabetic monozygotic cotwins [16]. The recipients were found to destroy selectively beta cells in the syngeneic graft within 6–10 weeks. Of special relevance is the finding that conventional immunosuppression was effective in either stopping ongoing beta-cell destruction or in preventing islet inflammation when given early enough. Thus the diabetic recipients have mounted an immune attack against beta cells within the transplanted organ. Immunosuppression was able to block this process.

We feel that if immunosuppression protects grafted islets from destruction in Type I diabetics there is substantial hope that immune intervention early after manifestation of the disease will also protect autologous beta cells and will help preserve endogenous insulin secretion.

References

1. Assan R, Debray-Sachs M, Laborie C, Chatenoud L, Feutren G, Quiniou-Debrie MC, Thomas G, Bach JF (1985) Metabolic and immunological effects of cyclosporin in recently diagnosed type 1 diabetes mellitus. Lancet I:67–71
2. Borch-Johnsen K, Kragh-Andersen P, Deckert T (1985) The impact of proteinuria on the relative mortality in patients with type 1 (insulin-dependent) diabetes mellitus. Diabetologia (in press)
3. Cahill GFJR, McDevitt HO (1981) Insulin dependent diabetes mellitus: the initial lesion. N Engl J Med 304:1454–1465
4. Cobb EW, Molitch M, Reichlin S (1980) Levamisole in insulin-dependent diabetes mellitus. N Engl J Med 303:1065–1066
5. Deckert T, Poulsen JE, Larsen M (1978) Prognosis of diabetics with diabetes onset before the age of thirty-one. Diabetologia 14:363–370
6. Elliot RB, Crossley JR, Berryman CC, James AG (1981) Partial preservation of pancreatic beta cell function in children with diabetes. Lancet II:1–4
7. Green A, Borch-Johnsen K, Kragh-Andersen P, Hougaard P, Keiding N, Kreiner S, Deckert T (1985) Relative mortality of type 1 (insulin-dependent) diabetics in Denmark 1933–1981. Diabetologia (in press)
8. Greulich B, Lander T, Standl E, Kolb H, Gerbitz KD, Kuschak D, Gries FA (1983) Immune intervention trial in newly diagnosed type 1 insulin dependent diabetes. Diabetologia 25:158
9. Koivisto VA, Aro A, Cantell K, Haataja M, Huttunen J, Karonen S-L, Mustajoki P, Pelkonen R, Seppälä P (1984) Remissions in newly diagnosed type 1 (insulin-dependent) diabetes: influence of interferon as an adjunct to insulin therapy. Diabetologia 27:193–197
10. Kolb H, Schernthaner G, Gries FA (1983) Diabetes and immunology: Pathogenesis and immunotherapy. Hans Huber, Bern Stuttgart Wien
11. Leslie RDG, Pyke DA (1980) Immunosuppression of acute insulin-dependent diabetics. In: Irvine WJ (ed) Immunology of Diabetes. Teviot Scientific Publications, Edinburgh, pp 345–347
12. Ludvigsson J, Heding L, Liedén G, Marner B, Lernmark Å (1983) Plasmapheresis in the initial treatment of insulin-dependent diabetes mellitus in children. Br Med J 286:176–178
13. Nerup J, Lernmark A, Scott J (1984) Autoimmunity. In: Gupta S (ed) Immunology of clinical and experimental diabetes. Plenum Medical Book Company, New York London, pp. 351–367
14. Rand KH, Rosenbloom AL, MacLaren NK, Silverstein JH, Riley WJ, Butterworth BE, Yoon JW, Rubenstein AH, Merigan TC (1981) Human leucocyte interferon treatment of two children with insulin-dependent diabetes. Diabetologia 21:116–119
15. Stiller CR, Dupré J, Gent M, Jenner MR, Keown PA, Laupacis A, Martell R, Rodger NW, von Graffenried B, Wolfe BMJ (1984) Effects of cyclosporine immunosuppression in insulin-dependent diabetes mellitus of recent onset. Science 223:1362–1367
16. Sutherland DER, Goetz FC, Najarian JS (1984) Pancreas transplants from related donors. Transplantation 38:625–633

Effects of Ciclosporin on Insulin Secretion in Recent Onset Type I Diabetes Mellitus

J. Dupre, C. R. Stiller, M. Gent, M. Jenner, N. W. Rodger, B. M. Wolfe, B. von Graffenried, D. Heinrichs, C. Purdon, R. Martell

In November 1982 a "pilot" (uncontrolled) clinical trial of the effects of the administration of ciclosporin to volunteer subjects with recent onset Type I diabetes mellitus was initiated. The rationale and preliminary findings in this study have been published earlier [1]. In this presentation we summarize further experience in this ongoing trial.

Consenting volunteers aged 9–49 years at onset of diabetes were recruited. Initially, subjects who had been treated with insulin for up to one year were considered, provided they exhibited basal or stimulated plasma immunoreactive C-peptide levels entering the normal range (0.18 pmol/ml). Conventional therapy with insulin was continued. The target for the control of glycemia was the maintenance of pre-meal levels of plasma glucose <7.8 mmol/l. Ciclosporin treatment was initiated with 10 mg/kg bodyweight/day, administered in two equal doses approximately 12 hours apart, and serum trough levels of immunoreactive ciclosporin were maintained at 100–150 ng/ml through most of the treatment period by adjustment of dosage. The volunteers were carefully followed for manifestations of toxicity of ciclosporin and dosage was reduced, or the drug withdrawn, when unacceptable adverse effects required. The intention was to treat with ciclosporin for at least 6 months, in the absence of contraindication, and to continue through 1 year if evidence of apparent benefit was obtained.

The assessment of the effects of ciclosporin on the course of the diabetes was based on the laboratory- and self-determined blood glucose levels, on the insulin dosage required for control of glycemia, and on serial measurements of the basal and glucagon-stimulated levels of immunoreactive C-peptide in the plasma. These C-peptide determinations were carried out after overnight fast in all patients, and before administration of insulin in those who continued to receive insulin therapy.

During the early months of recruitment to the study it appeared that striking reductions in daily insulin requirements were manifested by a majority of the patients with relatively recent onset of diabetes, i.e. those who had received insulin therapy for 6 weeks. A similar effect was much less frequent in subjects with diabetes of longer duration. Accordingly, after recruitment of 11 subjects with diabetes of 2–11 months' duration, entry of further volunteers with diabetes of 6 weeks' duration was discontinued. The 11 volunteers with diabetes of longer duration were designated Group II. The characteristics of these subjects are shown in Table 1. According to the agreed protocol, ciclosporin treatment was to be continued through 6 months in this group. This treatment was then terminated in the 7 of these 11 who had no obvious change in insulin requirement, but it was continued to approximately one year in 3 Group II subjects who exhibited very low insulin requirement (<2.0 U/kg/day: 2 of these 3 were transiently non-insulin-requiring).

Results

The recruitment of volunteers with diabetes who had received insulin therapy for <6 weeks at entry continued through February 1984, when 48 subjects had been entered. No subject was excluded because of low plasma C-peptide. We present here the data derived from experience in this group of subjects, designated Group I, for comparison with results in Group II subjects.

University Hospital, London, Canada

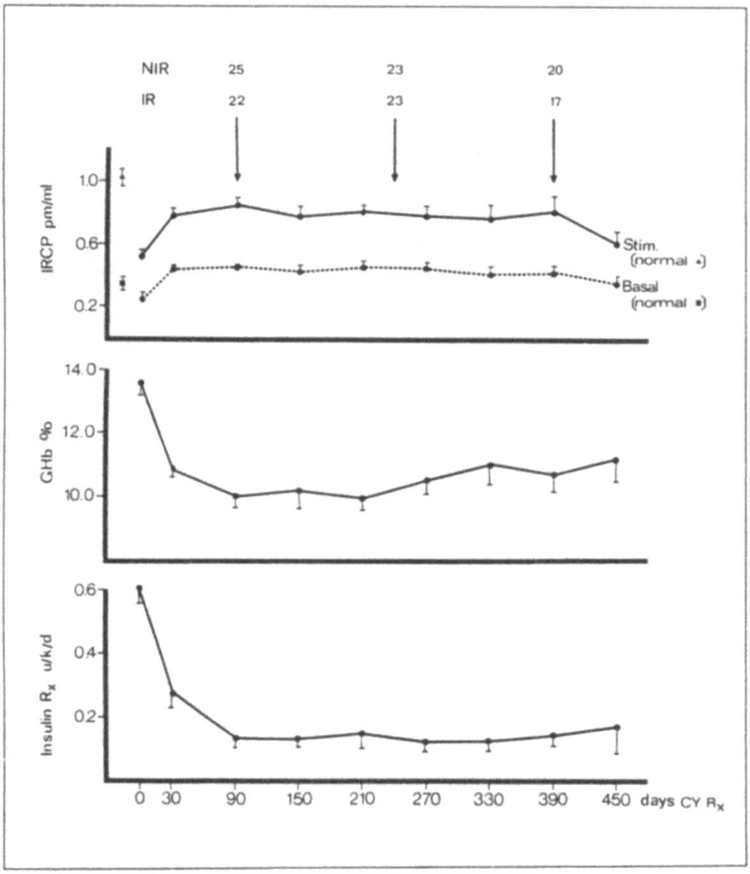

Fig. 1. Basal and glucagon-stimulated IRCP, gHb%, and insulin dose in all group I subjects who received CyA $R_x > 200$ days

Table 1. Group I subjects: IDDM, receiving insulin for < 6 weeks at entry, subjects with CyA $R_x > 200$ days at analysis: N = 47 (basal/stim CP) BCP/SCP

	D^NDM days	Age yrs	Sex (n)	Ins, at entry U/K/D	BCP/CP (pmol/ml)	
$\bar{X}$	17	15.6	M 30, F 17	0.60	0.24	0.51
± SEM	2	1.2		0.04	0.03	0.05

Group II subjects: IDDM, receiving insulin for > 8 weeks at entry CyA R_x > 180/7, n = 11 (basal/stim CP)

	D^NDM days	Age yrs	Sex (n)	Ins, at entry U/K/D	BCP/CP (pmol/ml)	
$\bar{X}$	164	16.9	M 7, F 4	0.51	0.19	0.32
± SEM	27	2.6		0.04	0.03	0.04

The results in Group I as a whole are presented in Figure 1, and the subjects' characteristics are shown in Table 1.

The mean daily insulin dosage of Group I patients is illustrated in Figure 1. This fell progressively, with an increasing number of patients maintaining glycemic control without administration of insulin. When this status was preserved for at least 2 weeks, the subjects were designated "non-insulin-requiring". The proportion designated "non-insulin-requiring" through the period of administration of ciclosporin from 6 months to 1 year was approximately 50%.

Not all patients maintained target control of glycemia. The mean glycohemoglobin level determined by a colorimetric method (by means of which 95% of normal subjects were determined to have values <9.7%) is shown in Figure 1. In the whole set of Group I patients mean glycosylated hemoglobin was maintained somewhat above the upper limit of normal. The mean basal and stimulated plasma C-peptide levels of the whole set of Group I patients are shown in Figure 1. It is apparent that these increased from subnormal levels at entry into the "low normal" range, and were preserved at these levels in the mean through 1 year during administration of ciclosporin.

Comparison of insulin-requiring (IR) and non-insulin-requiring (NIR) subjects

In Figure 2 the responses of NIR and IR patients are compared. The subjects' characteristics are shown in Table 2. This set of 38 patients from Group I comprises all those patients who reached 1 year of ciclosporin therapy at this analysis. In accounting for the total of 47 patients under consideration in Group I, it is noted that 4 volunteers did not reach 1 year from entry at this date. In 5 further volunteers administration of ciclosporin was interrupted. This decision was made on the basis of non-compliance with therapy and follow-up in 2 subjects; at the unexplained decision to withdraw by 1 subject; after the recognition of a thyroid adenoma (which proved to be benign) in a fourth subject;

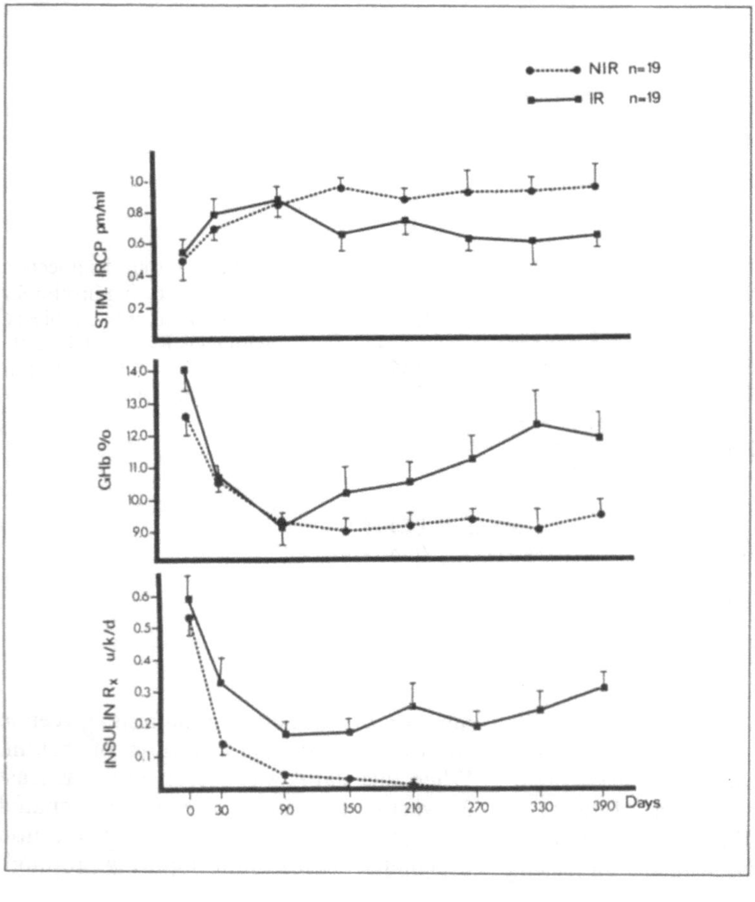

Fig. 2. All group I subjects with ciclosporin $R_x \geqq 1$ year (NIR set not requiring insulin $\geqq 1$ yr)

	CyA R_x > 1 yr			N=38 (basal/stim CP) BCP/SCP		
	D^NDM days	Age yrs	Sex (n)	Ins, entry U/K/D	BCP/SCP, entry (pmol/ml)	
NIR, at 1 yr	19	X̄ 18.3	M 11, F 8	0.55	0.27	0.52
(n=19)	4	±1.8		0.06	0.07	0.12
IR, at 1 yr	19	X̄ 15.4	M 12, F 7	0.60	0.27	0.57
(n=19)	2±SEM	2.2		0.08	0.03	0.06

Table 2. Group I subjects: receiving insulin <6 weeks at entry, and CyA for >1 year at analysis

and because of recurrent non-specific infections in the fifth subject. It can be seen that target control of glycemia was maintained in the NIR group, and that their mean IRCP level in the plasma was higher than that in the IR group in the latter period of treatment. The mean glycosylated hemoglobin level was in the normal range in the subset of patients who discontinued insulin therapy, but was higher in the IR group. Thus insulin was not withdrawn at the cost of optimal control of glycemia, and the continuing need for insulin in the group designated insulin-requiring is apparent. The characteristics of the IR and NIR sets of patients are shown in Table 2.

Effects of interruption of ciclosporin therapy in Type I diabetes

According to the protocol agreed for this study, administration of ciclosporin was to be continued for 6 months in the absence of contra-indication, and through 12 months if it was judged that there may be benefit to the subjects. In the event therefore, administration of ciclosporin was continued through 12 months and more in the Group I volunteers. It has been pointed out that, among the 47 volunteers in this group who reached 200 days or more of therapy with ciclosporin, the drug was withdrawn in 5 subjects before 1 year of therapy had been attained. The reasons for these discontinuations have been documented above. As volunteers in Group I reached approximately 1 year of therapy, the question of discontinuation was considered individually. It has now been agreed to continue the therapy to 18 months in those patients with perceived benefit who do not wish to discontinue earlier. However, administration of ciclosporin has been interrupted in a total of 24 subjects who received ciclosporin for a mean total of 369 days (Table 3), and who have been followed for 30 days thereafter. The serial determinations of basal and stimulated C-peptide and glycosylated hemoglobin, and the daily insulin requirement are illustrated in Figure 3. It can be seen that the mean values for C-peptide in the plasma declined after interruption of therapy. This was associated with increments of the mean glycohemoglobin levels, and of mean daily insulin dosage. Of the 7 volunteers who were non-insulin-requiring at discontinuation of ciclosporin therapy, 6 relapsed to insulin requirement within 160 days of interruption, and the 7th had been followed

(n=24)	Age	Sex (n)	Ins dose entry U/K/D	D^NDM days	At dc CyA BCP/SCP pmol/ml	
X̄	15.4	M 16, F 8	0.60	16.2	0.41	0.66
±SE	1.9		0.05	2.6	0.04	0.05

(Mean duration CyA R_x 369±18 days)

Table 3. Group I patients – follow-up of all subjects who discontinued CyA, after >200 days of this R_x (Patient characteristics for those with >30 days follow-up)

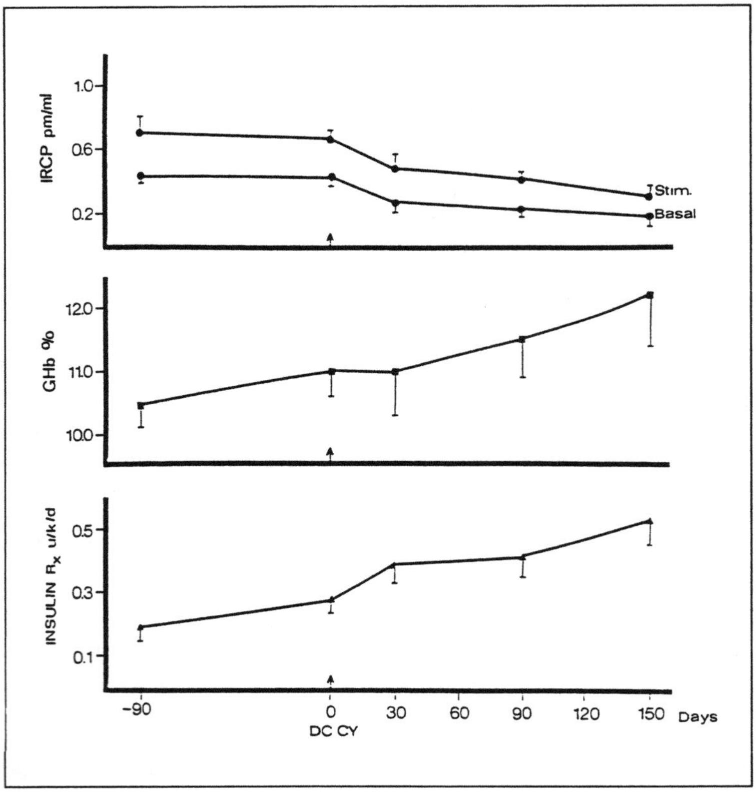

Fig. 3. Plasma IRCP, gHb%, and insulin dose in 24 subjects after DC CyA R_x (gpI) of >200 days duration (mean 369 ± 18)

for 90 days at this analysis. These observations suggest that progressive loss of B-cell function is resumed soon after discontinuation of ciclosporin under these conditions.

Adverse effects of ciclosporin

In the course of this pilot study the well-recognized adverse effects of ciclosporin were encountered, as documented elsewhere. These effects were not apparently different or more severe than those encountered in other experience with the drug. In addition, in this study the development of mild anemia was clearly documented for the first time. This effect was not progressive, and, like the other adverse effects, proved to be fully reversible on discontinuation of the drug. As discussed elsewhere in this symposium, the fall in creatinine clearance observed during ciclosporin treatment under these conditions was reversed within 60 days of discontinuation of the drug in subjects with diabetes who had been treated for up to 15 months.

Discussion

Although no experimental control subjects were entered in this pilot study, tentative comparisons can be made with historical experience of clinical remission to the NIR state in recent onset Type I diabetes mellitus. Historical control data also document the time-course of spontaneous partial recovery and subsequent decline of IR C-peptide levels in the blood in Type I diabetes mellitus. In addition, comparisons can be made within this pilot study in terms of observations of C-peptide levels in Group I and Group II subjects studied under the same conditions.

Apparent "complete" remission in Type I diabetes mellitus, recognized by maintenance of acceptable control of glycemia without continued administration of

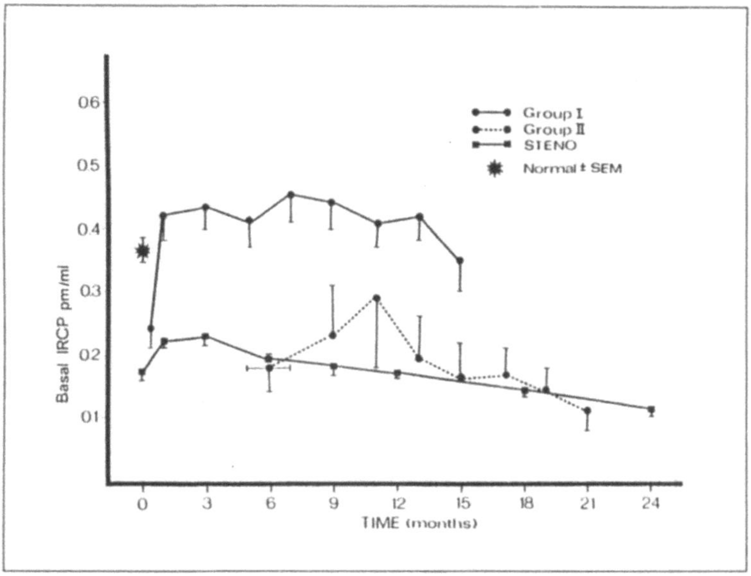

Fig. 4. Basal C-peptide (months post diagnosis)

insulin, has been documented in conventional clinical experience. In a large population-based record such remissions occurred in 5% of patients during the first year of diabetes [2]. However, in other circumstances higher remission rates have been observed. Notably, in the trial of treatment with interferon in newly diagnosed Type I diabetes in Helsinki, under double-blinded conditions approximately 50% of both placebo and interferon-treated subjects entered non-insulin-requiring remissions within 6 months, but in both groups relapse during the second 6 months reduced the incidence of non-insulin-requirement to approximately 15% at one year [3]. These observations contrast with the maintenance of non-insulin-requiring remission in 50% of ciclosporin-treated patients (and in 43% of the set, considered in the light of intention-to-treat) at 1 year of therapy in the present study. It may therefore be inferred that under controlled conditions the putative effect of ciclosporin on insulin requirement might not be apparent until after a period of treatment exceeding 6 months. For this reason the results of studies of shorter duration may be misleading.

The apparent enhancement and preservation of relatively high levels of C-peptide in the blood in basal and stimulated states in Group I subjects in the present study also contrast with other reports of the time-course of secretion of C-peptide in the early months of Type I diabetes. Figure 4 illustrates the basal C-peptide levels in the plasma of Group I and Group II subjects in the present study, in comparison with historical control values determined in a large-scale prospective study carried out at the Steno Hospital in Denmark [4]. It can be seen that C-peptide levels rose into the normal range in Group I subjects within a month of initiation of ciclosporin therapy and were maintained in this range through 15 months of immunosuppression. These values contrast with those determined in the Danish study. It is also apparent that at entry the Group II subjects in the pilot study had basal C-peptide levels in the plasma which were not significantly different from those of the historical control subjects. During administration of ciclosporin in these 8 subjects there was a mean (but not significant) rise in basal C-peptide levels, and after withdrawal of ciclosporin at approximately 12 months of diabetes the mean level declined, and remained close to the historical control levels of the Danish subjects. It is noted that the basal C-peptide data from the other 3 Group II patients in the pilot study have been omitted from this comparison. These 3 subjects received ciclosporin for 1 year, having developed basal C-peptide levels in the range encountered in Group I patients at 6 months of ciclosporin treatment. The selected set of Group II subjects presented in the figure provide local historical control data for subjects with Type I diabetes not receiving ciclosporin at the latest time-point indicated in the figure, when their mean basal C-peptide levels related to the duration of diabetes were significantly lower than those of the Group I subjects.

With regard to the response of non-insulin-requiring Group I subjects to ingestion of glucose during ciclosporin therapy, observations in a subset of these volunteers have demonstrated that they exhibit significant but subnormal release of C-peptide and free immunoreactive insulin after ingestion of glucose, whereas intravenous infusion of glucose resulting in simulation of the oral glucose tolerance curves is associated with little or no response of C-peptide or free immunoreactive insulin [5]. In this respect these volunteers resemble the siblings of patients with Type I diabetes studied in the prodromal phase before development of overt hyperglycemia [6]. It could therefore be suggested that under ciclosporin therapy the NIR subjects in the present study reverted to a status similar to that of subjects with pre-clinical Type I diabetes mellitus. It is apparent, however, that oral glucose tolerance is abnormal in these patients, who remain evidently diabetic by this criterion. It is also important to note that it is not possible to exclude effects of ciclosporin therapy on insulin secretion or intermediary metabolism. We have demonstrated that administration of ciclosporin by mouth in dogs, with maintenance of blood levels of the drug similar to those employed in human therapy, can lead to inhibition of release of insulin in response to intravenous administration of glucose, associated with impairment of glucose tolerance [7]. It is therefore important to examine the effects of ciclosporin on intermediary metabolism and insulin secretion in non-diabetic and diabetic states. It should be added that we have also reported that the presence or absence of islet cell cytoplasmic antibodies in the patients' serum did not predict the apparent response to ciclosporin [8].

Summary

The results of this pilot study suggest that initiation of immunosuppression with ciclosporin within 6 weeks of the start of insulin therapy in clinically diagnosed Type I diabetes mellitus results in enhancement and preservation of unexpectedly high levels of endogenous secretion of insulin. The patients' status seems to be similar to that of the relatively small proportion of patients with Type I diabetes who develop a prolonged clinical remission phase, in which control of glycemia is relatively easy with simple insulin regimens, or is maintained in some without administration of insulin. It is noted that under these conditions both insulin-requiring and non-insulin-requiring subjects appear to be free of hyperinsulinemia. Thus the risks of long-term hyperglycemia and hyperinsulinemia might be reduced, with improvement of the prognosis in diabetes, if this condition could be maintained. These plausible possible benefits of immunosuppression justify the performance of controlled clinical trials designed to confirm the apparent effects of administration of ciclosporin in recent onset Type I diabetes mellitus, and to assess the relative risks and benefits of conventional therapy by comparison with this experimental intervention.

References

1. Stiller CR, Dupre J, Gent M, Jenner MR, Keown PA, Laupacis A, Martell R, Rodger NW, v Graffenried B, Wolfe BMJ (1984) Effects of Cyclosporin Immunosuppression in insulin-dependent diabetes mellitus of recent origin. Science 223: 1362–1367
2. Drash AL, Leporte R, Daneman D, Fishbine H, Goldstein D, Becker D (1983) Insulin requirements in children with diabetes mellitus: Change of requirements by age and sex over the initial 5 years of therapy. In: Akerblom H (ed) The Remission Period: Pediatric and Adolescent Endocrinology. Karger, Basel
3. Koivisto VA, Aro A, Cantell K, Haataja M, Huttunen J, Karonen S-L, Mustajoki P, Pel-

konen R, Seppala P (1984) Remissions in newly diagnosed Type I (insulin-dependent) diabetes: Influence of interferon as an adjunct to insulin therapy. Diabetologia 27:193–197
4. Data communicated to the authors by Binder C, Nerup J et al. Steno Hospital, Gentofte, Denmark
5. Dupre J, Stiller CR, Behme M, Gent M, Jenner MR, Keown PA, Laupacis A, Martell R, Rodger NW, Wolfe BMJ (1984) Effects of ciclosporin in Type I diabetes: insulin secretion. Diabetes 33:157A
6. Srikanta S, Granda OP, Gleason RE, Jackson RA, Soeldner JS, Eisenbarth GS (1984) Pre-Type I diabetes: Linear loss of beta cell response to intravenous glucose. Diabetes 33:717–726
7. Unpublished observations of the authors
8. Mandrup-Poulsen T, Stiller CR, Bille G, Martell R, Keown PA, Rodger NW, v Graffenried B, Nerup J, Marner B, Heinrichs D, Dupre J, Jenner MR, Wolfe BMW, Binder C (1985) Disappearance and re-appearance of islet-cell cytoplasmic antibodies in ciclosporin-treated insulin-dependent diabetics. Lancet 1:599–602

Ciclosporin in Insulin-dependent Diabetes Mellitus: Design of Controlled Studies

B. von Graffenried

Based on the results of pilot studies from Stiller [2] and Assan [1] four large, placebo-controlled, double-blind studies have recently started in Canada, Europe and the US. The main characteristics of these studies are shown in the Table.

The aim of these studies is to test the hypothesis, generated from pilot studies, that immunosuppression with ciclosporin (CyA) arrests autoimmune isletitis and further destruction of pancreatic beta cells and induces and maintains clinical remission. The hope is that maintenance of endogenous insulin secretion will change the natural course of the disease and, by prevention of long-term vascular complications, provide relevant benefit to patients with acceptable risk. It must be realized that the currently ongoing studies are only the first, but nevertheless an essential, step to evaluating such benefit. The primary aim of the studies is to examine the question of remission-inducing efficacy in relation to the safety of the drug. The potential benefit of such an effect obviously requires many years of follow-up and larger patient numbers. The series of studies which have now started and which are very demanding for both patients and investigators will, however, enrol enough patients to prove or disprove efficacy. In the light of the potential risks of any form of immunosuppressive therapy and of the specific side effects of CyA, and in agreement with the conclusions of a recent Workshop on immunosuppression in the management of Type I diabetes [3], Sandoz Ltd. is of the opinion that, before results of the now ongoing studies become available, further studies are not justified. In this connection it also recommends not treating patients outside these studies.

Clinical Research Department, Sandoz Ltd., Basle, Switzerland

Table 1. Controlled studies with ciclosporin (CyA) in insulin-dependent diabetes mellitus

Studies
- Canadian-European Diabetes Study Group (11 centres)
- French multicentre study (6 centres)
- Two single-centre studies in USA
- In each study 100 – 200 patients

Design
- Randomized, stratified, controlled, parallel-group studies (insulin + CyA versus insulin + placebo)
- Stratification: Age, ketoacidosis at diagnosis
- Double-blind (2 separated teams: team 1 unmasked, responsible for dosage of CyA, safety monitoring; team 2 masked, responsible for diabetes therapy)

Entry criteria
- Recent-onset IDDM (entry to study within 4 – 12 weeks after diagnosis)
- Age: 9 – 40 years
- Strict exclusion criteria with respect to safety aspects
- Informed consent

Dosage, duration of therapy
- CyA: 7.5 – 10 mg/kg/day oral as initial dose. Dose adjustments according to CyA levels, renal function and other side effects/complications
- 6 – 18 months of therapy. Further therapy in remitters depending on results of continuing pilot studies.
- Early withdrawal of CyA in non-responders (switch to placebo)
- Follow-up: 5 years

End points
- Complete remission at defined points in time, defined by insulin requirement, blood glucose, glycosylated Hg and C-peptide
- Safety, side effects

Further investigations
- Extensive safety monitoring
- Immunological studies
- Metabolic studies

References

1. Assan R, Feutren G, Debray-Sachs M, et al. (1985) Metabolic and immunological effects of Cyclosporin in recently diagnosed type 1 diabetes mellitus. Lancet I:67
2. Stiller CR, Dupré J, Gent M, et al. (1984) Effects of Cyclosporin immunosuppression in insulin-dependent diabetes mellitus of recent onset. Science 223:1362
3. Summary of a Workshop on immunosuppression in the management of type 1 diabetes mellitus (IDD), Diabetes Research Program (1983) National Institute of Health. N Engl J Med 309:1199

4. Uveitis and Behçet's Disease

Effectiveness of Ciclosporin on Sight-threatening Endogenous Uveitis

R. B. Nussenblatt

Introduction

The term intra-ocular inflammatory disease or uveitis is a generalized term that in no way reflects the location, duration, etiology, or severity of a particular case. Indeed, the potential visual compromise resulting from uveitis is quite variable. Uveitis is the cause of about 10% of visual handicap in the U.S. [18], with an estimated cost of $ 10 million for the care of uveitis patients per year [19]. Though initially theorized as being due to infections, such as syphilis and tuberculosis, the causes of these intra-ocular inflammations are very varied, sometimes depending on a subtle yet complex combination of exogenous trigger mechanisms and endogenous immune dysregulation.

The disorders can be divided anatomically into two groups.

1. Anterior uveitis: This disorder primarily affects the front portion of the globe. One of the most common types of anterior uveitis is that which is HLA-B27 associated in about 80% of Caucasian patients [2]. This type of uveitis is usually unilateral in its presentation, but can re-appear in either eye. In the main this disorder is recurrent but will not cause irreversible visual loss in the majority of cases. However, anterior uveitis can lead to secondary sight-threatening conditions, which include glaucoma, band keratopathy, and cataract. On occasion, an anterior uveitis can be a manifestation of a severe inflammation located more posteriorly in the eye.

The etiology of this disorder has been associated with gram negative bacteria. Patients with active anterior uveitis as well as ankylosing spondylitis have been noted to have gram negative organisms in their gut more often than controls do [3]. Additionally, LPS injections into lower mammals at a site far from the globe will induce an anterior uveitis with some characteristics of the disease seen in man [16]. It has been suggested that an antigenic cross reactivity exists between the vitreous and gram negative bacterial cell walls, hence explaining the localization of the immune response to the eye [1]. It has been suggested that LPS may stimulate B-cell clonal expansion by an adjuvant effect which is capable of short-circuiting the T-cell's normally tight control on this part of the immune response. It is therefore felt that this disorder may be antibody or immune complex mediated.

2. Intermediate and posterior uveitis: These disorders mainly affect the vitreal cavity and posterior portion of the eye. They are usually painless at onset, with the patient noting hazy or blurred vision. These disorders can lead to many complications resulting in a marked drop in visual acuity. These complications include vitreal opacities, retinal vascular obstructions, retinal degenerative alterations, neovascularization of the retina and other areas, cystoid macula edema, and retinal detachment.

The etiology of posterior uveitis is known in some conditions, such as toxoplasmosis and cytomegalovirus retinitis, but speculative in others. Strong HLA associations have been noted in some of these disorders, such as birdshot retinochoroidopathy (HLA-A29) [7], a disease essentially localized to the eye, and Behçet's syndrome (HLA-B51) [13], a disease involving many organ systems. The four major criteria of Behçet's disease are mouth and genital ulcers, skin lesions, and usually severe anterior uveitis and/or a posterior obliterative type of uveitis [4]. The disorder appears to be more frequently seen in the Mediterranean basin and in Japan, with the risk of

---

Clinical Ophthalmic Immunology Section, National Eye Institute, Clinical Branch, NIH, Bethesda, MD blindness in these patients being quite high. Evidence for autoimmune retinal responses has been noted in posterior uveitis patients. Of particular note is that posterior uveitis patients' lymphocytes will frequently respond in culture to the highly uveitogenic purified retinal S-antigen [5, 7], a glycoprotein of 55,000 capable of inducing an experimental autoimmune uveitis in lower mammals and non-human primates [20]. Work has shown that this laboratory model for human disease requires the mandatory participation of T-cells [17], and by extension their role may be inferred in the human condition as well.

Treatment: For most cases of anterior uveitis, topical corticosteroid and mydriatic therapy will be quite effective. More severe cases may require peri-ocular or systemic corticosteroid administration. Nonsteroidal anti-inflammatory agents have not been found to be particularly effective. Uveitis affecting the posterior segment usually requires either periocular and/or systemic corticosteroid intervention. In severe cases, cytotoxic agents have been employed. For Behçet's syndrome, adequate treatments for the ocular manifestations have been lacking, with colchicine and cytotoxic agents until now being the only available therapeutic modalities [9].

Because of the particularly profound effects of ciclosporin (CyA) on the S-antigen-induced experimental autoimmune uveitis model [6], CyA therapy for selected uveitis patients with this drug was begun in the fall of 1981.

Effectiveness of ciclosporin in the treatment of endogenous intermediate and posterior uveitis

To date, over 70 patients have been treated in the open trial. The indications for therapy included a bilateral intermediate or posterior uveitis of noninfectious etiology [8, 10]. These individuals needed to have been actively treated with either systemic corticosteroids or cytotoxic agents, and must have been either a therapeutic failure or unable to continue because of intolerable side effects. The patients needed to have clinically active disease and a visual acuity of 20/40 (6/9) or worse in both eyes. All patients were carefully evaluated for evidence of systemic disease, particularly renal or hepatic, and underlying neoplasm or infection. Patients were begun on 10 mg/kg/day of ciclosporin orally, while any cytotoxic therapy was discontinued at least two weeks prior to therapy and corticosteroid therapy was tapered as rapidly as was medically indicated.

In some patients an increase in visual acuity could be noted within the first month after the initiation of therapy. This was followed by an improvement in the vitreal haze which dissipated before vitreal cellular activity did. This improvement was observed to be maintained for an extended period, with three-month and one-year visual acuities demonstrating similar improvements as noted earlier on in the therapeutic trial. Further, the continued effectiveness of this mode of therapy can be seen in the 35 patients who have reached an 18-month follow-up (Fig. 1). The comparison of visual acuities prior to the initiation of therapy to that at 18 months shows that most patients have maintained an improvement in vision. Further, a comparison of vitreal haze prior to CyA therapy and after 18 months of this treatment demon-

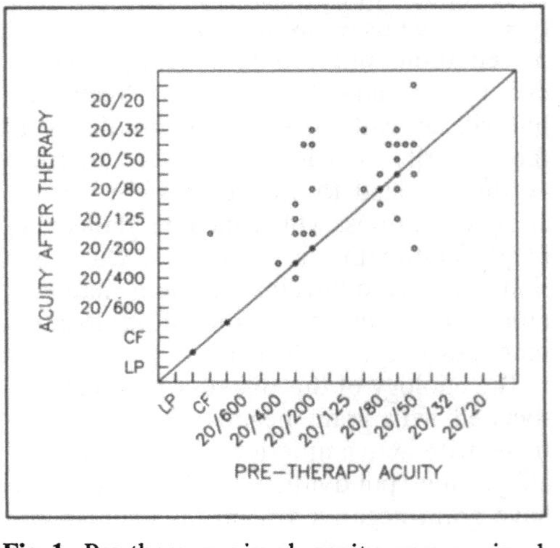

Fig. 1. Pre-therapy visual acuity versus visual acuity after 18 months of CyA therapy. All patients were steroid and/or cytotoxic agent failures.

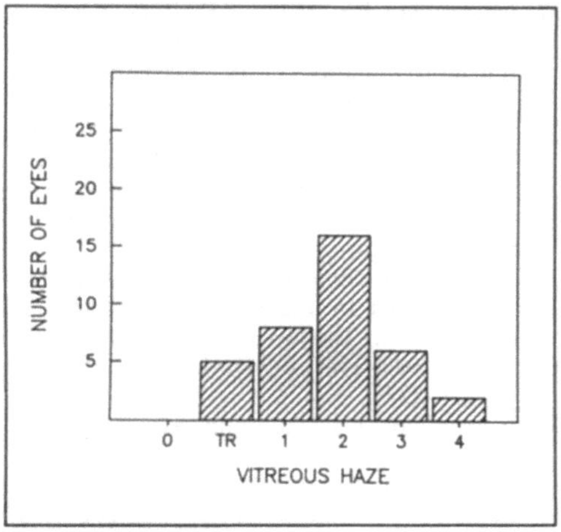

Fig. 2a. Vitreous haze before CyA therapy

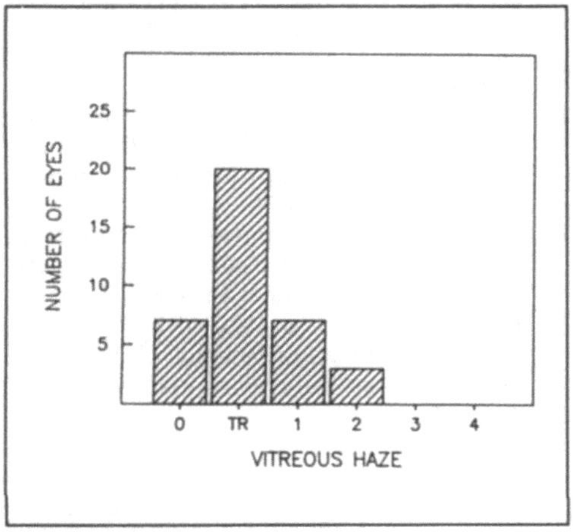

Fig. 2b. Vitreous haze after 18 months of CyA therapy

strates a dramatic difference (Fig. 2). The types of ocular conditions that have been treated at the National Eye Institute with ciclosporin include intermediate uveitis of both the non-pars planitis and pars planitis type, sarcoid uveitis, sympathetic ophthalmia, Vogt-Koyanagi-Harada's disease, birdshot retinochoroidopathy, serpiginous choroiditis and Behçet's disease. Patients with pars planitis and Behçet's disease appear to be particularly good candidates for this form of therapy. We have noted that the acute ocular episode of the posterior pole of Behçet's disease can be controlled. More importantly, the number of ocular attacks appears to be diminished considerably on ciclosporin therapy [12]. The recurrent attacks are accepted as the reason for the generally poor visual outcome of these patients. We have not noted that CyA has had any dramatic effect on the clinical course of serpiginous choroiditis.

These encouraging long-term results led to the initiation of a randomized double-masked study comparing the effectiveness of CyA to that of prednisone therapy in patients with severe sight-threatening endogenous uveitis. To date, over 50 patients have been enrolled in this study, but preliminary data are not yet available.

Several parameters, both clinical and immunologic, have been followed in the uveitis patients treated with ciclosporin. Cystoid macula edema that is noted in many uveitis patients may ultimately disappear with CyA therapy. However, an improvement in visual acuity was frequently noted before any dramatic changes of retinal vascular leakage could be identified with fluorescein angiography. We have found that the laser interferometer has been an effective tool to determine whose visual acuity may improve with CyA therapy.

Of interest has been the finding that the visually evoked response in an intermediate uveitis patient with concomitant optic nerve disease secondary to multiple sclerosis improved with CyA therapy. The changes in the latency period are characteristically found in the optic neuritis associated with multiple sclerosis. Interestingly, the visual evoked response returned to its original configuration once ciclosporin was discontinued.

All patients are tested for their S-antigen responses before the initiation of therapy. We have noted that both S-antigen "responders" and "non-responders" can have a beneficial response to ciclosporin therapy. Ciclosporin plasma levels are also followed in these patients. A direct relationship of therapeutic response or toxicity to specific plasma levels has not been readily noted by us, and requires further study.

As with all medications, secondary effects will be noted if used long enough and in a large enough number of patients. We have not, to date, observed ciclosporin-associated neoplasms in our patients. We have, however, noted significant renal toxicity in approximately 30% of our patients. Our patients have noted previously described cyclosporin-associated changes. These include transient fatigue, gingival changes, increased hair growth, and increased sensitivity to hot and cold stimuli [15]. To date, there have been no demonstrated opportunistic infections in the uveitis patients. We have reported that our patients have normal natural killer cell activity while taking ciclosporin [8]. A recent study completed by us would suggest as well that these patients are capable of responding both humorally and cellularly to new antigen challenges [14].

We have found that ciclosporin has been both a powerful immune probe as well as a potential new therapeutic modality for the treatment of severe noninfectious uveitis. Only under the stringent conditions of a double-masked randomized trial will a scientifically useful answer have an opportunity to be arrived at. Ciclosporin's contribution to our continuing attempt at understanding basic mechanisms and relating them to more rational therapy is well established, and has set the course for a most exciting future.

References

1. Avakian H, Abuknesha R, Welsh J, Fibringer A (1981) Uveitis, vitreous humor, and Klebsiella. I. Binding studies with rabbit antisera. Br J Ophthalmol 65:315
2. Brewerton DA, Caffrey M, Nicholls A, Walters D, James DCO (1973) Acute anterior uveitis and HL-A27. Lancet 2:994
3. Ebringer RW, Cawdell DR, Cowling P, Ebringer A (1978) Sequential studies in ankylosing spondylitis. Ann Rheum Dis 37:146
4. Editorial (1974) Jpn J Ophthalmol 18:291
5. Nussenblatt RB, Gery I, Ballintine EJ, Wacker WB (1980) Cellular immune responsiveness of uveitis patients to retinal S-antigen. Am J Ophthalmol 89:173
6. Nussenblatt RB, Rodrigues MR, Wacker WB, Cevario SJ, Salinas-Carmona MC, Gery I (1981) Inhibition of experimental autoimmune uveitis in Lewis rats. J Clin Invest 67:1228
7. Nussenblatt RB, Mittal KK, Ryan S, Green WR, Maumenee AF (1982) Birdshot retinochoroidopathy – an association with HLA-A29 and immune responsiveness to retinal S-antigen. Am J Ophthalmol 94:147
8. Nussenblatt RB, Palestine AG, Rook AH, Scher I, Wacker WB, Gery I (1982) Treatment of intraocular inflammatory disease with Cyclosporin A. Lancet I:235
9. Nussenblatt RB (1983) Treatment of autoimmune uveitis. In: Lichtenstein LM, Fauci AS (eds) Current Therapy in Allergy and Immunology 1983–1984. BC Decker, Philadelphia, pp 224–227
10. Nussenblatt RB, Palestine AG, Chan CC (1983) Cyclosporin A therapy in the treatment of intraocular inflammatory disease resistant to systemic corticosteroids and cytotoxic agents. Am J Ophthalmol 96:275
11. Nussenblatt RB, Palestine AG, Chan CC, Breen L, Caruso R (1984) Improvement of uveitis and optic nerve disease by Cyclosporine in a patient with multiple sclerosis. Am J Ophthalmol 97:790
12. Nussenblatt RB, Palestine AG, Chan CC, Mochizuki M, Yancey K (1985) Effectiveness of Cyclosporine therapy for Behçet's disease. Arthritis Rheum 28:671
13. Ohno S (1981) Immunological aspects of Behçet's and Vogt-Koyanagi-Harada's diseases. Trans Ophthalmol Soc UK 101:335
14. Palestine AG, Nussenblatt RB, Chan CC (1984) Side effects of systemic Cyclosporine in patients not undergoing transplantation. Am J Med 77:542
15. Palestine AG, Roberge F, Charous BL, Lane HC, Fauci AS, Nussenblatt RB (1985) The effect of Cyclosporine on immunization with tetanus and KLH in humans. J Clin Immunol, 5:115
16. Rosenbaum JT, McDewitt HO, Guss RB, Egbert PR (1980) Endotoxin-induced uveitis in rats as a model for human disease. Nature 286:611
17. Salinas-Carmona MC, Nussenblatt RB, Gery I (1982) Experimental autoimmune uveitis in the athymic nude rat. Eur J Immunol 12:480
18. U.S. DHEW: DHS, NIH (1976) Interim Report of the National Advisory Eye Council. Support for Vision Research, pp 20–22
19. Vision Research. A National Plan 1983–1987. Report of the Retinal and Choroidal Diseases Panel. Vol 2, 1983, p 33
20. Wacker WB, Donoso LA, Kalsow CM, Yankeelov Jr JA, Organisciak DT (1977) Experimental allergic uveitis. Isolation, characterization, and localization of a soluble uveitopathogenic antigen from bovine retina. J Immunol 119:1949

Treatment of Noninfectious Inflammatory Disorders of the Eye with Ciclosporin

P. Le Hoang and M. Fontaine

Since November 1983, we have been conducting an open pilot study in which we have treated 31 patients with various ocular inflammatory disorders of noninfectious origin. Previous studies have already shown the effectiveness of ciclosporin in the management of intra-ocular inflammation (1–5).

4 patients presented external inflammatory eye diseases:

- 2 Mooren's ulcer
- 2 ocular pemphigoid

27 patients had posterior uveitis. These comprised:

- 5 Behçet's disease
- 5 birdshot retinochoroidopathy
- 12 idiopathic retinal vasculitis
- 2 sarcoidosis
- 2 serpiginous choroiditis
- 1 sclerouveitis associated with polychondritis

26 out of 31 patients were either resistant to, intolerant to or dependent upon previous treatment with high doses of steroids, immunosuppressive cytotoxic agents or plasma exchanges. 5 patients were treated directly with ciclosporin. All the patients initially received 10 mg/kg/day of ciclosporin, the dose being adjusted according to plasma ciclosporin levels, serum creatinine levels, and of course clinical observations. The effectiveness of therapy was evaluated according to visual acuity, visual fields, inflammatory activity and fluorescein angiography.

Service d'ophthalmologie, Hôpital la Pitié Paris, France

Results

A) Results concerning posterior uveitis patients (n = 27): these patients can be divided into 3 groups:

1. *In the first group,* 12 patients were treated with ciclosporin alone (n = 12) and we observed positive results in 75% of the cases (9/12). This means that either visual acuity improved, or intraocular inflammation diminished, or both.
The period of follow-up ranged between 3 and 15 months. Indeed, for a majority of the responding patients (6/9) it was possible to decrease the necessary doses of ciclosporin to 5 mg/kg/day and sometimes to 3 mg/kg/day.
2. *In the second group,* 10 patients were treated with ciclosporin associated with steroids. Under this protocol, it was possible to significantly decrease or even eliminate (3 patients) concomitant steroid therapy. The doses of steroids could be reduced by 83%. All of these patients responded positively.
3. *In the third group,* 5 patients were treated with ciclosporin in conjunction with steroids but the dosage of the latter could *not* be reduced. Nonetheless, 3 of these patients maintained or improved their visual acuity.

No correlation could be found between our findings and the type of posterior uveitis or the immunological reactivity to retinal S-antigen. However, patients with birdshot retinochoroidopathy tend to respond consistently better regardless of the protocol followed.

B) Results concerning external inflammatory eye diseases:
In contrast, patients suffering from external inflammatory eye diseases did not respond to ciclosporin (n = 4).

Side Effects

In spite of the promising positive results obtained with ciclosporin we must take into consideration the side effects observed. Some of these were benign:

- asthenia (17)
- hyperesthesia (13)
- hirsutism (9)
- gingival hypertrophy (9)
- gastrointestinal intolerance (8)
- muscle spasms (7)
- headaches (6)
- backaches (2)
- gynecomastia (2)

Others however, were more serious:

- above all, nephrotoxicity in 16 cases, which has been shown to be reversible within 3 months after discontinuation of ciclosporin in all but one case
- 9 patients developed hypertension which was controllable
- mild hepatotoxicity was observed in 5 cases (as assessed by gamma glutamyl transferase serum levels)
- 3 cases of moderate anemia occurred.

It must be noted that all of these side effects regressed when ciclosporin was decreased or withdrawn. Therapy was interrupted in 4 cases owing to unpleasant side effects and in one case as a result of nephrotoxicity. No lymphomas were observed.

Conclusion

- 22 out of 27 posterior uveitis patients demonstrated positive results following ciclosporin treatment.
- However, the only valid method for defining the effectiveness of ciclosporin is that of the randomized study, in which connection a paper will be presented by our colleagues.

Reference

1. Graham EM, Sanders MD, James DG, Hamblin A, Grochowska EK, Dumonde D (1985) Cyclosporin A in the treatment of posterior uveitis. Trans Ophthalmol Soc UK 104:146
2. Le Hoang P, Fontaine M, Khalaf A, de Kozak Y, Debre P, Aupetit B, Thillaye B, Nussenblatt RB (1984) Treatment of severe posterior uveitis with cyclosporine A: preliminary results in France. 1st International Symposium on Uveitis, Hanasaari, Espoo, Finland, 16th–19th May 1984
3. Le Hoang P, Fontaine M, Khalaf A, Travers C, Saraux H, Loscas G, Massin M, Bernard JA, Gaudric A, de Kozak Y, Nussenblatt RB: Traitement des uvites non infectieuses par un nouvel immunomodulateur, la cyclosporine A. Société d'Ophthalmologie de Paris, France (Communication du 18 février 1984). Bull Soc Ophthalmol Fr (in press)
4. Nussenblatt RB, Palestine AG, Rook AH, Scher I, Wacker WB, Gery I (1982) Treatment of intraocular inflammatory disease with Cyclosporin A. Lancet I:235
5. Nussenblatt RB, Palestine AG, Chan CC (1983) Cyclosporin A therapy in the treatment of intraocular inflammatory disease resistant to systemic corticosteroids and cytotoxic agnet. Am J Ophthalmol 96:275

Ciclosporin (CyA) in the Treatment of Retinal Vasculitis

E. Graham [1], M. D. Sanders [1], A. Binder [2], A. M. Denman [2] and W. Dinning [3]

Summary

Seventeen patients with severe posterior uveitis and retinal vasculitis were treated with CyA. An initial improvement occurred in all cases and persisted until the dose was reduced or the drug withdrawn, when a rapid recurrence of symptoms was noted.

Ten patients did not complete the year of therapy, owing to deterioration of renal function (5 cases), severe malaise and nausea (4 cases) and blindness (1 case).

Patients and methods

Seventeen patients with severe posterior uveitis and retinal vasculitis were treated with CyA (Table 1). Patients 1–9 were treated in the Medical Eye Unit at St. Thomas' Hospital and patients 10–17 in Northwick Park Hospital and Moorfields Eye Hospital. There were 12 male and 5 female patients and their ages ranged from 16–47 years. Twelve patients had Behçet's disease, one had sarcoidosis, one had HLA B27 associated disease and three had idiopathic retinal vasculitis. All patients had active severe ocular inflammation and all except patient 11 had been previously treated with systemic steroids and immunosuppressives. The treatment had failed either because it was ineffective or because of intolerable side effects. All patients had a full clinical and ophthalmological examination before treatment, after 2 weeks of treatment and at 1, 3, 6, 9 and 12 months.

Ophthalmological assessment included visual acuity, grading of severity of inflammation [1] and indirect ophthalmoscopy. Fluorescein angiography was performed when possible prior to treatment, after 1 month and thereafter at 3-monthly intervals. Renal and liver function tests were performed before treatment and at monthly intervals thereafter. Only patients with normal renal function at the start were admitted into the study.

The drug was initially given in a dose of 10 mg/kg/day administered as an oily liquid (diluted with fruit juice if preferred) and taken once daily or in divided doses before breakfast and supper. All cytotoxic drugs were stopped prior to commencement of CyA and systemic steroids tailed off. Local steroids and other eye drops were given as clinically indicated. The follow-up period ranged from 2 weeks to 2 years and all patients were followed for at least 3 months after withdrawal of CyA therapy.

The parameters of efficacy were visual acuity, activity index of severity of inflammation and the number of relapses of both ocular and systemic symptoms and the daily steroid dose when compared to a similar period prior to treatment with CyA.

Results

Fifteen patients showed an initial improvement in visual acuity and a decrease in severity of ocular inflammation within 6 weeks of starting treatment. This improvement was maintained whilst the patients remained on a full dosage of CyA (10 mg/kg/day). The systemic features of Behçet's syndrome including oro-genital ulceration were also reduced during this time. Patient 5, developed hypopyon uveitis immediately prior to his first dose of CyA. The hypopyon did not resolve over 48 hours on CyA and consequently high dose prednisolone had to be added to the regime. Patient

1 Medical Eye Unit, St. Thomas' Hospital, London, SE1

2 Clinical Research Centre, Northwick Park Hospital, Harrow, Middlesex.

3 Moorfields Eye Hospital, City Road, London, EC1

Table 1. The effect of ciclosporin on visual acuity in 17 patients with posterior uveitis

	Age	Sex	Diagnosis	Length of time on CyA	PRE Rx VA		Post Rx VA		Side effects
					R	L	R	L	
1	47	F	Behçet's	5 months	1/60	CF	6/60	6/9*	Severe diarrhoea + vomiting
2	36	F	Idiopathic retinal vasculitis	22 months	6/36	6/12	6/24	6/9	'Rebound' uveitis
3	23	M	Sarcoidosis	22 months	6/9	6/60	6/18	CF	Hypertension, poor renal function, 'rebound' uveitis
4	23	M	Arthritis and uveitis (HLA B27)	5 months	6/5	HM	6/5	HM	Exacerbation of arthritis
5	36	M	Behçet's	5 months	6/36	6/60	3/60	3/60	Hypertension, poor renal function
6	38	M	Idiopathic retinal vasculitis	5 months	6/5	6/18	6/5	6/24	
7	26	M	Idiopathic retinal vasculitis	2 weeks	6/9	HM	6/9	HM	Severe hypertension, peripheral oedema
8	24	M	Behçet's	9 months	6/36	6/60	6/60	CF	Reduced renal function, 'rebound' uveitis
9	28	F	Behçet's	14 months	HM	6/60	6/36	6/36	
10	31	M	Behçet's	18 months	CF	PL	CF	PL	
11	16	M	Behçet's	10 months	CF	6/5	HM	6/5	Reduced renal function, 'rebound' uveitis
12	34	M	Behçet's	12 months	PL	6/12	6/36	6/5	Reduced renal function, 'rebound' uveitis
13	24	M	Behçet's	3 months	CF	PL	CF	PL	Severe vomiting
14	28	F	Behçet's	16 months	6/9	CF	6/9	6/24	'Rebound' uveitis
15	30	M	Behçet's	3 months	6/36	Pl	6/12	PL	Severe 'rebound' uveitis
16	35	F	Behçet's	10 months	PL	NPL	PL	NPL	
17**	40	M	Behçet's	12 months	6/24	–	6/12	–	

* = Cataract operation performed during Rx; ** = Left eye enucleated before Rx with CyA; VA = visual acuity; CF = counting fingers; PL = perception of light; NPL = no perception of light

6 showed no improvement at all and patient 7 developed severe side effects before the efficacy of the drug could be assessed.

Deterioration of vision occurred in 2 patients who suffered from vitreous haemorrhage in the absence of active inflammation. CyA was stopped for 48 hours in 4 patients (1, 13, 14, 15) because of severe malaise and nausea; uveitis, oro-genital ulceration and thrombophlebitis recurred immediately. In case 15, the uveitis could not be controlled by restarting CyA and permanent visual loss due to retinal vein occlusion ensued.

The uveitis recurred with a consequent drop in visual acuity in 6 patients (patients 2, 3, 5, 8, 11 and 12) when the dose of CyA was reduced because of impaired renal function. Inflammation could be controlled by a reduction in the dose of CyA in case 2 but in all the other patients this was impossible and conventional therapy was reestablished, but with only limited success in patients 11 and 12.

Seven patients completed twelve months of treatment and the daily dose of CyA was then reduced by 50 mg each month but symptoms recurred in all patients when the dose reached 7 mg/kg/day. All these patients chose to remain on 8 mg/kg/day after 12 months as the uveitis had been well controlled on this dose.

Sixteen patients (all except patient 11) were on regular steroid therapy before the start of the study: the daily steroid requirement was halved in fourteen patients from the start to the end of CyA therapy and the relapse rate was halved in all patients when compared to a similar period before treatment with CyA.

Side Effects (Table 2)

Common complaints were a burning sensation in the throat after swallowing the medicine, paraesthesias, and difficulties with body temperature regulation. Eight patients developed gingivitis despite alteration to dental hygiene, but all these patients took the medicine in divided doses. Renal toxicity was the most important side effect: twelve patients developed impaired renal function with a rise in serum creatinine to above 130 μmol/l, a fall in creatinine clearance to less than 40 ml/minute and an increase in urinary N-acetyl glucosaminidase (NAG) excretion to more than 30 μmol creatinine. Five patients had therapy stopped for this reason. Renal function returned to normal in all patients within one month of stopping the drug. Seven patients became hypertensive. Patient 7 developed severe hypertension and peripheral fluid retention within 3 days of starting CyA: the drug was stopped for 48 hours and a diuretic given. CyA therapy was re-established at half the original dose but the symptoms recurred immediately and the drug was withdrawn after only 12 days' therapy. Malaise, vomiting and diarrhoea occurred in eight patients and resulted in withdrawal of therapy in four (patients 1, 13, 14 and 15). One patient developed candida oesophagitis, and six patients minor abnormalities of liver function. Patient 4 had a severe relapse of his arthritis although his ocular inflammation remained well controlled. All these side effects resolved after CyA was stopped, although "rebound" uveitis was often severe and difficult to control with steroids and immunosuppressives.

Table 2. Side effects of ciclosporin therapy in seventeen patients

Side effect	Number of patients
Renal toxicity	12
Malaise and nausea	8
Gingivitis	8
Hypertension	7
Liver toxicity	6
Haemoglobin ↓ (> 2 g/dl)	11
ESR ↑ (> 20 units)	11

Haematological and immunological investigations

The haemoglobin (Hb) concentration decreased by more than 2 g/dl and the ESR increased by more than 20 units in eleven patients during the course of therapy. There was no change in white blood count or lymphocyte count during the study and the immunoglobulin and complement levels were also unaffected. Three patients had elevated circulating immune complexes. Five patients had antibodies to retinal S antigen measured by passive haemagglutination or by immunofluorescence. The lymphocytes of 2 patients (1 and 8) showed positive in vitro transformation to retinal S antigen, both before and during treatment. The reactivity of the lymphocytes of the other patients did not alter during the course of therapy.

Discussion

This uncontrolled study confirms earlier reports that CyA has beneficial effects in the management of severe posterior uveitis and retinal vasculitis irrespective of aetiology [3]. Fifteen of our seventeen patients showed an initial reduction in ocular inflammation accompanied generally by an improvement in visual acuity. However, in the majority of patients this improvement was difficult to maintain because the toxic effects of CyA necessitated reduction of the dose, which provoked relapse of the inflammation.

There are great difficulties in assessing these results: for ethical reasons patients were entered into the trial only if conventional therapy (steroids and immunosuppressives) had failed to control their ocular inflammation. Consequently irreversible retinal damage and vitreous haemorrhage sometimes obscured any benefit produced by CyA. In addition all the conditions studied have a fluctuating course and no control group was included in the trial.

The high incidence of side effects which required the drug to be withdrawn in thirteen patients is worrying; the nature of the renal toxicity is not fully elucidated and although permanent damage has been reported [2], the renal function reverted to normal in all our patients within 2 weeks of reducing the dose below 8 mg/kg/day; in seven patients the inflammation was then difficult to control with conventional therapy. All of these ten patients had shown a substantial drop in haemoglobin concentration and a rise in ESR during CyA therapy; perhaps these features should alert the clinician to impending relapse since only one of the seven patients who did not relapse following reduction of dose showed similar changes in haematological data.

Ciclosporin is a powerful immunosuppressive agent which is effective in the management of inflammatory eye disease. The duration of such benefit is unknown and further controlled studies are being performed to establish the best way to use the drug.

References

1. Dumonde DC, Kasp Grochowska E, Graham E, Sander MD, Faure JP, Kozak Y de, Tuyen V van (1982) Antiretinal autoimmunity and circulating immune complexes in patients with retinal vasculitis. Lancet I:787
2. Myers BD, Ross J, Newton L, Luetscher J, Perlroth M (1984) Cyclosporine associated chronic nephropathy. N Engl J Med 331:699
3. Nussenblatt RB, Palestine AG, Chan C (1983) Cyclosporin A therapy in the treatment of intraocular inflammatory disease resistant to systemic corticosteroids and cytotoxic agents. Am J Ophthalmol 96:172

Ciclosporin Treatment of Autoimmune Inflammatory Disorders of the Eye

K. Bendtzen, C. Nissen, N. Tvede and V. Andersen

The mainstay of the management of sight-threatening, intraocular inflammatory disease of unknown infectious origin is systemic corticosteroids. Unfortunately, moderate doses of these drugs are often not able to control disease activity, and the high doses then necessary lead to intolerable side effects and the prescription of cytotoxic drugs for these often young patients. However, with the advent of ciclosporin (CyA), an alternative to present therapies seems at hand.

CyA is a selective inhibitor of the interleukin 1-mediated activation signal to T-lymphocytes [1, 2]; it has been shown to be effective in the prevention of experimental autoimmune uveitis in rats [5]. Furthermore, the studies by Nussenblatt et al. [6] indicate that CyA may be clinically beneficial in selected cases of autoimmune uveitis.

We report here on our experience with CyA treatment of severe, inflammatory eye disease of presumed autoimmune pathogenesis.

Patients and methods

The study included 17 adults with intraocular inflammatory disease, in whom tests for possible underlying infections were negative. All had verified or potentially sight-threatening disease that had required therapy with corticosteroids or cytotoxic agents (Table 1). Eight had bilateral disease, and one of these patients had already lost an eye as a result of chorioretinitis (No. 10). The clinical diagnoses of the patients are shown in Table 1.

Medical Department TA and Ophthalmic Department E, Rigshospitalet University Hospital, Copenhagen, Denmark

The patients were started on 7.5 mg/kg/day of oral CyA, and adjustments were frequently made to obtain trough serum CyA levels of 100–200 ng/ml. In our experience, however, these measurements were not very helpful and despite low serum CyA levels, dose reductions were often necessary because of side effects, mainly renal dysfunction. To see whether initial disabling of the immune function might improve the long-term immunosuppressive effect of CyA, 11 patients also received oral prednisolone 80 mg/day for the first 5 days on CyA. This dose was rapidly reduced (over 2 to 4 weeks) to maintenance doses of less than 15 mg/day. The majority of the patients were continued on prednisolone at doses of 2.5 to 10 mg/day. Table 1 shows a summary of the individual clinical data.

Results and discussion

The 17 patients treated with CyA ranged in age from 19–66 years (mean 34). Of these, 11 had previously been treated with glucocorticoids only, whereas 6 had received a combination of glucocorticoids and cytotoxic agents (azathioprine or cyclophosphamide). Average follow-up on CyA was 10.7 months (range 2–22).

Clinical response

As shown in Table 2 and Figure 1, the group as a whole had a positive therapeutic response as measured by improvements in visual acuities. The improvements were seen within a month of treatment and remained after 4 months. The condition of the 10 patients treated for a year or longer remained stable except for one (No. 17). In this patient, an intraocular haemorrhage obscured the view of the fundus and thus impeded evaluation of the inflammatory

Table 1. Patient characteristics

No.	Age	Sex	Diagnosis	Abbr. case history
1	24	M	Iritis rec. o.s.	6 months, steroids not tolerated
2	42	M	Iritis rec. o.u.	8 years, relapse on AZA
3	32	F	Iridocycl. chron. o.u.	5 years, relapses
4	24	F	Pars planitis o.u.	7 years, relapse on AZA, fam. hist.
5	19	M	Panuveitis o.d.	2 years, relapses
6	27	F	Panuveitis o.d.	2 years, steroids no effect
7	28	M	Chor. retinitis exud. o.u.	1½ years, macul. oedema
8	58	M	Chor. retinitis exud. o.u.	Detachment on steroids ×2
9	27	M	Chor. retinitis o.u.	Relapses on steroids, AZA and cyclophosph.
10	32	M	Chor. retinitis exud. o.s.	One eye lost due to chor. retinitis
11	35	F	Chor. retinitis o.u.	Relapses on steroids and AZA
12	28	F	Chor. retinitis o.s.	Relapses on steroids
13	25	F	Chor. retinitis o.d.	Relapse on high-dose steroid
14	59	F	Chor. retinitis (panuveitis) o.u.	Relapses on steroids and AZA
15	28	M	Behçet's syndrome o.s.	Relapses on steroids and cyclophosph.
16	66	M	Vasculitis o.d., ulcerative colit.	Relapses on high-dose steroids
17	37	F	Vasculitis (chor. retinitis) o.d.	Relapses on steroids and AZA

Table 2. Results and side effects

No.	Duration (mo.)	V.A.: before	–1 mo. after	–4 mo. after	–last	Princ. side effects
1	4 (S.E.)	1.0	1.0	1.0	1.0	EBV infection
2	8	1.0	1.0	1.0	1.0	Renal, muscle pain, fatigue
		0.33	0.8	1.0	1.0	
3	11 (pregnancy)	0.25	0.67	0.85	0.3	Hirsutism
		0.67	0.67	0.67	0.7	
4	12	1.0	1.0	1.0	1.0	Hirsutism, gingivitis
		0.67	1.0	1.0	1.0	
5	12 (S.E.)	0.67	1.0	0.5	0.67	Hypertension, tremor
6	4 (S.E.)	0.16	0.25	0.1	0.1	Hirsutism
7	14	0.25	0.4	0.35	0.33	Hypertension
		0.16	0.16	0.16	0.1	
8	6	0.67	1.0	1.0	1.0	Hypertension
		1.0	1.0	1.0	1.0	
9	14	0.16	0.25	0.33	0.33	None
		0.16	0.25	0.33	0.33	
10	16	0.1	0.33	0.5	0.5	Hypertension, herp. zoster
11	22	0.5	0.67	0.67	0.5	Renal, hypertension
12	12	0.5	1.0	1.0	1.0	Renal, dysaesthesia
13	4	1.0	1.0	1.0		Hirsutism, hypertension
14	2+1	0.25	0.45		0.33	Severe tremor, comb. Hydergine®
		0.5	0.5		0.5	
15	13	0.1	1.0	1.0	1.0	Tremor
16	13	1.0	1.0	0.67	1.0	None
17	15	0.1	0.33	0.67	L.P.	Gingivitis

S.E.: CyA-treatment withdrawn because of side effects.
L.P.: Light perception.
V.A.: Visual acuities

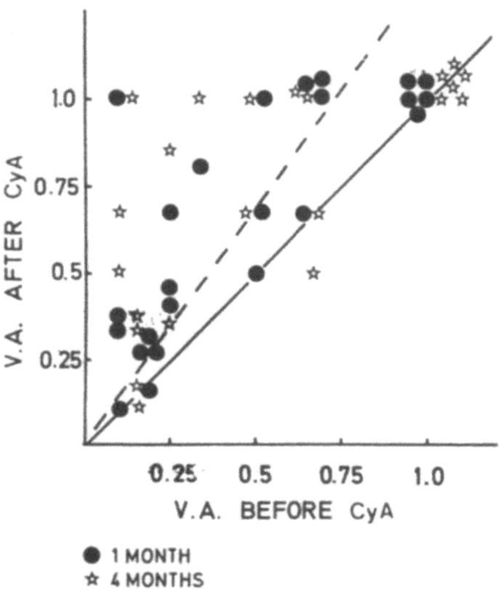

Fig. 1. Improvements in visual acuity (V.A.) after treatment with ciclosporin (CyA). The number of eyes examined after 1 month on CyA was 24; 22 eyes were examined after 4 months. The broken line corresponds to improvements of one line on the Snellens chart

activity. Ultrasonic scans excluded detachment of the retina. In all other cases, the improvement in visual acuity was accompanied by diminution in the inflammatory activity as judged by ophthalmoscopy, slit-lamp examination, and in most cases also by fluorescein angiography.

Momentary relapses occurred in 8 patients (Nos. 1, 4–6, 10–12 and 17) but all responded well to transient increases in prednisolone doses (> 15 mg/day); in 2 cases (Nos. 11 and 17), local steroid injections were given with a definite improvement in one. Since most of these relapses came in patients who had been tapered out of prednisolone, we now recommend concomitant low-dose prednisolone treatment for at least 4 months. The relatively poor response of patients 3, 5 and 7, as determined by visual acuities before and after CyA therapy, might to some extent be explained by the presence of cataract, probably contributed by the previous steroid medication.

The 6 patients who were initiated on CyA without concomitant high-dose prednisolone treatment (Nos. 1, 2, 4, 8, 13 and 14) did not perform worse than those receiving CyA plus 80 mg/day of prednisolone. Thus, initial high-dose glucocorticoid treatment does not seem to be justified.

Ciclosporin toxicity and patient compliance

In 10 patients (59%), renal dysfunction occurred (defined as increases in serum creatinine above 50% over baseline or above 0.15 mmol/l). In all cases renal functions normalized with dose reductions, but slight increases in serum creatinine and urea levels had to be accepted in most patients.

One patient (No. 11) was particularly sensitive in this regard. Several attempts to increase CyA doses above 2–3 mg/kg/day resulted in immediate 50–100% increases in serum creatinine and urea levels despite low or unmeasurable serum CyA levels. Interestingly, these findings were always accompanied by a peculiar pressing sensation in both renal regions, but underlying renal disease was not found. The abnormalities always disappeared within a few days after dose reductions. Phenobarbitone treatment allowed a higher dosage of CyA but, as expected, the serum CyA values did not reach therapeutic levels. Despite this, however, her clinical condition seemed to improve while on phenobarbitone. Recently, concomitant treatment with co-dergocrine (Hydergine®) has allowed a doubling of the CyA dose with retained renal function. Decreased inflammatory activity and vitreous haze were seen at the latest eye examination. Thus Hydergine may offer some protection against side effects in these patients apparently without influencing the immunosuppressive property of CyA. In rats, Hydergine also prevents CyA-induced adverse general and renal effects [7]. In this context, it is interesting that a recent lithium clearance and micropuncture study in rats shows that the early, CyA-induced nephrotoxicity is due to a hemodynamic effect, probably as a result of afferent arteriolar vasoconstriction [4].

In another patient (No. 14), a preexisting fine tremor of the hands was severely intensified along with aggravation of hypertension and a secondary glaucoma. CyA treatment was discontinued after 2 months, and the condition improved within a week. Significant alterations in blood calcium and magnesium levels were not seen. At this point, CyA therapy was considered contraindicated. However, we were forced to renew the CyA medication because of continued eye inflammation, a marked drop in visual acuities in both eyes (<0.25), and aggravation of the glaucoma, along with severe side effects with even moderate doses of prednisolone. The initial dose of CyA was low (1.2 mg/kg/day), but after doubling this dose, all the side effects recurred. Concomitant therapy with Hydergine was therefore initiated (4 (6) mg/day), and a month later she was able to tolerate CyA doses of 5–7.5 mg/kg/day. At this time, the acute eye inflammation had improved.

Ten patients experienced moderate gingival hyperplasia, and in an advanced case the hyperplasia assumed the appearance of an epulis [3]. In 2 patients gingivectomy had to be done. One patient (No. 1) had a febrile illness 5 months after initiation of CyA therapy. A positive test for heterophil antibodies indicated that Epstein-Barr virus was the causative agent. CyA was discontinued, and the febrile illness followed an uneventful clinical course. Continued remission in the underlying inflammatory disease was noted at follow-up examinations 2 and 4 months after. No malignancies have been observed.

The compliance of these patients was generally very good, probably because of the grave prognosis if the therapy failed. However, one patient (No. 5) had to be taken off CyA therapy because of lack of compliance and another patient with unilateral uveitis (No. 6) wished to stop CyA treatment because of moderate to severe hirsutism. Finally, one patient (No. 3) became pregnant during therapy despite the presence of an IUD (does CyA interfere with IUD-induced endometrial inflammation thus allowing implantation of a fertilized egg?). The pregnancy was terminated, but CyA was withdrawn on the patient's request because of a wish for a renewed pregnancy.

Conclusion

We believe that ciclosporin is an important alternative to conventional therapy in the management of selected cases of noninfectious, intraocular, inflammatory diseases. In the first 4–6 months, CyA should be used as an adjunct to glucocorticoid therapy, and only if the patient responds poorly or has intolerable side effects associated with prolonged treatment with glucocorticoids at moderate maintenance doses. At present we advocate the use of CyA before cytotoxic drugs but only if close supervision is guaranteed. Unfortunately most patients on CyA experience serious and potentially dangerous side reactions, but some of these effects may be ameliorated by concomitant Hydergine treatment.

References

1. Bendtzen K (1984) Ciclosporin (cyclosporin A). Prototype of a new generation of immunosuppressive drugs. Allergy 39:565
2. Bendtzen K, Dinarello CA (1984) Mechanism of action of cyclosporin A. Effect on T-cell-binding of interleukin 1 and antagonizing effect of insulin. Scand J Immunol 20:43
3. Brandt K, Pindborg JJ, Bendtzen K (1984) Gingival hyperplasia in patients treated with ciclosporin (cyclosporin A). Tandlaegebladet 88:677 (summary in english)
4. Dieperink H, Leyssac PP, Starklint H, Kemp E: The nephrotoxicity of cyclosporin A. A lithium-clearance and micropuncture study in rats. (Submitted for publication)
5. Nussenblatt RB, Rodrigues MR, Wacker WB, Cevario SJ, Salinas-Carmona MC, Gery I (1981) Inhibition of experimental autoimmune uveitis in Lewis rats. J Clin Invest 67:1228
6. Nussenblatt RB, Palestine AG, Chan C-C (1983) Cyclosporin A therapy in the treatment of intraocular inflammatory disease resistant to systemic corticosteroids and cytotoxic agents. Am J Ophthalmol 96:275
7. Siegl H, Ryffel B, Donatsch P (1984) Prevention of Sandimmune R induced adverse general and renal effects by Hydergine® in rats. Sandoz Pharmaceutical Division

Treatment of Ocular Involvement in Behçet's Disease with Ciclosporin (Preliminary Report)

Asuman Ü. Müftüoğlu, H. Pazarlı, S. Yurdakul, H. Yazıcı, B. Ülkü, Y. Tüzün, S Serdaroğlu, Y. Özyazgan, E. Altuğ and H. Bahçecioğlu

Introduction

Behçet's disease is a multisystem disease characterized by oral and genital ulcers, ocular involvement in various forms, arthritis, thrombophlebitis and neurological involvement. The ocular involvement in Behçet's disease, encountered in about 50% of the cases, constitutes a major hazard because it may lead to blindness especially in young patients [5]. The ocular disease was first described by Behçet [1] as iridocyclitis sometimes associated with hypopion. In addition to the originally described lesions, conjunctivitis, episcleritis, keratitis, hemorrhage and cellular infiltrations into the vitreous body, retinitis, retinal thrombophlebitis, optic atrophy, macular and papilla-edema have been described [2].

There is indirect evidence that the retinal S antigen stimulated T-cells are important in experimental and clinical uveitis [3, 4]. In this investigation ciclosporin (CyA), a T-cell modulator, has been used in the treatment of patients with sight-threatening posterior uveitis of Behçet's disease.

Material and methods

Seven patients with Behçet's disease received a total of ten 3-month courses of ciclosporin oral solution 10 mg/kg/day. If side effects were observed the dose was adjusted to 6–8 mg/kg/day. Five of the seven patients received one course each, one patient received two courses and one patient received three separate courses of treatment. All patients were able to complete the therapy schedule. The patients were followed initially at weekly and later at monthly intervals at the Behçet's Disease Outpatient Clinic under the care of an internist (S.Y.) and the ophthalmological examinations were carried out by two ophthalmologists not directly involved with patient care.

Departments of Medicine, Ophthalmology, and Dermatology of the Cerrahpaşa Medical School of Istanbul University, Istanbul, Turkey

Results (Table 1)

1. Anterior chamber: The anterior chamber had not been involved in 11 eyes before therapy. Chronic sequelae of anterior uveitis were observed in 5 eyes, and 4 eyes had had attacks of uveitis before therapy without chronic sequelae. At the end of the 3-month treatment period, 3 eyes were better, 6 eyes were worse and 11 eyes were unchanged (Table 2).

2. Vitreous body: 1+ to 2+ vitreous opacities were present in 14 eyes before treatment. 4 eyes were intact and two eyes were difficult to evaluate. After treatment 8 eyes were better, 10 eyes were unchanged, one eye was worse and one eye could not be evaluated.

3. Retina: Retinal involvement had been present in 17 eyes before therapy, one eyeground was normal and two could not be evaluated. 10 eyes showed improvement on CyA therapy: within a period of two weeks macular edema disappeared in 4 eyes, papilla-edema regressed in two eyes, exudates and hemorrhages improved in 4 eyes. Optic atrophy, chronic sequelae of venous thromboses and periphlebitis were unchanged in 8 eyes.

4. Visual acuity: Visual acuity improved in 16 of 20 eyes. Improvement was thought to be due to the regression of both retinal vasculitis and vitreal opacities in 4 eyes, regression of the vitreal opacities only in 4 eyes, regression of the retinal findings in 8 eyes. In addition, in one eye with cataract, light perception improved to finger count-

Table 1. The effect of ciclosporin on ocular findings in Behçet's disease

Case	Anterior chamber		Vitreum		Retina		Visual acuity	
	Before	After	Before	After	Before	After	Before	After
H.T. Rt	0	Synechiae	2+	1+	Vasculitis	Idem	2/10	9/10
(1) Lt	0	Synechiae	2+	1+	Vasculitis	Idem	8/10	9/10
H.T. Rt	3+	Sequelae	2+	1+	Optic atrophy	Idem	CF 3m	3/10
(2) Lt	2+	Sequelae	2+	1+	Periphlebitis	Idem	5/10	6/10
H.T. Rt	Sequelae	3+	1+	1+	Optic atrophy	Idem	CF 3m	2/10
(3) Lt	Sequelae	3+	1+	1+	Periphlebitis	Idem	6/10	1/10
K.E. Rt	0	Synechiae	1+	1+	Macular edema	Disappeared	5/10	10/10
(1) Lt	0	Synechiae	1+	0	Macular edema	Disappeared	2/10	10/10
K.E. Rt	1+	1+	1+	1+	Hemorrh. + exudat.	Idem	CF 4m	2/10
(2) Lt	1+	1+	1+	1+	Macular edema	Cicatrix	CF 3m	CF 4m
N.P. Rt	0	0	0	2+	Vasculitis	Disappeared	7/10	10/10
Lt	0	0	0	0	Vasculitis	Disappeared	10/10	10/10
Ö.D. Rt	0	0	2+	±	Papilledema	Regressed	4/10	9/10
Lt	0	0	1+	0	Papilledema	Regressed	5/10	9/10
S.D. Rt	Synechiae	0	0	0	Vasculitis	Regressed	3/10	5/10
Lt	0	0	0	0	Not seen	Not seen	CF 4m	CF 4m
B.P. Rt	Seclusion	Seclusion	?	?	Subhyaloid hem.	Regressed	LP	CF 2m
Lt	Synechiae	Idem	?	?	Not seen	Not seen	CF 0.5m	CF 2m
S.T. Rt	0	0	1+	1+	Normal	Normal	10/10	10/10
Lt	0	0	1+	0	Macular edema	Disappeared	1/10	10/10

Table 2. The summary of ciclosporin effects on various ocular findings

Anterior chamber	Better	3
	Unchanged	11
	Worse	6
Vitreous body	Better	8
	Unchanged	10
	Worse	1
Retina	Better	10
	Unchanged	9
	Worse	0
Visual acuity	Better	16
	Unchanged	3
	Worse	1

ing at two meters and in one eye with subhyaloid hemorrhage finger counting range improved from 0.5 m to 2 m.

5. Relapse on cessation of CyA treatment: An acute relapse was observed in 14 eyes, occurring within one week in 11 and within two weeks in 3. An acute increase in the inflammatory activity in all the segments resulted in a significant decrease in visual acuity. Figure 1 illustrates the regression and progression of the inflammatory activity on three separate courses of CyA treatment. The only patient in whom no relapse occurred upon the cessation of CyA had been on chronic immunosuppression with corticosteroids and cyclo-

Table 3. Relapse phenomena after the cessation of ciclosporin therapy

Chamber	Relapse +	Relapse −	Not known
Anterior chamber	14	4	2
Vitreous body	12	4	4
Retina	14	4	4

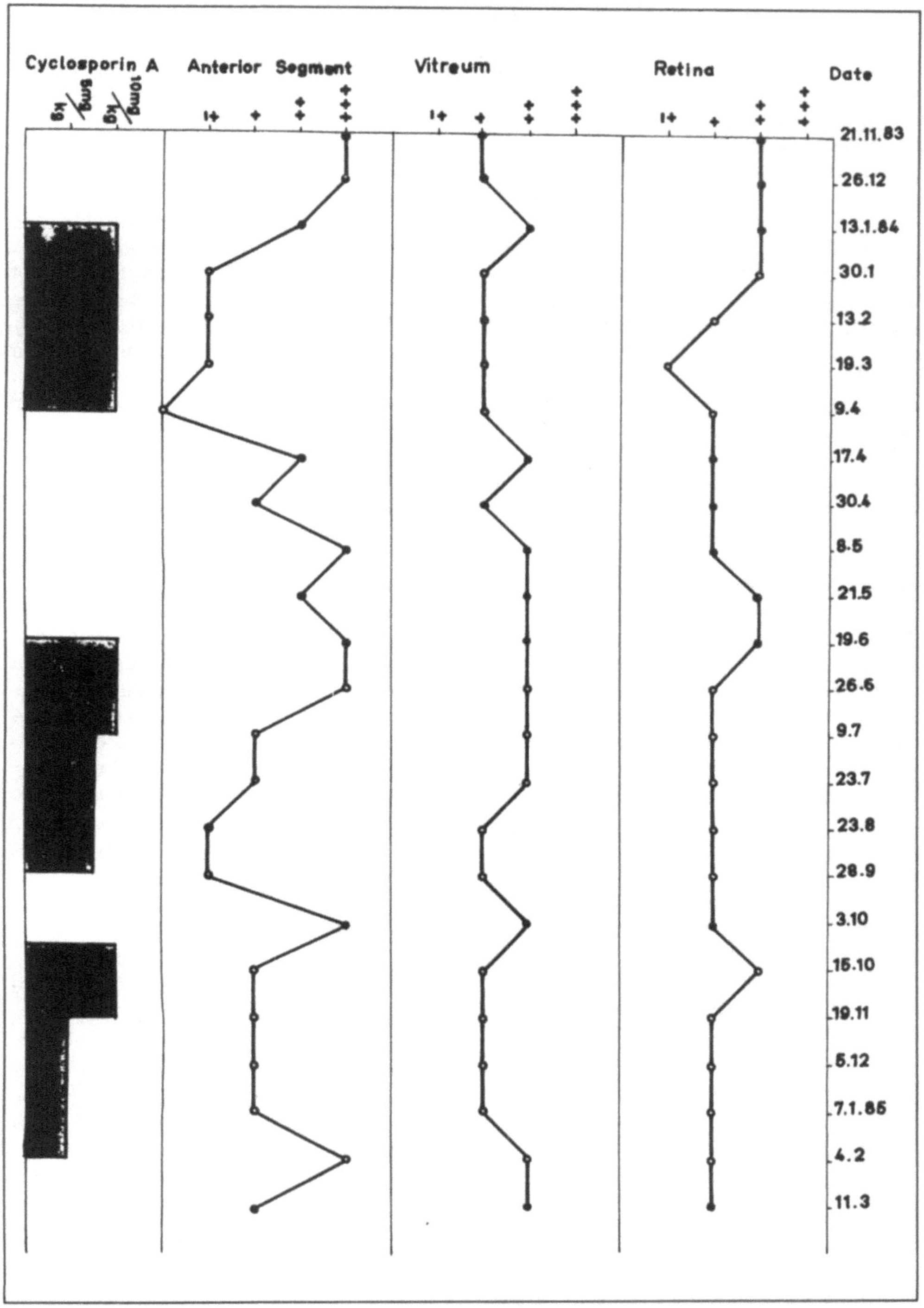

Fig. 1. The effect of 3 separate courses of CyA on the ocular findings of H.T.

phosphamide which were continued at a lower level during CyA therapy (Table 3).

6. The effect of CyA treatment on extra-ocular manifestations of Behçet's disease: During CyA therapy the muco-cutaneous manifestations were encountered less frequently than before in all cases except one. In two cases arthralgias recurred as before. No other major manifestations were encountered in the short 3-month therapy period. All patients reported an increase in the number, severity and frequency of muco-cutaneous manifestations such as aphthous stomatitis, genital ulcers, osteofolliculitis and erythema nodosum-like lesions immediately upon the cessation of CyA treatment.

7. Side effects: Paresthesias and hyperesthesias were the most frequent complaints, encountered in 5 of 7 cases. Epigastric discomfort on ingestion of the drug, flatulence, and nausea which rarely culminated in vomiting, were reported by 4 patients. Hirsutism was the major complaint in all the three female patients. One patient complained of a decrease in libido and burning sensations in the penis during intercourse. All complaints except hirsutism disappeared immediately on cessation of therapy.

Serum bilirubins were slightly elevated in two cases and BUN was elevated in one patient, both returning to normal levels when the CyA dose was decreased to 8 mg/kg/day. One patient exhibited a slight but progressive decrease in his hematocrit towards the end of the 3-month period. This may be partly due to the extensive investigations necessitating repeated venipunctures several times a week. No concomitant decreases were observed in his leukocyte and platelet counts. One patient had mild diastolic hypertension, which returned to a normal level at the end of therapy.

Discussion

Ciclosporin was found to be effective in the control of acute attacks of posterior uveitis in Behçet's disease. The rapid decrease in the inflammatory acitivity in the vitreous body and the retina was accompanied by a significant increase in visual acuity 1–2 weeks after the beginning of therapy. CyA did not seem to influence disease activity in the anterior chamber.

The effective dose of CyA in the control of inflammatory activity in the eyes of Behçet's patients was 10 mg/kg/day in this study. One patient suffered an acute exacerbation when the drug was reduced to 6 mg/kg/day because of undesirable side effects during the third 3-month period. CyA 10 mg/kg/day for 3 months did not cause significant side effects necessitating its withdrawal, but it is probable that a longer duration of therapy might result in increased toxic effects.

A definite relapse was observed in most of the cases 1–2 weeks after cessation of CyA therapy. Increased inflammatory activity was present not only in the posterior but also in the anterior segment. Disease activity in the eye was also accompanied by an increased number, frequency and severity of mucocutaneous lesions in all patients upon cessation of therapy.

In conclusion, it can be stated that ciclosporin in a dose of 10 mg/kg/day orally is effective in the control of inflammatory activity in the eyes of Behçet patients. This control is temporary and a relapse was observed upon the withdrawal of the drug. Therefore, CyA therapy should be maintained for longer than three months in order to be effective in the protection of the eye in Behçet's disease. Its combined use with other immunosuppressive agents should also be investigated.

Acknowledgements

The Behçet's Disease Study Group at the Cerrahpaşa Medical School is partially supported by the Scientific and Technical Research Council of Turkey (TAG-337, 386, 484).

References

1. Behçet H (1937) Über die rezidirende Aphthose durch ein Virus verursachte Geschwüre am Mund, am Auge und an den Genitalien. Dermatol Wochenschr 105:1152

2. Bietti GB, Bruna F (1966) An ophthalmic report on Behçet's disease. International Symposium on Behçet's Disease. Karger, Basel New York, p 79
3. Nussenblatt RB, Gery I, Ballintine EJ, Wacker WB (1980) Cellular immune responsiveness of uveitis patients to retinal S-antigen. Am J Ophthalmol 89:173
4. Nussenblatt RB, Rook AH, Wacker WB, Palestine AG, Scher I, Gery I (1983) Treatment of intraocular inflammatory disease with Cyclosporin A. Lancet II:235
5. Yazıcı H, Tüzün Y, Pazarlı H, Yurdakul S, Özyazgan Y, Özdoğan H, Serdaroğlu S, Ersanlı M, Ülkü BY, Müftüoğlu AÜ (1984) Influence of age of onset and patient's sex on the prevalence and severity of manifestations of Behçet's syndrome. Ann Rheum Dis 43:783

Preliminary Results of a Randomized Prospective Study on Treatment of posterior Uveitis with Ciclosporin or Prednisolone

M. Wiederholt [1, 2], C. Kämpe [1], L. L. Hansen [1], and G. Hövener [1]

Summary

In a controlled study eight patients with active non-infective posterior uveitis were treated with either ciclosporin (CyA) or prednisolone. Both drugs were administered for at least three months. The initial visual acuity was between 0.4 (20/50) and 0.1 (20/200). Three months after starting the treatment one of four patients with CyA showed a better visual acuity (change of at least two lines on the test card), while in one patient visual acuity deteriorated. In the prednisolone group visual acuity improved in one patient and did not change in three. In the CyA group, in three patients a disease relapse was observed during or shortly after CyA therapy. In one patient vitrectomy had to be performed. Thus a beneficial effect of CyA on posterior uveitis cannot so far be demonstrated.

Introduction

The current therapy for posterior uveitis is either high-dose systemic corticosteroids or immunosuppression. Neither approach is very effective and both are fraught with serious complications. With CyA a new and promising immunosuppressive principle has been introduced. Initial CyA studies in patients with sight-threatening, corticosteroid-resistant posterior uveitis have yielded very promising results [3, 4].

Patients and methods

All adult patients with uni- or bilateral active non-infectious posterior uveitis referred to our hospital from February 1984 to December 1984 were considered for the randomized, controlled, prospective trial. Only patients entered the study in whom the clinical symptoms were so severe that oral corticosteroids were indicated and whose visual acuity at entry to study was equal to or worse than 0.5 (a criterion which excluded the majority of patients referred to the hospital).

During the initial ophthalmological evaluation, the following examinations were performed: Visual acuity (Snellen chart, fully refracted), slit lamp examination, fundus biomicroscopy (direct and indirect), applanation tonometry, visual fields, photography of the fundus. All visual acuity measurements were performed under strictly standardized conditions by an investigator who was not involved in patient care. Inflammatory activity of uveitis was assessed by two investigators according to the schema used by Nussenblatt et al. [3, 4] and introduced by Hogan et al. [1] and Kimura et al. [2]. The classification was as follows: anterior chamber (0 = no cells; 1 = 5–10; 2 = 10–20; 3 = 20–50 cells per field; 4 = hypopyon), vitreous opacity (0 = not present; 1 = few scattered fine and coarse opacities, fundus clearly seen; 2 = fundus details somewhat obscured; 3 = many opacities with marked blurring of the fundus; 4 = dense opacities which prevent a view of the fundus). Concerning the diagnosis of the uveitis all patients also exhibited an anterior inflammatory activity. Thus the disease was declared as panuveitis and included such conditions as chorioretinitis, uveitis with retinal necrosis, pars planitis, vitritis, etc. No case of Behçet's disease was included. An infectious origin of the uveitis was excluded by routine laboratory methods. After complete medical and ophthalmological examination and after informed consent had been ob-

Departments of Ophthalmology [1] and Clinical Physiology [2], Klinikum Steglitz, Freie Universität Berlin, Hindenburgdamm 30, 1000 Berlin 45, FRG.

tained from the patient, each patient was randomly assigned to either a CyA group or a prednisolone group.

Patients were treated with 8–10 mg/kg per day of CyA mixed with milk. This dosage was titrated after one week to obtain whole blood CyA concentrations in the range of 400 to 1000 ng/ml for at least three months. Since the total dosage was given in two portions, the trough level of CyA was determined 12 hours after the last dose (the CyA measurements were kindly performed by Mrs. Braun, Nephrological Laboratory, Klinikum Steglitz). Tablets of prednisolone were administered in the following manner: 80–100 mg/day for 2 weeks, then slowly tapering off to zero at three months by drug administration every second day. Usually, the patients stayed in the hospital for the first three weeks.

Results and discussion

The development of visual acuity and vitreous opacity in four patients treated with CyA is summarized in Figure 1 and Figure 2. Case 01 is a patient with a history of chorioretinitis 12 years ago. Vitreous opacity improved within one week after CyA and the severe hypopyon disappeared after 2 days. Two months after stopping therapy, she developed a relapse which again responded positively to CyA. In patient 02 vision had gradually decreased in spite of therapy with systemic corticosteroids for more than two years. She gained weight (104 kg body weight at admission to our hospital) and became depressed while taking steroids. During an acute relapse of the disease she responded slightly to CyA. However, on continuing CyA therapy visual acuity and vitreous opacity in both eyes became worse. Thus the patient was withdrawn from CyA therapy after 7 months. In patient 07 the vitreous body became clearer, but visual acuity did not improve due to a cystoid macular oedema in both eyes. Patient 08, with a four-year history of chorioretinitis/vitritis did not improve after 3 months of therapy with CyA. Moreover, at a whole blood concentration of CyA of ap-

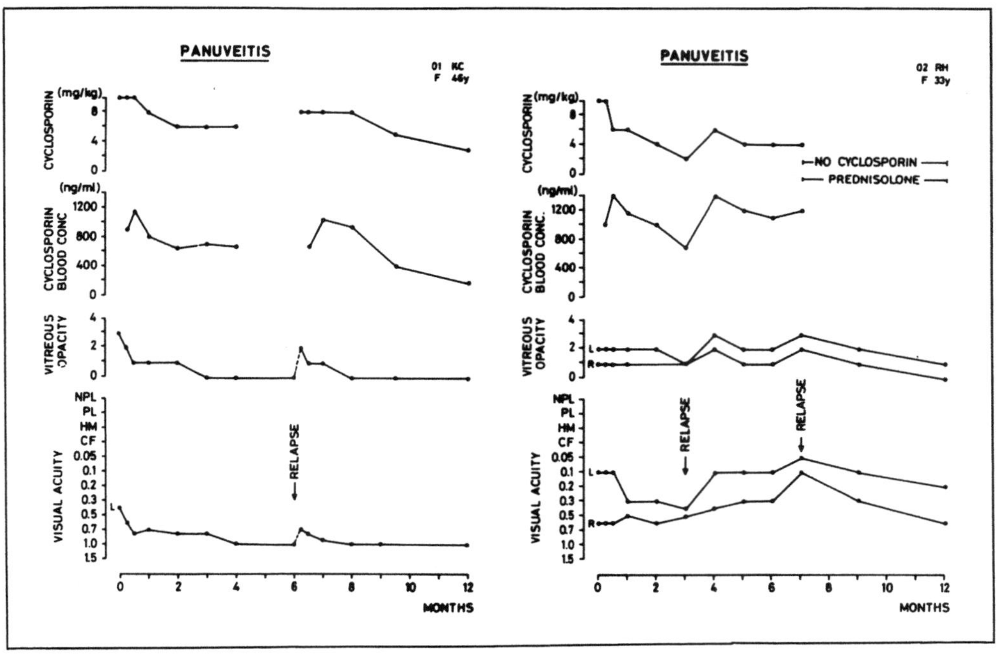

Fig. 1. Progress of visual acuity (CF = counting fingers; HM = hand movement; PL = perception of light; NPL = no perception of light), inflammatory activity of the vitreous body, ciclosporin whole-blood concentration and ciclosporin dosage in patients with uveitis. R = right eye; L = left eye. The number of the case, initials, sex and age of the patients are given at the top of the figure

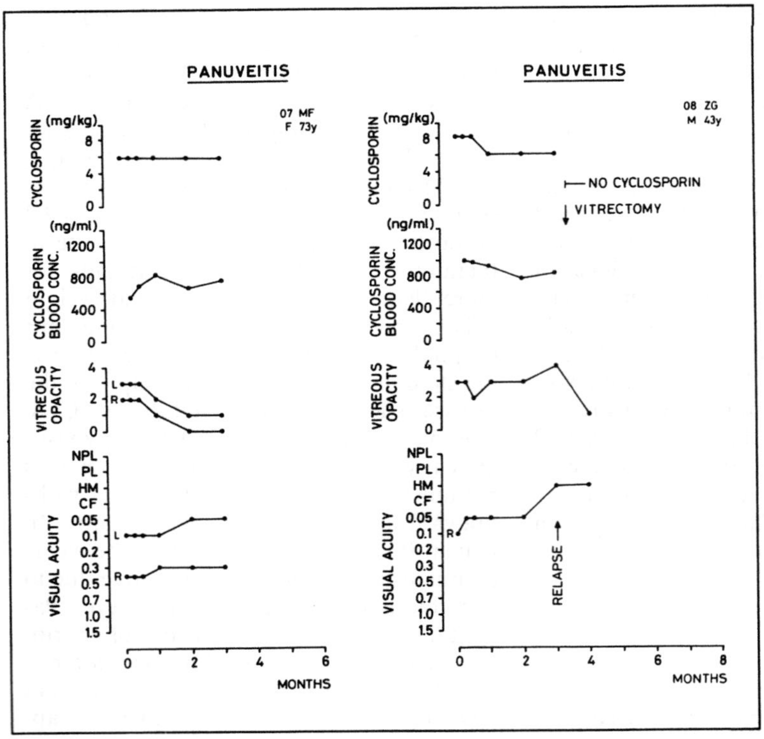

Fig. 2. Patients with uveitis treated with CyA

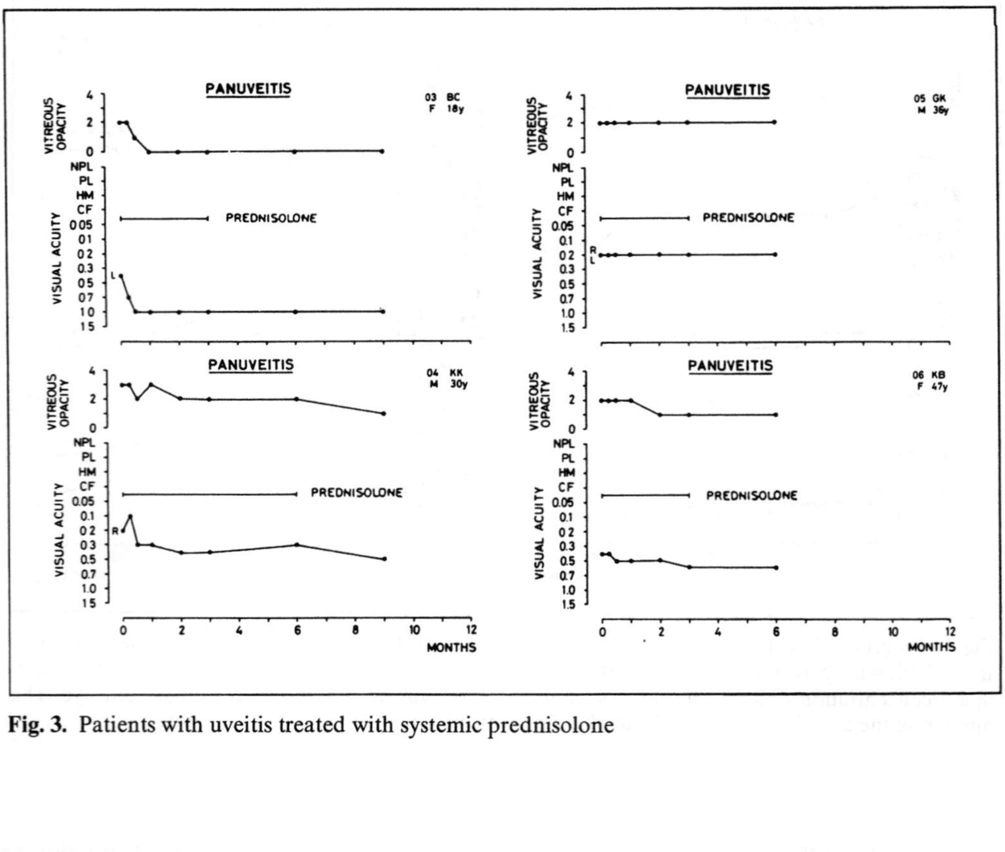

Fig. 3. Patients with uveitis treated with systemic prednisolone

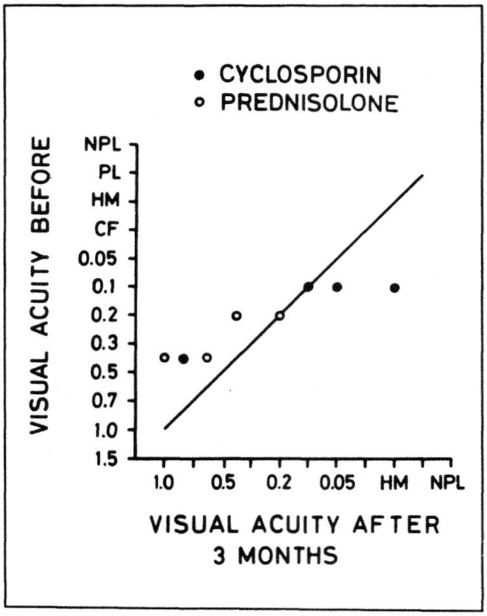

Fig. 4. Visual acuity before and three months after starting therapy

prox. 800 ng/ml both visual acuity and vitreous opacity deteriorated within a few days. CyA therapy was discontinued and vitrectomy was performed. From the material harvested by vitrectomy and aqueous humor puncture, no indication for an infectious etiology of the disease could be obtained.

Figure 3 summarizes data of four patients treated with systemic prednisolone over a period of three to six months. The most important difference as compared to the CyA group seems to be the lack of a true relapse with deterioration of visual acuity and inflammatory activity in the anterior and posterior chamber. On the other hand visual acuity improved in one patient only.

Because CyA is known to produce adverse reactions, all patients were carefully followed up for possible side effects. As described earlier in patients with uveitis [5], we observed a slight but reversible increase of the serum creatinine level (maximum 121 μmol/l). Other side effects of CyA therapy were paresthesias, tremor, increased hot and cold sensations, fatigue and mild hirsutism. One patient developed hypertension which had to be treated.

The visual acuity results three months after commencement of therapy are shown in Figure 4. A change in visual acuity was considered to be present when the patient could read at least two lines more or less on the test card. Among the CyA group, one improved, two remained unchanged and one deteriorated. On the other hand, in the prednisolone group, one patient improved and three remained unchanged. The visual outcome of posterior uveitis in general is very poor. Thus it was very promising that patients resistant to corticosteroids responded with an improvement in visual acuity when treated with CyA [3, 4]. However, in another pilot study [6] in 6 patients with posterior uveitis no such effect of CyA could be observed. Our initial results from this controlled study suggest that CyA is not an effective treatment of severe posterior uveitis.

References

1. Hogan MJ, Kimura SJ, Thygeson P (1959) Signs and symptoms of uveitis. I. Anterior uveitis. Am J Ophthalmol [Suppl] 47:155
2. Kimura SJ, Thygeson P, Hogan MJ (1959) Signs and symptoms of uveitis. II. Classification of the posterior manifestations of uveitis. Am J Ophthalmol [Suppl] 47:171
3. Nussenblatt RB, Palestine AG, Rook AH, Scher I, Wacker WB, Gery I (1983) Treatment of intraocular inflammatory disease with cyclosporin A. Lancet II:235
4. Nussenblatt RB, Palestine AG, Chan CC (1983) Cyclosporin A therapy in the treatment of intraocular inflammatory disease resistant to systemic corticosteroids and cytotoxic agents. Am J Ophthalmol 96:275
5. Palestine AG, Nussenblatt RB, Chan CC (1984) Side effects of systemic cyclosporine in patients not undergoing transplantation. Am J Med 77:652
6. Radda TM, Gnad HD (1984) Cyclosporin A in der Augenheilkunde. Klin Monatsbl Augenheilkd. 185:441

Ciclosporin in Idiopathic Posterior Uveitis; Interim Report of a Randomized Double-masked Study

J. de Vries[1], G. S. Baarsma, P. J. Kruit, T. N. Boen-Tan, A. Rothova, H. J. Buitenhuis and A. Kijlstra

The study is being conducted by the Rotterdam Eye Hospital, and the Ophthalmological departments of the Free University and the Amsterdam Medical Centre in cooperation with the Netherlands Ophthalmic Research Institute.

Patients and methods

Patients are eligible for admission to the study if they have active idiopathic posterior uveitis, an insufficient response to systematic corticosteroids and a best corrected visual acuity of 0.5 or less in their best eye. This last criterion does not apply for patients with Behçet's disease or sympathetic ophthalmia. Exclusion criteria are: Age under 18, presumed infectious uveitis, corneal or lens opacities preventing the evaluation of the efficacy parameters, anticipated intra-ocular surgery, pregnancy, impaired kidney or liver function, concomitant therapy with nephrotoxic antibiotics or cytostatic agents, contraindications to corticosteroids or immunosuppressives, malabsorption syndrome and drug or alcohol abuse.

Two groups of patients are compared with regard to visual acuity, inflammatory activity, number of relapses, number of patients taken out of study because of side effects or treatment failure, and a number of safety parameters (i.e. CyA blood level, serum creatinine, BUN, SGOT, SGPT, bilirubin, hemoglobin, WBC and differential, platelets, ESR, urinalysis, urine sediment, blood pressure, pulse rate and body weight).

At the start all patients receive a low dose of prednisone (i.e. 0.3 mg/kg/day to a maximum of 20 mg/day). In one group this treatment is combined with CyA (i.e. 10 mg/kg/day) while the second group receives a placebo instead. In case of a satisfactory effect after two weeks of therapy the prednisone dosage is reduced by a maximum of 2.5 mg per week and eventually stopped.

The dosage of CyA (or placebo) remains constant for up to 3 months provided the pré-dose whole-blood concentration does not exceed 1000 ng/ml.

Each patient is monitored by two investigators. A first investigator, with no previous information, evaluates the visual acuity and inflammatory activity, and decides about possible changes in therapy. The second investigator knows the assigned treatment and checks the safety parameters. Patients are evaluated at one-month intervals or more frequently when necessary. Allocation to either group is done according to a randomisation list in a strictly consecutive order.

Results

Up to now 10 patients have entered the study. The following diagnoses have been made: panuveitis (3×), uveitis posterior (3×), pars planitis (1×), birdshot choroidopathy (1×), Behçet's disease (1×) and necrotizing vasculitis (1×).

Nine of the patients have been followed up for at least 3 months. The results are based on these 9 patients. In order to safe-

Table 1. Visual acuity

Month	0	1	2	3
Placebo + prednisone	7	8	8	7
CyA + prednisone	7	7	8	9

1 Rotterdam Eye Hospital, Schiedamse Vest 180, 3000 LM Rotterdam, The Netherlands

Table 2. Inflammatory activity

Month	0	1	2	3
Placebo + prednisone	12	9	8	9
CyA + prednisone	14	8	7	4

Table 3. Safety parameters

Month	Placebo		Ciclosporin	
	0	3	0	3
Creatinine	90	109	79	119
SGOT	15	12	13	14
SGPT	14	14	14	13
WBC	8.1	10.2	10.0	11.3
Platelets	190	176	277	269
Hemoglobin	7.9	9.1	8.8	8.7
ESR	8	8	19	12
Body weight	72	72	69	73
Diastolic BP	80	80	85	85

guard the double-masked design of the study the results are expressed as mean values. Individual patients are not analysed.

The development of visual acuity is shown in Table 1. The visual acuity of each patient was given a ranking number in order to compare the ordinal scale of the Landolt optotypes with the semi-quantitative scale of finger counting, hand movements and light perception.

Table 2 shows the results relating to inflammatory activity. The inflammatory activity was assessed according to a modified Hogan-Kimura scale [1] and expressed as a score. A comparison of some safety parameters is shown in Table 3. The main side effects have been an increase in body weight and a decrease in renal function.

No statistically founded statement can be made on the basis of these initial results, but so far the efficacy parameters show a trend in favour of CyA.

Acknowledgements

We thank M.R. Beintema, G. Dijkman, R. v. d. Gaag, S.N. Meriwani, R. de Keizer, Z. Timmermans and L.A.M. de Vries for their constructive criticism.

Reference

1. Kimura SK, Thygeson P, Hogan MJ (1959) Signs and symptoms of uveitis. Am J Ophthalmol 47: 155–176

Ciclosporin (CyA) Versus Conventional Therapy in Behçet's Disease: Preliminary Observations of a Masked Study

D. BenEzra [1], M. Brodsky [1], J. Pe'er [1], T. Hajek [2], S. Pizanti [3], E. Vertman [4] and U. Sachs [1]

Behçet's disease is characterized by a widespread inflammation of the blood vessels in many organs. It has been classically diagnosed by the triad manifestations of recurrent iridocyclitis with or without hypopyon, aphthous ulcerations of the mouth and ulcers of the genitalia [1]. The large variability of manifestations observed among individual patients, the unpredictable acute exacerbation of the ocular inflammatory reactions and the length of remissions hamper the adequate evaluation of treatment efficacy [2]. Reliable controlled studies of the many modalities of treatment are not available, for which reason success or failure has depended largely on the subjective evaluations of the treating physician. Nevertheless, treatment with large doses of steroids, chlorambucil or colchicine are being used in many centers with variable degrees of satisfaction while others have used levamisole or transfer factor with great enthusiasm [3]. With the emergence of CyA, the treatment of a few patients with Behçet's disease was followed by a spectacular improvement of the ocular and systemic condition [4, 5]. We have been conducting a controlled masked study comparing conventional therapy to treatment with CyA in Behçet's disease, and here report our preliminary observations concerning the intensity of ocular inflammation and visual acuity in the first twelve patients of this study.

The Immuno-Ophthalmology Unit, Departments of Ophthalmology [1], Internal Medicine B [2], Oral Medicine [3] and Neurology [4], Hadassah Hebrew University Hospital, Jerusalem, Israel.

Correspondence should be addressed to D. BenEzra, M.D., Ph.D., The Pediatric and Immuno Ophthalmology Unit, Department of Ophthalmology, Hadassah University Hospital, P.O. Box 12000, 91120 Jerusalem, Israel.

Materials and methods

Diagnosis. Candidates with uveitis underwent thorough initial internal, ophthalmological and neurological clinical examinations. The diagnosis of Behçet's disease was based solely on the findings of the classical triad of ocular inflammation (iridocyclitis with or without hypopyon, vasculitis retinae with or without pipe-stem sheathing), aphthous ulcerations of the mouth and genital ulcers. Although the above triad of clinical findings was a sine qua non for the diagnosis of Behcet's disease in our study, not all patients had to present the three symptoms at the time of examination. The diagnosis of Behçet's disease was made if active ocular inflammation and either aphthous stomatitis or genital ulcers were found and evidence of the missing third symptom was obtained from the patient's statements on his past history or from patient record data. In most cases other signs of the generalized vasculitis were present and recorded; however, these were not considered for the diagnosis.

Selection of patients. When the clinical diagnosis of Behçet's disease was made, patients underwent chest X-ray and thorough hematological, biochemical and immunological tests. Clinical and laboratory data were evaluated for inclusion in the study during a staff meeting of an ophthalmologist, an internist, a neurologist and dentist. If diagnostic criteria were undoubtedly present and there were no abnormalities of kidney or liver function and no major hematological or immunological abnormalities, the patient was admitted.

Treatment. If a patient fulfilled all criteria for inclusion in the study, the coordinator and/or one of the physicians explained the study to the patient, who signed the consent forms. The coordinator then drew a sealed envelope for treatment assignment prepared by Sandoz and the patient with the sealed envelope was referred to the internist. The latter explained the treatment to the patient. The internist was responsible for the modulation of the drug regimen according to side effects and laboratory data.

Follow-up. After inclusion in the study, each patient was re-examined and his findings recorded openly by the internist in the "Internist file" and in a masked manner by the ophthamologist in the "Ophthalmologist file". The ophthalmologists had no knowledge of the treatment. Examinations were scheduled according to protocol: 1st, 2nd and 4th week and every month thereafter for a total of six months. After this period, the visits were scheduled for three-month intervals.

During the period beginning September 1984 to March 1985, 12 patients had fulfilled the inclusion criteria. They had been followed for a period ranging from 3 to 18 weeks and are the subject of this preliminary report.

Table 1. Patients randomly assigned to the conventional therapy regimen

Age	Sex	Initial VA	Weeks	VA	Interim inflam.	Condition*
28	F	6/15, J2 6/7.5, J1	18	6/30, J7 6/21, J6	++	Worse
34	M	6/60, J12	18	6/60, J<14	++	Worse
21	M	6/240, J<14 6/240, J<14	10	6/90, J12 6/200, J<14	+	No change
40	F	6/9, J1 6/21, J4	14	6/6, J1 6/7.5, J2	±	Improved
29	M	6/240, J<14 6/60, J7	13	6/180, J<14 6/60, J3	±	Improved

* Objectively recorded by coordinator from records data and subjective assessment of patient.

Table 2. Patients randomly assigned to the CyA therapy regimen

Age	Sex	Initial VA	Weeks	VA	Interim inflam.	Condition*
33	F	6/15, J2 6/9, J1	18	6/9, J1 6/6, J1	–	Improved
30	M	6/7.5, J1 6/360, J<14	14	6/6, J1 6/360, J<14	++	No change
40	M	6/180, J<14 LP	15	6/90, J<14 HM	++	No change
42	F	6/9, J2 6/18, J3	3	6/9, J6 6/9, J1	+	Dropped
27	M	6/12, J1 HM	10	6/7.5, J1 6/400	+	Improved?**
36	F	6/30, J10 6/6, J1	6	6/12, J3 6/6, J1	±	Improved
46	F	F.C. 0.5 6/30	3	F.C. 0.5 6/21	+	Improved?

* Objectively recorded by coordinator from records data and subjective assessment of patient.
** Questionable improvement was recorded when the improvement in visual acuity did not correlate with the unchanged inflammatory ocular reaction and the subjective feeling of the patient.

Results

Of the 12 patients with Behçet's disease participating in this study, 5 (3 males and 2 females) were randomly assigned to conventional therapy and 7 (3 males and 4 females) were assigned to CyA treatment. Tables 1 and 2 illustrate the initial acuity of distant and near vision before treatment and the findings on the last visit for both groups of patients. During the period of follow-up, two of the patients on conventional therapy worsened, with a decrease in vision and an increase in the ocular inflammation. One patient had no noticeable changes and two improved slightly with a marked decrease in inflammatory signs and an improvement of visual acuities (Table 1). Among the patients on CyA therapy, none showed any worsening, two patients clearly improved, two were unchanged, two had a questionable improvement and one patient stopped her participation in the study after three weeks for personal reasons (Table 2). The changes in acuity of distant vision and the intensity of ocular inflammatory reaction recorded on each visit for case 001 are illustrated in Figure 1. This patient was randomly assigned to the conventional therapy group and treated with changing doses of steroids for 18 weeks. Because of the worsening of her symptoms, she was removed from the masked study and crossed over to CyA treatment with a dramatic improvement in her visual acuity and a marked decrease in the ocular inflammatory signs.

Discussion

Due to the great variability of the individual clinical course in Behçet's disease, it is difficult to draw definite conclusions from the data of our first 12 patients enrolled in the masked study. Nonetheless, some of these preliminary observations deserve attention. In our opinion, the fact that under the CyA treatment none of the patients showed any worsening of the ocular con-

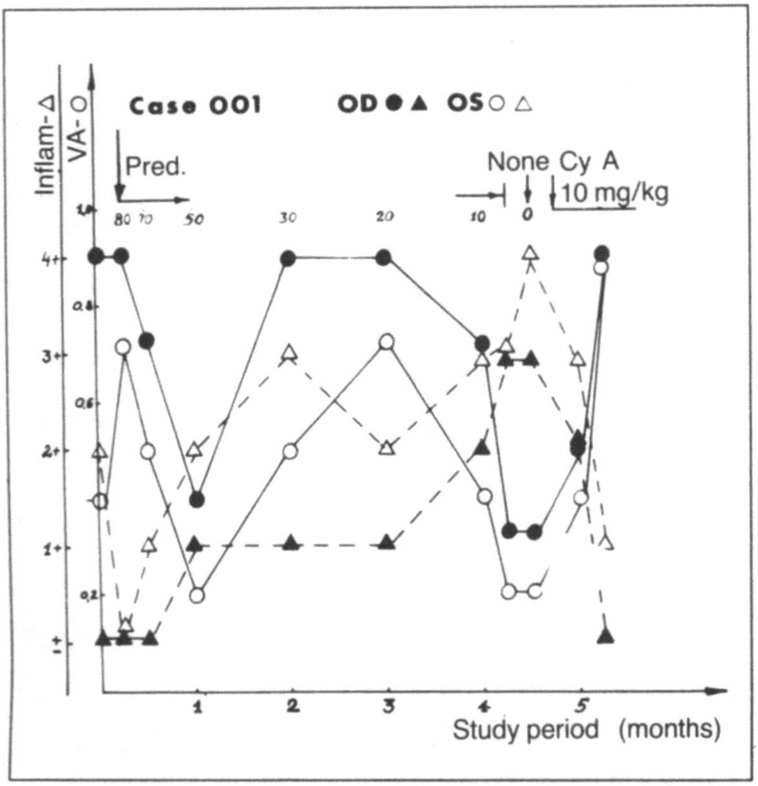

Fig. 1. Visual acuity and ocular inflammatory reactions recorded from a patient randomly assigned to the steroid treatment regimen and switched openly to CyA treatment

dition and that two of them demonstrated a clear improvement might be of some significance if confirmed on further follow-up. In comparison, two patients under the conventional regimen of treatment with high doses of steroids showed a worsening of their ocular condition. One of these had to be withdrawn after 18 weeks and switched openly to treatment with CyA. This patient had a dramatic improvement with recovery of visual acuity of 6/7.5 in both eyes and a marked decrease of the ocular inflammatory signs within a few days. It should be stressed, however, that these are individual cases and the period of follow-up is short. There is a need for a larger number of patients and a longer follow-up period before any adequate conclusions can be drawn regarding the influence of CyA on the ocular manifestations of Behçet's disease.

From our experience with patients suffering from various uveitides as exemplified by the one case of this study shown in Figure 1, it is clinically evident that although a remission of the inflammatory signs with a favorable influence on visual acuity is recorded early during the treatment, an "escape phenomenon" with a relative insensitivity to the initial drug regimen is observed on a longer follow-up. In these cases, crossing over from treatment with steroid to treatment with CyA induces dramatic effects on the ocular inflammatory signs. The marked changes are observed within a few days and in some cases during the first 24 hours of the treatment switch. The combination of "escape" on the one hand and hypersensitivity on the other might be the result of cell population selection during the chronic treatment and is under investigation.

Summary

Twelve patients with Behçet's disease have been enrolled in a masked study designed to compare conventional therapy to CyA treatment in this disease. Preliminary data on visual acuity and ocular inflammatory signs during the period of follow-up appear to be in favor of the CyA treatment. However, due to the small number of patients and the short period of follow up, operative conclusions should be deferred until a larger number of patients is studied.

Acknowledgements

We are grateful to Ms. Genia Maftzir, Evelyne Cohen, Leora Vikert and Judith Fisher and to Mr. Arie Zelikovitch for their help.

References

1. Behçet H (1937) Über rezidivierende, aphtose, durch ein Virus verursachte Geschwüre am Mund, am Auge und an den Genitalien. Dermatol Wochenschr 105:1152
2. BenEzra D, Nussenblatt R (1978) Ocular manifestations of Behçet's disease. J Oral Pathol 7:431
3. BenEzra D (1980) Diseases of the choroid and anterior uvea, in Michaelson's Textbook of the Fundus of the Eye, 3rd edn. Churchill Livingstone, Edinburgh, p 703
4. Ffrench-Constent C, Wolman R, James DG (1983) Cyclosporin in Behçet's disease. Lancet 2:454
5. Nussenblatt RB, Rook AH, Wacker WB, Palestine AG, Scher I, Gery I (1983) Treatment of intraocular inflammatory disease with Cyclosporin A. Lancet 2:235

A Double-masked Study of Ciclosporin Treatment in Behçet's Disease

K. Masuda [1] and A. Nakajima [2]

Methods and subjects

A double-masked study of the use of ciclosporin (CyA) in Behçet's disease was carried out for 4 months beginning in March 1984 in various uveitis clinics in Japan. Informed consent was obtained from all patients.

The subjects of this study were patients with Behçet's disease in the active phase. The total number of patients participating in this trial was 96; 47 patients were in the CyA group and 49 patients in the colchicine group. There were no differences between the two groups in sex, age, type of disease, the affected eye side, duration of the disease, duration of the eye involvements, complications, the number of the ocular attacks for 4 months before the trial, the drugs used before the trial and visual acuity before the study.

The initial dose of CyA was 10 mg/kg/day and that of colchicine was 1.0 mg/day. The dose was reduced according to the side effects during the trial.

It was reasonable to choose colchicine as a control in this study because its effectiveness on Behçet's disease is already established.

The routine ophthalmological examinations – liver function, renal function, erythrocyte sedimentation rate and the immunological laboratory tests including immunoglobulins, T- and B-cell population, T-cell subpopulation, blast formation in the lymphocytes by PHA or Con A, immune complexes and complement fractions in serum – were carried out at least once every 4 weeks.

1 Department of Ophthalmology, Branch Hospital of Tokyo University, Mejirodai 3-26-8, Bunkyo-ku, Tokyo, Japan

2 Department of Ophthalmology, Juntendo University, Hongo 3-1-3, Bunkyo-ku, Tokyo, Japan

Results

1 The ocular symptoms

The frequency of the ocular attacks was markedly reduced. The reduction was greater in the CyA group than in the colchicine group, as shown in Table 1. There was a statistical significant difference in the two groups ($p < 0.001$).

The same tendency was found in the severity of the ocular attacks; the ocular attacks in the CyA group became much less severe during the study than in the colchicine group. There was also a statistically significant difference between the two groups ($p < 0.001$).

Visual acuity was improved more in the CyA group than in the colchicine group but there was not a significant difference between the two groups.

2 The cardinal symptoms other than the ocular symptoms

The oral aphthae decreased much more in the CyA group than in the colchicine group ($p < 0.001$). The skin lesions also decreased more in the CyA group than in the other group ($p < 0.01$).

3 Overall evaluation

The final improvement rate is summarized in Table 2. In the CyA group, 89% of the patients showed amelioration compared with 31% of the patients treated with colchicine. There was a signficant difference between the two groups ($p < 0.001$). Deterioration was found in 18% in the colchicine group while there was no de-

Table 1. Incidence of ocular attacks

	Markedly improved	Moderately improved	Slightly improved	Unchanged	Slightly aggravated	Moderately aggravated	Markedly aggravated	Drop-out	Total
Ciclosporin	22 (47)	13 (74)	7 (89)	3	0	1 (2)	0	1	47
Colchicine	6 (12)	2 (16)	9 (35)	23	0	5 (12)	1	3	49
Test χ^2 / F	***	***	***			N.S.			U test ***

***: $p<0.001$
( ): %

Table 2. Final global improvement rate

	Markedly improved	Moderately improved	Slightly improved	Unchanged	Slightly aggravated	Moderately aggravated	Markedly aggravated	Drop-out	Total
Ciclosporin	17 (36)	18 (74)	7 (89)	4	0	0 (0)	0	1	47
Colchicine	4 (2)	3 (14)	8 (31)	22	4	4 (18)	1	3	49
Test χ^2 / F	**	***	***			**			U test ***

**: $p<0.01$
***: $p<0.001$
( ): %

Table 3. Side effects in double masked study of Ciclosporin in Behçet's disease (%)

	Ciclosporin n=47		Colchicine n=49		Test
Renal dysfunction	11	(23)	2	(4)	*
Hepatic dysfunction	3	(6)	3	(6)	
Hirsutism	23	(49)	2	(4)	***
Body heat sensation	5	(11)	1	(2)	
Numbness	2	(4)	0	(0)	
GI disorders					
Loss of appetite	5	(11)	1	(2)	
Nausea, vomiting	4	(9)	1	(2)	
Others	5	(11)	4	(8)	
General malaise	3	(6)	0	(0)	
Gingival hypertrophy	3	(6)	1	(2)	
Others	10	(21)	0	(0)	

*: $p<0.05$
***: $p<0.001$

terioration in the CyA group. There was a significant difference between the two groups ($p < 0.01$).

The safety evaluation (based on side effects and abnormal laboratory values) showed almost complete safety in 96% in the colchicine group while 79% of the CyA group showed almost complete safety. There was a significant difference between the two groups ($p < 0.01$).

21% in the CyA group were problem cases while only 4% of the colchicine group showed problems and there was a significant difference between the two groups ($p < 0.01$).

However, the final efficacy of CyA in Behçet's disease was evaluated at 87%, while colchicine was rated at only 51%. There was a significant difference ($p < 0.001$).

4 Side effects

Many patients complained about the side effects of CyA. The side effects are summarized in Table 3. In each item, the number of patients in the CyA group was more than in the colchicine group. Especially renal dysfunction and hirsutism were found more frequently in the CyA group than in the colchicine group ($p < 0.05$ and $p < 0.001$ respectively). These symptoms diminished gradually after the decrease of the drug dosage.

5 The laboratory tests

There were no significant differences in the immunological tests except the OKT4/OKT8 ratio. The ratio decreased more in the CyA group than in the colchicine group. There was a significant difference between the two groups ($p < 0.05$).

Discussion

In Japan the visual prognosis of Behçet's disease has been reported to be very bad and 12% of aquired blindness is due to Behçet's disease. There have been many papers reporting that colchicine is the most effective drug for suppressing the frequency of the ocular attacks. Colchicine is now the first choice for treating patients with ocular involvements, especially of the chorioretinal type. However, almost 10% of the patients with ocular involvements have shown resistance to colchicine treatment and become blind within several years. We call this the severe type of Behçet's disease.

Nussenblatt et al. reported that CyA was very effective in patients with posterior uveitis including Behçet's disease. We used CyA in the severe type of Behçet's disease and obtained encouraging results in suppressing the eye involvements.

This double masked trial clearly verified that the usefulness of CyA is superior to that of colchicine not only in the suppressing of ocular involvements but also in other systemic symptoms.

As far as the side effects were concerned, more appeared in the CyA group than in the colchicine group. Creatinine levels in serum increased significantly in the CyA group in 2 ($p < 0.01$), 4 ($p < 0.001$), 8 ($p < 0.001$), 12 ($p < 0.001$) and 16 weeks ($p < 0.001$) compared with the pretreatment levels, while no significant increases were observed in the colchicine group in this period. The maximum level (1.27 ± 0.07, maximum value 2.5 mg/dl) was reached at 12 weeks and remained stable up to 16 weeks. Almost all of them diminished, however, when the drug dose was decreased. No malignancy was reported in this study.

5. Primary Biliary Cirrhosis – Crohn's Disease

Primary Biliary Cirrhosis

Roger Williams, J. Neuberger, M. R. Lucey [1]

During the last few years, understanding of the natural history of primary biliary cirrhosis (PBC) has undergone considerable revision, with realisation of the great variability of presentation and progression. The majority of patients are middle-aged women who present with a history of gradual onset of pruritus, increasing skin pigmentation and subsequently signs and symptoms of cholestatic liver disease. Others will present with a history of portal hypertension with gastrointestinal haemorrhage, or as a consequence of hypersplenism. Others, with a poorer prognosis, present with signs of decompensated liver disease. It is becoming increasingly recognised that there is a substantial pool of patients, who present either with some of the associated conditions of PBC (such as sicca syndrome, sclerodactyly or Raynaud's phenomenon) or who are truly asymptomatic and who are detected because of abnormal liver function tests or antimitochondrial antibodies (AMA) on routine screening. Most, but not all, present with early histological disease; some, at presentation, have an established cirrhosis. In this asymptomatic group, life expectancy is probably not significantly different from that of a normal, matched population [6, 11]. Thus, despite the lack of proven effective specific treatment for the disease, due to recognition of patients at an earlier stage there has been an apparent improvement in prognosis from 5 years twenty-five years ago [14] to over 10 years currently [2].

Attempts to assess the prognosis of individual patients within these four broad groups have emphasised the importance of the serum bilirubin. Longitudinal studies have indicated that once serum bilirubin has exceeded 100 μmol/l, life expectancy is limited to two years. More recently, based on an analysis of patients participating in an international trial assessing the therapeutic benefit of azathioprine [1], it has been possible to provide a more quantitative assessment of prognosis at the time of diagnosis. This index (PI) is based on six independent variables, of which the major component is the serum bilirubin (Table). Thus, a PI of 3 approximates to a median estimated survival time of 60 months and a PI of 6 to about 12 months.

Table 1. Calculation of prognostic index (PI) at presentation in PBC

2.5 × log serum bilirubin (μmol/l)
+ exp ((age in years − 20)/10)
+ 0.88 (if cirrhosis present)
− 0.05 × serum albumin (g/l)
+ 0.68 (if central cholestasis present)
+ 0.52 (if not treated with azathioprine)

Immune abnormalities

A number of abnormalities of the immune system have been documented in patients with PBC. On the humoral side these patients have elevated levels of serum immunoglobulins, especially IgM and IgG, and increased levels of autoantibodies. Classically the autoantibody of PBC is the antimitochondrial antibody, which is present in 80–100% of cases. A number of different specificities have been described and PBC is associated with the M2 antibody reacting with a component on the inner mitochondrial membrane, possibly the translocator enzyme [13].

Another feature of these patients is the reported presence of circulating immune

1 The Liver Unit, King's College School of Medicine and Dentistry, Denmark Hill, London SE5 8RX, U.K.

complexes; indeed dissection of these complexes has shown the presence of mitochondrial and of biliary antigens. These immune complexes mainly of large size (>19 S) have been detected using the C1q assay and the Raji cell assay. However, some doubt has been cast on the validity of these assays, which may have been false positives due to the activation of complexes by these macromolecules, possibly aggregated immunoglobulin, and by anti-lymphocyte antibodies. A recent attempt to show immune complexes using monoclonal assays has failed to confirm these findings [3]. It may be that the large circulating immune complex-like material is responsible for activation of complement. Patients with PBC have normal C3 levels, but measurements of complement activation (such as C3d and C1q) and fractional rates of complement degradation have shown hypercatabolism of complement by the classical pathway. Such findings have not been reported in autoimmune chronic active hepatitis. In addition hepatic clearance of C3b opsonised particles is reduced and implies selective C3b receptor dysfunction of Kupffer cells; we have recently shown that this defect is due to serum factors.

On the cellular side, T helper, T suppressor/cytotoxic and plasma cells have been identified around the portal tracts and IgM plasma cells cluster around the bile ducts [2]. In the parenchyma, $OKT8^{+}$ cells (suppressor/cytotoxic) predominate. These patients have evidence of anergy to a variety of agents and in vitro tests show impairment of mitogen-induced transformation, altered responsiveness to the liver specific lipoprotein complex (LSP) and bile duct antigens. That these abnormalities are secondary to a generalised disorder of immune regulation is suggested by a number of findings including a reduced responsiveness in the autologous mixed lymphocyte reaction, although the allogeneic mixed lymphocyte reaction is normal. Concanavalin A (Con A)-induced suppression of mitogen-induced T cell proliferation is abnormal in both autologous and allogeneic systems. Studies on regulation of immunoglobulin secretion are less clearly defined. Thus, some studies have shown defective T cell regulation of suppression of allogeneic but not autologous B cells; others have shown that Con A activated T suppressor cells were able to regulate autologous B cells from normal subjects [7]. However, Miller, Sepersky, Bronn et al. [9] showed defective Con A-induced suppression of autologous lymphocytes in most patients with PBC, independent of stage of disease; their findings were seen in some close relatives. Our own findings on immunoregulation are presented subsequently.

Pathogenesis of PBC

A number of theories on the pathogenesis of PBC have been developed; these are briefly outlined below. For full reviews, see reference [7].

Infective: One of the theories for the origin of AMA is cross-reactivity between mitochondrial antigens and certain micro-organisms: some of these may be expected to induce granuloma formation and some of the immunologic features of PBC. However there is no proof of this hypothesis and direct evidence is lacking.

Immune complex disease: This hypothesis is based on the concept that antibody, derived either from the portal tract plasma cells or from the portal blood, combines with an antigen possibly derived from bile or biliary epithelium, to form large immune complexes which will activate complement, inducing both tissue injury and granuloma formation. Excess immune complexes would spill over into the circulation. However, controversy still exists over the actual existence of immune complexes in PBC. D-penicillamine, which will lower immune complex-like activity in the serum of patients, is not associated with therapeutic benefit, as will be discussed later.

T cell mediated cytotoxicity. PBC and acute and chronic graft versus host disease (GVHD) share some clinical and serological features, such as scleroderma. Raynaud's phenomenon, hyperglobulinaemia, formation of auto-antibodies and immune complex-like material, anergy and bile duct destruction. This has led to the suggestion that the hepatic lesions of PBC may be due to an autoimmune response to histocompatibility antigens or biliary antigens on biliary epithelium, or to a T cell mediated cytotoxicity reaction. However, there is no evidence to date that, in PBC, T cells are sensitised to altered histocompatibility antigens or fail to recognise normal HLA antigens. Furthermore, close histological examination shows that the histological lesion in PBC differs from GVHD [8].

Defective immunoregulation. Jones [7] has postulated that the fundamental defect in PBC is a defect in the interaction of autoreactive T cells and surface antigens or autologous non-T cells, i.e. a defective autologous mixed lymphocyte reaction. This might be expected to lead to defective activation of suppressor T cells, leading to increased immune responsiveness and could permit cell-mediated autologous immune responses and perpetuate tissue injury.

Specific therapies for PBC

Therapeutic trials in PBC, usually of immunologically active drugs, are difficult to organise. Because of the long natural history and variety of patterns of progression, useful answers can be obtained only if large numbers of patients are followed for a suitable length of time. In practice, multicentre trials are required. It may be necessary to stratify patients to ensure that treated and untreated groups are equal in the proportion of asymptomatic cases. Randomisation will ensure against bias but will not necessarily ensure similarity between groups. It is paradoxical that results will be obtained most readily in the illest patients who may benefit least from therapy, whereas obtaining definitive results in those who may benefit most – those at early stages of the disease – is more difficult.

Corticosteroids: There have been a number of uncontrolled studies [4, 7], but while some of these have shown a transient improvement in serum biochemistry, no convincing effects on either survival or progression have been apparent. Any potential benefit of corticosteroids must be balanced against their propensity to exacerbate osteoporosis. Indeed, a recent study showed that in patients with PBC, severe osteoporosis was present only in those who had received corticosteroids [15].

Alkylating agents: Cyclophosphamide and chlorambucil have both been used in preliminary studies in PBC; although preliminary published results appear encouraging, it is too early to anticipate definitive results.

Colchicine: Preliminary studies in a limited number of patients have suggested a benefit but again long-term results are awaited.

Azathioprine: Although a preliminary study showed that azathioprine 2 mg/kg/day was of no significant benefit, a larger multi-centre study has raised the possibility that azathioprine at 1 mg/kg/day may improve survival [1]. 236 patients were followed for up to 10 years, and although no significant effect on survival of the treated group was seen when the two groups were corrected for imbalance in prognostic variables, azathioprine was shown to exert a beneficial effect, prolonging survival on average by 18 months.

D-penicillamine: This agent was introduced on the basis that it would reduce liver copper which is now thought to be secondary to cholestasis and not toxic, and to reduce CIC (circulating immune complex)-like material. Although initial studies were encouraging, a number of multicentre trials have confirmed the toxicity of the agent but failed to show any significant overall effect [5].

Use of ciclosporin (CyA)

With a daily dose of 10 mg/kg/day in an eight-week study of 6 patients, there were significant reductions in serum aspartate aminotransferase and alkaline phosphatase levels [12]. It was also noted that use of CyA was associated with improvement in the helper/inducer: cytotoxic/suppressor cell ratio. However, use of CyA was discontinued because of a high incidence of nephrotoxicity. No blood levels of CyA were measured. Other studies have shown that CyA at a dose of 3 mg/kg/day in patients with PBC is associated with therapeutic levels of the drug [10]. On the basis of this study, further work both in vivo and in vitro was carried out to determine the effect of CyA in PBC and the results are described in the following two chapters.

References

1. Christensen E, Neuberger J, Crowe J et al. (in press) Beneficial effect of azathioprine and prediction of prognosis in primary biliary cirrhosis. Final results of an international trial. Gastroenterology
2. Eggink HF, Houthoff HJ, Huitema S, Gips CH, Poppema S (1982) Cellular and humoral reactions in chronic liver disease. I. Clin Exp Immunol 50:17
3. Goldberg MJ, Kaplan MM, Anderson CL (1982) Evidence against an immune complex pathogenesis of primary biliary cirrhosis. Gastroenterology 83:677
4. Howat HT, Ralston AJ, Varley H, Wilson JAC (1966) The late results of long-term treatment of primary biliary cirrhosis by corticosteroids. Revue Internat. d'Hepatologie 16:227
5. James OFW (1985) D-penicillamine for primary biliary cirrhosis. Gut 26:109
6. James OFW, Macklon AF, Watson AJ (1981) Primary biliary cirrhosis: a revised clinical spectrum. Lancet i:1278
7. Jones EA (1985) Primary biliary cirrhosis: potential pathogenic mechanisms and the effects of therapies on the disease process. In: Thomas HC, MacSween RNM (eds) Advances in Hepatology, vol 1. Churchill-Livingstone, Edinburgh, p 131
8. MacSween RNM, Sumithran E (1981) Histopathology of primary biliary cirrhosis. In: Jones EA (ed) Seminars in Liver Diseases, vol 1. Thieme-Stratton, New York p 282
9. Miller KB, Sepersky RA, Bronn KM, Goldberg MJ, Kaplan MM (1983) Genetic abnormalities and immunoregulation in primary biliary cirrhosis. Am J Med 75:75
10. Robson S, Neuberger J, Keller HP, Abisch E, Niederberger W, Graffenried B von, Williams R (1984) Pharmacokinetic studies of Cyclosporin A (Sandimmun) in patients with primary biliary cirrhosis. Br J Clin Pharmacol 18:627
11. Roll J, Boyer JL, Barry O, Klatskin G (1983) The prognostic importance of clinical and histological features in asymptomatic and symptomatic primary biliary cirrhosis. N Engl J Med 308:1
12. Routhier G, Epstein O, Janossy G, Thomas HC, Sherlock S, Kung PC, Goldstein G (1980) Effects of cyclosporin on suppressor and inducer T lymphocytes in primary biliary cirrhosis. Lancet 2:1223
13. Schultheiss HP, Berg P, Klingenberg M (1983) The mitochondrial adenine nucleotide translocator is an antigen in primary biliary cirrhosis. Clin Exp Immunol 54:648
14. Sherlock S (1959) Primary biliary cirrhosis (chronic intrahepatic obstructive jaundice). Gastroenterology 37:574
15. Stellon AJ (personal communication)

Effect of Ciclosporin (CyA) on Suppressor Cell Function in Patients with Primary Biliary Cirrhosis

J. Neuberger, G. Alexander, M. N. Al-Aghbar, M. R. Lucey, Roger Williams [1]

Introduction

As indicated in the previous chapter, the pathogenesis of primary biliary cirrhosis (PBC) remains to be established. Host factors have been implicated and several workers have described defective regulation of antibody production in patients with this disease [5, 9]. We have assessed concanavalin A (Con A) induced T suppressor cell regulation of immunoglobulin-producing cells using an haemolytic plaque assay and have studied the effect of CyA after in vivo and in vitro administration.

Suppressor cell assay

Venous blood was mixed with 6% dextran (1 ml/10 ml blood) and preservative free heparin (100 U/10 ml blood), and suspended for 45 minutes at 37 °C to allow sedimentation of red cells. The leucocyte enriched plasma was centrifuged on Ficoll-Triosil for 20 minutes at 400 *g* and partial monocyte depletion was carried out by incubation in plastic Petri dishes for 45 minutes at 37 °C. The non-adherent cells were washed three times in Hanks balanced salt solution (HBSS); the cells were resuspended in RPMI-1640 (containing 2 mM glutamine, 200 U/ml penicillin, 20 U/ml streptomycin and 2 µg/ml amphotericin B) and 20% heat inactivated foetal calf serum (FCS), at a concentration of 10^6 cells/ml. Peroxidase staining was 3–5%. 200 µl of the cell suspension was added to a minimum of 20 wells in a flat bottomed microplate (Sterilin): to 10 of these wells, 20 µg pokeweed mitogen/well (PWM, Sigma) was added. The cells were cultured at 37 °C in an atmosphere of 5% carbon dioxide in air for 7 days. For Con-A activation 5 ml of the cell suspension was incubated with 100 µg Con A (Sigma) for 24 hours at 37 °C and then washed three times in HBSS containing 0.3M α-methyl-D-mannoside to remove Con A. 100 µl of the Con A treated lymphocytes at 10^6 cells/ml was then added to an equivalent volume of untreated lymphocytes in a minimum of 10 wells and PWM added. The lymphocytes were then incubated as above. Viability, assessed by trypan blue exclusion, exceeded 93% after Con A incubation.

After 7 days the PBMC were harvested by centrifugation and washed three times in RPMI, then resuspended at 10^5 cells/ml. Viability ranged from 66–96%. 50 µl of PBMC were mixed with an equal volume of sheep red blood cells coated with staphylococcal protein A, together with an equal volume of an appropriately diluted IgG fraction of rabbit antihuman IgG and 500 µl of agarose indubiose. The mixture was then poured into plastic Petri dishes and incubated at 37 °C for four hours. 1 ml of guinea pig complement diluted 1 : 25 in RPMI was added to each dish, which was then incubated for a further two hours. Discrete concentric areas of haemolysis were counted visually by indirect light and the result expressed as the number of IgG-producing cells per 10^6 viable lymphocytes. The results of the suppressor cell assay were expressed according to the following formula

$$\%\ \text{suppression} = \left(1 - \frac{\text{No. of IgG-producing cells with PWM and Con A}}{\text{No. of IgG-producing cells in PWM alone}}\right) \times 100$$

1 JN is a Wellcome Senior Clinical Research Fellow
The Liver Unit King's College Hospital and School of Medicine and Dentistry, Denmark Hill, London SE5 8RX, UK.

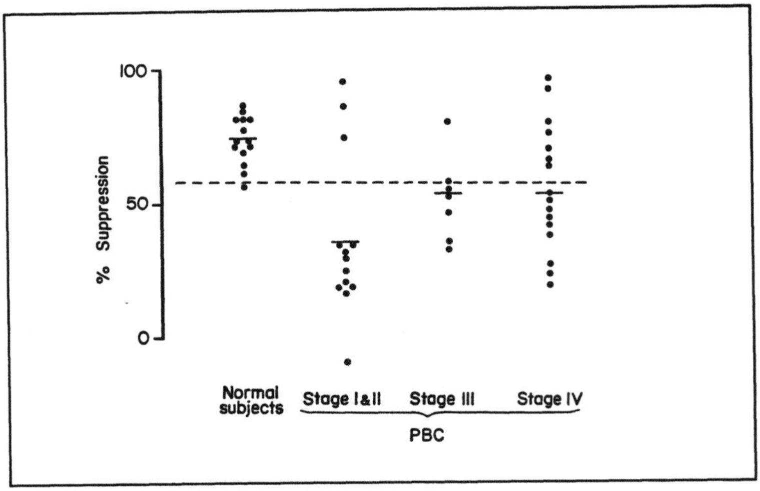

Fig. 1. Con A activated suppressor cell function in normal controls and patients with PBC. Dotted line indicates the lower limit of normal (Submitted for publication in Gut)

Suppressor cell function in normals and patients with PBC

Using the suppressor cell assay, Con A activated suppressor cell function was studied in 14 healthy subjects and 36 patients with histologically diagnosed PBC. At the time of testing, 13 patients had early disease (Stage I/II) and 23 late stage (III/IV). None were taking any specific therapy for PBC. The normal range was defined as the mean ± 2SD of control subjects (Fig. 1). While there was considerable overlap between the supressor cell function of normals and patients, suppressor cell function was decreased in the patients with PBC. Furthermore, this defect was detected in all stages of the disease.

Effect of CyA in vivo on suppressor cell function

The subjects under study were the first 20 patients in the open study of the effects of CyA on patients with PBC described by Dr Lucey in the next chapter. Of these, ten patients had Con A induced T suppressor cell function on IgG production assessed before treatment and during the first six months of therapy with CyA. Suppression of IgG production prior to therapy was 33 ± 22% (mean ± SD) (Fig. 2). After six months of therapy suppressor cell function improved to 68 ± 8%. In contrast, no changes were observed in untreated patients. Thus, in vivo administration of CyA is associated with a significant improvement in the Con A induced suppressor cell function in patients with PBC.

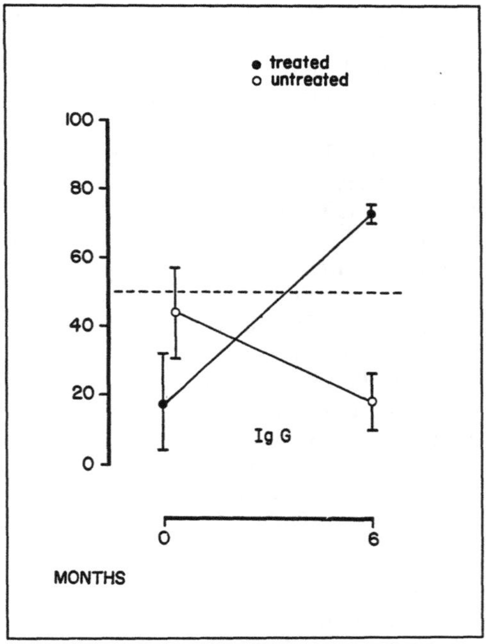

Fig. 2. Suppressor cell function on IgG production before and after 6 months of treatment with CyA (●) and in controls (○)

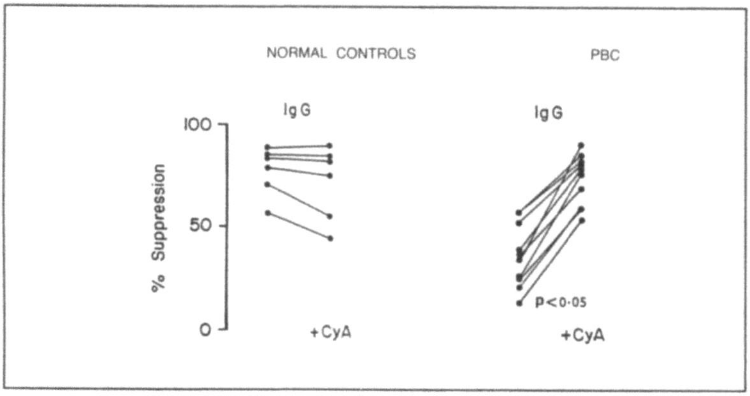

Fig. 3. Suppressor cell function on IgG production in 16 patients with PBC before and after incubation with CyA prior to activation by Con A

Effect of CyA in vitro on suppressor cell function

To assess the effect of in vitro incubation of PBMC with ciclosporin, PBMC were incubated with CyA, dissolved in 0.15% ethanol and RPMI-1640 at 300 ng/ml for 30 minutes at 37 °C. The cells were then washed in HBSS three times and suspended in 20% FCS at 10^6 cells/ml. As a control CyA solvent (donated by Sandoz), was dissolved in ethanol and RPMI-1640 as above. Mean viability after incubation with either CyA or control, assessed by trypan blue exclusion, was greater than 98%. PBMC, isolated from 16 patients and laboratory personnel, were incubated with either CyA or control medium either prior to culture with Con A or after stimulation with Con A. In subsequent experiments varying doses of CyA were used prior to incubation with Con A.

Preincubation of PBMC with CyA, prior to incubation with Con A, increased suppression of IgG-producing cells in patients with PBC (Fig. 3) from 35.7 ± 14% to 73.7 ± 12% (mean ± SD). ($p < 0.01$). In contrast, preincubation of PBMC from normal subjects with CyA, prior to Con A activation, had no effect on suppressor cell function. Similarly, preincubation of PBMC from patients with PBC had no effect on IgG suppressor cell activity when performed after Con A activation. Incubation of PBMC with the solvent alone had no effect on suppressor cell activity.

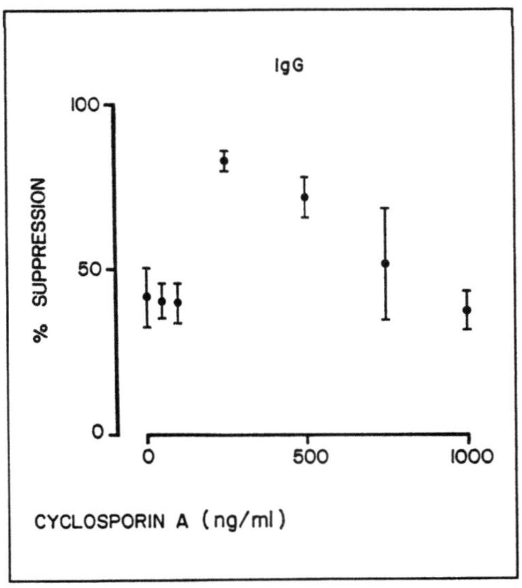

Fig. 4. Effect of varying concentrations of CyA on suppressor cell function on IgG production. PBMC were incubated with CyA prio to Con A activation (Submitted for publication in Gut)

The effect of concentration of CyA on Con A induced suppression

PBMC isolated from 6 patients with a suppressor cell defect were incubated prior to Con A activation with CyA at concentrations of 0, 50, 100, 250, 750 and 1000 ng/ml. Since it was not possible to obtain enough cells from one individual to test at all concentrations of CyA, each patient was studied at alternate concentrations. Viability of cells was greater than 96% at all concentrations of CyA. As shown in Figure 4, increasing the concentration of CyA resulted in increased Con A suppressor cell function up to a concentration of 250 ng/ml; increasing concentrations of CyA were thereafter associated with a loss of this effect.

Discussion

These results, obtained with the above assay, show that patients with PBC have defective Con A induced suppressor cell activity and that this can be corrected in vivo by treatment with CyA. Clearly, until the results of long term clinical trials are available, it is impossible to establish the relevance of the improvement in this defect for the pathogenesis and progression of the disease. Furthermore, the assay employed measures only one aspect of suppressor activity and the system used is antigen nonspecific. However, the target of immune-mediated damage in PBC has yet to be defined, so that assays of antigen specific cells are not feasible. Ideally the suppressor cell activity of the lymphocytes in liver tissue should be studied, but suitable techniques for obtaining adequate numbers of lymphocytes from biopsy samples have not yet been developed. The mode of action of CyA in this system may be related to inhibition of the earliest stages of lymphocyte activation. Thus CyA, while allowing expression of the Tac receptor, interferes with the secretion of IL-1 and IL-2 and the expression of T9, T10 and DR antigens [2, 8, 10, 11] and may be related to inhibition of protein synthesis by unstimulated lymphocytes [3, 7]. This would explain the failure of effect of CyA after Con A exposure.

Con A activated cells are the most likely targets for CyA in this study and this is the lectin most sensitive to CyA [4]. Other studies [1] have shown that CyA can inhibit T-helper cell activity and that in the mixed lymphocyte reaction, CyA selectively inhibits cytotoxic cells, sparing suppressor cells [12]. This explanation is consistent with the finding by Kahan and colleagues [6] that CyA binds more avidly to T-helper cells than to T-suppressor cells.

The rationale for the use of CyA is that correction of the suppressor cell defect will lead to improvement in the immunoregulation and thus retard progression of the disease. In view of the dose-response effect of varying concentrations of CyA on suppressor cell function, in contrast to graft recipients high levels of CyA should be avoided in these patients.

References

1. Borel JF, Weisinger D, Gubler HV (1978) Effects of the anti-lymphocyte agent Cyclosporin A. Eur J Rheumatol and Inflamm 1:327
2. Bunjes D, Harot C, Rollinghoff M, Wagner H (1981) Cyclosporin A mediated immunosuppression of primary cytotoxic T cell response impairing the release of interleukin I and interleukin 2. Eur J Immunol 11:657
3. Elliott JF, Lin Y, Mizel SB, Bleakley RC, Harnish DH, Paetru C (1984) Induction of interleukin 2 messenger RNA inhibited by Cyclosporin A. Science 226:1439
4. Hess AD, Matyas JR, Tutschka PJ (1979) Inhibition of in vitro lymphocyte responses to Cyclosporin A. Exp Hematol 7:104
5. James SP, Elson CO, Jones EA, Strober W (1980) Abnormal regulation of immunoglobulin synthesis in vitro in primary biliary cirrhosis. Gastroenterology 79:242
6. Kahan BD, Kerman RH, Agostino G, Preinoman A, Lrgrue SJ (1983) In: White DJG (ed) Cyclosporin A. Elsevier, Amsterdam, p 281
7. Kay JR, Benzie CR (1983) Effects of cyclosporin A on metabolism of unstimulated and mitogen activated lymphocytes. Immunology 49:153
8. Larsson E-L (1980) Cyclosporin A and dexamethazone suppress T cell responses by selectively acting at distinct sites of the triggering process. J Immunol 124:2828
9. Miller KB, Seperesky RA, Bronn KA, Goldberg MJ, Kahan MM (1983) Genetic abnormalities of immunoregulation in primary biliary cirrhosis. Am J Med 75:75
10. Miyakawi T, Yachie A, Ohzeki S, Nagaoki I, Taniguchi N (1983) Cyclosporin A does not prevent expression of Tac antigens, a probable TCGF receptor molecule, on mitogen stimulated T cells. J Immunol 130:2737
11. Palacios R, Moller S (1981) Cyclosporin A blocks the receptors for HLA-DR in T cells. Nature 290:792
12. Wang BS, Heacock EH, Collins KH, Hutchinson IC, Tilney NF (1981) Suppressive effects of cyclosporin A on the induction of alloreactivity in vitro and in vivo. J Immunol 127:89

Treatment of Primary Biliary Cirrhosis with Ciclosporin (CyA): Pilot Study

M. R. Lucey [1], J. M. Neuberger, G. J. M. Alexander, S. Robson, Roger Williams [2]

Introduction

Primary biliary cirrhosis (PBC) is accompanied by disturbances of the immune system [6]. Thus, although it is unclear whether these disturbances have any significance in the aetiopathogenesis of PBC, many immunomodulatory drugs have been used to treat PBC [8]. Administration of corticosteroids has been associated with improvement of liver function tests but there has been no controlled trial of their efficacy.

Azathioprine is associated with a moderate increase in life expectancy in PBC. However, initial reports of increased life expectancy with use of d-penicillamine have not been confirmed by long-term studies [5]. The advent of the novel immunosuppressive agent ciclosporin (CyA) has provided a new opportunity to ameliorate PBC by interfering with the immune system. This paper reports initial observations on a pilot study of CyA in PBC.

Subjects and methods

Patients

All patients gave fully informed consent. The diagnosis of PBC was based on a combination of clinical and laboratory observations. All patients had liver histology showing features compatible with or diagnostic of PBC in the absence of other liver diseases. In addition there was one or more of the following: serum alkaline phosphatase in excess of twice the upper limit of normal, raised serum IgM, antimitochondrial antibody.

Study protocol

Open treatment: The initial 10 subjects were recruited to an open trial of CyA.

Single-blind study: Thereafter 19 subjects were recruited to a single-blind placebo-controlled study in which 9 received the active agent and 10 received the vehicle solution. The following patients were excluded: those in whom serum creatinine exceeded 150 µmol/l, those in whom survival prognosis was adjudged to be less than 6 months, and asymptomatic patients with early histological disease.

Dosage regimen

The starting dose of CyA was 3 mg/kg/day. Patients were assessed monthly for the initial 3 months and thereafter at 3-monthly intervals. When the whole-blood trough CyA level measured by radioimmunoassay was less than 150 ng/ml the dose of CyA was increased by 50 mg/day. When serum creatinine exceeded 170 µmol/l or when other marked side effects occurred, the CyA dose was reduced by 50 or 100 mg/day. Patients underwent an annual liver biopsy.

Results

As shown in Table 1, the sex distribution and mean age at entry were similar in CyA-treated and placebo-treated patients. The median duration of follow-up was longest in patients treated with open CyA (27 months, range 4–30) and of similar duration in the single-blind study in both CyA (18 months, range 2–24) and placebo-treated (21 months, range 12–24) subjects. Four

1 Gastroenterology Division, Dept. of Int. Medicine University of Michigan Ann Arbour 48109

2 The Liver Unit, King's College School of Medicine and Dentistry, Denmark Hill, London SE5 8RX, U.K.

Table 1. Clinical features and outcome in pilot study of ciclosporin in PBC

	Open CyA	Single blind CyA	Single blind placebo
M/F	1/9	2/7	1/9
Mean age (range)	50 years (35–60)	55 years (42–66)	58 years (42–67)
Median duration of follow-up (range)	27 months (4–30)	18 months (2–24)	21 months (12–24)
Deaths	1	3	2

Table 2. Severe side effects in 19 patients treated with ciclosporin

Side effect	No. of patients	No. to stop CyA
Raised serum creatinine	5 (2–21 months)	1
Raised BP	2	1
Headaches	1	
Acne rosacea	1	1
Total	9 (47%)	3 (16%)

(21%) CyA-treated and 2 (20%) placebo-treated patients died.

The serial changes in serum bilirubin are shown in Figure 1. Pre-treatment serum bilirubin levels were similar in all groups and there were no significant differences in serial serum bilirubin levels between the CyA-treated and placebo-treated patients.

Table 2 shows the incidence of severe side effects in CyA-treated patients. CyA had to be reduced or stopped in 9 (47%). In 5 subjects serum creatinine rose after 2–21 months of treatment. In 4 subjects serum creatinine fell on reducing the dose of CyA. The fifth patient was mildly hypertensive and had a high serum creatinine level prior to treatment. She remained hypertensive and serum creatinine rose further after 2 months of therapy. CyA was then stopped. Subsequently the patient had a cerebrovascular accident, but was alive 30 months later. Two patients became hypertensive, requiring dosage reduction in one and withdrawal in the other. Hypertension has persisted in the latter patient. In toto CyA was withdrawn in 3 patients (16%).

Discussion

This is the first report of the long-term administration of CyA in PBC. PBC displays a wide spectrum of clinical manifestations and some patients may remain asymptomatic for many years [1]. Thus, as the recent experience with d-penicillamine in PBC has shown [5], the efficacy in PBC of therapies under study can be established only by clinical trials which include many patients followed for many years. Hence one cannot deduce, from the small numbers in the present pilot study, whether CyA is an effective remedy for PBC.

The present study does however indicate that CyA can be used safely in PBC. Routhier et al. previously reported that nephrotoxicity, as shown by a rising serum creatinine level, occurred in 5 of 6 patients with PBC treated with CyA (dose 10 mg/kg/day) for 8 weeks [7]. Recently structural renal damage has been described in the recipients of heart [4] and renal [3] transplants treated with CyA for one year or more. In each of these reports the dose of CyA was considerably greater than that in the present study. It has been suggested that nephrotoxicity is related to a high in-

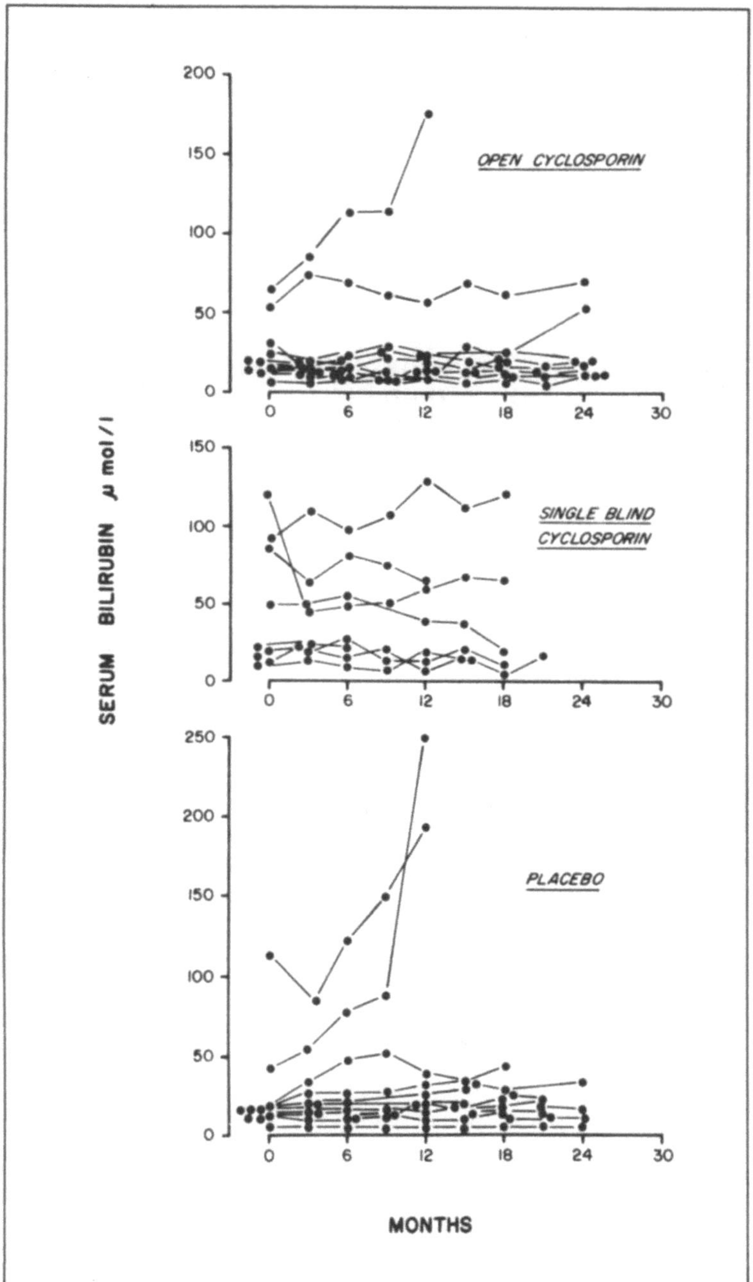

Fig. 1. Serial serum bilirubin in ciclosporin- and placebo-treated patients

itial dose of CyA [3]. In common with other workers [2] we have found in the present study that a reduction of the CyA dose was sufficient to correct the rise in serum creatinine in most affected individuals. Further follow-up will be necessary to show whether the restoration of a normal serum creatinine continues in these patients treated with low-dose CyA. However on the evidence available at present we suggest that when serum creatinine and blood pressure are carefully monitored and the dose of CyA adjusted accordingly, low dose CyA is a safe for long-term use in PBC.

References

1. James OFW, Macklon AF, Watson AJ (1981): Primary biliary cirrhosis: a revised clinical spectrum. Lancet i: 1278–1281
2. Klintmalm GBG, Iwatsuki S, Starzl TE (1981) Nephrotoxicity of cyclosporin A in liver and kidney transplant patients. Lancet 1:470–471
3. Klintmalm G, Bohman SO, Sundelin B, Wilczek H (1984) Interstitial fibrosis in renal allografts after 12 to 46 months of cyclosporin: beneficial effect of low doses in early post-transplantation period. Lancet 11:950–954
4. Myers BO, Ross J, Newton L, Luetscher J, Perlroth M (1984) Cyclosporin-associated chronic nephropathy. N Engl J Med 311:699–705
5. Neuberger J, Christensen E, Portmann B, Caballeria J, Rodes J, Ranek L, Tygstrup N, Williams R (1985) Double-blind controlled trial of d-penicillamine in patients with primary biliary cirrhosis. Gut 26: 114–119
6. Neuberger J, Alexander GJM, Al-Aghbar MN, Lucey MR, Williams R (1985) Effect of cyclosporin A on suppressor cell function in patients with primary biliary cirrhosis. International Workshop on Ciclosporin in autoimmune diseases, Basel 1985
7. Routhier G, Epstein O, Janossy G, Thomas HC, Sherlock S (1980) Effects of Cyclosporin A on suppressor and inducer T lymphocytes in primary biliary cirrhosis. Lancet i: 1223–1226
8. Williams R, Neuberger J, Lucey MR (1985) Primary biliary cirrhosis – introduction. International Workshop in Ciclosporin in auto-immune diseases, Basel 1985

Ciclosporin Therapy in Primary Biliary Cirrhosis (PBC): A Pilot Study in 10 Patients

R. Beukers, S. W. Schalm [1]

Patients and methods

Ten symptomatic patients with PBC (9 women, 1 man; median age 47.5 years) were treated with ciclosporin (CyA) in an initial dose of 5 mg/kg/day for 6 months. The diagnosis of PBC was established according to classic criteria (i.e. alkaline phosphatase in excess of twice the upper limit of normal, positive antimitochondrial antibodies and typical bile duct lesion in liver biopsy). The median duration of the disease was 7.5 years. Five patients were icteric (all stage IV PBC), the other five anicteric (stage I–IV PBC).

The efficacy of CyA treatment on symptoms (general well being, fatigue, pruritus), biochemical (alk. phosphatase, bilirubin, aspartate aminotransferase (AST)) and immunological (IgM, IgG, circulating immune complexes, T lymphocyte subtypes) parameters was evaluated.

The CyA dose was adjusted according to CyA plasma levels and clinical and biochemical side effects. CyA was measured in plasma (separated from cells at 37 °C [1]) and in blood by the Sandoz radioimmunoassay.

Results

The results of 9 patients are presented. One icteric patient was withdrawn from the study after 4 months of therapy because of chronic diarrhoea associated with the absence of therapeutic CyA levels, possibly related to malabsorption of the drug. No obvious immediate effect of CyA treatment on general well being (expressed as a capacity index) or on fatigue was observed. In the icteric patients pruritus appeared to become less prominent.

The most striking effect was seen in serum alkaline phosphatase values, which showed a significant decrease of 16.1% ($p < 0.05$, Wilcoxon test). Bilirubin values were not influenced in the whole group, but a decrease was observed in the icteric patients (number of patients in this subgroup too small for meaningful statistical analysis). No effect on AST levels was seen.

Serum levels of IgM decreased from an average of 7.2 to 5.9 grams per litre ($p = 0.05$). No effect was observed on serum IgG levels and circulating immune complexes as determined by the C 1q-binding test. Because of difficulties with the determination of T-cell subtypes with OKT monoclonal antibodies, no evaluable results were obtained. The main side effect was nephrotoxicity (as indicated by a rise in serum creatinine), necessitating a dose adjustment to an average of 2.6 mg/kg/day. Impairment of renal function was dose dependent and reversible. The degree of nephrotoxicity at a given measured CyA level was individually different. Figure 1 shows a typical example of the relationship between serum creatinine, CyA blood and plasma levels and CyA dose. Other side effects included hirsutism, gingival hyperplasia and tremor each occurring in one patient and gastro-intestinal complaints in four.

Discussion

Ciclosporin treatment for 6 months in this group of patients with different stages of PBC had no obvious immediate effect on symptoms. A significant decrease of alkaline phosphatase values and an obvious effect on serum IgM levels was observed.

---

1 Department of Internal Medicine II, University Hospital Dijkzigt, Erasmus University, Rotterdam, the Netherlands.

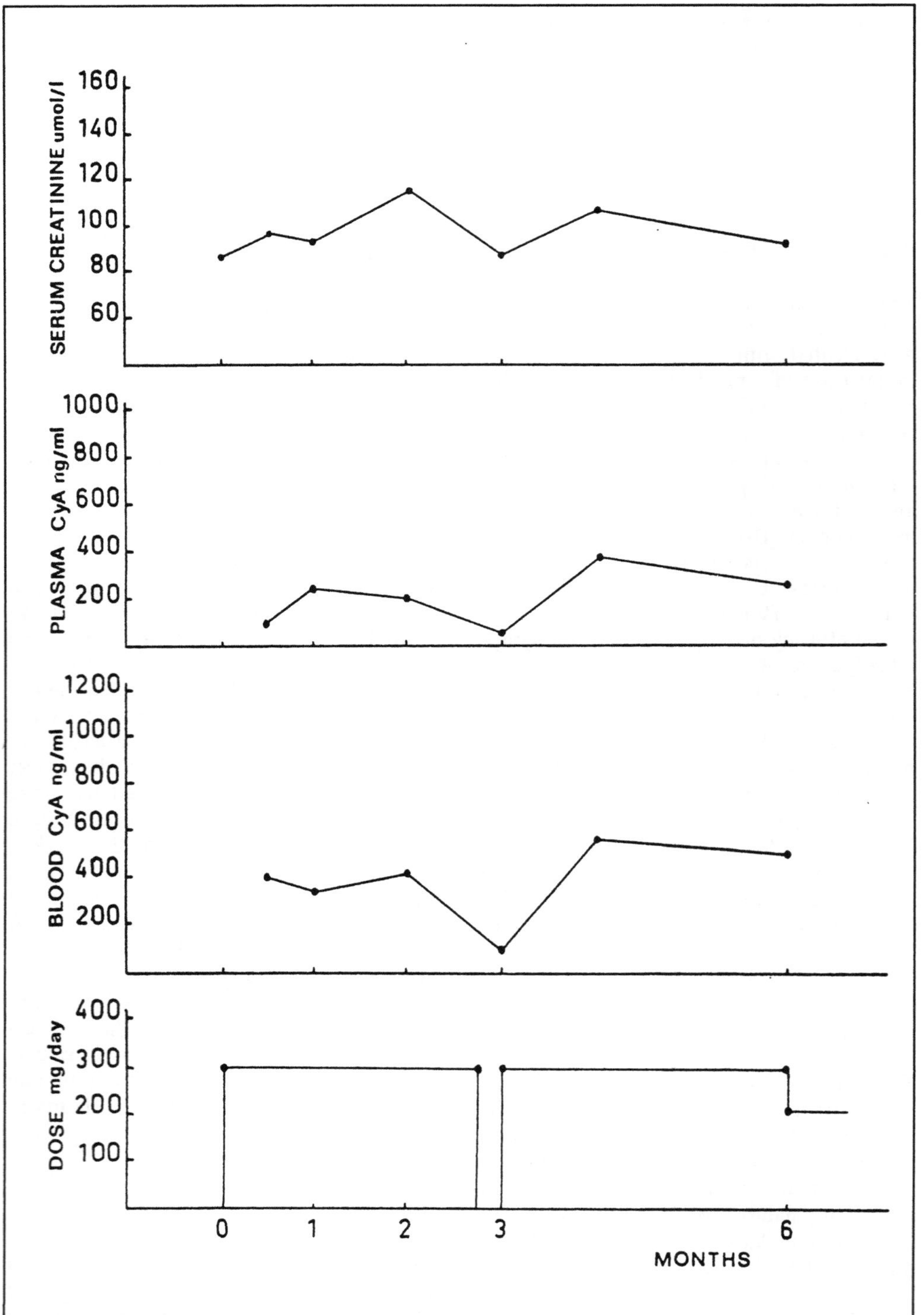

Fig. 1. Relationship between CyA dose, CyA blood and plasma levels and serum creatinine in a 50-year-old woman with stage IV PBC

Nephrotoxicity was the main side effect of CyA treatment in PBC, as reported by other authors [2]. The degree of nephrotoxicity was variable but individually dose-dependent and reversible. CyA therapy did not prevent further clinical deterioration in patients with end-stage PBC. However, in some patients with earlier stages of the disease a decrease was observed in alkaline phosphatase, AST, serum IgM, serum IgG and circulating immune complexes.

We conclude that CyA treatment is of no value in end-stage PBC, but a positive effect is potentially present in earlier stages. Our results warrant more extensive studies on the effects of CyA treatment in earlier stages of this chronic liver disease.

References

1. Berg JWO van den, et al. (1985) Cyclosporin A assay: conditions for sampling and processing of blood. Clin Chim Acta, 147:291–297
2. Routhier G, et al. (1980) Effects of cyclosporin A on suppressor and inducer T lymphocytes in primary biliary cirrhosis. Lancet II:1223–1226

Ciclosporin (CyA) in Primary Biliary Cirrhosis (PBC): A Multicentre, Double-blind, Placebo-controlled Long-term Therapeutic Study. The Study Design

N. Tygstrup[1], L. Ranek[1], E. Juhl[1], S. Keiding[1], E. Christensen[1], R. Williams[2], J. Neuberger[2], J. Rodes[3]

Primary biliary cirrhosis (PBC) is a chronic inflammatory disease involving the intrahepatic bile ducts and progressing to cirrhosis, liver failure and variceal hemorrhage. Sjögren's syndrome and pancreatic hyposecretion occur in up to 70% of patients with PBC, thus accounting for the "dry gland syndrome". The incidence of PBC is approximately 50 per million population [5] and PBC is more common in females aged 40–60 years. The mean duration of survival of symptomatic patients is approximately 11.9 years [2], but symptom-free patients appear to have a similar life expectancy to age-matched and sex-matched controls from the general population of the USA [3].

The etiology and pathogenesis of PBC is still unclear and several hypotheses including chronic "graft versus host reaction" have been put forward. PBC is associated with some specific and nonspecific immunological features: elevated IgM levels (nonspecific), circulating antibodies which react with the cytoplasm of bile ductule cells in 75% of patients with PBC (nonspecific), periductal IgM-forming lymphocytes in liver biopsy, impaired lymphocyte transformation and autoantibodies, particularly antimitochondrial autoantibodies (AM-AB).

Further investigations on the ability of Con-A-generated suppressor T-cells to inhibit mitogen response of allogenic responder cells in PBC [6] and the T-cell mediated help and suppression of PWM-induced IgM and IgG synthesis in vitro [1], were suggestive of an abnormal T-cell function in PBC.

1 The Copenhagen Liver Units at Rigshospitalet and Hvidovre, Copenhagen/DK
2 The Liver Unit, King's College Hospital, London/UK
3 The Liver Unit Hospital Clinic, Barcelona/Spain

Therapy for PBC including azathioprine, d-penicillamine and colchicine has not had a clear effect on the survival of patients with PBC and has been associated with numerous side effects. CyA has been found to reduce inflammatory activity in PBC at a dosage of 10 mg/kg/day [4]. There was also an increase in the T-suppressor to -helper cell ratio in peripheral blood lymphocytes. However, CyA therapy had to be discontinued in view of the reversible deterioration of renal function observed in all cases.

Published data of concise clinical studies regarding the therapeutic value of CyA in PBC are still very limited and patient numbers are small.

The data of an unpublished pilot-study performed in a collaborating liver centre suggested a better risk-benefit ratio following low dose CyA treatment in patients with PBC. This encouraged us to investigate the efficacy, safety and tolerability of a long-term therapy with CyA in a double-blind, randomized, placebo-controlled multicentre study. The study design and the first impressions of the still ongoing investigation are reported in brief.

According to statistical calculations, about 200 patients (100 patients per therapy group) with an entry time of 3 years are needed to demonstrate clearly a significant (80% probability on the 5% level, one-sided significance test) and clinically relevant therapeutic effect of CyA within 5 years of start of the study, including an accrual phase of 3 years and a follow-up period of 2 years. The observation period per patient is therefore 2 years at the minimum and 5 years at the maximum. A 50% reduction in mortality was considered to be the most relevant primary study parameter (Table 1). The final statistical analysis consists of multivariate log-rank analysis (Cox regression) including model-building pro-

Table 1. Study variables

Primary variables	– Mortality, directly or indirectly due to PBC Major complications: encephalopathy ascites collapse of vertebrae gastrointestinal bleeding
Secondary variables	– Changes in liver histology Clinical symptomatology of PBC Biochemical variables of PBC (bilirubin, alanine- or aspartate-aminotransferase, alkaline phosphatase, gamma-GT, protein, albumin, prothrombin) Subjective and objective tolerability (plasma and/or whole blood concentrations of CyA) Immunological variables (IgM, IgG, IgA, AM-AB, ANF)

cedures, goodness-of-fit-tests, estimation, and testing with respect to the primary end points. Secondary parameters are analysed, being considered as response variables as well as time-dependent risk variables (see Table 1).

Persons eligible for the study are patients with liver histology compatible with PBC. Numerous exclusion criteria were formulated to limit the influences of age (< 20 years, > 75 years), severity of PBC (end-stage disease), patient compliance and pre-existing disease which might lead to an increased incidence of side effects. Furthermore, patients having no signs and symptoms of PBC, and other confirmed causes of liver disease, e.g. hepatitis-B, alcoholic hepatitis or hemochromatosis, as well as patients suffering from serious non-hepatic diseases which reduce the life expectancy to less than one year, were kept apart from the study. Pregnancy, the wish to conceive and contraindications for immunosuppressive treatment (recent malignant tumors, uncontrollable infections) completed the exclusion criteria. All previous therapy, whether steroids, d-penicillamine, azathioprine or CyA, was discontinued before admission to the study. Corticosteroid treatment was only allowed if indicated for conditions other than hepatic disease.

CyA and a CyA placebo of identical appearance was given in a single daily dose of 3 mg/kg/day for patients assigned to CyA. CyA trough levels were measured 3 months after the start of the treatment. The measurements were repeated at 6-monthly intervals for dosage control and adjustments, which were made if pre-dose whole-blood levels of CyA were below 150 ng/ml and non-compliance was excluded or serum creatinine levels were above 170 μmol/l. Therapy was withheld in case of disease and events which contraindicate immunosuppressive therapy.

The patients were examined before entry to the study and at months 1 and 2 for side effects and serum creatinine, at months 3 and 6, and thereafter at 6-monthly intervals according to the initial examination procedure. IgM, IgG and IgA were repeated every 6 months and AM-AB and ANF at yearly intervals. Liver biopsy is performed at yearly intervals.

95 patients with PBC have entered the study since 1983. Only preliminary results are available on the still running and unblinded investigation. The age distribution shows a peak in the 5th and 6th decades of life with a preponderance of the female sex (80%). Side effects and discontinuation of treatment have been documented in 3 and 4 patients in the placebo and CyA therapy groups respectively. The total number of drop-outs is similar. Though a total of seven patients have died since 1983, namely 2 and 5 patients in each group, the estimation of survival using the life-time table method is only speculative.

The end of this blind and controlled study is scheduled for 1986. Preliminary descriptive data analyses are made at yearly intervals. The first full analysis will be available at the end of 1988.

References

1. James S. P., et al. (1980) Gastroenterol 79:242
2. James O., et al. (1981) Lancet i:1278
3. Roll R. K., et al. (1983) N Engl J Med 1:1–7
4. Routhier G, et al. (1980) Lancet II: 1223–1226
5. Triger D. R. , et al. (1980) Br Med J 281:772–775
6. Zetterman R. K., et al. (1980) Dig Dis Sci 25:104

Ciclosporin for Crohn's Disease

M. C. Allison, R. E. Pounder [1]

Corticosteroids are the mainstay of the pharmacological management of active Crohn's disease. Alternative immunosuppressive agents, such as azathioprine and its metabolite 6-mercaptopurine, are of proven effectiveness only in combination with prednisolone [3].

We have already reported our experience with ciclosporin (CyA) in a 20 year-old woman with severe extensive Crohn's disease [1]. She had developed a severe psychotic reaction to prednisolone: her Crohn's disease remained active for a year after the prednisolone was withdrawn. We treated her with CyA alone for eight weeks, initially at a dose of 16 mg/kg/day. Her response to CyA is shown in Figure 1. Her abdominal pain and diarrhoea disappeared while she was taking CyA, and she gained 5 kg in weight with a return of menstruation. We observed an improvement in the markers of disease activity: the erythrocyte sedimentation rate (ESR) and C-reactive protein (CRP) – both of which had been grossly elevated for the preceding year – decreased during treatment with CyA. The serum albumin rose from 24 g/l to 39 g/l (normal range 30–50 g/l). The patient felt much better during her course of treatment with CyA.

The object of the present pilot study was to ascertain whether the favourable experience with CyA in our first patient could be repeated in patients with active Crohn's disease.

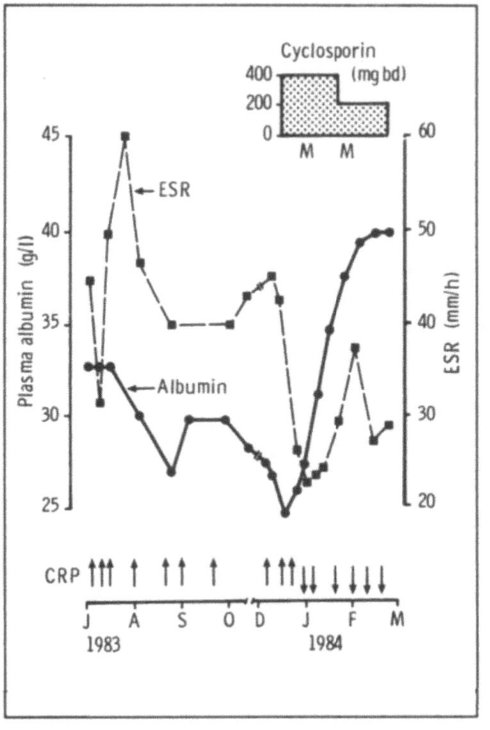

Fig. 1. Treatment of index patient with CyA (2): CRP ↑ = > 5 μg/ml CRP↓ = ≦ 5 μg/ml

Patients and methods

A group of patients was selected who had failed to respond to treatment with prednisolone and azathioprine, or had developed unacceptable side effects from such treatment. The patients had at least three of the following six criteria for active Crohn's disease: recent weight loss, elevated modified Crohn's Disease Activity Index (Table 1) [2]; hypoalbuminaemia; a raised ESR, CRP or platelet count. The six patients (one male and five female) had a median age of 21 years (range 18–26 years) and a median weight of 47.7 kg (range 39

1 Academic Department of Medicine, Royal Free Hospital, Pond Street, London, NW3 2QG.

Table 1. Crohn's disease activity index[3]

◆ General well-being yesterday	0 = very well 1 = slightly unwell 2 = poor 3 = very poor 4 = terrible	◆ Abdominal pain	0 = none 1 = mild 2 = moderate 3 = severe
◆ Number of liquid stools yesterday			
◆ Abdominal mass	0 = none 1 = dubious 2 = definite 3 = definite and tender	◆ Complications: arthralgia eye skin aphthous ulcers anal fissure new fistula abscess	1 per item

–55 kg). One patient had only large bowel disease, and five had disease affecting both small and large bowel.

The design of the study is summarised in Figure 2. At each visit throughout the study the following measurements were made: Crohn's Disease Activity Index, blood pressure, weight, full blood count, ESR, plasma electrolytes, urea, creatinine and liver function tests, helper and suppressor T lymphocyte subsets, serum CRP, and trough (12-hour) plasma CyA concentration.

The patients were observed on their existing therapy for at least five weeks. All treatment was then stopped for two weeks except in those patients who had been taking corticosteroids, who were continued on a small dose of prednisolone (6–8 mg daily) to prevent adrenal failure; this dose was continued throughout the remainder of the study.

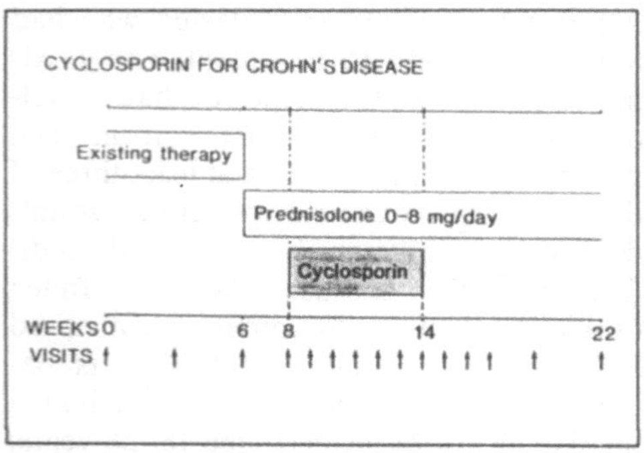

Fig. 2. Design of present study

All patients were then treated with oral CyA (2.5–10 mg/kg/day taken in two divided daily doses) for six weeks. The dose was adjusted to maintain a trough (12-hour) plasma CyA concentration of 70–100 ng/ml (determined by high performance liquid chromatography by Dr Z. Varghese, Royal Free Hospital, London). CyA was stopped after six weeks of treatment and the patients were followed for a further six weeks.

A pharmacokinetic study was performed in all patients before starting treatment. CyA was given as a single dose of 5 mg/kg in milk after an overnight fast. Venous blood was taken for plasma CyA concentration before and at 1, 2, 3, 4, 6, 8, 12 and 24 hours after administration. Plasma CyA concentration was measured by high performance liquid chromatography.

Results

Pharmacokinetic study: We demonstrated considerable variations in the time taken to reach peak plasma CyA concentration and in the height of this peak level. There was no correlation with the site of the disease: patients with extensive small bowel involvement were neither "better" nor "worse" at absorbing CyA than those with primarily large bowel Crohn's disease. However, smaller doses of CyA were required to achieve satisfactory trough CyA concentrations during the treatment period

Table 2. Side effects reported by six patients in trial. The brackets indicate side effects requiring treatment

Side effects	
Hirsutism	5 (1)
Fine tremor	3
Tingling hands	2
Upper respiratory infections	2
Headaches	2
Slight ↑ diastolic BP	2
Worsening acne	1 (1)
Fibroadenoma	1 (1)

by those patients who achieved peak plasma concentrations greater than 200 ng/ml in the pharmacokinetic study.

Response to treatment: During the six-week treatment period the mean dose of CyA was 8.2 mg/kg/day (range 2.5 –10 mg/kg/day).

Five of the six patients noticed a considerable improvement in symptoms during treatment with CyA. Diarrhoea disappeared in four of the five patients who had this symptom. Abdominal pains abated in four patients. The three patients in whom recent weight loss was a feature gained weight during the six weeks of treatment.

Indices of disease activity showed different responses to treatment with CyA. There was no improvement in the ESR, but the C-reactive protein concentration fell in all patients, with a return to normal in four. No clear trends were seen in helper or suppressor T-lymphocyte subsets.

All six patients relapsed within six weeks of stopping CyA. These relapses were accompanied by abrupt rises in serum CRP concentration.

Side effects: CyA was generally well tolerated (Table 2), and all patients were able to complete the six weeks' course of treatment. Five patients experienced an increase in body hair, but only one patient required specific treatment. Another patient developed worsening acne, which required a course of oxytetracycline after withdrawal of the CyA. This patient also noticed a breast lump two weeks after stopping CyA; histological examination of the excised lump showed a fibroadenoma. This benign form of breast disease has been reported in patients taking CyA [4]. There was no deterioration of renal function in any patient during the study. High trough plasma CyA concentrations (233–246 ng/ml) were associated with a mild increase of diastolic blood pressure in two patients; their blood pressure returned to normal after a decrease in the dose of CyA.

Discussion

This study suggests that ciclosporin may be an effective treatment for active Crohn's disease. There was an improvement in five of six patients who had either failed to respond to, or were unsuitable for, conventional pharmacological treatment. The observation of a marked relapse after stopping CyA lends further support to the belief that the drug is effective in patients with Crohn's disease.

The apparent benefit of CyA needs to be confirmed by controlled clinical trials. If this benefit is confirmed, further work will be necessary to define the optimum dose of CyA and duration of therapy. The role of CyA as a maintenance therapy for Crohn's disease in remission remains to be assessed.

References

1. Allison MC, Pounder RE (1984) Cyclosporin for Crohn's disease. Lancet 1:902
2. Harvey RF, Bradshaw JM (1980) A simple index of Crohn's disease activity. Lancet 1:514
3. Lennard-Jones J (1983) Sulphasalazine, corticosteroids, and immunosuppressive drugs in the treatment of Crohn's disease. In Allan RN, Keighley MRB, Alexander Williams J, Hawkins C (eds) Inflammatory bowel diseases. Churchill Livingstone, Edinburgh
4. Rolles K, Calne RY (1980) Two cases of benign lumps after treatment with cyclosporin A. Lancet 2:795

Controlled Study of Ciclosporin versus Corticosteroids in Acute Crohn's Disease: Methodology and Early Findings

U. A. Marbet, K. Gyr, G. A. Stalder [1]

Methodology

Stimulated by positive therapeutic effects of ciclosporin (CyA) in various autoimmune diseases, we have started a single blind randomised pilot study of CyA versus prednisone/salazopyrine in patients with Crohn's disease (CD) in addition to the uncontrolled use of CyA in patients with severe Crohn's disease not responding to treatment with high doses of steroids. It is planned to include 40 patients (age 18–60 years) with acute CD defined by a Crohn's disease activity index (CDAI) according to Best [1] of 150 to 350. The diagnosis of CD is established by the criteria used in the European Cooperative Crohn's Disease Study (ECCDS) [2]. The patients are stratified with regard to 1) the presence or absence of a previous maintenance therapy with steroids (patients previously treated with doses of steroids exceeding the equivalent of 20 mg prednisone are excluded from the study) and 2) the need for hospitalisation on entry into the study.

The effect of CyA is being compared with prednisone alone in CD patients with large and/or small intestinal involvement, and with the combination of prednisone and salazopyrine in CD patients with isolated involvement of the colon. Prednisone and salazopyrine are used in the doses employed in the ECCDS [2]. CyA is started in a dose of 5 mg/kg bodyweight/day and adjusted thereafter to obtain trough blood levels of 200–500 ng/ml. CyA is reduced if the serum creatinine exceeds 150 μmol/l.

The effects on CD activity of the different medications are evaluated after 6, 12, and 18 weeks of treatment using the activity index of Best [1] and of van Hees [3]. Additionally, the endoscopic and/or radiologic changes of the involved intestine are ascertained at the end of the study and the effects of the medications compared. Side effects of the different drugs are also noted.

The study is terminated if the Best CDAI falls below 150 at the evaluation after 6 or 12 weeks or after 18 weeks if it does not. Premature termination is envisaged primarily in the following cases: increase in Best CDAI of more than 100 over baseline at any time, fever of 39 °C or more for longer than 2 weeks, severe complications of the disease requiring surgery, or severe side effects of the medications which do not improve after appropriate dose reduction.

Early findings

We cannot as yet draw any conclusions. However, we would like to highlight two problems we have encountered during our limited observation time:

Oral administration of CyA: The obtaining of therapeutic blood levels in CD by oral administration of CyA may involve special problems, as illustrated by the following patient (not included in the prospective CD study): A 29-year-old hospitalised man with Crohn's colitis persistently suffered from bloody diarrhoea (9 times daily with need of blood transfusions of 800 cc per week) and severe abdominal cramps. Despite treatment with oral prednisone (7 weeks 40–60 mg daily), parenteral steroids (100 mg hydrocortisone tid 16 days) and hospitalisation with total parenteral nutrition (4 weeks), he lost 10 kg of weight (normal weight 57 kg), his serum albumin fell to 20 g/l, and the Best CDAI was elevated to 398. In this situation we decided to start a therapeutic trial with CyA (5, later 8 mg/kg bodyweight orally per day), while the steroids were discontinued gradually. During the following 3 weeks of treatment, the patient showed neither an

---

1 Division of Gastroenterology, University Hospital, CH-4031 Basel, Switzerland

improvement nor a deterioration of his disease. In view of the fact that the CyA trough blood levels remained below 135 ng/ml despite an increase of dosage, we started intravenous administration of 2 and later 4 mg CyA i.v./kg bodyweight daily in 2 doses, which resulted in CyA trough blood levels above 300 ng/ml. This change of administration form evoked a dramatic change in the disease activity with the CDAI falling to 170 after 3 weeks of therapy. The patient gained 6 kg of weight during this time, serum albumin increased from 20 to 30 g/l, and no further blood transfusions were needed. Nutrition could be changed to an oral low residue diet (3000 kcal daily).

Weak antipyretic effect of CyA: The second problem which may be encountered is the possibly weaker antipyretic effect of CyA compared to that of steroids. As demonstrated by another patient (19 years) this may mask a favorable effect of CyA on CD activity. The patient in question had a second flare-up of CD with small and large intestinal involvement and was treated with CyA according to our protocol. During the first 5 weeks of treatment the patient showed a partial response with an improvement in abdominal pain, diarrhoea, and general condition (fall of the Best CDAI from 318 to 249). However, the temperature remained around 39 °C and the study had to be terminated prematurely for this reason. Retrospectively, we learned that the CyA trough blood level never exceeded 200 ng/ml. The patient was treated thereafter with 60 mg oral prednisone per day, resulting in a rapid deterioration of his disease with the return of severe abdominal pain, diarrhoea, and a 4 kg weight loss in 11 days (increase of Best CDAI to 354). Only the temperature returned to normal. The patient finally improved after hospitalisation and the addition of a low residue diet (3000 kcal daily), the high dose prednisone therapy being continued. The therapeutic effect of CyA was apparently better than that of steroids alone although the effect of CyA was not sufficient during this therapeutic trial of 5 weeks. This patient had to be regarded as a premature therapeutic failure, probably due to the weaker antipyretic effect of CyA. Additionally, it has to be mentioned that the CyA trough blood levels were below 200 ng/ml. Since continuous high fever can be a sign of abscess formation or unrecognized superinfection, we do not think that we can for the time being drop this criterion for premature interruption of the study. Additionally, we cannot rule out that the response to treatment with steroids was diminished by the preceding therapy with the more strongly immunosuppressive CyA.

Conclusions

According to our limited experience with CyA in CD, CyA trough blood levels above 200 ng/ml seem to be necessary to obtain full therapeutic activity.

It may be difficult to obtain therapeutic blood levels in patients with CD by oral administration of CyA, possibly because of absorption problems or because of increased clearance due to enzyme inductions by previous medications. Therefore, measurements of CyA trough blood or serum concentrations twice weekly at the beginning with rapid reporting of the results is advisable in order to adjust the dosage optimally.

The probably weaker antipyretic effect of CyA compared to steroids may mask a positive therapeutic response to CyA treatment in CD. This has to be taken into account in the evaluation.

Further experience is needed to determine whether previous treatment with CyA may diminish the therapeutic effect of later treatment with steroids in CD and vice versa.

References

1. Best WR, Becktel JM, Singleton JW, Kern F (1976) Development of a Crohn's disease activity index. National Cooperative Crohn's Disease Study. Gastroenterology 70:439–444
2. Malchow H, Ewe K, Brandes JW, Goebell H, Ehms H, Sommer H, Jesdinsky H (1984) European Cooperative Crohn's Disease Study (ECCDS): Results of drug treatment. Gastroenterology 86:249–266
3. Hees PAM van, Elteren PH van, Lier HJJ van, Tongeren JHM van (1980) An index of inflammatory activity in patients with Crohn's disease. Gut 21:279–286

6. Sarcoidosis – Dermatology

Ciclosporin (CyA) in the Treatment of Pulmonary Sarcoidosis

A. S. Rebuck, C. R. Stiller, A. C. Braude, A. Laupacis, R. D. Cohen, K. R. Chapman [1]

Much progress has recently been made towards a better understanding of the pathogenesis of sarcoidosis [5, 9]. The fundamental role of the T lymphocyte has been highlighted by the observation of Pinkston et al. [9] that interleukin-2 has a central role in increasing the number of T cells in active pulmonary sarcoidosis. The activated alveolar macrophage also plays a crucial role not only in propagating the alveolitis associated with this condition, but also in initiating the progressive interstitial fibrosis that sometimes results. Recent work has demonstrated the importance of alveolar macrophage derived growth factor in causing fibroblast stimulation in pulmonary fibrosis [1].

Cyclosporin A is an 11-amino acid cyclic peptide metabolite of two fungi that suppresses T helper lymphocytes [4], blocks the release of interleukin-2 [4] and thereby prevents primary responses, but also terminates secondary T dependent responses [6]. It may also have an inhibitory effect on certain metabolic functions of rat alveolar macrophages, both in vivo and in vitro [7]. Its use in humans thus far has been largely limited to immunosuppression in the setting of organ transplantation [11] but recent reports in juvenile diabetes [12], posterior uveitis [8] and Graves' ophthalmopathy [13] suggest it has a role in autoimmune disease. We wish to report on three patients with active, biopsy proven pulmonary sarcoidosis who were treated with CyA.

1 Division of Respiratory Medicine, Toronto Western Hospital and Nephrology and Transplantation Unit, University Hospital, London, Ontario

Patient 1

A 28-year-old Caucasian male presented with shortness of breath and cough of six months duration. His chest X-ray showed bilateral hilar adenopathy, partial collapse of the right upper lobe and diffuse pulmonary infiltrates (Fig. 1). The vital capacity was reduced to 2.50 l (54% of predicted value), the flow rates at all lung volumes being reduced. At bronchoscopy the mucosa of the major airways was found to be edematous and friable, with the right upper lobe bronchus 90% occluded by massive mucosal swelling. Biopsies of bronchial mucosa, lung parenchyma and mediastinal nodes showed non-caseating granulomata. Gallium^{67} scan was diffusely positive, and the bronchoalveolar lavage differential cell counts from multiple sampled segments yielded an average of 50% T lymphocytes, with a relative increase in the percentage of helper T cells (T4/T8 = 1.2).

In view of his obesity (weight 350 lbs) and hypertension, the option of CyA therapy was offered. Informed consent was obtained; CyA was administered in a dose sufficient to maintain serum levels of 150–400 ng/ml for eight weeks (initial dose 17.5 mg/kg/day, adjusted to 5.3 at 8 weeks). Gradual clinical, radiological and physiological improvement was recorded. On cessation of therapy, vital capacity had increased by 650 ml, chest X-ray showed aeration of the right upper lobe (Fig. 2) and bronchoscopic appearance was normal. Parameters of disease activity confirmed suppression of the alveolitis [negative Ga^{67} scan and BAL lymphocyte count 20% (T4/T8 = 0.76)].

Long-term follow-up was not possible as 3 weeks after cessation of therapy the patient died at home of aspiration of gastric contents. Autopsy demonstrated persistence of multiple organ granulomata, but patency of major bronchi.

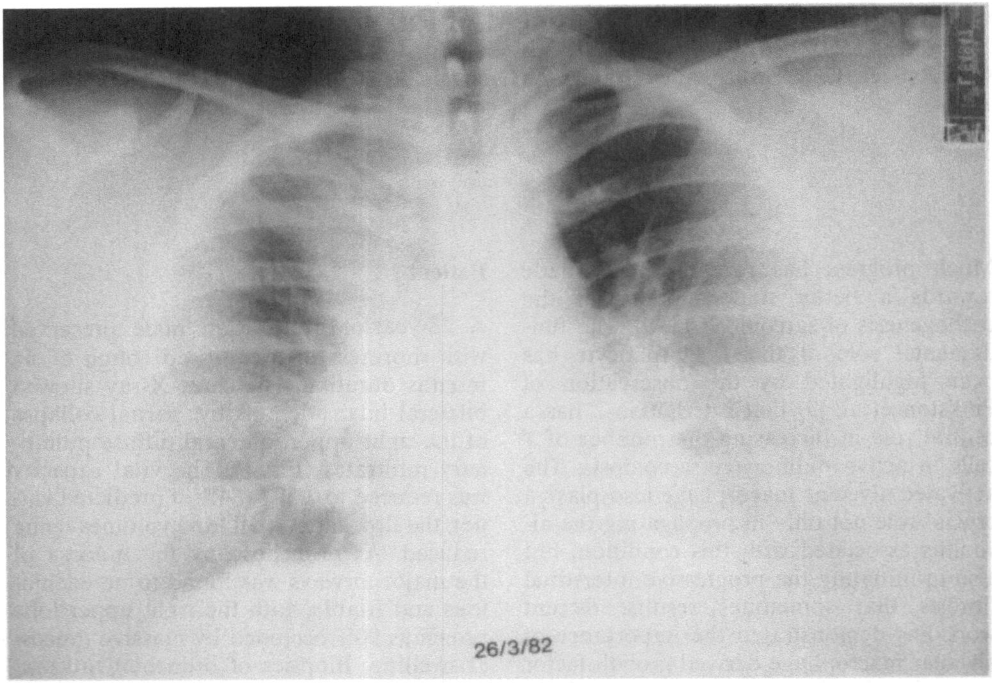

Fig. 1. Chest X-ray of Patient 1 at time of presentation with pulmonary infiltrate

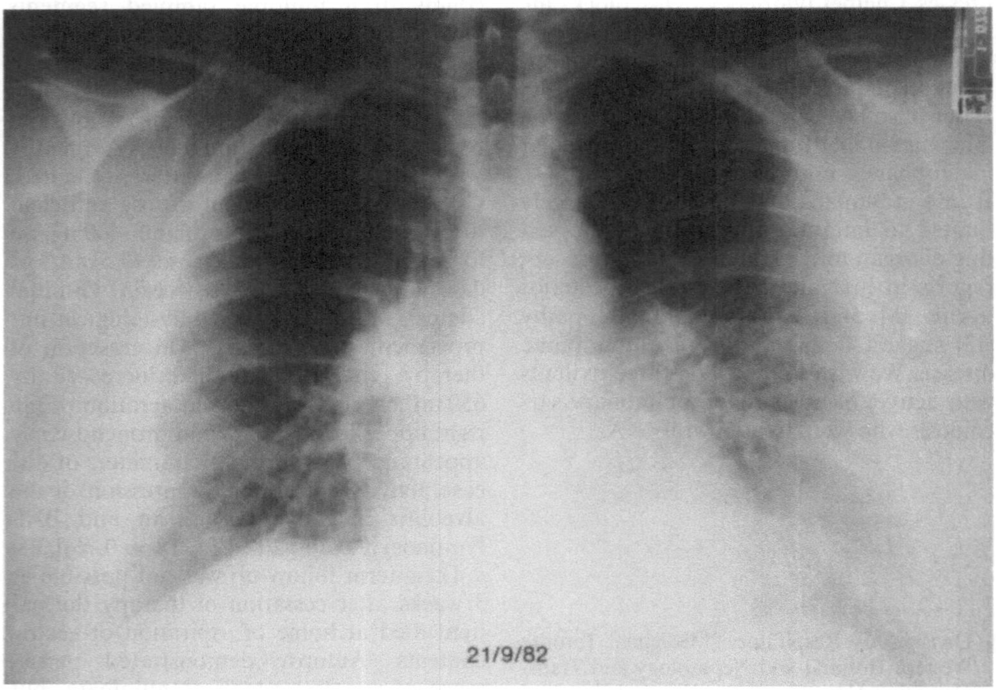

Fig. 2. Chest X-ray of Patient 1 following two months of ciclosporin therapy

Patient 2

A 27-year-old Italian woman had been treated unsuccessfully for lung biopsy proven sarcoidosis for two years. Disease activity, judged by strongly positive gallium^{67} scintigraphy and a BAL differential lymphocyte count consistently >40% T cells, had failed to respond to prolonged therapy with prednisone >0.75 mg/kg and the patient had become profoundly cushingoid. Dramatic relief of her cough and exertional dyspnea was achieved with an eight-week course of CyA (serum level 150–520 ng/ml; initial dose 17.5 mg/kg/day, adjusted to 7.3 at 10 weeks) complicated only by mild, transient gingival hypertrophy. Aside from radiographic improvement, vital capacity increased by 250 ml, diffusion capacity rose from 10.6 to 15.7 ml/min/mmHg (73% of predicted). There was suppression of the previous active alveolitis such that the Ga^{67} scintigram became normal and the BAL proportional lymphocyte count fell to 12%. During CyA therapy, the prednisone dose was reduced to a maintenance dose of 0.18 mg/kg. During the three-month follow-up period she has remained symptom-free, with stable lung function.

Patient 3

A 39-year-old Black male had been treated for 12 months with up to 50 mg/day of prednisone for biopsy proven pulmonary sarcoidosis. Treatment was stopped because of a lack of discernible effect on disease activity, as judged by a persistently positive gallium^{67} lung scintigram (lung/thigh ratio 9.1) and a proportional BAL lymphocyte count of >65% on repeated testing. Twelve months after steroids had been discontinued, CyA was administered for a total of 10 weeks (serum level 110–660 ng/ml; initial dose 17.5 mg/kg/day, adjusted to 9.1 at 10 weeks), the only complication being a mild deterioration in renal function which reversed once the drug was discontinued. The BAL proportional lymphocyte count decreased slightly to 55%. There was a progressive improvement in both the chest X-ray and gallium^{67} scintigram. Gallium scintigraphy showed the lung/thigh ratio falling to 4.3 after three weeks and to 2.8 at the completion of therapy. Pulmonary function studies remained within normal limits, apart from a mildly reduced CO diffusion capacity (87% predicted). The patient remained asymptomatic throughout the treatment period.

Discussion

This report describes our initial promising experience with ciclosporin in treating the alveolitis of active sarcoidosis. We were able to demonstrate a symptomatic radiographic and physiological improvement in two of our patients, and the third demonstrated a decrease in intensity of one component of his alveolitis, as evidenced by a significant improvement in his gallium^{67} scintigram and chest X-ray. Apart from the first patient, where corticosteroids were potentially hazardous because of extreme obesity, CyA was only administered when first line therapy with prednisone had failed. Side effects were minimal at the blood levels obtained.

Although the ultimate mechanism of action of CyA in producing immunosuppression is not known [2], two possible explanations might account for its observed beneficial effect in the alveolitis of active sarcoidosis. First, it inhibits the release of interleukin-2 from activated T-lymphocytes [4]. Secondly, it has been demonstrated to have an effect against selected metabolic functions of alveolar macrophages in an animal experimental model [6]. As gallium^{67} is taken up in the lung primarily by alveolar macrophages [3], the significant improvement in the scintigram of all three patients strongly suggests that CyA suppressed the macrophage-mediated component of the alveolitis either directly or by way of T-cell lymphokine inhibition. This demonstration of possible benefit without untoward toxicity of CyA merits a properly controlled trial of CyA in sarcoidosis.

Following our initial pilot study in the three patients reported here [10] we propose to extend the first phase to 10 patients. The study patients will have evidence of active sarcoidosis despite treatment with prednisone therapy (prednisone failure study). The second phase phase of the study (with the additional collaboration of Drs. P. Keown, S. G. Carruthers, D. Ahmad, D. Heinricks, R. Begin and S. F. P. Man) will compare the effect of ciclosporin therapy and high dose methylprednisolone pulse therapy, the design of which is to be randomized and double-blind.

References

1. Bitterman P, Adelberg S, Crystal R (1983) Mechanisms of pulmonary fibrosis: spontaneous release of the alveolar macrophage derived growth factor in the interstitial lung disorders. J Clin Invest 72:1801–1813
2. Borel JF (1981) Cyclosporin-A, present experimental status. Transplant Proc xiii:344–346
3. Braude AC, Chamberlain DW, Rebuck AS (1982) Pulmonary disposition of Gallium ^{67} in humans: Concise communication. J Nucl Med 23:574–576
4. Bunjes D, Hardt C, Rollinghoff M, Wagner H (1981) Cyclosporin-A mediates immunosuppression of primary cytotoxic T cell responses by impairing the release of interleukin 1 and interleukin 2. Eur J Immunol 11:657–661
5. Crystal RG, Roberts WC, Hunninghake GW, Gadek JE, Fulmer JD, Line BR (1981) Pulmonary sarcoidosis: a disease characterized and perpetuated by activated lung T-lymphocytes. Ann Intern Med 94:73–94
6. Drath DB, Kahan BD (1983) Alterations in rat pulmonary macrophage function by the immunosuppressive agents Cyclosporin, Azathioprine, and Prednisolone. Transplantation 35:588–592
7. Keown PA, Essery GL, Stiller CR, Sinclair NR, Mullen R, Ulan RA (1981) Mechanisms of immunosuppression by Cyclosporin. Transplant Proc 13:386
8. Nussenblatt RB, Palestine AG, Rook AH, Scher I, Wacker WB, Gery I (1983) Treatment of intraocular inflammatory disease with Cyclosporin A. Lancet II:235–238
9. Pinkston P, Bitterman PB, Crystal RG (1983) Spontaneous release of interleukin-2 by lung T-lymphocytes in active pulmonary sarcoidosis. N Engl J Med 308:793–800
10. Rebuck AS, Stiller CR, Braude AC, Laupacis A, Cohen RD, Chapman KR (1984) Cyclosporin-A in the treatment of pulmonary sarcoidosis. Lancet I:1174
11. Stiller CR (1985): Cyclosporin Therapy in Perspective. In: Morris PJ, Tilney NI (eds) Progress in Transplantation. Vol. 1 Churchill Livingstone, Edinburgh in press
12. Stiller C, Dupre J, Gent M, Jenner MR, Keown PA, Laupacis A, Martell R, Rodger NW, Graffenried B von, Wolfe BMJ (1984) Effects of Cyclosporin in insulin dependent diabetes mellitus of recent onset. Science 223:1362–1367
13. Weetman AP, McGregor AM, Ludgate M, et al. (1983) Cyclosporin improves Graves' ophthalmopathy. Lancet II:486–489

Ciclosporin (CyA) as an Alternative to Steroids in the Treatment of Sarcoidosis and Cryptogenic Interstitial Lung Disease

J. R. Joubert, G. Burger

Treatment of sarcoidosis and cryptogenic interstitial lung disease involves high doses of corticosteroids. This treatment is frequently not curative and a high incidence of undesirable side effects, such as tuberculosis, osteoporosis and hypertension is incurred. The immune pathogenesis of sarcoidosis and cryptogenic interstitial lung disease (CILD) is unknown but could be susceptible to the inhibitory effect of CyA. A pilot study was conducted in which the therapeutic efficacy and side effects of CyA, at its initial dose of 10 mg/kg/day, were compared with those of the conventional prednisone therapy. Two groups of 4 patients each, with either sarcoidosis (total 8) or CILD (total 8) were randomly allocated to either prednisone or CyA study groups. Prior to the start of treatment, patients were evaluated for the correct diagnosis by clinical investigation, radiology, alveolar lavage and open lung biopsy. The activity of the disease process was assessed before commencement of treatment and at three-monthly intervals for the 9-month period of treatment. Only patients with active disease were admitted to the study. Determination of activity included alveolar lavage analysis, serum angiotensin converting enzyme (SACE) values, clinical and radiological evaluation. The progression of the disease process was assessed by serial lung function studies. Four patients with CILD who had been treated extensively with corticosteroids and in whom the disease had reactivated subsequent to cessation of treatment were included in an open CyA trial. At the present time four patients with sarcoidosis have completed the full course of treatment, two of them having been treated with prednisone and two with CyA. Another two sarcoid patients on CyA have completed the first three months of treatment. In the CILD group, three patients have completed the CyA treatment, and one patient the corticosteroid treatment. Another three patients are in the process of completing the prednisone and CyA regimes.

The results of the sarcoid group indicate that clinical and radiological improvement was noted in patients on both therapeutic regimes. One patient on steroids and one on CyA remained unchanged, but no deteriorations were noted on either treatment regimens. Both forms of treatment suppressed abnormally high lymphocyte counts in the alveolar lavage.

In the CILD group, CyA induced a clinical improvement in all five patients but no significant radiological changes. Lung function improvement was noted on CyA treatment in four patients, while one remained unchanged. On completion of the CyA therapy a resumption of active disease was recorded in two patients.

In the steroid group the disease process relapsed in one patient when the dose was tapered. This patient subsequently improved again when he joined the open CyA study group.

Side effects recorded in patients on corticosteroid treatment included emotional disturbance, obesity and increased susceptibility to infections. Well-known and reversible side-effects were recorded in CyA therapy groups, and included hirsutism, paraesthesia and reversible elevation of serum creatinine levels.

Conclusion

Ciclosporin inhibits disease activity in patients with sarcoidosis and CILD. It does

---

Department of Internal Medicine and Allergy Clinic, Medical Faculty, University of Stellenbosch, Tygerberg Hospital not appear to inhibit all aspects of the immune pathogenesis of these diseases. It represents a feasible alternative to corticosteroids in selected patients, specifically those prone to the dangerous side effects of corticosteroids. The safety and efficacy of long-term therapeutic regimens which include CyA need to be studied. Accurate monitoring of kidney function is essential in patients in whom this tends to be impaired by the underlying disease.

This study is being conducted within the Diffuse Obstructive Pulmonary Disease Research Unit of the Medical Research Council of South Africa and in conjunction with Sandoz (SA).

Ciclosporin in the Treatment of Progressive Systemic Sclerosis

J. Knop and G. Bonsmann[1]

In this pilot study we plan to investigate the therapeutic effect of ciclosporin in the treatment for one year of 10 patients with progressive systemic sclerosis (PSS).

Study protocol

All patients entering the study had definite scleroderma as defined by ARA criteria and the disease was of more than three years' standing. Besides history and physical examination a full clinical status was performed including pulmonary function, roentgenogram of chest and upper gastrointestinal tract, in addition to renal and liver function tests, laboratory values, CBC and differential and evaluation of skin changes as monitored by using biomechanics testing parameters at multiple skin sites. Patients were further seen by a cardiologist and by a neurologist to evaluate heart, muscular and neurological involvement. Immunological parameters included antinuclear antibodies (ANA), ENA anti-n-DNA, complement CH50. The determination of T and B cells and T cell subset will also be studied.

During follow-up CBC, laboratory parameters, ESR were repeated regularly, skin changes were monitored again after 6 months, immunological parameters after 3 months. At termination of the study after one year all tests are to be repeated, including complete clinical status and monitoring of skin changes.

Ciclosporin was given orally, initially at 10 mg/kg/day in two divided doses. After 4 weeks the dose was reduced to about 4–5 mg/kg and adjusted to a blood trough level between 200 and 600 ng/ml. The drug level was monitored using a radioimmune assay* initially 2 times a week, later every 4 weeks.

Results

At this stage, 5 patients entered the study. No patient has completed the study, and 4 patients are still on ciclosporin. One patient took the drug very irregularly and has therefore been excluded from the study. Another patient has been on ciclosporin for one month only and can therefore not be evaluated. Three patients have now been on ciclosporin treatment for 8–10 months.

Patient Sch. F.: This 75-year-old woman had had PSS for about 4 years, with sclerosis of her hands, palms, face and anterior chest. The skin thickness on both hands before treatment was approximately 60 units and on the anterior chest about 70 units. She had mild interstitial fibrosis and pulmonary function was slightly affected. Raynaud's phenomenon was present. The pathological laboratory parameters were a ESR of 42 mm for the first hour, ANA 1 : 64 and an increase of IgG, IgA and IgM. After about 10 months of treatment a softening of the skin, particularly of the anterior chest and the hands, was observed. Skin thickness as measured on the hands was 26 units and on the anterior chest 23 units. The motility of the fingers was improved. No data are yet available with respect to the interstitial fibrosis and pulmonary function. The Raynaud symptoms occurred less frequently. No change of the pathological laboratory parameters was observed. After 9 months of treatment an increase of serum creatinine was observed which was reversible after reducing the ciclosporin dose. No further side effects were observed.

1 Universitäts-Hautklinik Münster

* (kindly performed by Prof. Lison, Medizinische Klinik, University of Münster)

Patient R. U. is a man aged 30 years who has now been treated with ciclosporin for 10 months. Two years before the first signs of scleroderma he had a myocarditis. At the time of hospital admission his hands were puffy with some sclerosis. His face and arms were swollen and the skin indurated. Skin thickness of the hands and arms was 70 units. He also complained of Raynaud symptoms. All laboratory parameters were normal. After 10 months of ciclosporin treatment there was a significant softening of the skin and a reduction of its thickness on the hands to 40 units and on the arms to 50 units. Raynaud symptoms occurred less frequently. No side effects were observed.

Patient E. B. is a 42-year-old women who has been treated for 9 months with ciclosporin. Before commencing the treatment she presented with scroscleroderma of the hands, arms and face which was partially softening. She further complained of Raynaud symptoms. She also had muscular involvement and her pulmonary function was impaired. The muscle enzymes were slightly increased. Anti-nuclear antibodies were found after 10 months of treatment, and the scleroderma improved further. No change in the Raynaud symptoms and muscular weakness was observed, and pulmonary function has not been evaluated. Muscle enzyme levels (aldolase, CPK) were also unchanged. She felt very well during ciclosporin treatment and no side effects were observed.

Summarizing the results of these preliminary observations, it can be said that neither a progression of PSS nor a marked improvement of the disease was observed. Under therapy, the sclerosis of the skin improved and Raynaud phenomena were less frequently observed. It should be mentioned, however, that softening of the skin may occur spontaneously and we are not able to say whether this is definitely due to the ciclosporin treatment. We cannot yet evaluate the effect of ciclosporin on internal organ involvement. Ciclosporin had no effect on pathological laboratory parameters such as ANA, immunoglobulins and ESR. Serious side effects were not observed (1 patient had renal side effects, 1 nausea and 1 gingivitis). Further data are required to evaluate the effectiveness of ciclosporin in the treatment of PSS.

Ciclosporin Inhibits the Effector Function of the T Effector Cell of Delayed Type Hypersensitivity

M. Braida and J. Knop [1]

Introduction

A substantial body of data demonstrates the immunosuppressive properties of the fungal metabolite cyclosporin A (CyA). Several T cell responses such as a mixed leukocyte reaction and lectin mitogenesis are blocked by this drug. It has been suggested that CyA inhibits the first stages of the T cell responses by suppressing the T cell stimulatory signals leading to activation and proliferation. It has been shown that CyA prevents the expression of receptors for T cell growth factor interleukin 2 [5] and in addition depresses the production of IL2 via a pathway involving inhibition of IL 1. The delayed type hypersensitivity reaction to various antigens is usually depressed by CyA, particularly if it is administered during the induction phase [2]. However, recent investigations have shown that in various in vivo delayed type hypersensitivity models cyclosporin A may even enhance the immune response, depending on the time of administration [6]. We have used contact sensitivity to 2,4-dinitrofluorobenzene (DNFB) in mice as a model of delayed type hypersensitivity to study the effects of CyA on this reaction. By transferring T effector cells of delayed type hypersensitivity (T_{DH} cells) to naive recipients we were able to show that CyA does not inhibit the induction of this T subpopulation but very efficently blocks its functional expression in the recipient animal. CyA may even enhance the immune response if a suppressive dose (antigen overload) of the contact sensitizer is applied to the skin.

1 Universitäts-Hautklinik Münster

Material and methods

Female BALB/c mice were sensitized to DNFB by two daily paintings on the shaved abdomen with 15 µl of 0.5% DNFB in an acetone/olive oil solution. Five days after the last painting 20 µl of a 0.3% solution was applied to the right ear. One day later, ear swelling was measured as a difference between the left and right ear thickness [3]. T effector cells of delayed type hypersensitivity (T_{DH} cells) were prepared from regional lymph nodes of sensitized animals in MEM Dulbecco. 5×10^7 cells were injected i.v. into normal syngeneic recipients which were ear challenged within 2 hours after injection. CyA was given orally in olive oil. The following dosages (mg/kg/bw) were used: 3.1, 6.2, 11.7, 23.3, 45.0 and 67.0. All the methods have been described in more detail in a recent publication [4].

Results

CyA given orally at a dose of 2 mg per animal at the time of sensitization (one day before and at days 0 and 1 of sensitization) suppressed the contact sensitivity response as measured 4 days later. Feeding the same dose one day before elicitation and at the day of elicitation of contact sensitivity also blocked the ear swelling response (result not shown). However, feeding 1.35 mg CyA one day before and during sensitization did not suppress the ear swelling response, although a significant suppression was observed when this dose was applied during elicitation (days 3 and 4; Fig. 1).

In the following experiment CyA at a dose of 2.0 and 1.35 mg/animal was fed during the sensitization phase. Lymph node cells containing T_{DH} cells were transferred from these animals to naive syngeneic recipients which were challenged

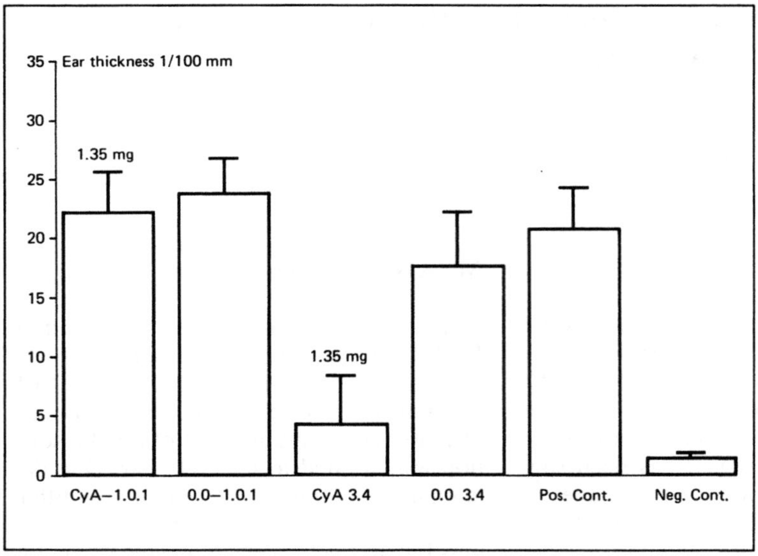

Fig. 1. Effect of CyA on the induction and effector phase of contact sensitivity. CyA was given orally one day before (day –1) and on two days of sensitization (days 0 and 1) or one day before (day 3) and on the day of elicitation (day 4) of contact sensitivity. Ear swelling was measured 24 h later. Positive control: sensitized animals. Negative control: non-sensitized animals painted at day 4 with DNFB. CyA = cyclosporin A; O.O. = olive oil control

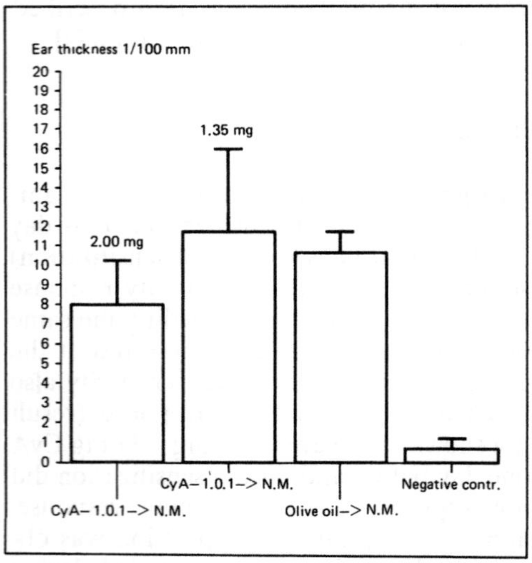

Fig. 2. Effect of CyA on the induction of T effector cells of delayed hypersensitivity (T_{DH}). Mice were treated with CyA on days –1, 0, 1 (see legend Fig. 1). At day 4 lymph node cells containing T_{DH} were prepared and transferred to non-sensitized, normal animals. These were painted on the ear 1 h later. Ear swelling was measured 24 h later. N.M. = normal mice

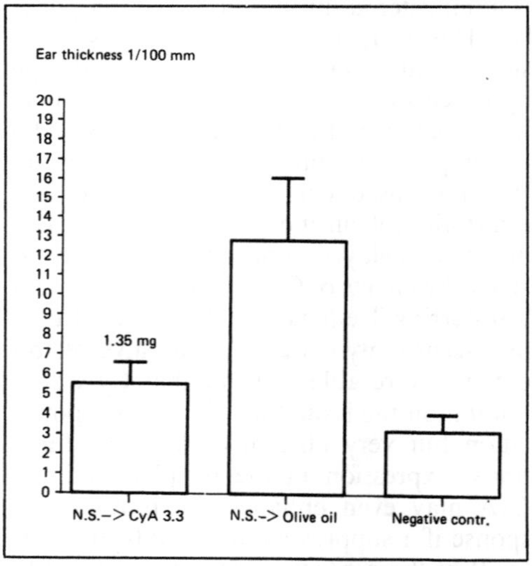

Fig. 3. Effect of CyA on the effector function of T_{DH} cells. T_{DH} cells were induced by sensitization with DNFB and transferred to recipient animals treated with CyA or olive oil one day before and on the day of transfer. Ear challenge was performed after transfer and ear swelling measured 24 h later. N.S. = normal sensitization

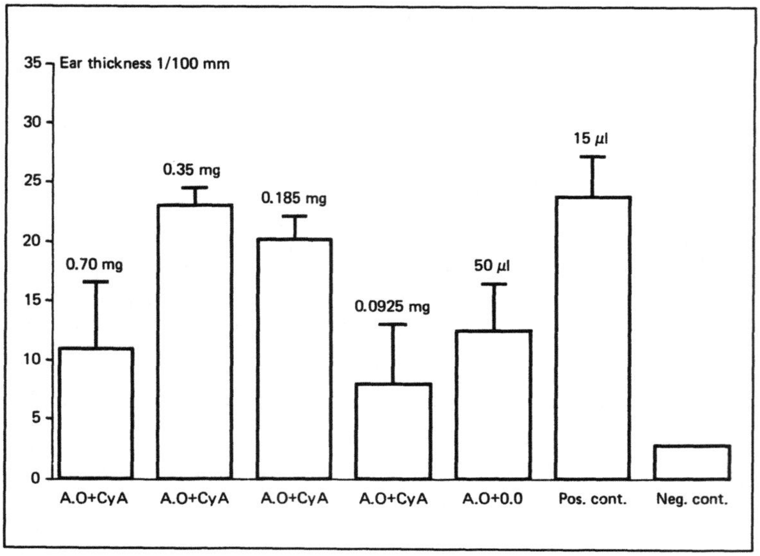

Fig. 4. Effect of CyA on contact sensitivity in animals sensitized with an DNFB antigen overload. CyA was given orally on days −1, 0, 1 (see legend Fig. 1). All animals (except pos. control) were sensitized with 50 µl DNFB instead of 15 µl. Ear challenge was performed as usual on day 4, ear swelling measured 24 h later. N.M. = normal mice

within one hour after transfer. 24 hours later the ear swelling was measured. Treatment with CyA during the sensitization phase had no effect on the generation of active transferable T_{DH} cells since all groups of recipients showed a significant ear swelling response (Fig. 2). Transfer of lymph node cells from DNFB-sensitized animals which had been treated with CyA one day before and on the day of the lymph cell preparation again resulted in a significant immune response in the recipient animals as compared with the controls, indicating that CyA must be present in order to be inhibitory.

In the following experiment the recipient animals of T_{DH} cells were treated one day before and on the day of lymph node cell transfer. As shown in Figure 3 the ear swelling response was clearly inhibited by the CyA treatment.

Increasing the dose of the contact sensitizer DNFB during sensitization to 50 µl instead of 15 µl of 0.5% DNFB (antigen overload) results in a diminished immune response which has been shown to be due to T suppressor lymphocytes. We treated animals sensitized with an antigen overload with various doses of CyA one day before and on the two days of sensitization. As shown in Figure 4, application of a sensitization dose of 50 µl (instead of 15 µl) resulted in a significantly reduced immune response. This was reversed by feeding 0.35 or 0.185 mg of CyA to the animals during sensitization. This result indicates that CyA can enhance a non-optimal immune response.

Discussion

The results presented demonstrate that:

1. CyA does not block the generation of T_{DH} cells when administered during sensitization.
2. CyA very efficiently inhibits the effector function of the T_{DH} cells.
3. The blocking effect of CyA on the effector function of the T_{DH} cell is reversible, i.e. CyA must be present in order to inhibit the functional expression.
4. CyA even may enhance a suboptimal immune response, indicating that at low concentrations it probably blocks the T suppressor cell pathway.

We have preliminary results from transfer experiments showing that CyA does indeed block the T_s cell. Similar results have been obtained in guinea pigs, using ovalbumine immunization [6] or the delayed hypersensitivity immune response to herpes simplex virus [1]. These results therefore strongly suggest that the T suppressor cell of delayed type hypersensitivity (at least one type out of several of these cells) is very sensitive to the action of CyA. Since this is a highly proliferative T cell subpopulation, it is tempting to speculate that CyA may act by inhibiting IL 2 receptor expression and IL 2 delivery to this cell type. Another possibility may be that CyA blocks the secretion of T cell suppressor cell factors. These experimental findings may be of clinical importance.

References

1. Altmann DM, Blyth WA (1985) The effects of cyclosporin A on the induction, expression and regulation of the immune response to Herpes simplex virus. Clin Exp Immunol 15:17
2. Borel JF, Lafferty KJ (1983) Cyclosporin A: speculation about its mechanism of action. Transplant Proc XV:1881
3. Knop J, Riechmann R, Macher E (1981) Modulation of suppressor mechanisms in allergic contact dermatitis: 1. Effect of C. parvum on the induction phase of contact allergy. J Invest Dermatol 76:193
4. Knop J, Stremmer R, Taborski U, Freitag W, De Maeyer-Guignard J, Macher E (1984) Inhibition of the T-suppressor circuit of delayed-type hypersensitivity by interferon. J Immunol 133:2412
5. Larsson EL (1980) Cyclosporin A and dexamethasone suppress T-cell responses by selectivity acting at distinct sites of the triggering process. J Immunol 124:2828
6. Thomson AW, Moon DK, Inoue Y, Geczy CL, Nelson DS (1983) Modification of delayed-type hypersensitivity reactions to ovalbumin in cyclosporin A-treated guinea-pigs. Immunology 48:301

Treatment of Pemphigus with Ciclosporin

G. Tappeiner, M. D. and V. Groh, M. D.

Case reports

Case 1

This was a 43-year-old Caucasian woman who was referred to our department with a 6-week history of a rapidly spreading bullous rash accompanied by fever and malaise.

On physical examination she showed numerous flaccid blisters as well as denuded and occasionally bleeding erosions involving large areas of the skin and mucous membranes. Nikolski's sign was positive. Except for a high sedimentation rate (40 mm in the first hour) and moderate leukocytosis (13,600), routine laboratory evaluation was non-contributory. Histological examination of a skin biopsy revealed intraepidermal suprabasal cleft formation. Deposition of IgG and complement within the intercellular spaces in diseased as well as in adjacent skin having a clinically normal appearance was demonstrated by direct immunofluorescence studies. The initial titer of circulating autoantibodies was 5120.

Based on these findings, the patient's disease was diagnosed as pemphigus vulgaris. After steroid pulse therapy (day 1–4, 100 mg 6-methylprednisolone/day) had failed to alter the disease activity, immunosuppressive therapy with CyA was initiated on day 5. A regimen of 500 mg/day CyA (≙ 10 mg/kg body weight) in a single daily dose was begun and monitored daily by whole-blood CyA level determinations. Within one week of this therapy, neither clinical activity nor titers of circulating autantibodies had changed; therefore, concomitant plasmapheresis was started (4 cycles/week, exchange of 3 litres of plasma per cycle). However, no decrease of clinical activity or serum auto-antibody titers could be obtained. On day 22, CyA was therefore replaced by 6-methylprednisolone, 300 mg/day. The patient's condition further deteriorated and she eventually succumbed to side effects of immunosuppressive therapy.

Case 2

This 30-year-old Libyan woman was hospitalized in our department from July 1984 to January 1985 because of a skin disease from which she had been suffering for the last two years. The patient had previously been treated with large doses of systemic corticosteroids and she already presented cushingoid features. A diagnosis of pemphigus foliaceus was made by histopathology and immunofluorescence in several skin biopsies as well as by the demonstration of circulating pemphigus autoantibodies. The major problem encountered with this patient was her poor response to treatment. First, combined therapy with 6-methylprednisolone, 200 mg/day and azathioprine, 200 mg/day was given. The patient tolerated the therapy well and showed prompt clinical improvement which permitted tapering the dose of 6-methylprednisolone down to 40 mg/day, at which point a rebound of the skin condition occurred. Seven plasmaphereses were therefore performed. After the last of these the patient showed another flare-up so that a trial of CyA was initiated. Corticosteroids and azathioprine were stopped and the patient received 600 mg of ciclosporin (≙ 10 mg/kg body weight) for 10 days. There was no favourable response but, if anything, a deterioration of the disease. Therefore, corticosteroids (60 mg fluocortolone/day) plus cyclophosphamide 100 mg/day were reinstated. However, no

---

Department of Dermatology I, University of Vienna, Vienna, Austria

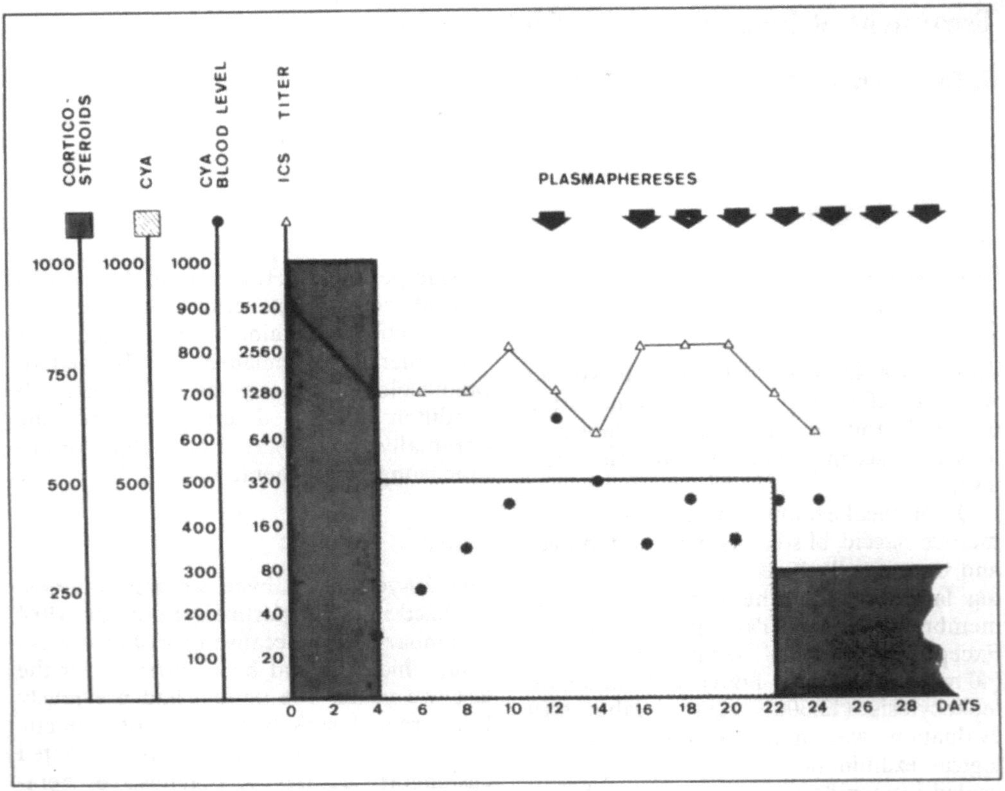

Fig. 1. Treatment of pemphigus with CyA, patient 1. Dark shaded areas indicate corticosteroids, given intravenously on days 0–4 and in a single oral dose after day 22. Light shaded area shows CyA, round dots CyA whole-blood levels. Pemphigus antibody titer is indicated by triangles and plasmaphereses by arrows. There was no clinical improvement of the disease over the observation period

marked improvement of the disease could be obtained.

Discussion

Pemphigus is a rare autoimmune disease of the skin in which an autoantibody directed against a cell surface glycoprotein of keratinocytes (pemphigus antibody) [1] causes loss of epidermal cohesion and blister formation [2, 3].

The introduction of glucocorticosteroids and immunosuppressive agents has vastly improved the management of this previously almost intractable and frequently fatal disorder [4, 5]. In spite of these advances, the treatment of pemphigus is not effective in all patients and the side effects of immunosuppression and cortisone therapy are themselves major causes of morbidity and mortality [6, 7, 8].

Therefore, a preliminary trial of CyA in the management of pemphigus was initiated. Because of the possibility of cumulative effects and particularly the induction of lymphoma, and because we wanted to obtain a clear picture of the effectiveness of CyA in this disease, no concomitant immunosuppresive or cortisone therapy was to be given. The doses administered were similar to those used in allograft rejection; CyA blood levels, monitored in one patient, were in the therapeutic range.

In the two patients reported on here, there was no favourable clinical response within the treatment period of two to two and a half weeks. Moreover, titers of circulating pemphigus antibody, which is thought to be indicative of disease activity,

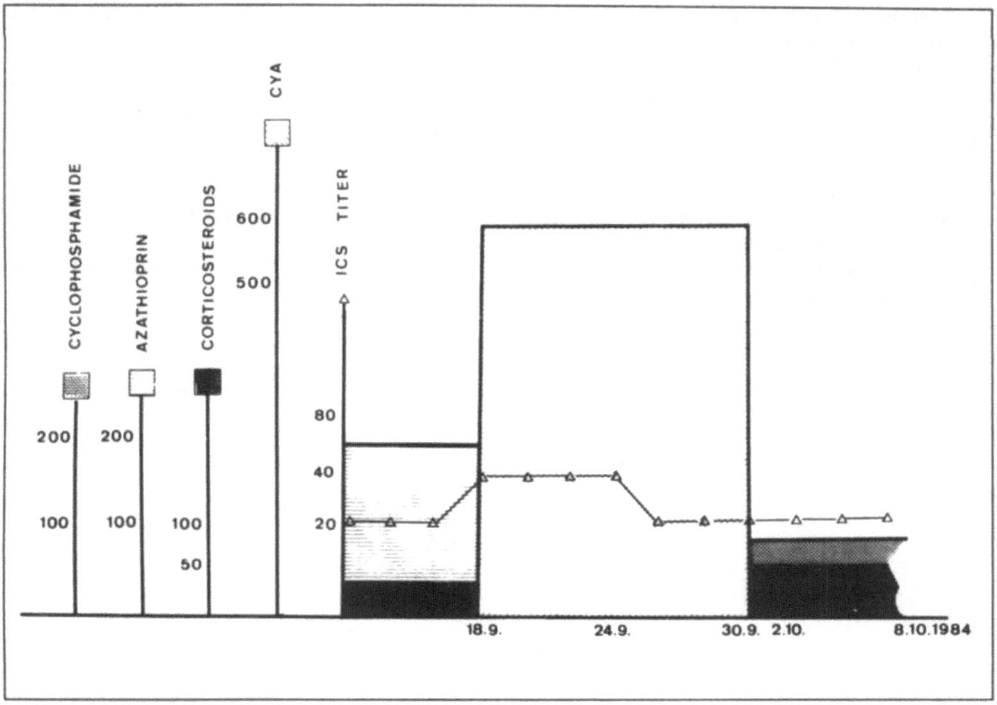

Fig. 2. Treatment of pemphigus with CyA, patient 2. Dark shaded areas indicate corticosteroids, light shaded area above it azathioprine and cross-hatched area above it cyclophosphamide, all administered orally; dosages to be read starting from the base line. Light horizontally shaded area shows CyA dosage, triangles indicate pemphigus antibody titers. There was no clinical improvement over the observation period. Plasmaphereses prior to CyA therapy not shown

did not change appreciably within the treatment period, even though plasmaphereses were started in one patient after the first week of CyA administration.

Because of the infrequent occurrence and heterogeneity of pemphigus, formal studies on patient groups of adequate size are not easily conducted. From the observation of these two patients we conclude that CyA, given as the sole immunosuppressive therapy or together with plasmapheresis, has no beneficial effect in pemphigus. Moreover, it does not seem to influence autoantibody production much, as evidenced by the failure of plasmapheresis and CyA therapy to decrease autoantibody titers. This agrees well with the new experimental data demonstrating little or no effect of CyA on B cells [9, 10].

It remains to be seen whether CyA combined with other modes of treatment may be of value in the management of pemphigus.

References

1. Stanley JR, Yaar M, Hawley-Nelson P, Katz SI (1982) Pemphigus antibodies identify a cell-surface glycoprotein synthesized by human and mouse keratinocytes. J Clin Invest 70:281
2. Farb RM, Dykes R, Lazarus GS (1978) Anti-epidermal-cell surface pemphigus antibody detaches viable epidermal cells from culture plates by activation of proteinase. Proc Natl. Acad Sci USA 75:459
3. Anhalt GJ, Labib RS, Vorhees JJ, Beals TF, Diaz LA (1982) Induction of pemphigus in neonatal mice by passive transfer of IgG from patients with the disease. N Engl J Med 306:1189
4. Fellner MJ, Katz JM, McCabe JB (1978) Successful use of cyclophosphamide and

prednisone for the initial treatment of pemphigus vulgaris. Arch Dermatol 114:889
5. Wolff K (1976) Immunosuppressive Therapie bullöser Dermatosen. Hautarzt 25 [Suppl 1]:25
6. Savin JA (1979) The events leading to the death of patients with pemphigus and pemphigoid. Br J Dermatol 101:521
7. Savin JA (1981) Some factors affecting prognosis in pemphigus vulgaris and pemphigoid. Br J Dermatol 194:415
8. Ahmed AR, Moy R (1982) Death in pemphigus. J Acad Dermatol 7:221
9. Borel JF (1985) Mechanism of action of CyA and rationale for use in autoimmune diseases. In: Schindler R (ed) Ciclosporin in Autoimmune Diseases. 1st International Symposium, Basle, March 18–20, 1985. Springer, Berlin Heidelberg New York Tokyo
10. Bach JF (1985) Contrasting effects of CyA on humoral and cell mediated immunity in patients with atuoimmune diseases. In: Schindler R (ed) Ciclosporin in Autoimmune Diseases. 1st International Symposium, Basle, March 18–20, 1985. Springer, Berlin Heidelberg New York Tokyo

Treatment of Bullous Dermatoses with Ciclosporin (CyA)

B.-R. Balda, D. Rosenzweig[1]

Today pemphigus vulgaris, including its clinical variants pemphigus foliaceus, pemphigus erythematosus Senear-Usher etc., is generally accepted to be an autoimmune disease with intraepithelial IgG antibodies. For that reason treatment aims at achieving the most effective immunosuppression possible by the systemic administration of steroids and azathioprine and occasionally also methotrexate [7]. If the course of the disease is particularly severe and serum antibody levels are high, plasmapheresis is tried as an additional means of treatment [7, 8]. However, this form of therapy involves considerable side effects because the immunosuppression is not selective. Almost all proliferative cell systems are more or less equally affected by the cytotoxic effects of the above-mentioned drugs, and in particular the immunocompetent cells and the haemopoietic system. A number of authors also report an increased incidence of malignant tumours in patients who receive such immunosuppressive treatment over a prolonged period [6]. In addition there are always patients whose bullous condition cannot be arrested or healed despite the prolonged use of immunosuppressives in high doses.

In the field of organ transplantation, a compound known as ciclosporin has been used for some time and can evidently suppress both humoral and cell-mediated immunity solely or at least preferentially through the suppression of certain T-helper cell populations, but does not impair the important macrophage function or have a myelotoxic effect [4]. We believed it would be useful to study the possible applications of this substance in so-called problem patients with bullous dermatoses, and report below on the successful use of ciclosporin in four patients with these diseases.

Cases

1. Patient F. B., female, born 29. 03. 1933. Diagnosis: Pemphigus foliaceus.

Case history: Several admissions to various hospitals over the past seven years for bullous eruptions on all parts of the integument. Freedom from symptoms not achieved despite continuous treatment with steroids and azathioprine in various doses. First admitted to our hospital on 20. 02. 1984 because of progressive deterioration of condition.

General condition: Fatigue, moderately severe moon face, slight bull neck and truncal obesity as signs of incipient drug-induced Cushing's syndrome.

Skin findings: All areas of the skin affected, including the scalp: Multiple lentil- to coin-sized erosions tending to merge in patches and covered with crusts, some haemorrhagic. Efflorescences of the same type also present on the face with a butterfly form of distribution.

Histology: In accordance with the clinical diagnosis.

Direct immunofluorescence: Characteristic for the clinical diagnosis with clear IgG and C3 deposits along the epidermal cell boundaries.

Indirect immunofluorescence (Dermatological Clinic and Out-Patient Clinic of the Ludwig Maximilian University, Munich, Director: Prof. Dr. Dr. med. h. c. O. Braun-Falco): Pemphigus antibody titre 640.

---

1 Dept. of Dermatology and Allergology, Augsburg, W. Germany, Stenglinstr. 1, D-8900 Augsburg, W. Germany

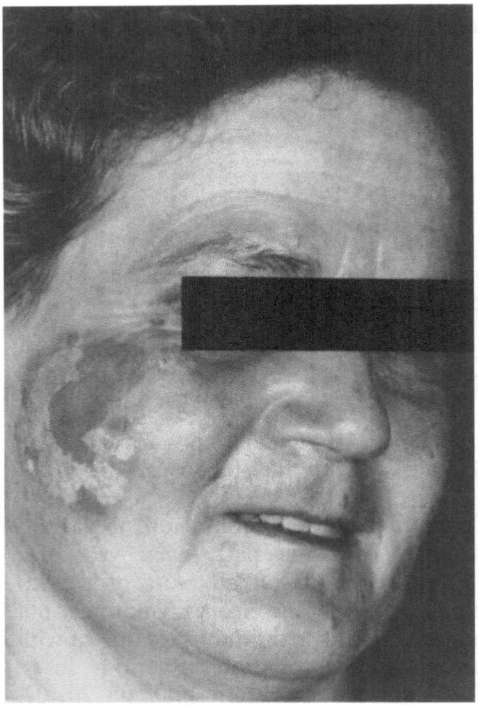

Fig. 1.

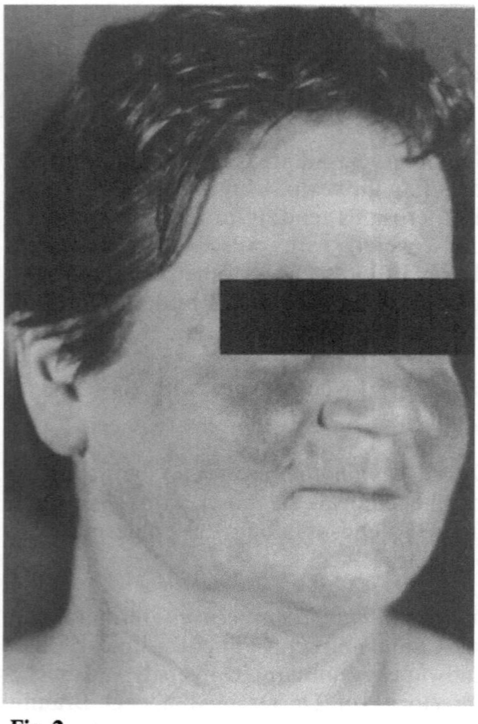

Fig. 2.

Other clinical and laboratory studies: No special abnormalities.

Therapy and course: Prednisone 100 mg/day and azathioprine 150 mg/day had no effect. Azathioprine was discontinued and replaced with oral ciclosporin in a dosage of 10 mg/kg/day. The steroid was reduced to 40 mg/day within 10 days, followed by a further gradual reduction to 10 mg on alternate days. Since then continuous treatment over one year with a ciclosporin dosage of 5.5 to 6.5 mg/kg/day and 7.5 to 10 mg prednisone on alternate days. On this treatment the patient has been virtually free of symptoms and has remained well with normal laboratory values. A further reduction of one of the two drugs was tried, but immediately led to "unrest in the skin" and itching, and to new skin eruptions after a few days. In the same way two trial withdrawals of ciclosporin were immediately followed by eruptions of the disease. Irrespective of the clinical disease pattern and the subjective condition of the patient, under this therapy the pemphigus antibody titre varied between 320 and 40.

2. Patient T. K., female, born 27. 05. 1929.
Diagnosis: Pemphigus erythematosus.

Case history: Bullous skin disease since 1981. Never free from symptoms despite treatment with azathioprine and steroids in various doses.

General condition: Fatigue, marked moon face, truncal obesity, and moderate bull neck as manifestations of drug-induced Cushing's syndrome.

Skin findings: Trunk, face and scalp affected: Poorly demarcated multiple areas of erythema, approximately coin-sized but sometimes as large as the palm of the hand, haemorrhagic crusts and yellowish, serous squamous crusts (Fig. 1).

Histology: In accordance with clinical diagnosis.

Direct immunofluorescence: IgG deposits along epidermal cell boundaries.

Indirect immunofluorescence (Dermatological Clinic and Out-Patient Clinic of the Ludwig Maximilian University, Munich, Director: Prof. Dr. Dr. h.c. O. Braun-Falco): Pemphigus antibody titre 80.

Other clinical and laboratory findings: Virtually normal throughout.

Therapy and course: Azathioprine stopped, prednisone reduced to 40 mg/day. Oral administration of ciclosporin started at 10 mg/kg/day, briefly increasing to 12 mg/kg. After clear clinical improvement prednisone reduced to 7.5 mg on alternate days and ciclosporin to 5 mg/kg/day. On this dose almost complete freedom from symptoms except for slight residual desquamation of the scalp and discrete erythema on the face (Fig. 2). Development of slight hypertrichosis on the cheeks. After a few weeks a further dose reduction was tried, but was followed by a new exacerbation of the disease. For one year now the patient has therefore been treated continuously with 3.5 to 4.5 mg/kg/day ciclosporin and 7.5 mg prednisone on alternate days. She is both subjectively and objectively well.

3. Patient M. H., female, born 28. 01. 1941.
Diagnosis: Mixed bullous disease.

Case history: Erosions of the buccal mucosa for 1½ years. Unsuccessfully treated with steroids and azathioprine and later also with dapsone. Extension of lesions to pharyngeal area and larynx, leading to marked hoarseness.

General condition: Clear drug-induced Cushing's syndrome with truncal obesity and moon face, fatigue, marked hoarseness. Incipient steroid-induced cataract and intraocular pressure at the upper limit of normal.

Skin findings: Multiple, sharply demarcated, yellowish-coated approximately pea- to coin-sized erosions and ulcers on the palate, the tongue and the buccal mucosa opposite the molars. Also small erosions in the lower pharyngeal area and at the inlet of the larynx. Small ulceration on the genital mucosa.

Histology: Suprabasal acantholytic and in parts subepidermal cleavage.

Direct immunofluorescence: Intra-epidermal IgG deposits, likewise intra-epidermal C3 and fibrin deposits. Also C3 and fibrin fluorescence along the basal membrane zone.

Indirect immunofluorescence (Dermatological Clinic and Out-Patient Clinic of the Ludwig Maximilian University, Munich, Director: Prof. Dr. Dr. med. h.c. O. Braun-Falco): Pemphis antibody titre 10.

Other clinical and laboratory findings: Largely free from abnormality.

Therapy and course: Steroids reduced to present dose of 10 mg prednisone/day, all other drugs discontinued. Since January 1985 initially 10 mg/kg/day ciclosporin, gradually reducing to present dose of 4.5 mg. Clear improvement in condition but slight rise in serum creatinine and blood pressure. After the ciclosporin dose was split into 2 daily portions, these symptoms returned to normal with a complete resolution of the mucosal changes and only occasional "thickness" of the voice. Marked regression of the cushingoid appearance, patient well.

4. Patient M. G., male, born 21. 03. 1923.
Diagnosis: Pemphigus vulgaris.

Case history: Bullous eruption over whole integument for seven years, resulting in hospitalisation in 1979 and 1983. Continuous treatment with methotrexate since 1978, also methylprednisolone in various doses. Largely free from symptoms under this treatment, except for occasional relapses. However, lesions had again been present on the buccal mucosa for four months.

General findings: Largely normal.

Skin findings: Small ulceraton with yellowish coatings on the right side opposite the lower molars.

Table 1. Ciclosporin (CyA) in patients with bullous dermatoses

Pat. No. Sex	Initials Date of birth	Diagnosis duration	Diagnosis made by	Unsuccessful previous treatment	Side effects	Treatment	Effects
1 Female	F. B. 29. 3. 33	Pemphigus foliaceus for 7 years	Clinical symptoms histology, DIF, IIF	Azathioprine, steroids	Initial Cushing syndrome, fatigue	5.5 – 6.5 mg/kg/day CyA, 7.5 – 10 mg prednisone every 2 days for 1 year	Free of symptoms
2 Female	T. K. 27. 5. 29	Pemphigus erythematosus for 4 years	Clinical symptoms, histology, DIF, IIF	Azathioprine, steroids	Initial Cushing syndrome, fatigue	3.5 – 4.5 mg/kg/day CyA, 7.5 mg prednisone every 2 days for 1 year	Free of symptoms, residual erythemas, transient initial hypertrichosis of the face
3 Female	M. H. 28. 1. 41	Mixed bullous disease for 18 months	Clinical symptoms, histology, DIF, IIF	Azathioprine, steroids, dapsone	Cushing syndrome, cataract, fatigue	4.5 mg/kg/day CyA, 10 mg prednisone daily for 3 months	Impressive improvement, transient hypertrichosis on legs and face as well as transient hypertension
4 Male	M. G. 21. 3. 23	Pemphigus vulgaris for 7 years	Clinical symptoms, histology, DIF, IIF	Methotrexate, methylprednisone	None	6.1 mg/kg/day CyA, 4 mg methylprednisone daily	Free of symptoms

Histology: In accordance with the clinical diagnosis.

Direct immunofluorescence: Unequivocal intra-epidermal IgG deposits.

Indirect immunofluorescence (Dermatological Clinic and Out-Patient Clinic of the Ludwig Maximilian University, Munich, Director: Prof. Dr. Dr. med. h.c. O. Braun-Falco): No evidence of pemphigus or pemphigoid antibodies.

Other clinical and laboratory findings: Diffuse damage to the liver parenchyma, but no other abnormalities.

Therapy and course: Methotrexate discontinued and methylprednisolone reduced to 4 mg/day. Additional 6.1 mg ciclosporin /kg/day in 2 portions. After 14 days on this treatment the lesions had regressed completely, and the patient was well with no demonstrable clinical or laboratory abnormalities.

These data are presented in summarised form in Table 1.

Discussion

The compound ciclosporin, its structural formula, its mode of production and its biological effects have already been presented in detail elsewhere in this monograph. Although its interactions at the molecular level are still largely unknown, it seems to be established that there is a selective inhibition of T-helper cells in the G_0 or G_1 phase and consequently of the formation of humoral antibodies and sensitised lymphocytes. For the clinical application of the substance it is particularly important that it is evidently not myelotoxic and that macrophage function is unaffected. The effects of ciclosporin are dose-dependent and reversible [4], as are the undesirable side effects such as nephro- and hepatotoxicity, hypertrichosis, tremor, hyperaesthesias, gingival hypertrophy, and, occurring very rarely and evidently only with the concomitant use of other immunosuppressives, lymphomas. However, the last-mentioned case applies only to extremely high dosages which are not normally used even in organ transplantation [2, 3].
Outside the field of organ transplantation there are a sporadic series of reports on the use of ciclosporin, primarily in non-dermatological conditions, in which connection the indications have not so far been clearly established (for overview see [1]).

The patients presented here are highly refractory cases of pemphigus in whom what in some cases was long-term therapy with immunosuppressives brought no improvement in the disease but led to considerable side effects. We therefore decided to administer ciclosporin in order to determine whether there was a demonstrable therapeutic effect and in order to avoid further risks to the patients resulting from their therapy. The previously administered immunosuppressives were stopped with the exception of steroids, which were initially continued in a medium dosage. The maximum initial dose of ciclosporin was 10 mg/kg/day, and this could rapidly be reduced to maintenance doses of 3.5 to 6.5 mg/kg/day. This resulted in active substance levels in the serum of 200 to 400 ng/ml. Under these conditions the steroids could also be reduced to small dosages ranging from 5 to a maximum of 10 mg per day, administered in most cases only on alternate days.

All patients showed a rapid improvement of their condition and finally a healing of the lesions. The side effects of the previous treatment disappeared. A few patients showed mild side effects of ciclosporin in the form of slight hypertrichosis and a small rise in blood pressure. However, these side effects regressed immediately after the ciclosporin dose was split into 2 portions per day. We have now observed two of the patients for more than a year, during which time they have remained symptom-free.

The drug's oral mode of administration proved to be a particularly pleasant feature. It enabled the patients to be rapidly discharged, attending only for ambulatory checks. Attempts to discontinue steroid administration completely proved a failure. We consider it a very important observation that minimal steroid doses around or below the Cushing threshold are mandatory for the successful use of ciclosporin in this indication. We cannot at present offer a satisfactory explanation for this phenomenon.

According to this limited experience, ciclosporin seems to be an effective medication for pemphigus vulgaris and its clinical variants when standard methods of treatment fail or have given rise to complications. It is very well tolerated in correct dosages and with adequate monitoring of the active substance levels. Nevertheless a warning should be given against the indiscriminate use of this mode of treatment. In our opinion careful clinical and laboratory checks and reliable patient cooperation are essential requirements, and it is no less important for the therapist to have adequate experience with the use of cytostatics and immunosuppressives. The determinations of blood ciclosporin levels must also be reliable, in particular because in a number of methods various metabolites are included in the result of measurement.

It will be important in future to carry out additional studies relating to dosage, in particular with regard to the possibility of combination with other drugs. However, the use of ciclosporin could help to improve our understanding of the pathological mechanism of these conditions.

References

1. Beveridge T (1982) Treatment of auto-immune conditions with Cyclosporin A. In: White DG (ed) Cyclosporin A. Elsevier Biomed Press, Amsterdam New York Oxford, pp 561–564
2. Beveridge T (1983) Cyclosporin A: An Evaluation of Clinical Results. Transplant Proc XV:433–437
3. Beveridge T, Krupp P, McKibbin C (1984) Lymphomas and lymphoproliferative lesions developing under Cyclosporin therapy. Lancet 8380/I:788
4. Borel JF, Lafferty KJ (1983) Cyclosporine: Speculation about its mechanism of action. Transplant Proc 15:1881–1885
5. Borel JF, Stähelin H (1983) Cyclosporin A – Geschichte und Bedeutung seiner Entdeckung. Sandorama 2:4–8
6. Kinlen LJ, Sheil AGR, Peto I, et al. (1979) Collaborative United Kingdom-Australasian study of cancer in patients treated with immunosuppressive drugs. Br Med J ii:1461–1466
7. Lever WF, Schaumburg-Lever G (1984) Treatment of pemphigus vulgaris. Arch Dermatol 120:44–47
8. Ruocco V, Astarita C, Pisani M (1984) Plasmapheresis as an alternative or adjunctive therapy in problem cases of pemphigus. Dermatologica 168:219–223

Ciclosporin (CyA) in Pemphigus and Bullous Pemphigoid

H. Barthélémy, J. Thivolet

Pemphigus and bullous pemphigoid are two models of autoimmune skin diseases. In these two dermatoses fixed and circulating antibodies directed against skin structures can be demonstrated.

Patients with bullous pemphigoid have type IgG anti-skin basement membrane antibodies. Fixed antibodies are invariably present but circulating antibodies may be absent. Pemphigus is manifested by the presence of auto-antibodies directed against the intercellular substance of the epidermis. The level of these circulating antibodies is generally well correlated with the development of the disease. Both these diseases are responsive to steroid therapy. The usual dose is 1 mg/kg/day of prednisone for bullous pemphigoid and 2 mg/kg/day for pemphigus. The classic treatment is difficult to carry out because of the side effects such as diabetes, heart failure and gastric ulcer occurring in these often elderly patients [1].

Patients

We treated seven patients with bullous pemphigus and eight with pemphigus. The patients had either received no treatment or were on steroid therapy. In this second group we took patients who were not controlled by steroids or had relapsed while taking them.

Therapeutic protocol

Whatever the treatment on entry into the protocol the patients were given 6 to 8 mg/kg of CyA daily in 2 doses. This dose was adjusted to obtain a residual serum level of CyA between 150 and 220 μg/l.

Where treatment was combined with steroid therapy from the onset, this was reduced by 5 mg prednisone equivalent per week as soon as clinical improvement was evident. For patients on CyA alone, prednisone was introduced at a dose of 0.5 mg/kg/day if there was no clinical improvement at the end of two weeks. On clinical improvement, cortisone was tapered off in line with the protocol as previously.

Subjects refractory to the combined treatment were removed from the test. All patients were treated for at least two months. Several patients have at present been on CyA for five and a half months.

Surveillance and criteria of assessment

All the patients were monitored every week for liver and kidney function (SGOT, SGPT, GT, alkaline phosphatases, bilirubin, creatinine, creatinine clearance) and blood count. If creatinine rose above 160 mmol/l, the daily dose of CyA was reduced by 20%. Blood pressure and pulse were checked twice a day.

In both diseases circulating antibody titres were rated every week. Wherever possible, a direct immunofluorescence examination was made after clinical cure. Efficacy was checked every week by evaluation of the functional signs (pruritus, dysphagia) and assessing the severity of the lesions (cutaneous and mucosal bullae, erythematous area).

A patient was judged to be cured when clinical lesions and functional signs had disappeared.

Clinique Dermatologique, Hópital E. Herriot, Pav. R, 69374 Lyon Cedex 08, France

Table 1. Bullous pemphigoid

Case	Fixed antibodies		Circulating antibodies		Age	Associated diseases	Results with CyA alone	Results with combinated treatment	CyA treatment duration (weeks)	Treatment at the time of workshop
	Before	After	Before	After						
1	DEJ	None	0	0	61	Obesity Diabetes Hypertension	Healing	–	16	Stop
2	DEJ	ND	0	0	46	Hemodialysed	Healing	–	18	Continuous
3	DEJ	DEJ	100	0	77	–	Failure	Healing	14	Continuous
4	DEJ	DEJ	0	0	81	Hypertension Obesity Stomach ulcer	ND	Healing	17	Continuous
5	DEJ	ND	1600	100	73	–	ND	Healing	22	Continuous
6	DEJ	0	0	0	80	Diabetes Hypertension	ND	Healing*	16	Stop
7	DEJ	ND	50	100	90	Cardiac failure Renal failure	Failure	Failure	9	Stop

* Relapse 10 days after treatment stopped
DEJ Dermo-epidermal junction
ND Not done

Results

1. Bullous pemphigoid (Table 1)

Four patients were treated with CyA alone. Two were cured in three and four weeks (cases 1 and 2). On clinical improvement failing to materialize, one patient was given prednisone, and her eruptions were controlled within a week. At present, after 14 weeks' treatment, she shows no signs of recurrence (case 3). The last patient did not respond to CyA treatment alone, or to combined treatment, or to prednisone alone in the usual dosage, and died. This resistance may be explained by age and especially the poor general state of health (case 7).

Three other patients (cases 4, 5, 6) relapsed or were not controlled by prednisone. The addition of CyA brought about a cure in every case within one to three weeks. In cases 4 and 5 this cure is stable after 18 and 22 weeks of treatment.

Patient 6 relapsed 5 weeks after steroid therapy was discontinued and 10 weeks after suspension of CyA. Resumption of CyA treatment enabled the disease to be controlled in an initial stage but the onset of moderate renal failure dictated the discontinuation of CyA.

In conclusion we obtained two good results with CyA alone and our patients receiving combined treatment were cured. We had one failure where evaluation was difficult due to the patient's advanced age.

2. Pemphigus (Table 2)

The patients were given first-line therapy with CyA alone. One case (case 1) was cured both clinically and immunologically in two weeks. He had a moderate pemphigus.

In two others (cases 2 and 4) the symptoms disappeared one week after the addition of prednisone at a dosage of 1 mg/kg/day for case 2. This undisciplined patient broke off treatment at the end of 15 weeks and relapsed eight weeks later. Resumption of therapy was unsuccessful and plasmapheresis had to be instituted.

In case 3 we obtained a marked improvement in the initial stage followed by a relapse. On ethical grounds the treatment was then discontinued and successfully replaced by prednisone at a dosage of 2 mg/kg/day, which was followed by serious side effects.

Patient 8 relapsed on low-dose prednisone. The addition of CyA was effective during an initial phase but then proved inadequate and the patient was then given combined treatment and was cured.

Cases 5, 6, 7 are the most noteworthy. These were patients who were resistant to steroid therapy in the usual dosage and in each case their symptoms disappeared in three to five weeks. In all these cases the cortisone has been discontinued or is being tapered off without a clinical or immunological relapse.

In conclusion, as in bullous pemphigoid, CyA, used alone, has no or only a limited effect (one success, four failures). On the other hand, combined treatment has always been successful and, in particular, CyA made it possible to cure patients who did not respond to steroids.

Tolerance

The overall tolerance of the drug was invariably good. We did not observe any arterial hypertension or changes in liver function.

Blood creatinine rose in four patients but in each case was normalized by reduction of the CyA dose. It is noteworthy that, even in one patient with a slightly impaired renal function (pemphigoid 7), CyA treatment could be given.

Four patients had infectious skin episodes. Cases 5 and 7 with bullous pemphigoid had two attacks and one attack of erysipelas respectively. In each case streptococcus A 12 was involved. Patient 5 had a generalized bullous infection due to a staphylococcus.

Patients 2 and 3, suffering from pemphigus, likewise had episodes of superinfection on their bullous lesions. All these bacterial skin infections responded well to appropriate antibiotic treatment.

These episodes are normally rare in pemphigus and bullous pemphigus and CyA may be a predisposing factor.

Table 2. Pemphigus

Case	Fixed antibodies		Circulating antibodies		Age	Associated diseases	Results with CyA alone	Results with combinated treatment	CyA treatment duration (weeks)	Treatment at the time of workshop
	Before	After	Before	After						
1	IC	IC	200	0	30	–	Healing	–	16	Continuous
2	IC	ND	100	0	20	–	Failure	Healing*	15	Stopped
3	IC	ND	100	800	54	–	Healing and relapse	ND	12	Stopped
4	IC	ND	0	0	76	Stomach ulcer Hypertension	Failure	Healing	6	Continuous
5	IC	ND	0	0	52	–	ND	Healing	5	Continuous
6	IC	0	200	0	59	Obesity	ND	Healing	24	Continuous
7	IC	IC	400	0	48	Rhumatoid arthritis Parkinson	ND	Healing	12	Stopped
8	IC	IC	100	0	48	Diabetes Psychosis	ND	Healing	18	Continuous

* Relapse in 8 weeks
IC Intercellular
ND Not done

Conclusion

CyA is not a first-line treatment for pemphigus and bullous pemphigus. In combination with low-dose corticotherapy (0.5 mg/kg/day of prednisone) it is regularly effective. It has been of particular value in controlling steroid-resistant pemphigus and, in every case, in reducing the duration and dosage of prednisone treatment. It is therefore a supportive drug of great interest.

It was excellently tolerated during our study and in this respect was greatly superior to corticotherapy at the usual dosage which gives rise to very severe side effects in these aged patients.

Our study is of a purely preliminary nature and calls for confirmation by a randomized multicentre study in which the therapeutic regimen would be as follows:

- the first month prednisone 0.5 mg/kg/day combined with CyA at a dosage of 7 mg/ kg/day.
- dose of prednisone tapered off and discontinued during the second month
- overall treatment with CyA for six months.

References

1. Levene GM (1982) The treatment of pemphigus and pemphigoïd. Clin Exp Dermatol 7:643–652
2. Palestine AG, Nussenblatt RB, Chan CC (1984) Side effects of systemic cyclosporine in patients not undergoing transplantation. Am J Med 77:652–656

7. Endocrine Ophthalmopathy

Endocrine Ophthalmopathy

R. Volpé [1], MD, FRCP(C), FACP

Endocrine ophthalmopathy is one of a triad of features including hyperthyroidism and pretibial dermopathy which characterize Graves' (Parry's, Basedow's) disease [4–6, 13]. The ophthalmopathy occurs in clinically recognizable form in about half of the patients with the hyperthyroidism of Graves' disease, is severe in perhaps 3–5%, and may be present in an occult form in many (but not all) of the remainder of the patients with Graves' disease. Conversely, it may occur in the absence of hyperthyroidism, and in many of these patients there is evidence of either overt or occult autoimmune thyroiditis. In still another small group with the same type of oculopathy, no evidence whatever of any thyroid disturbance is revealed by even the most sophisticated testing [15].

The ocular symptoms and signs vary [16, 17] (Table 1). On the one hand the patients may have no symptoms whatever, or conversely may present with manifestations due to inflammation, vascular congestion, proptosis, extraocular muscle involvement or optic neuropathy. Signs relating to these elements include conjunctival injection and oedema, periorbital oedema, photophobia, excessive lacrimation, discomfort in the eyes, blurring of vision, corneal ulceration, diplopia, diminution of visual acuity, or even blindness.

Pathology

Many tissues in the orbit seem to be involved in the lesion of endocrine ophthalmopathy, most particularly the extraocular muscles. The degree of ocular proptosis has been shown to be directly proportional to the extent of orbital filling [4–6]. Since the extraocular muscles of patients with ophthalmopathy may be enlarged to as much as eight times their normal size, it is not difficult to comprehend how the volume of the orbits in markedly increased.

The extraocular muscles are firm, rubbery, and markedly thickened on gross inspection. The medial and inferior recti are often more extensively involved than the other groups of muscles and asymmetrical involvement is common. Histological examination demonstrates widespread infiltration with mononuclear cells, particularly lymphocytes, plasma cells and macrophages. In addition, interstitial oedema is constant. The muscle fibres themselves appear normal. Fibrosis and fatty infiltration (but not myopathy) result in restriction of eye movements and diplopia. It is curious that only extraocular muscles are involved in this disorder, as skeletal muscles do not manifest this infiltration. There are structural differences and presumably antigenic differences between these two groups of muscles.

While there may be an increase in orbital fat, this finding is in dispute. In any event, muscle involvement seems to be the most significant abnormality since the ratio of muscle volume to fat volume increases with increasing proptosis. There is also an increased deposition of mucopolysaccharides which may be a by-product of the inflammatory reaction. The optic neuropathy has now been shown to be due to mechanical compression of the nerve by means of markedly enlarged medial rectus muscles at the apex of the orbit [4–6].

Investigations

In patients with obvious hyperthyroidism due to Graves' disease, the relationship of

1 Professor, Department of Medicine, University of Toronto; Physician-in-Chief, The Wellesley Hospital, Toronto, Ontario, Canada

Table 1. A detailed classification of the eye changes of Graves' disease
From Werner, S.C. [16, 17]

Class	Grade	Suggestions for Grading
0		No physical signs or symptoms
1		Only signs
2		Soft tissue involvement with symptoms and signs
	0	Absent
	a	Minimal
	b	Moderate
	c	Marked
3		Proptosis 3 mm or more in excess of upper normal limit, with or without symptoms
	0	Absent
	a	3 to 5 mm increase over upper normal
	b	5 to 7 mm increase over upper normal
	c	8 mm or more increase
4		Extraocular muscle involvement (usually with diplopia, other signs and symptoms)
	0	Absent
	a	Limitation of motion at extremes of gaze
	b	Evident restriction of motion
	c	Fixation of a globe or globes
5		Corneal involvement (primarily due to lagophthalmos)
	0	Absent
	a	Stippling of cornea
	b	Ulceration
	c	Clouding, necrosis, perforation
6		Sight loss (due to optic nerve involvement)
	0	Absent
	a	Disc pallor or choking, or visual field defect; vision 20/20–20/60
	b	Same, but vision 20/70–20/200
	c	Blindness i.e. failure to perceive light, vision less than 20/200

the exophthalmos in Graves' disease will be virtually beyond dispute. However, even in patients with ophthalmopathy in whom thyroid disease is not overt, testing the thyroid for the presence of autoimmune thyroid disease is essential in order to establish the association between the thyroid and eye disease (Fig. 1). This is therefore useful diagnostically in order to determine the nature of the ophthalmic disease where doubt may otherwise exist. Thus, levels of circulating thyroid hormones and TSH will be important to determine the presence of thyroid dysfunction, and a T3 suppression test may also provide useful information. The presence of thyroid autoantibodies and most particularly thyroid stimulating antibodies will also indicate the presence of autoimmune thyroid disease, although there is no correlation between the presence of thyroid stimulating antibody and the presence of exophthalmos in euthyroid patients ("euthyroid ophthalmic Graves' disease") [15].

More recently antibodies against extraocular muscles have been demonstrated to correlate with the presence of clinical exophthalmos; while this will be discussed further below, these antibodies have not yet been utilized for diagnostic purposes.

Measurements of intraocular pressure on upward gaze have been said to correlate well with exophthalmos and may be elevated even in the absence of clinical exophthalmos [3]. However, this point is in some dispute. Finally, visualization of the retro-orbital muscles, either by B scan ultrasonography or computerized axial tomograpy, has demonstrated the marked swelling of the extraorbital muscles, most particularly the medial rectus muscle [4–6]. These procedures have been exceedingly

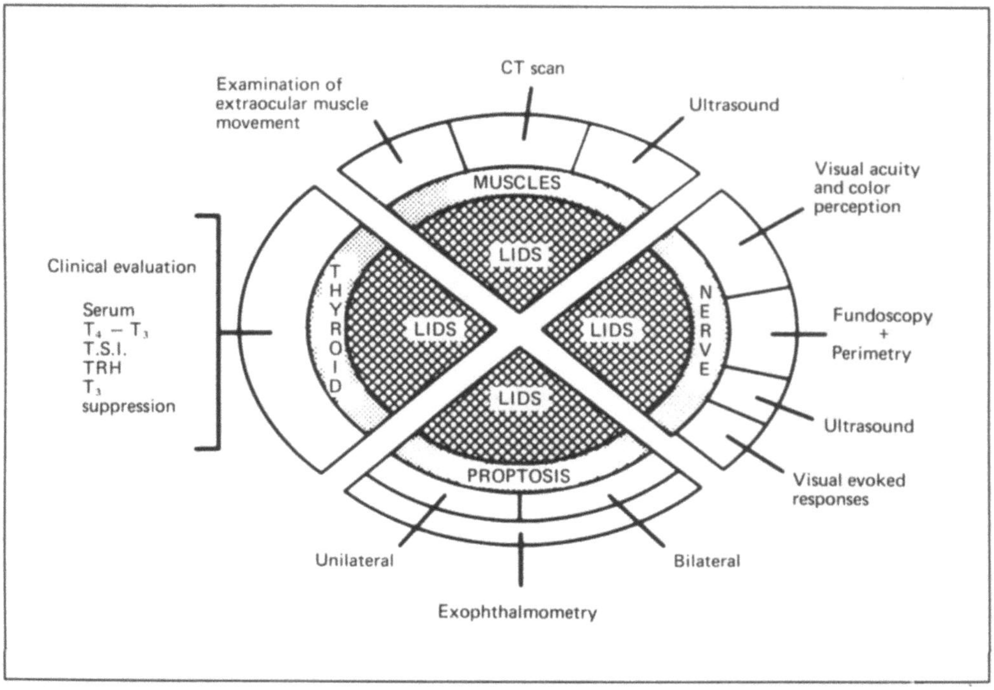

Fig. 1. Clinical and laboratory findings associated with endocrine ophthalmopathy. When all features are present, the diagnosis is assured. When all features displayed in one quadrant are present, the diagnosis is likely. Isolated involvement of the eyelids, muscles or nerves leaves the diagnosis open to question. Reprinted with permission from C.A. Gorman. Extrathyroidal manifestations of Graves' disease. In: The Thyroid, edition 5, ed. by SH Ingbar and L.E. Braverman. J.B. Lippincott, Philadelphia (in press)

useful in demonstrating the presence of the disorder, even in some patients with no obvious clinical exophthalmos.

Pathogenesis

Despite the apparently immune nature of the lesions of exophthalmos, the precise pathogenesis of exophthalmos remains controversial and unclear. The most interesting group of patients to study in this respect are those with "euthyroid" endocrine exophthalmos ("euthyroid ophthalmic Graves' disease") who have no clinical evidence of overt thyroid disease. Immunological testing of thyroid gland function in many of these patients may show evidence of some minimal thyroid dysfunction (see above). Thyrotropin binding inhibitory immunglobulin (TBII) or thyroid stimulating antibody (TSAb) may be present or absent in patients with ophthalmopathy who are clinically euthyroid [15]. If present, this is clear evidence of autoimmune thyroid disease and may be accompanied by other evidence such as antithyroglobulin or antimicrosomal antibodies, nonsuppressibility of thyroid function with T3 or an abnormal TSH response to thyrotrophin releasing hormone (TRH). Patients who are negative for TBII or TSAb may have clinical Hashimoto's thyroiditis (with or without hypothyroidism), may have occult autoimmune thyroid disease with thyroid antibodies, *or may lack all evidence of a thyroid disorder, no matter how tested* [15].

Studies of cell-mediated immunity in exophthalmos are of interest. Whole leukocyte preparations from patients with both ocular and thyroidal autoimmune disease

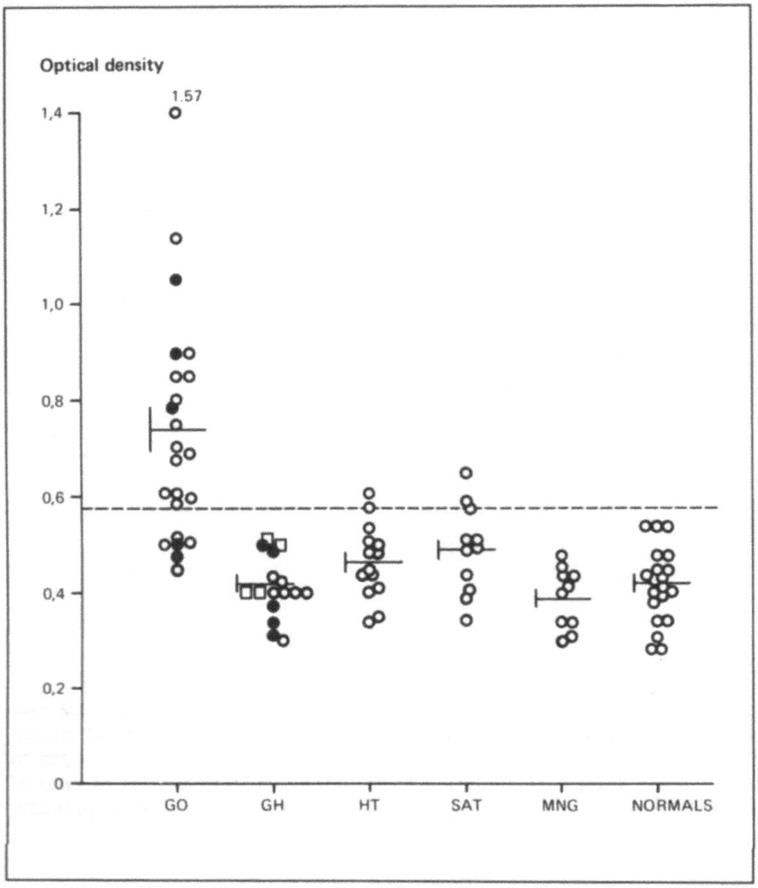

Fig. 2. Serum antibodies against a soluble antigen obtained from human eye muscle, measured by an enzyme-linked immunosorbent assay in patients with (a) active Graves' ophthalmopathy (GO) (● = euthyroid ophthalmic Graves' disease); (b) Graves' hyperthyroidism without eye disease (GH); (c) Hashimoto's thyroiditis (HT); (d) subacute thyroiditis (SAT); (e) multinodular goitre (MNG); and (f) age/sex matched normal subjects. Serum dilution 1/100. Results expressed as optical density. Horizontal lines represent means (± SE). Broken line (0.58) represents upper limit of normal. Reprinted with permission from Kodama et al. [10]

will exhibit migration inhibition factor (MIF) activity in response to retro-orbital muscle antigen. Patients with thyroid disease alone usually have a positive test in response to thyroid antigen but negative in response to retro-orbital mucsle antigen. Conversely if the patient with ophthalmopathy is devoid of any evidence of thyroid disease, MIF will be found only for retro-orbital muscle antigen [14].

It may be assumed that immunoglobulins (antibodies) play a role in exophthalmos; the serum of some patients with exophthalmos can cause the lesions experimentally. Cooperation between antibodies and lymphocytes in the production of exophthalmos has been demonstrated, and plasmapheresis has been used successfully to treat some patients with rapidly progressive exophthalmos and coincidental dermopathy [15]. While other authors have reported some successes with this modality, the overall view is that plasmapheresis is of little value in the treatment of exophthalmos.

Interestingly, Kodama et al. [8] have been able to demonstrate a circulating autoantibody against a soluble eye muscle antigen in Graves' ophthalmopathy (Fig. 2). These antibodies were detected in 17 of 23 patients with Graves' ophthalmopathy but in only 1 of 14 patients with Hashimoto's thyroiditis, in 2 of 11 patients with subacute thyroiditis, in no patient with Graves' hyperthyroidism without eye disease and in none with multinodular goitre. Similar findings have been reported by Kendall-Taylor et al. [7] and Faryna et al. [2].

Gamblin et al [3] have suggested that there may be a common pathogenesis for the orbital and thyroidal abnormalities in Graves' disease, even though some patients with hyperthyroidism of Graves' disease have no exophthalmos and despite the lack of parellelism between exophthalmos and Graves' hyperthyroidism as noted above. Early reports that total removal of thyroid tissue, (i.e. thyroid antigen) would result in improvement of the Graves' ophthalmopathy have not been confirmed [8]. However, two groups of investigators demonstrated that retro-orbital muscle has an affinity for thyroglobulin and thyroglobulin antibody-antigen immune complexes [15]. Kriss and Mehdi [12] demonstrated that lymphocytes from patients with exophthalmos will injure cell membranes from extraocular muscle when the muscle is first exposed to thyroglobulin. In addition, Kriss [11] was able to demonstrate lymphatic connections between the thyroid region and the retro-orbital area. Thus these authors postulated that thyroglobulin, immune complexes and lymphocytes from the thyroid gland reached the eyes via the lymphatics and there set up an immune reaction in the retro-orbital muscles. However, several groups studying immune complexes in the circulation of patients with Graves' disease with or without exophthalmos, have been unable to find any correlation between the presence of immune complexes and either the presence or the severity of the exophthalmos [15]. Moreover this hypothesis fails to explain the lack of relationship between exophthalmos and thyroid status in the absence of thyroid disease. In addition, Kodama et al. [9] could not confirm that human eye muscle membranes contain thyroglobulin, nor could they find binding sites for human thyroglobulin on human eye muscle membranes. Finally, Blau et al. [1] were able to demonstrate a thyroglobulin-independent, cell-mediated cytotoxicity of human eye mucsle cells in tissue culture of lymphocytes of a patient with Graves' ophthalmopathy. It would therefore seem that the hypothesis that the thyroid gland is in some way directly related to the exophthalmos does not constitute an adequate explanation or at least not an explanation for all cases, and it thus suffers as a unitary hypothesis.

Kohn and Winand [10] have suggested that TSH or fragments of TSH may be important etiological factors. Although TSH has been shown to be exophthalmogenic in animal studies, there is really no evidence to suggest an etiological role in man. On the contrary, TSH is reduced and its α and β subunits are suppressed in Graves' disease. Moreover, severe exophthalmos has been reported after an apparently total hypophysectomy [15]. Furthermore, in the MIF studies of Munro et al., TSH was ineffective as both antigen and enhancer of migration inhibition [14].

With the evidence demonstrated by Munro et al. [14], namely that patients with exophthalmos but no thyroid disease whatever will have leukocyte MIF activity in response to retro-orbital muscle antigen only whereas patients with thyroid disease alone without exophthalmos usually have a positive test for thyroid antigen only, a case could be made that the two entities, exophthalmos on the one hand and hyperthyroidism or Graves' disease on the other, represent very closely related but separable organ-specific autoimmune diseases. Moreover, as noted above, the studies of Kodama et al. [8], Kendall-Taylor et al. [7], and Faryna et al. [2], also suggest that patients with Graves' hyperthyroidism who do not have exophthalmos also do not have antibodies to soluble eye muscle membrane, once again suggesting that Graves' hyperthyroidism and endocrine ophthalmopathy do not share a completely common pathogenesis and thus could be classified as separable (albeit extremely closely related) organ-specific autoimmune diseases as originally proposed by our group [14]. There does not appear to be a separate

HLA marker for this disorder, although this has been disputed [15].

The proposal that exophthalmos may be a closely related but separate and overlapping organ-specific autoimmune disease is by no means accepted by all. While this author feels that the proposal best fits the clinical and immunological observations, it is clear that much more investigation is necessary before this field is finally illuminated. Gorman [4–6] certainly has a different perspective, suggesting that there could be a common pathogenesis for both thyroid disease and the eye disease, but the present author feels that this view is unjustified in the light of the available clinical and immunological observations, as summarized in this section.

Finally, medical therapy directed at the immune disturbance has, in the past, been disappointing. Large dosage corticosteroid therapy, while effective, is attended by unacceptable side effects [4–6]. Benefits from orbital irradiation, immunosuppressive drugs, and plasmapheresis have been variable. We anxiously await a new and promising initiative.

References

1. Blau HN, Kaplan I, Tao GW, Kriss, JP (1983) Thyroglobulin-independent cell mediated cytotoxicity of human eye muscle cells in tissue culture by lymphocytes of a patient with Graves' ophthalmopathy. Life Sci 32:54
2. Faryna M, Naumann J, Gardas A (1985) Measurement of autoantibodies against human eye muscle plasma membranes in Graves' ophthalmopathy. Br Med J 290:191
3. Gamblin GT, Harper DG, Galentine P, Buck DR, Chernow B, Eil C (1983) Prevalence of increased intra-ocular pressure in Graves' disease: Evidence of frequent subclinical ophthalmopathy. N Engl J Med 308:420
4. Gorman CA (1983) Ophthalmopathy of Graves' disease. N Engl J Med 308:453
5. Gorman CA, Waller RR, Dyer JA (1984) The eye and orbit in thyroid disease. Raven Press, New York, pp 1–341
6. Jacobson DH, Gorman CA (1984) Endocrine ophthalmopathy: Current ideas concerning etiology, pathogenesis and treatment. Endocr Rev 5:200–220
7. Kendall-Taylor P, Atkinson S, Holcombe M (1984) A specific IgG in Graves' ophthalmopathy and its relation to reto-orbital and thyroid autoimmunity. Br Med J 288:1183
8. Kodama K, Sikorska H, Bandy-Dafoe P, Bayly R, Wall JR (1982) Demonstration of a circulations autoantibody against a soluble eye muscle antigen in Graves' ophthalmopathy. Lancet 2:1353
9. Kodama K, Sikorska H, Bayly R, Bandy-Dafoe P, Wall JR (1984) Use of monoclonal antibodies to detect a possible role for thyroglobulin in the pathogenesis of Graves' ophthalmopathy. J Clin Endocrinol Metab 59:67
10. Kohn LD, Winand RJ (1971) Relationship of thyrotropin to exophthalmos-producing substance. Formation of an exophthalmos producing substance by pepsin digestion of pituitary glycoprotein containing both thyrotropic and exophthalmogenic activity. J Biol Chem 246:6570
11. Kriss JP (1970) Radio isotopic thyroidolymphography in patients with Graves' disease. J Clin Endocrinol Metab 31:315
12. Kriss JP, Mehdi SO (1979) Cell mediated lysis of lipid vessicles containing eye muscle protein. Implications regarding pathogenesis of Graves' ophthalmopathy. Proc Natl Acad Sci USA 76:2003
13. Lewis M, Topliss DJ, Okita N, How J, Row VV, Volpé R (1983) The etiology of endocrine exophthalmos. In: Franklin EC (ed) Clinical Immunology Update 1983. Elsevier Biomedical, New York, pp 261–280
14. Munro RE, Lamki L, Row VV, Volpé R (1973) Cell mediated immunity in the exophthalmos of Graves' disease as demonstrated by the migration inhibition factor (MIF) test. J Clin Endocrinol Metab 37:286
15. Volpé R (1985) Autoimmune thyroid disease. In: Volpé R (ed) Autoimmunity and endocrine diseases. Marcel Dekker New York, pp 225–231
16. Werner SC (1977) Modification of the classification of the eye changes of Graves' disease. Recommendation of the ad hoc Committee of the American Thyroid Association (Editorial). J Clin Endocrinol Metab 44:203
17. Werner SC (1978) Eye changes. In: Werner SC, Ingbar SH (eds) The thyroid, a fundamental and clinical text, edn 4. Harper and Row, Hagerstown, Maryland, pp 655

Ciclosporin in the Management of Graves' Ophthalmopathy

A. M. McGregor, M. Beck [1], A. P. Weetman, R. Hall

Introduction

Whilst the symptoms and signs of Graves' ophthalmopathy occur particularly commonly in patients with hyperthyroid Graves' disease and less commonly in eu- or hypothyroid individuals, they are usually benign and self-limiting [4]. In a small percentage of these patients the disease is progressive and disfiguring, and may threaten vision if left untreated. The pathogenesis is uncertain [4, 9, 10]. With poor understanding as to what causes the disease coupled with access to only small numbers of patients in individual centres, management is unsatisfactory.

Immunosuppressive therapy, orbital irradiation and orbital decompression have been used widely but never in a controlled trial situation. Having previously relied on high dose steroid regimens to control the disease, we remained concerned about the side effects associated with this mode of therapy and keen to seek an alternative but nevertheless equally effective treatment. In studies using a rat model of experimental autoimmune thyroid disease (EAITD) we had previously shown the ability of ciclosporin (CyA) to reduce the severity of EAITD, both once established [5] and during the period of its induction [2]. On the basis of these results we felt that a trial of CyA in Graves' ophthalmopathy was indicated and were able to report most encouraging results in our first two patients [8]. Eleven patients have now been treated and the results obtained with them are reported in this paper.

1 Departments of Medicine and Ophthalmology, University of Wales College of Medicine, Heath Park, Cardiff CF4 4XN, Wales, UK

Protocol

Criteria for entry to the study were that patients with progressive Graves' ophthalmopathy should have evidence of worsening congestion, ophthalmoplegia, or compromised visual tract function. Age, sex, duration of eye disease, thyroid status and previous therapy for ophthalmopathy were not considered as grounds for exclusion of patients from the study. The only patients excluded were those with systemic diseases other than thyroid disease. Informed consent was obtained, as was ethical committee approval. As a result of the decision made by the latter committee no patient was permitted to receive CyA in conjunction with any other immunosuppressive agent as combined therapy. Patients received 10 mg/kg/day of CyA orally. Prior to commencement of therapy blood was taken to assess haematological, hepatic, renal and thyroid function. Thereafter these parameters were measured regularly throughout the three-month course of treatment with CyA.

Ophthalmic assessment prior to and during treatment with CyA took into consideration alterations in both symptoms (Table 1) and objective signs of the disease (Table 2). Both subjective and objective criteria for disease severity prior to and in response to CyA were scored on a scale from 0 (nil) to 3 (severe) for the benefit of this

Table 1. Symptoms

Pain/grittiness
Watering
Photophobia
Double vision
Blurred vision
Protrusion
Difficulty closing eyes

presentation, so as to make the data more comprehensible. In addition, all patients were assessed prior to treatment and wherever possible post-treatment by orbital CT scanning for any alteration in eye muscle size.

Table 2. Objective assessment

Visual acuity
Visual fields (± scotomata)
Colour vision
Eye movements
Proptosis
Periorbital oedema
Chemosis
Intraocular pressure (upward gaze)

Table 3. Trial patients

Patient number	Age (years)	Sex	Disease duration (months)	Previous steroid treatment
1	59	M	1	–
2	58	M	9	–
3	51	F	7	–
4	35	F	5	–
5	48	F	4	–
6	41	F	20	+
7	59	F	24	+
8	49	M	11	–
9	51	F	36	+
10	58	M	3	–
11	46	F	14	+

Table 4. Concurrent steroid treatment

Patient number	Steroid treatment
1	Nil
2	Nil
3	Nil
4	Nil
5	Nil
6	Hydrocortisone 15 mg
7	Prednisolone 10 mg reducing
8	Nil
9	Prednisolone 15 mg reducing
10	Nil
11	Nil

Results

The eleven patients studied are shown in Table 3. The seven women and four men ranged in age from 35 to 59 (50.5 ± 7.5 years, mean ± SD) with a disease duration which ranged from 1 to 36 months (12.2 ± 10.2). Four had been treated previously (all with steroids) and of these 3 were still reducing their dose of steroid at commencement of their CyA therapy (Table 4). Nine had a previous history of hyperthyroidism (Table 5) and of these 7 were taking either antithyroid drugs or thyroxine replacement therapy during their course of CyA. Their symptoms at presentation are listed in Table 6.

Following commencement of treatment regular monitoring showed early evidence of impaired renal function in 4 patients (Table 7). In 3 the dose was reduced because of rising serum creatinine levels. Other side effects noted are listed (Table 8). In one woman hypertrichosis was so severe that, despite improvement in her ophthalmopathy, she insisted on discontinuing her CyA. All side effects were reversible either on reducing the CyA dose or on completion of the course of therapy. Patient number 6 had a complicated course. She was treated initially with CyA, but this was stopped after 4 weeks because of disease progression and she was transferred to high dose steroids. Once stable and on a reducing dose of steroid she was restarted on CyA and 10 days later developed pyrexia and an atypical pneumonia which was shown to be Legionnaire's disease. Steroids and CyA were stopped and she responded well to therapy for her Legionnaire's disease. Four patients failed to complete the 3-month course of treatment, namely patients number 5 (hypertrichosis, stopped at 8 weeks), 6 (progression of ophthalmopathy and Legionnaire's disease, stopped at 4 weeks in first course and ten days in second), 10 (progression of ophthalmopathy and renal impairment, stopped at 4 weeks) and 11 (progression of ophthalmopathy, stopped at 2 weeks).

Assessment of response to CyA treatment in the group as a whole was based on the patients' own subjective impressions, with the data obtained for each patient being

Table 5. Graves' ophthalmopathy/ciclosporin trial – thyroid status

Patient number	Thyroid history	Current thyroid treatment
1	Euthyroid, Flat TRH test	Nil
2	Hyperthyroid	Carbimazole
3	Hyperthyroid, Carbimazole, ^{131}I	Thyroxine
4	Hyperthyroid, Thyroidectomy	Nil
5	Hyperthyroid	Nil
6	Hyperthyroid, Thyroidectomy	Carbimazole Thyroxine
7	Hyperthyroid	Carbimazole Thyroxine
8	Hyperthyroid, $^{131}I \times 2$	Carbimazole
9	Hyperthyroid, Thyroidectomy, ^{131}I	Thyroxine
10	Euthyroid	Nil
11	Hyperthyroid, ^{131}I	Carbimazole Thyroxine

Table 6. Presentation

Patient	Eye presentation
1	Watering, Diplopia, Periorbital oedema, Proptosis
2	Diplopia, Proptosis, Periorbital oedema, Chemosis
3	Impaired visual acuity, Field defect, Loss of colour vision, Pain
4	Proptosis, Chemosis, Diplopia
5	Proptosis, Diplopia
6	Grittiness, Proptosis, Impaired lid closure, Diplopia, Periorbital oedema, Impaired acuity
7	Steroid sparing
8	Photophobia, Pain, Diplopia, Proptosis, Impaired acuity
9	Profuse watering, Pain, Photophobia, Impaired acuity, Incomplete lid closure, Periorbital oedema, Chemosis, Proptosis
10	Diplopia, Periorbital oedema, Impaired acuity, Minimal proptosis
11	Diplopia, Periorbital oedema, Chemosis, Proptosis

shown prior to and on completion of their course of treatment (Table 9). On the basis of these criteria it is apparent that in all patients except number 11 there was an impressive symptomatic improvement. The same could not be said for the objective criteria used to assess the response to CyA treatment. Whilst most patients showed some improvement in the criteria used (Table 10) it was only in patients 1, 3 and 4 that this could really be said to be dramatic. It is noticeable too that, apart from these 3 patients and patient number 5, all the remaining 7 patients required steroids on completion of their trial of CyA (Table 10). Assessment of eye muscle involvement by CT scan showed enlarged muscles in all patients prior to treatment (Table 11), except for patient 7 who never underwent CT scanning and patient 5 who had normal extraocular muscles. Following completion of treatment 7 patients were re-examined; 2 showed a decrease, 1 an increase and 4 no change in their extraocular muscle size.

Table 7. Serum creatinine level prior to and during treatment with ciclosporin

Patient number	Serum creatinine (mmol/l)							
	Pre-treatment	Weeks post treatment						
		2	4	8	12	16	24	30
1	90	88	116	110	110	87	82	74
2	94	139	159**	165	214	88	82	90
3	90	205**	90	95	139	100	93	91
4	106	79	87**	104	118	96	90	81
5	65	65	61	69*	71	80	69	64
6	104	90	84*	80	82	88	92	–
7	78	94	108	121	119	78	81	64
8	110	104	108	109	115	108	101	104
9	87	88	79	90	88	84	–	–
10	101	136	178*	191	198	141	111	98
11	84	96*	–	90	78	81	–	–

Normal range 60–120 mmol/l
Treatment ceased after 12 weeks

* CyA stopped
** CyA dose reduced to 5 mg/kg/day

Table 8. Side effects

Side effects	Number of patients	Outcome
Renal impairment	5	reversible
Hypertrichosis	5	reversible
Peripheral neuropathy	1	reversible
Abdo. pain and nausea	2	reversible
Legionnaire's disease	1	treated
Abnormal liver function	2	reversible

Table 9. Symptomatic alteration on treatment

Patient	Pre-treatment score	Post-treatment score
1	6	0
2	3	2
3	4	1
4	2	0
5	13	0
6	14	6*
7	5	3
8	9	4
9	14	5
10	5	2*
11	5	6*
	80	29

* Received only 4 weeks of ciclosporin

Table 10. Objective response

Patient	Pre-treatment score	Post-treatment	
		score	steroids
1	15	0	–
2	12	13	+
3	9	1	–
4	7	0	–
5	10	5	–
6	16	16*	+
7	5	3	+
8	12	11	+
9	18	16	+
10	9	9*	+
11	9	13*	+
	122	87	

* Received only 4 weeks of ciclosporin

Conclusions

In a trial in which we planned to treat patients with severe, progressive Graves' ophthalmopathy with a 3 month course of CyA (10 mg/kg/day) alone, eleven patients were studied. Four patients failed to complete the course of therapy because of worsening ophthalmopathy or unacceptable side ef-

Table 11. Eye muscle assessment by CT scan

Patient number	Pre-treatment scan	Post treatment	
		scan	outcome (muscle size)
1	+	+	decrease
2	+	+	increase
3	+	+	decrease
4	+	+	N/C
5	+ (normal muscles)	N/D	–
6	+	+	N/C
7	N/D	N/D	–
8	+	+	N/C
9	+	+	N/C
10	+	N/D	–
11	+	N/D	–

N/C = no change; N/D = not done

fects. But for a single patient who developed Legionnaire's disease whilst being treated with CyA and required specific treatment for this, all side effects were reversible and their complete resolution was observed on CyA dose reduction or cessation of therapy. The commonest problems noted were evidence of renal impairment and hypertrichosis. Evaluation of the effectiveness of CyA therapy was based on both subjective and objective criteria. Whilst most patients reported marked improvement in their symptoms, ophthalmological and radiological assessment did not support their enthusiasm. In only 3 patients was there really convincing evidence of improvement in their ophthalmopathy and but for these 3 patients and one other, all patients required steroid treatment on completion of their course of CyA. Furthermore, in only 2 patients of the 7 tested by orbital CT scanning before and after CyA could any reduction in extraocular muscle size be demonstrated. In 4 there was no change and in the 5th extraocular muscle size increased. On the basis of these results it would seem that CyA could be shown to be of benefit in the management of 4 of the 11 patients studied. Our initial impression, [8, 10] that CyA might be particularly effective in those with disease of relatively recent or even acute onset, ideally without previous treatment, in which one might expect the aberrant autoimmune response still to be ongoing, rather than in those with more chronic disease in whom fibrotic change would be likely to predominate [4, 6], has not been substantiated. On these grounds we would have expected an excellent response in patient 10, who gave a very short history and yet in fact developed worsening ophthalmopathy despite CyA and required subsequent high dose steroid treatment.

Whilst considerable interest has focussed on the potential use of CyA in the treatment of Graves' ophthalmopathy, it is much too early to assess its effectiveness. Small studies, like our own, have reported both a total lack of effect [1, 3] and extremely encouraging results [7, 11]. Whilst our own initial successes with CyA [8] have been somewhat altered by enlargement of our patient group, it is clear that a group of patients may exist in whom CyA is of benefit and as such may control their disease without the need for steroids. Until such time as we understand the disease better, and larger multicentre studies are performed in which increased numbers of patients are available and comparisons of therapeutic regimens (including CyA) in matched groups of patients is possible, the management of Graves' ophthalmopathy will not improve. In the meantime, however, individual units will continue to exhibit their own particular therapeutic biases and for the moment anyway CyA will continue to feature in ours.

References

1. Brabant G, Peter H, Becker H, Schwarzrock R, Wonigeit K, Hesch RD (1984) Cyclosporin in infiltrative eye disease. Lancet i: 515
2. Hassman RA, Dieguez C, Rennie DP, Weetman AP, Hall R, McGregor AM (1985) The influence of cyclosporin A on the induction of experimental autoimmune thyroid disease in the PVG/c rat. Clin Exp Immunol 59: 10
3. Howlett TA, Lawton NF, Fells P, Besser GM (1984) Deterioration of severe Graves' ophthalmopathy during cyclosporin treatment. Lancet ii: 1101
4. Jacobson DH, Gorman CA (1984) Endocrine ophthalmopathy: current ideas concerning

etiology, pathogenesis and treatment. Endocr Rev 5:200
5. McGregor AM, Rennie DP, Weetman AP, Hassman R, Foord SM, Dieguez C, Hall R (1983) The influence of cyclosporin A on experimental autoimmune thyroid disease in the rat. Life Sci 32:97
6. Trokel SL, Jakobiec FA (1981) Correlation of CT scanning and pathologic features of ophthalmic Graves' disease. Ophthalmology 888:553
7. Utech CH, Brunk G, Wulle K (1984) Treatment of severe Graves' ophthalmopathy with cyclosporin A. Ann Endocrinol 45, 14th Annual Meeting, European Thyroid Association, Rotterdam, p 14, Abstract no 11
8. Weetman AP, McGregor AM, Ludgate M, Beck M, Mills PV, Lazarus JH, Hall R (1983) Cyclosporin improves Graves' ophthalmopathy. Lancet ii:486
9. Weetman AP, McGregor AM (1984) Autoimmune thyroid disease: developments in our understanding. Endocr Rev 5:309
10. Weetman AP, McGregor AM, Hall R (1984) Ocular manifestations of Graves' disease: A review. J R Soc Med 77:936
11. Witte A, Landgraf R, Markl A, Boergen K-P, Hasenfratz G, Pickardt CR (1984) Treatment of Graves ophthalmopathy with cyclosporin A Acta Endocrinol (Copenh) 105, [suppl 264] 83, Abstract no 97

Treatment of Graves' Ophthalmopathy with Ciclosporin

R. Landgraf, A. Witte, A. Markl [1], K. P. Boergen [2], G. Hasenfratz, C. R. Pickardt

Introduction

Graves' ophthalmopathy is likely to be the result of autoimmune processes associated with autoimmune thyroid disease (for review see [8]). Whereas the eye signs do not require special treatment in most cases because they resolve spontaneously, in some patients extraocular tissue involvement is progressive with occasionally severe impairment of muscle function and loss of vision. In these cases immunosuppressive treatment [2], orbital irradiation [14], plasmapheresis [9], thyroidectomy [10] and surgical decompression [4] have been applied with contradictory results.

Recently ciclosporin has been reported to be beneficial in the treatment of a variety of autoimmune disorders [1]. Weetman et al. published two cases of endocrine ophthalmopathy which improved rapidly during ciclosporin treatment [16], and Utech and co-workers also reported an improvement of this condition [15]. Moreover, beneficial effects of ciclosporin on experimental autoimmune thyroid diseases in the PVG/c rat have been published [6, 12].

For these reasons, we felt justified in using ciclosporin in a group of patients whose eye disease could not be adequately controlled by the usual mode of treatment with steroids and radiotherapy.

Patients

Thirteen patients with a mean age of 51 ± 9 years were included in this study (Table 1). The clinical manifestation of thyroid disease ranged in duration between 1 and 42 months. All patients were euthyroid at the time of the study, and were receiving or had received treatment for hyperthyroidism. The eye symptoms occurred 6–18 months before initiation of ciclosporin treatment. All patients had severe class IV–VI ophthalmopathy according to the classification of Werner [17]. Ciclosporin treatment was preceded by steroid administration in 9 patients (Table 1), and in 4 of them steroids were continued. Previous orbital radiotherapy had been performed without success in 7 patients. The start of ciclosporin coincided with radiotherapy in patient No. 8 (Table 1).

The initial dose of ciclosporin was 10 mg/kg bodyweight per day in two divided doses with subsequent reduction in accordance with the CyA blood levels in order to obtain a range of 200–500 ng/ml 12 hours after the last dose. The duration of therapy was 4–7 months, with 3 exceptions in whom treatment had to be stopped or interrupted due to side effects. Follow-up investigations were performed initially every two weeks and then at monthly intervals.

Investigation methods

Thyroid function, renal function, hematological parameters and liver function were tested by routine assays.

TSH-displacing activity (TDA) was measured in a radioreceptor assay using crude human thyroid membranes, membrane purified iodinated TSH and IgG purified from patients' serum with PEG-precipitation followed by anion exchange chromatography [18].

Complete ophthalmological investigation (Hertel ophthalmometer, visual field,

Medizinische Klinik Innenstadt der Universität München, Ziemssenstrasse 1, D-8000 München 2

1 Klinik und Poliklinik für Radiologie der Universität Innenstadt, Ziemssenstrasse 1, D-8000 München

2 Augenklinik der Universität, Mathildenstr. 8, D-8000 München 2

Table 1. Summary of clinical data of 13 patients, with regard to hyperthyroidism and ophthalmopathy

No.	Sex	Age	Hyperthyroidism			Ophthalmopathy		
			duration (m)	treatment	present thyr. fct.	duration (m)	previous treatment	present treatment
1	f	51	15	med.	eu	9	steroids, irrad.	steroids
2	f	54	12	surg.	eu, TSH suppr.	9	steroids	–
3	m	61	24	surg.	eu, (med.)	13	steroids, irrad.	steroids
4	f	38	34	surg., ^{131}I	eu, TSH suppr.	16	steroids, irrad.	–
5	f	47	18	med.	eu, (T_4)	12	steroids, irrad.	steroids
6	f	50	9	surg.	eu	9	steroids	steroids
7	m	52	13	med.	eu, (med.)	6	steroids, irrad.	–
8	f	43	23	med.	eu, (med.)	9	–	irrad.
9	f	53	42	med.	eu	6	–	–
10	f	47	6	med.	eu, (med.)	11	–	–
11	f	40	13	surg.	eu, (T_4)	13	steroids, irrad.	–
12	f	70	1	surg.	eu, (med.)	1	–	steroids, irrad.
13	f	63	10	med.	eu	10	steroids, irrad.	–

abbreviations: med. = medical treatment (carbimazole), surg. = surgical treatment, ^{131}I = radioiodine treatment, eu = euthyroid, TSH-suppr. = TSH refractory to TRH, T_4 = thyroid hormone treatment, irrad. = orbital irradiation

Table 2. Characteristics of the "ophthalmopathy index" (I)

> "sandy" feeling	> proptosis
> retrobulbar discomfort	> conjunctival injection
> increased lacrimation	> upper lid retraction
> painful eye movement	> lid lag
> diplopia	> puffiness
> blurring	> chemosis
> photophobia	> restriction of eye movement

0 = not present; 1 = mild; 2 = moderate; 3 = severe

intraocular pressure in primary position and on upgaze, visual acuity) was performed at monthly intervals. Orbital ultrasonography was obtained by A and B ultrasonogram [13].

Two dimensional computed tomography [5] of the orbits, using axial, transverse and coronary sections, was performed before and after treatment. In computed tomography the area of the muscle cross sections, which were corrected for perpendicular angles in relation to the course of the muscle, were measured according to the assumption of the corrected cross sections being ellipsoid: $a/2 \times b/2 \times \pi$ (mm^2).

Proptosis was calculated from the computerized tomography as the maximum distance of the corneal peak from line joining the medial and lateral orbital edges.

Signs and symptoms of the disease were monitored using a scale of 0–3 as detailed in Table 2.

Results

Clinical signs and symptoms improved in all 8 patients, whose data were summarized by the "ophthalmopathy index" (Fig. 1). The decrease was most striking in the patient with simultaneous radiotherapy (No. 8). There was no correlation between the improvement of the "ophthalmopathy index" and the previous duration of the eye signs.

The ophthalmological parameters (Table 3) did not change during ciclosporin treatment.

Ultrasonographic investigations demonstrated the typical asymmetrical involvement of the different extraocular muscles. In most cases a slight decrease in muscle diameter was found during treatment (Fig. 2), but it is noteworthy that different muscles in one individual did not behave uniformly: an increase in one muscle diameter and a decrease in another could be observed simultaneously.

Computerized tomography was performed in 11 patients prior to ciclosporin and repeated in 7 after discontinuation of this drug. All but 3 patients (Nos. 1, 5, 9,

Table 3. Changes of ophthalmological parameters during ciclosporin treatment

	n	improved	unchanged	deteriorated
proptosis	13	2	10	1
visual field	3	–	3	–
intraocular pressure	7	2	5	–
visual acuity	4	1	3	–

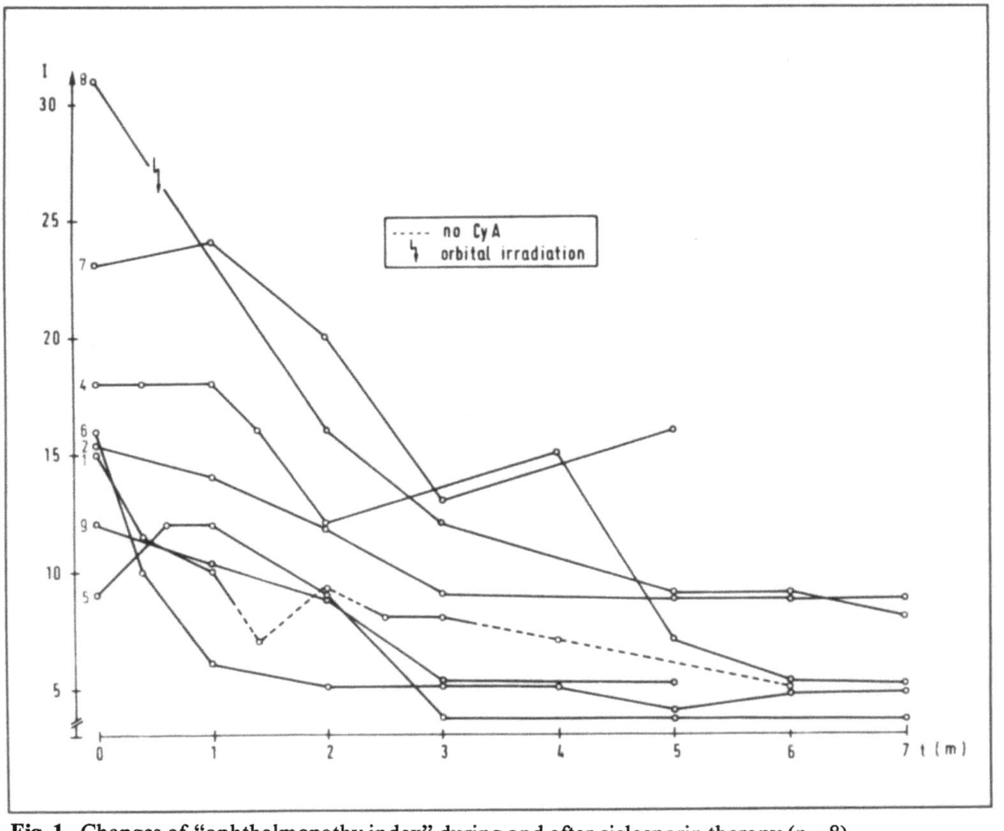

Fig. 1. Changes of "ophthalmopathy index" during and after ciclosporin therapy (n = 8)

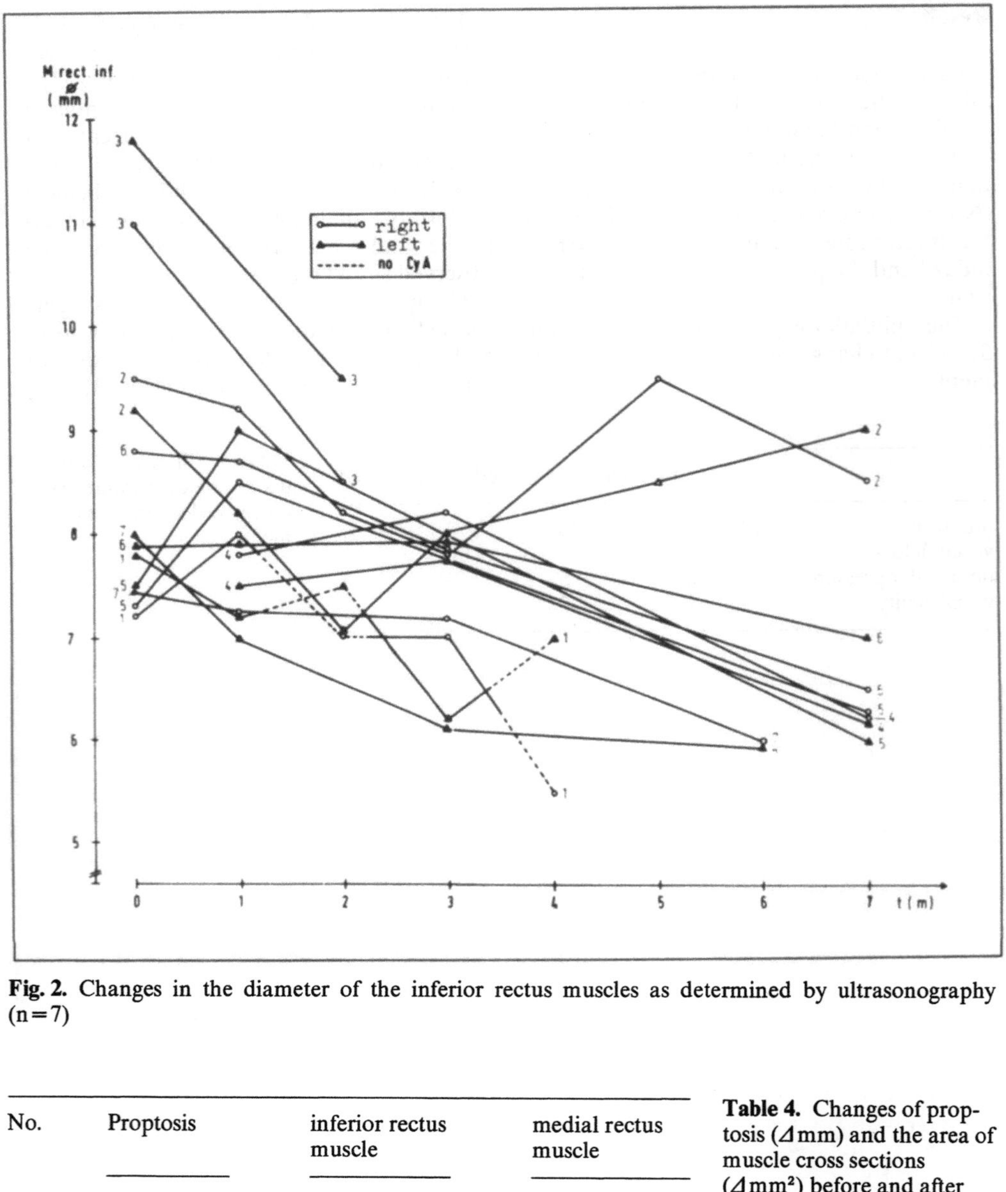

Fig. 2. Changes in the diameter of the inferior rectus muscles as determined by ultrasonography (n=7)

No.	Proptosis		inferior rectus muscle		medial rectus muscle	
	r	l	r	l	r	l
1	±0	+3	− 1	−19	−10	− 9
2	+2	+2	+38	+10	−16	+ 4
3	±0	±0	−22	+ 4	+13	+13
4	+1	+1	+12	± 0	−16	−27
6	+2	+1	+23	− 2	+29	− 9
7	+8	±0	+27	−25	+75	+50
8	+4	+1	− 5	+10	+ 4	+40

Table 4. Changes of proptosis (Δmm) and the area of muscle cross sections (Δmm^2) before and after ciclosporin as determined by CT scan

Table 5. Microsomal antibodies during and after ciclosporin

No.	before	1	2	3	4	6 m.	after (2–3 m.)
1	0	400	400	100	–	–	100
2	0	0	0	100	–	100	400
3	0	0	100	100	100	–	
4	400	400	100	100	–	100	
5	100	100	100	100	–	0	400
6	0	0	0	0	0	100	100
7	100	0	0	0	–	0	100
8	6,400	–	6,400	6,400	–	6,400	6,400
9	400	0	0	0			
10	25,600	102,400	102,400	102,400	102,400	102,400	6,400
11	0	0	0	0			0

Table 6. TSH-displacing activity on ciclosporin (%)

Patient	Months						
	0	1	2	3	4	5	6
1	100	–	59	100	–	–	–
2	–	44	16	47	–	51	44
3	–	119	–	92	98	–	104
4	22	–	29	30	–	25	–
5	102	–	110	100	–	51	–
6	83	54	59	67	–	–	44
7	40	55	–	49	–	55	–
8	37	–	23	42	–	26	28
9	88	101	113	109	–	–	–
10	68	82	78	–	–	90	–

Positive < 80%

Table 7. Incidence of side effects of ciclosporin (n = 13)

Gastrointestinal intolerance Gum hypertrophy Edema
Hypertension
Increase in – creatinine (> 1.1 mg/dl) – bilirubin (> 1.1 mg/dl) – alkaline phosphatase (> 180 U/l)

Table 4) had an enlargement of extraocular muscles. In 2 cases with a normal CT finding, ultrasonography revealed thickening of the superior rectus muscles. During treatment muscle thickness (Table 4) declined in only one individual (No. 1), whereas there was a predominant increase in muscle area in the remaining cases. Moreover, proptosis did not improve, but even deteriorated in half of the patients (1, 2, 7, 8). Thyroid function, thyroid autoantibody titers (Table 5) and TSH-displacing activity (Table 6) did not change during treatment. Side effects (Table 7) were frequent but completely reversible. Treatment had to be discontinued after 10 days in 1 patient due to gastrointestinal symptoms and interrupted after 4 weeks in another patient because of hypertension and increase in creatinine levels. In patient No. 12 treatment was discontinued after 2.5 weeks because of progressive loss of visual acuity and CT-indicated compression of the orbital nerve. In Table 8 the course of creatinine levels before, during and 1 month after ciclosporin treatment is given in detail.

Table 8. Serum creatinine levels (mg/dl) before, during and after ciclosporin treatment

Patient No.	Before	During months				After
		1	2	3	6	1
1	0.8	2.0	–	–	–	1.0
2	0.7	0.8	0.7	0.7	0.7	0.7
3	1.0	1.4	1.0	–	1.5	1.0
4	0.7	0.8	0.7	–	1.0	1.0
5	0.8	1.2	1.1	–	0.8	0.8
6	0.9	0.9	0.9	–	–	0.7
7	0.9	1.0	1.0	1.2	1.2	1.1
8	1.0	1.1	1.0	0.8	0.8	1.1
9	0.8	0.9	0.9	–	–	–
10	0.7	1.2	1.1	–	0.9	0.8
11	0.8	0.8	0.9	–	–	0.8

The mean follow-up period after ciclosporin treatment was 3.6 months (range 1–12 months). In eight patients no significant change in the "ophthalmopathy index" and muscle involvement was observed. In 3 patients a unilateral and bilateral increase of proptosis and in 1 patient severe periocular edema led to further steroid medication with orbital decompression surgery in two cases.

Conclusion

The interpretation of these results is difficult because the patients included in the study represent a heterogenous group with long-standing severe and pretreated ophthalmopathy. The observed improvement of clinical signs and symptoms in most patients contrasts with the more objective criteria. Visual field impairment remained unchanged in all 3 cases with class VI signs.

The severe eye muscle involvement improved in only one patient. Thus the concomitant diplopia did not resolve in any of the other patients.

On the basis of these results we were unable to confirm previously published data [16, 17]. We therefore conclude that, despite some slight effects on the soft tissue, ciclosporin was unable to correct the involvement of extraocular tissue in Graves' disease in patients who had not responded sufficiently to glucocorticosteroids and radiotherapy [7].

Moreover, ciclosporin had no effect on the antibody activity in serum, despite normalization of cellular immunity reported by other investigators [3, 11].

In conclusion, this study revealed no beneficial effect of ciclosporin on the orbital disease of patients who were unresponsive to conventional treatment.

References

1. Beveridge T (1982) Treatment of autoimmune conditions with Cyclosporin A. In: White DG (ed) Cyclosporin A. Elsevier Biochemical Press, Amsterdam, pp 561–564
2. Bigos St, Nisula BC, Daniels GH, Eastman RC, Johnston HH, Kohler PO (1979) Cyclophosphamide in the management of advanced Graves' ophthalmopathy. Ann Intern Med 90:921–923
3. Brabant G, Peter H, Becker H, Schwarzrock R, Wonigeit K, Hesch RD (1984) Cyclosporin in infiltrative eye disease. Lancet 1:515–516
4. DeSanto LW, Gorman CA (1973) Selection of patients and choice of operation for orbital decompression in Graves' ophthalmopathy. Laryngoscope 83:945–952
5. Enzmann DR, Donaldson SS, Kriss JP (1979) Appearance of Graves' disease on orbital computed tomography. J Comput Assist Tomogr 3 (6):815–819
6. Hassmann RA, Dieguez C, Rennie DP, Weetmann AP, Hall R, McGregor AM (1985) The influence of cyclosporin A on the induction of experimental autoimmune thyroid disease in the PVG/c rat. Clin Exp Immunol 59:10

7. Howlett TA, Lawton NF, Fells P, Besser GM (1984) Deterioration of severe Graves' ophthalmopathy during cyclosporin treatment. Lancet II: 1101
8. Jacobson DH, Gorman CA (1984) Endocrine ophthalmopathy: current ideas concerning etiology, pathogenesis and treatment. Endocr Rev 5:200–220
9. Kelly W, Longson D, Smithard D, Fawcitt R, Wensley R, Noble J, Keeley J (1983) An evaluation of plasma exchange for Graves' ophthalmopathy. Clin Endocrinol 18:485–493
10. Kirmse L, Lahrtz H-G, Schemmel K, Waschulzik G (1975) Totale Thyreoidektomie bei progredienter endokriner Orbitopathie. Dtsch Med Wochenschr 100:535–537
11. Markl A, Boergen KP, Hasenfratz G, Mayr B, Fink U, Lissner J (1984) Computerized tomography in the evaluation of endocrine ophthalmopathy. Acta Endocrinol [Suppl] (Copenh) 264, Vol 105, p 84
12. McGregor AM, Rennie DP, Weetmann AP, Hassmann R, Foord SM, Dieguez C, Hall R (1983) The influence of cyclosporin A on experimental autoimmune thyroid disease in the rat. Life Sci 32:97–108
13. Ossoinig KC (1971) Echo-orbitography – a reliable method for the differential diagnosis of endocrine exophthalmos. In: Fellinger K, Höfer R (eds) Further advances in thyroid research. Verlag Wiener Med Akademie, Wien, p 871
14. Teng CS, Cormbie AL, Hall R, Ross WM (1980) An evaluation of supervoltage orbital irradiation for Graves' ophthalmopathy. Clin Endocrinol 13:545–551
15. Utech ChH, Wulle KD, Kiefer H (1985) Cyclosporin A-Behandlung bei schwerer endokriner Ophthalmopathie (Leserzuschrift). Dtsch Med Wochenschr 110:155–156
16. Weetman AP, McGregor AM, Ludgate M, Beck M, Mills PV, Lazarus JH, Hall R (1983) Cyclosporin improves Graves' ophthalmopathy. Lancet II:486–489
17. Werner SC (1977) Modification of the classification of the eye changes of Graves' disease: recommendations of the ad hoc committee of the American Thyroid Association (editorial). J Clin Endocrinol Metab 44:203–204
18. Witte A, Habermann J, Pickardt CR (1982) Is TSH-displacing activity a helpful parameter in diagnosis and follow-up of Graves' disease. Acta Endocrinol [Suppl] 246:73

A Pilot Study of Ciclosporin in Endocrine Ophthalmopathy

F. A. Karlsson [1], P. A. Dahlberg [1], R. Jansson [1], P. Enoksson [2], E. Thorgeirsson [2], T. Tötterman [3]

Positive [3] and negative [1, 2] reports concerning ciclosporin A (CyA) therapy in endocrine ophthalmopathy have recently appeared. In the present paper, we describe our experience of CyA therapy in 9 cases with severe endocrine ophthalmopathy. The ophthalmopathy was associated with Graves' disease in 7 cases, with Hashimoto's thyroiditis in 1 case, whereas in 1 case no thyroid disease was found. All patients had local symptoms (such as conjunctival injections, eyelid retraction, periorbital swelling etc) and eye muscle involvement as assessed by computerized orbital tomography (CT-scan); in 5 cases bulb protrusion was 20–23 mm and in 4 cases > 25 mm; 4 cases had optic nerve involvement (visual loss and/or reduced visual field) and in 1 additional case papillary oedema was present. The histories of disease, previous and ongoing therapy in the 9 cases are shown in Table 1. In general, the patients had had eye symptoms for a few years. As the disease had passed into an active phase or gradually progressed, the patients were referred to our hospital. Four of the 7 patients with Graves' disease had received radioiodine therapy, 2 had undergone surgery and 1 had received long-term thyrostatic drug therapy. During treatment of the thyroid disease, the eye disease had worsened and was accompanied by hypothyroid episodes in 4 instances and hyperthyroid episodes in 2 instances.

CyA therapy

When CyA therapy was initiated 3 of the 9 patients were on prednisolone (7.5, 7.5 and 30 mg daily), 3 patients were receiving methimazole and 8 patients were on thyroxin medication. This ongoing drug therapy was not changed when CyA therapy was started, except for the patient with 30 mg prednisolone, which was reduced to 15 mg daily. In 5 cases CyA was instituted together with 15 mg prednisolone daily, while the 3 cases already on prednisolone stayed on this drug and one case (GP), with a history of psychiatric disorder, received CyA alone.

The initial CyA dose of 10 mg/kg/d was subsequently reduced to a mean maintenance dose of 6 mg/kg/d; on this dosage the serum CyA levels averaged 90 ng/ml (range 20–140 ng/ml). The basic plan was 6 months therapy with a gradual reduction of CyA and steroids. When well tolerated the therapy was prolonged (4 cases). The CyA and prednisolone doses given are shown in Figure 1. As can be seen, the duration of therapy ranged between 1 and 9 months, mean 6 months. In one case (GP) CyA alone was given for 3 months, and in one other case (KAA) CyA + 15 mg prednisolone was stopped after one month and changed to prednisolone 80 mg daily because of lack of response.

In 4 patients serum creatinine levels increased after initiation of CyA therapy, and diminished on reduction of the dose (Fig. 2). No change in blood pressure was noted when values prior to and following CyA therapy were compared (140/80, 110–200/60–90 vs. 130/80, 110–180/60–90 mean and range values respectively). Two patients developed slight facial hirsutism and in one case pathological liver enzymes were observed. It was, however, not necessary in any case to stop therapy because of side effects.

Departments of Internal Medicine [1] and Ophthalmology [2] and Clinical Immunology Section [3], University Hospital, 751 85 Uppsala, Sweden

Table 1. Patients with severe endocrine ophthalmopathy included in a pilot study of ciclosporin therapy

Patient	Sex	Age	History	Active eye disease prior to CyA	Ongoing therapy	Change in therapy at time of initiation of CyA (10 mg/kg/d)	CyA therapy (months)
KEJ	M	62	Left eye involvement –78, acute bilateral worsening –84, no thyroid disorder	2 months	0	15 mg prednisolone	9
KP	F	30	Graves' disease –81, operation –82, eye disease since –82, hypothyroid phase. Steroids, azathioprine tried	2 years	Prednisolone 7.5 mg Methimazole 20 mg Thyroxin 0.25 mg		9
AM	F	58	Graves' disease –83, methimazole therapy. Bilateral eye disease, worsened during hypo- and hyperthyroid episodes	10 months	Methimazole 20 mg Thyroxin 0.15 mg		8
VS	F	72	Insulin-dep. diab. since –68, Graves' disease –79, radioiodine –79. Prednisolone since –82.	3 years	Prednisolone 7.5 mg Methimazole 15 mg Thyroxin 0.15 mg		7
GJ	M	64	Graves' disease –71, radioiodine –71, bilateral eye disease –81, local injections of steroids –81	3 years	Thyroxin 0.20 mg	15 mg prednisolone	6
SM	F	39	Graves' disease –82, operation –82, eye disease –83, worsened during hyperthyroid episode. Steroids tried, cushingoid	1½ years	Methimazole 20 mg Thyroxin 0.15 mg	15 mg prednisolone	6
GBN	F	37	Right eye disease –72, Hashimoto's thyroiditis –76, left eye disease –83, steroids given	1½ years	Prednisolone 30 mg Thyroxin 0.15 mg	–15 mg prednisolone	4.5
GP	F	41	Graves' disease –83, radioiodine –83, hypothyroid phase, eye disease since –83	1 year	Thyroxin 0.25 mg		3
KAA	M	49	Graves' disease –79, radioiodine –82, hypothyroid episode, eye disease since –83, steroids tried	1½ years	Thyroxin 0.10 mg	15 mg prednisolone	1

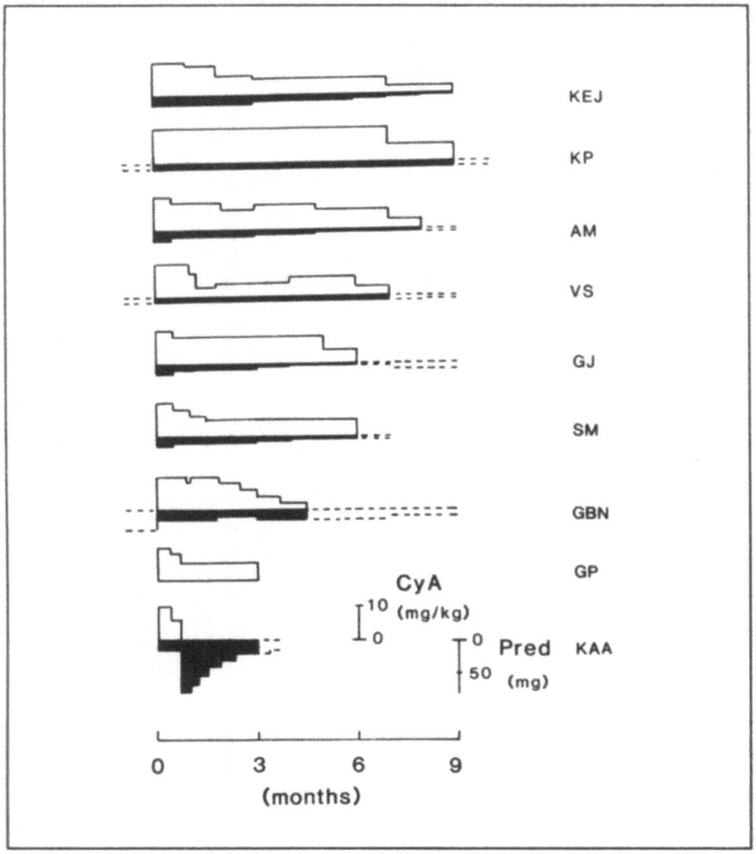

Fig. 1. Ciclosporin and prednisolone therapy in 9 patients with severe endocrine ophthalmopathy. The dashed lines indicate therapy prior to or following the period of CyA therapy

Changes in signs and symptoms

During the periods when CyA was included in the treatment of the 9 patients with severe endocrine ophthalmopathy changes in signs and symptoms occurred as shown in Table 2. The relative distribution of purified circulating lymphocyte subpopulations was studied in 3 cases using monoclonal antibodies before and 1–3 weeks after initiation of CyA therapy. The percentage of HLA-DR-expressing non-B, non-phagocytic cells (=mainly activated T cells) dropped from 13% (5–23%) to 1% (0–3%). The helper/suppressor-T cell ratios were low (0.72; 0.62–0.84) and remained unaltered. The clinical response varied from apparently good to nil. In one case (KEJ) with active eye disease of short duration the response was very good, an impaired visual activity (0.6/1.0) and a reduced visual field being normalized within one month of therapy. However, in the majority of cases small to moderate changes were observed. A reduction of bulb protrusion was observed in 2 additional cases, and in another 2 patients optic nerve function was improved. In one case (KAA) who had a visual field defect and reduced visual acuity (0.4/0.5), one month of CyA therapy with 15 mg prednisolone did not result in improvement. Following a change to 80 mg prednisolone daily the optic nerve function was normalized. Antibodies against the TSH receptor, the thyroid microsomal antigen and thyroglobulin were found in 6, 4 and 2 cases, respectively. The changes that occurred were small and should be considered not significant.

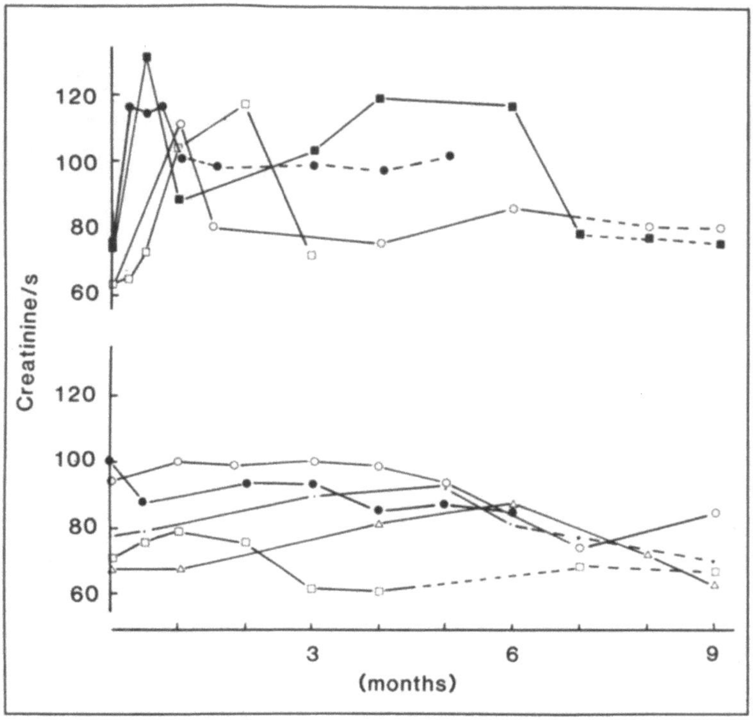

Fig. 2. Serum creatinine values in 9 patients with severe endocrine ophthalmopathy who received CyA therapy. The broken lines indicate changes following cessation of CyA therapy

Table 2. Changes in signs and symptoms[1] of endocrine ophthalmopathy in 9 patients during a period of treatment when ciclosporin was included

Patient	Duration of CyA (months)	Local symptoms	Bulb protrusion	Visual field, visual acuity, pap. oedema	Eye muscle enlargement (CT scan)	TRAK[2]	MsAb[3]	TgAb[3]
KEJ	9	2→1	3→1	2→0	3→1	0	0	0
KP	9	1→1	2→1	0	2→1	0	400→ 100	0
AM	8	2→1	3→3	0	3→3	150→160	0	0
VS	7	1→0	0	3→2	2→2	100→120	0	10→20
GJ	6	2→1	3→3	0	3→3	57→ 34	1600→ 400	0
SM	6	2→1	1→1	2→0	3→2	95→ 42	0	0
GBN	4.5	2→1	1→0	0	2→2	0	400→ 100	0
GP	3	2→2	1→1	0	1→1	160→150	400→1600	10→20
KAA	1	1→1	1→1	2→2	2→2	12→ 17	0	0
Reduction		6/9	3/8	3/4	3/9	3/6	3/4	0
Increase		0	0	0	0	3/6	1/4	2/2
No change		3/9	5/8	1/4	6/9	0	0	0

[1] Signs and symptoms, severe = 3, moderate = 2, mild = 1, none = 0

[2] TRAK, i.e. TSH receptor antibodies (reference range 0–2 TRAK U/l), determined with TRAK-kit (Henning Berlin, West Germany)

[3] MsAb, TgAb, i.e. antibodies against thyroid microsomal antigen or thyroglobulin, determined with haemagglutination kits (Wellcome Ltd, England). Titres are 100, 400, 1600 etc and 10, 20, 40 etc, respectively; reference range < 100 and < 10, respectively

Conclusions

The results of this open trial suggest limited usefulness of CyA in endocrine ophthalmopathy. The drug may have a place in cases where the disease is of short duration or high doses of steroids are not tolerated.

References

1. Brabant G, Peter H, Becker H, Schwarzrock R, Wonigeit K, Hesch RD (1984) Cyclosporin in infiltrative eye disorder. Lancet ii:515
2. Howlett TA, Lawton NF, Fells P, Besser GM (1984) Deterioration of severe Graves' ophthalmopathy during cyclosporin treatment. Lancet ii:1101
3. Weetman AP, McGregor AM, Ludgate M, Beck L, Mills PV, Lazarus JH, Hall R (1983) Cyclosporin improves Graves' ophtalmopathy. Lancet ii:486

Ciclosporin Treatment in Severe Graves' Ophthalmopathy

C. Utech, K. G. Wulle, H. Kiefer, N. Panitz

Graves' ophthalmopathy is currently considered to be caused by autoimmunological processes. Weetman and his colleagues [9, cf. also 1, 2, 10] have shown in two patients that this disease can be successfully treated with ciclosporin. We therefore examined the efficacy of this immunosuppressive drug in a group of ten patients with severe Graves' eye disease, who were treated for six months and have so far been followed up for another six months [5–8].

Another four patients have been treated for six months but have not yet been followed up for such a long period.

In all ten patients of the first group previous treatment with corticosteroids had been unsuccessful. In nine patients retroorbital irradiation had not brought any improvement, and in one of them the ophthalmic disease had even worsened following irradiation therapy. Three patients had had several plasma exchanges with additional corticoid and azathioprine treatment without noticeable improvement. When ciclosporin medication was started all patients were euthyroid having received drug therapy either alone or together with surgery or radioiodine.

The duration of ophthalmic disease in our ten patients ranged from one to three years. All patients suffered from lid oedema, conjunctivitis sicca, chemosis, exophthalmus, limitation of bulbar motility, increased ocular tension on elevation of the bulbus and oedema of orbital muscles. Three patients exhibited corneal erosions and three partial loss of sight in addition to the above impairments.

Prior to ciclosporin treatment all other immunosuppressive medication was stopped but the local therapy with eyedrops and ointments was continued.

Deutsche Klinik für Diagnostik, 6200 Wiesbaden

The initial dose of ciclosporin was 10 mg/kg/day. The ciclosporin level in peripheral blood was measured weekly, using a specific radioimmunoassay, to ascertain the maintenance of a concentration between 200 and 500 ng/ml which is considered therapeutic.

In five patients the initial dose had to be reduced by half because of side effects such as diarrhoea, paraesthesia of the oral region and finger and toe tips and inflammatory changes of the gums. In three patients blood pressure increased under treatment. After reducing the ciclosporin dose all of these symptoms disappeared. In one patient antihypertensive medication had to be administered.

A routine laboratory work-up was performed weekly, comprising in particular urinalysis, creatinine, alkaline phosphatase, transaminases and thyroid parameters including thyroid antibodies and thyrotropin receptor antibodies.

Every month the ophthalmological parameters were evaluated:

1. Vision and refraction to exclude any significant hyperopia and myopia.
2. Bulbar motility, exophthalmometry by the method of Hertel and measurement of the width of the interlid space.
3. Tonometry with measurements of interocular pressure in primary position and on attempted bulbar elevation.
4. Visual field test to exclude any vision defects.
5. Examination with slit lamp to diagnose erosions of the cornea and chemosis, and, after staining with Bengal rose, to recognize conjunctivitis sicca.
6. Ophthalmoscopic examination.

Before and after therapy computerized tomography of the retroorbital region and electrophoresis of urinary proteins were performed.

Results

After one to four weeks of ciclosporin treatment seven patients of our group felt a subjective amelioration of their eye symptoms. In five of them a clinical improvement could be documented. In two other patients additional corticoid medication was initiated after four months because of progressive severe chemosis. In both patients combined treatment resulted in an impressive improvement. Only one of the ten patients did not attain a therapeutic level of ciclosporin determined in blood by radioimmunoassay.

Conjunctivitis sicca and chemosis regressed in all patients; lid oedema, however, did not change in two of the ten patients (Fig. 1).

The increase of intraocular pressure on bulbar elevation diminished in nine patients. This decrease was statistically significant. Normally intraocular pressure in primary eye position does not exceed 18 mmHg and does not increase on bulbar elevation by more than 5 to 6 mmHg (Fig. 2).

Proptosis decreased in five patients and bulbar motility improved (Table 1). In one patient in whom no relevant level of ciclosporin could be obtained, bulbar protrusion increased during the period of observation and surgical decompression was necessary on the right side.

Table 1. Measurements of exophthalmos according to Hertel (data in mm) before and after 6 months of treatment with ciclosporin.

Patient No.	Right eye		Left eye	
	Before	After	Before	After
1	20	18	20	18
2	20	20	20	20
3	18	18	19	19
4	21	24	17	19
5	22	21	22	21
6	20	19	21	18
7	19.5	19.5	19.5	19.5
8	22	21	22	21
9	24	23	26	23
10	19	19	19	19

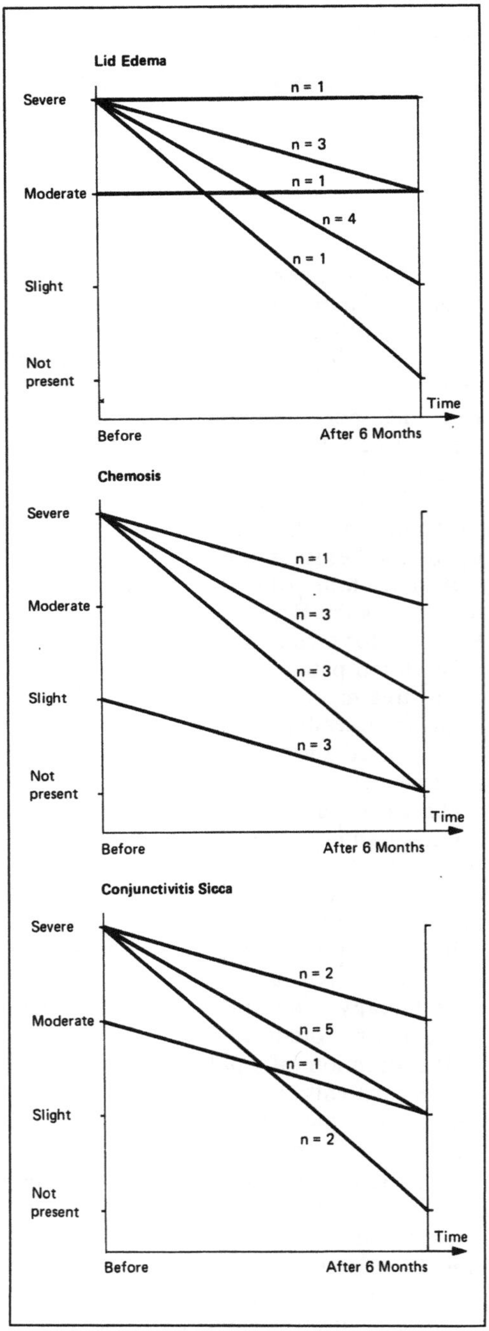

Fig. 1. Changes of severity of soft tissue involvement after 6 months of treatment with ciclosporin: n = number of patients

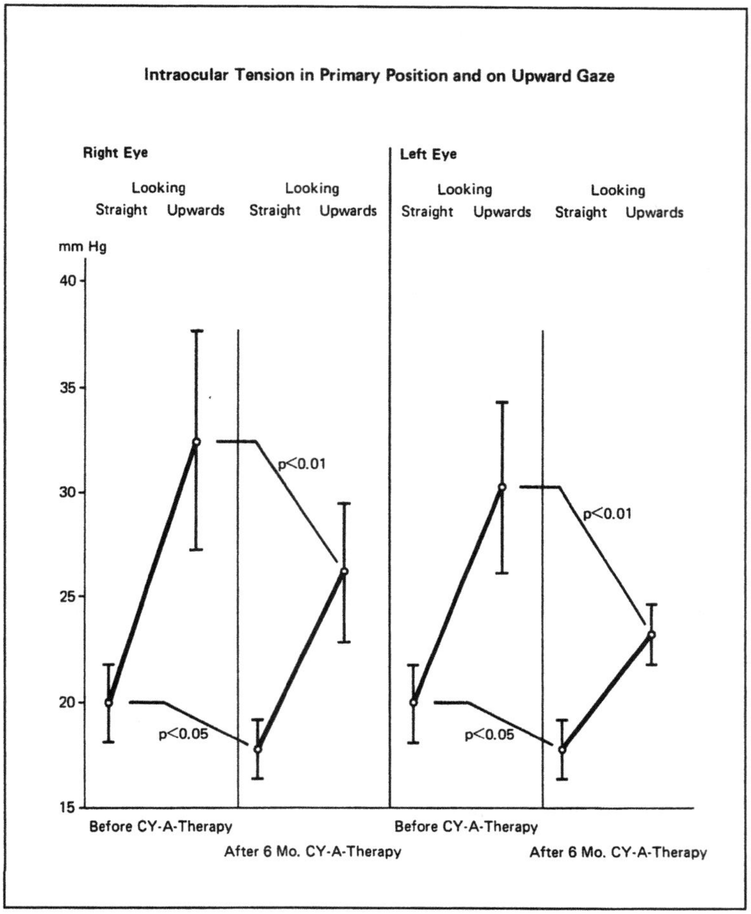

Fig. 2. Mean values (± SD) of intraocular tension of right and left eye before and after 6 months of treatment with ciclosporin. Significant differences were observed in nine patients

Table 2. Maximum thickness of ocular muscles determined by computerized tomography of retrobulbar space before and after 6 months of treatment of cyclosporin. The decrease of thickness reached statistical significance ($p < 0.05$) for the medial rectus muscle. (INF = M. rect. inf. – MED = M. rect. med.) Computerized tomography (mm)

Pat. No.	Right eye				Left eye			
	Before		After		Before		After	
	INF	MED	INF	MED	INF	MED	INF	MED
1	11	5	8	3	11	3	8	3
2	14	8	8	3	14	11	8	5
3	11	10	11	8	11	11	11	8
4	11	3	14	5	3	3	8	5
5	11	8	11	8	11	8	11	8
6	8	5	8	3	8	5	8	3
7	8	5	8	5	8	5	8	3
8	8	5	5	3	8	5	5	3
9	14	11	8	5	14	11	8	5
10	8	3	8	3	8	5	8	5

Table 3. Titers of antibodies against thyroid microsomes (MAb, Fujizoki kit) and thyroglobulin (TAb) and thyrotropin receptor antibodies (TBIAb, TRAK assay, Henning, Berlin) before and after therapy with ciclosporin

Patient No.	Thyroid microsomes		Thyroglobulin		TSH-receptor of the thyrocyte	
	Before 6 mo. CyA	After therapy	Before 6 mo. CyA	After therapy	Before 6 mo. CyA	After therapy
1	1: 100	1: 400	O	O	O	O
2	1: 1600	1:1600	O	O	O	O
3	1: 1600	1:6400	O	O	O	O
4	1: 1600	1:1600	O	O	O	O
5	1:25600	1:6400	1:1600	1:1600	62	62
6	1: 6400	1:6400	O	O	27	41
7	1:25600	1:6400	O	O	O	O
8	1: 1600	1:1600	O	O	O	O
9	1: 400	1:1600	O	O	50	30
10	1: 400	1:1600	1: 100	O	37	20

In six patients orbital CT examination revealed a decrease of muscular thickness. The decrease in thickness of the medial rectus muscle was statistically significant (Table 2).

Antibodies against thyroid microsomes were found positive in nine of ten patients while antibodies against thyroglobulin were found positive in only one patient. There was no significant influence of ciclosporin on thyroid antibodies. Thyrotropin receptor antibodies were found positive in only four patients. These likewise were not significantly influenced by ciclosporin treatment (Table 3).

No significant changes in laboratory parameters, and creatinine in particular were observed in any patient. Traces of protein were detectable in the urine of three patients during the initial high dosage treatment with ciclosporin. However, this minimal urinary protein loss ceased on reduction of ciclosporin.

Two patients developed moderate arterial hypertension and in a third patient antihypertensive medication had to be administered.

Follow-up

In three of these ten patients, Nos 1, 2 and 7 (Fig. 3), low dose treatment could be stopped after six months because of satisfactory results. At follow up examination the ophthalmic findings remained stable up to six months after ciclosporin treatment.

In patient No. 4 no relevant ciclosporin level could be obtained, and this patient finally agreed to decompressive surgery on the right eye.

In patient No. 10, who was treated over a seven-month period, the eye findings deteriorated again one month after withdrawal of ciclosporin.

In five of the ten patients of the first group, Nos 3, 5, 6, 8 and 9, corticosteroids were added after four to seven months of monotherapy with ciclosporin because of unsatisfactory results relating to soft tissue involvement including chemosis. All five patients improved under combined treatment. This effect remained stable in patients No. 3 and 8 after withdrawal of the combined therapy.

In patients No. 5 and 6 a slight increase of the retroorbital process was apparent after three months. In the fifth patient, No. 9, a rapid deterioration was observed after termination of ciclosporin and corticosteroids and he then also agreed to decompressive surgery on both eyes.

In addition to the first group of ten patients, another four patients were treated starting in July 1984. The initial dose of ciclosporin was 5 mg/kg/day. No side ef-

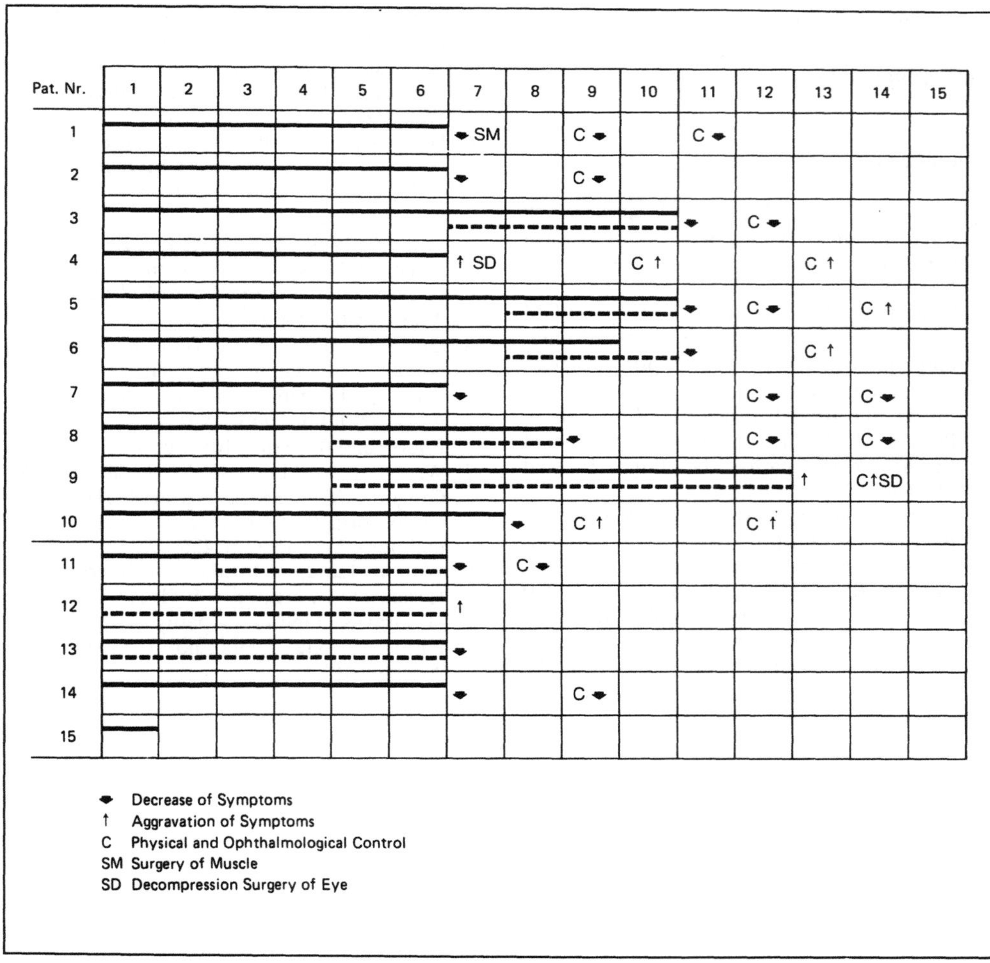

Fig. 3. Duration (months) of treatment with ciclosporin (–) and corticosteroids (- - -)

fects were noted with this dosage. Three out of these four patients, Nos 11, 12 and 13, received additional corticosteroids, patients No. 12 and 13 from the beginning and patient No. 11 from the third month, because of severe chemosis. Improvement was seen in two of them, Nos 11 and 13, while the third patient, No. 12, did not respond to ciclosporin or to corticosteroids.

One patient, No. 14, receiving ciclosporin alone, improved and was still in a stable condition three months after the end of the therapy.

In conclusion, ciclosporin is effective in severe Graves' ophthalmopathy. However, for the time being it should be reserved for patients with more advanced stages of the disease who have not responded to any other form of treatment and who have refused decompressive surgery. A randomized control group would also have been desirable but we could not decide to withhold any of these patients with severe eye changes – some threatened with loss of sight – from the therapeutic trial with ciclosporin.

A low dose of ciclosporin as used in our trial was already effective in Graves' ophthalmopathy without major side effects [but cf. 3, 4]. If this beneficial effect is also confirmed in extensive studies over longer periods, ciclosporin treatment might prove a valuable addition to the means of therapy in Graves' ophthalmopathy, especially in more advanced stages.

References

1. Brabant G, Peter H, Becker H, Schwarzrock R, Wonigeit K, Hesch RD (1984) Cyclosporin in infiltrative eye disease. Lancet I:515–516
2. Howlett TA, Lawton NF, Fells P, Besser GM (1984) Deterioration of severe Graves' Ophthalmopathy during Cyclosporin A Treatment. Lancet II:1101
3. Myers BD, Ross J, Newton L, Luetscher J, Perloth M (1984) Cyclosporin – associated chronic nephropathy. N Engl J Med 311:699–705
4. Starzl TE, Nalesnik MA, Porter KA, Ho M, Iwatsuki S, Griffith BP, Rosenthal JT, Hakala TR, Shaw jr BW, Hardesty RL, Achison RW, Jaffe R, Bahnson HT (1984) Reversibility of lymphomas and lymphoproliferative lesions developping under cyclosporin-steroid therapy. Lancet I:583 –587
5. Utech C, Pfannenstiel P, Brunk G, Wulle KG, Adam W, Maier R, Bieler EU, Simon RS (1980) Diagnostik und Therapie der endokrinen Ophthalmopathie. Internistische Welt 8:285–291
6. Utech C, Brunk B, Wulle K (1984) Treatment of severe Graves' Ophthalmopathy with Cyclosporin A. Abstract: Ann Endocrinol 45:14
7. Utech C, Wulle KG, Bieler EU, Pfannenstiel P, Panitz N, Kiefer H: Treatment of severe Graves' Ophthalmopathy with Cyclosporin A. (Submitted for publication)
8. Utech C, Bieler EU, Wulle K, Kiefer H (1985) Treatment of Graves' Ophthalmopathy with Cyclosporin A alone and in combination with corticosteroids. Acta Endocrinol (Copenh) 108 [Suppl 267]:72
9. Weetman AP, Ludgate M, Mills PV, Mc Gregor AM, Beck L, Lazarus JH (1983) Cyclosporin A improves Graves' Ophthalmopathy. Lancet II:486–489
10. Witte A, Landgraf R, Markl A, Boergen KP, Hasenfratz G, Pickardt CR (1983) Treatment of Graves' Ophthalmopathy with Cyclosporin A. Acta Endocrinol (Copenh) 105 [Suppl 264]:83

8. Hematology

Ciclosporin (CyA) as Primary Treatment for Severe Acute Aplastic Anaemia*

P. Jacobs, L. Wood, R. W. Martell

Summary

In adult patients with severe acute aplastic anaemia, primary therapy with CyA alone (n = 6) was compared in a prospective randomised trial to an equivalent amount of this immunosuppressive agent in combination with antilymphocyte serum (n = 6). At minimum follow-up of 36 months no response could be attributed to either regimen. Thus, the use of CyA, either on its own or in combination with antilymphocyte serum, cannot be recommended for this indication.

Introduction

Allogeneic bone marrow transplantation is the preferred treatment for patients under the age of 45 with severe acute aplastic anaemia having a suitable donor [3]. Without this option, supportive care [16] is essential, but anabolic androgens do not significantly alter the course of the disease [3]. The demonstration that antilymphocyte serum or antithymocyte globulin [6, 11] produced variable response rates suggested that in some individuals an immunologic mechanism may be active in pathogenesis. To further explore this possiblity the immunosuppressive agent, CyA [14], was randomly given to consecutive patients with severe acute aplastic anaemia, either alone or in combination with antilymphocyte serum.

The Leukaemia Centre and Department of Haematology, University of Cape Town and Groote Schuur Hospital, Observatory, Cape, South Africa.

* Based on a publication in press and cited with acknowledgement and permission for its use to Blackwell Scientific Publications Limited and the Editor of the British Journal of Haematology.

Materials and methods

Twelve patients with severe acute aplastic anaemia [2] were randomised to receive either CyA alone (n = 6) or the same schedule of this agent with concurrent infusion of antilymphocyte serum (n = 6). The trial was approved by the Ethics Committee of the University of Cape Town and Groote Schuur Hospital, and informed consent obtained from each patient. CyA was given at a loading dose of 25 mg/kg/day in two divided doses for one week, followed thereafter by a daily split schedule, with dosage adjustment using radioimmunoassay (Ciclosporin RIA Kit, Sandoz, Switzerland) [12] to maintain peak levels 4 hours after the dose between 300 and 500 ng/ml and trough levels between 200 and 400 ng/ml. Antilymphocyte serum (Merrieux, France) was administered by intravenous infusions over half an hour, at a dose of 15 mg/kg on each of 4 consecutive days: The CyA was continued for a minimum period of 3 months unless undesirable side effects necessitated withdrawal.

Patients who failed to respond after 3 months continued receiving CyA and, in addition, were given oral prednisone (0.5 mg/kg/day) in combination with oral oxymetholone (2 mg/kg/day), the latter being increased to the maximum tolerated dosage. All patients received standard supportive care in the form of red cell and platelet transfusion; appropriate antibiotics were given for infections.

Hematologic response was defined as a rise in platelet count above $50 \times 10^9/l$, absolute granulocytes above $1 \times 10^9/l$, and no red cell transfusion requirement [8].

Results

The median age of the patients was 27 years (range 12–49); there were 8 males and 4 females. In none was there any ascertainable cause for the aplastic anaemia. The period from diagnosis to commencement of CyA varied from 1 month to 2 years. Three patients were lost to follow-up; one at 2 months and two at 18 months. One patient subsequently received bone marrow from an HLA identical and MLC non-reactive sibling, having initially elected to enter the trial of immunosuppressive therapy. Patients have been followed for a minimum of 36 months.

There was no sustained response in either group.

Two patients responded to therapy during the second phase of the study whilst receiving additional prednisone and oxymetholone. In one patient the remission was sustained until he was lost to follow-up after 18 months. A second patient achieved a transient response only and died after 18 months of treatment, at which time she was again aplastic.

All patients are accounted for, having either died or been lost to follow-up; median survival was 8 months (3–36 months).

Some degree of toxicity occurred. With CyA administration, an elevation of serum creatinine and diminishing clearance was recorded in 6 of the 12 patients but was reversed following dosage adjustment in all but one, in whom the drug was discontinued. Tremor developed in 2, hirsutism in 1, hypertension in 1, and transient elevation of the serum bilirubin level in 3 patients. The antilymphocyte globulin resulted in serum sickness in one individual, and generalised convulsions occurred in a second patient.

Discussion

Severe acute aplastic anaemia may occur as a result of irreversible damage to the haematopoietic stem cell [1] although an indistinguishable syndrome can arise on an immunologic bases [15]. Most established cases do not respond to standard forms of immunosuppressive therapy, including adrenocorticosteroids and additional cyclophosphamide administration [7], but there have been reports of significant improvement following antilymphocyte serum and antithymocyte globulin [6, 11]. The decision to undertake this trial, evaluating CyA in previously untreated patients with severe acute aplastic anaemia, remains largely empirical. Available evidence for the action of this agent suggests that maximum efficiency would be anticipated at the time when antigen exposure first occurs [9] and this may account for the apparent lack of response in our patients.

The combination with antilymphocyte serum, anticipated to be additive to the functional lesions produced by CyA in abrogating a potentially cellular mechanism in the aplastic patients, was equally unsuccessful. The results of treatment with both antilymphocyte serum and antithymocyte globulin are variable and may reflect differences in dosage, duration of therapy, quality, and type of protein used [5, 15]. Because of the small number of patients in our series, it is not possible to draw any conclusions about the effect of either this particular product or the schedule used for its administration. However, the dosage was lower than had been reported in some trials, where a more favourable outcome was achieved [4]. Alternatively, the failure to obtain any response may be due to concurrent administration of CyA which modified the protein or its action, thereby rendering it ineffective. The subsequent administration of adrenocorticosteroids and anabolic androgens was included to ensure that any patients with hypoplasia rather than aplasia would not be compromised [13]. This approach would appear to be justified in view of the two patients where a response was documented.

CyA is acknowledged to have a range of toxic effects [10] and patients receiving this agent require scrupulous clinical and biochemical monitoring.

It is concluded from this data that CyA either as a single immunosuppressive agent or when used in combination with antilymphocyte serum has no place in treating patients with severe acute aplastic anaemia. The two responses in the present series are attributable to the subsequent administration of adrenocorticosteroids and anabolic androgens. It can, however, not be discounted that in one of these individuals the antilymphocyte serum may have had a minor or contributing role in the response.

References

1. Boggs DR, Boggs SS (1976) The pathogenesis of aplastic anemia: a defective pluripotent hematopoietic stem cell with inappropriate balance of differentiation and self-replication. Blood 48:71
2. Camitta BM, Rappeport JM, Parkman R, Nathan DG (1976) Selection of patients for bone marrow transplantation in severe aplastic anemia. Blood 45:355
3. Camitta BM, Thomas ED, Nathan DG, Gale RP, Kopecky KJ, Rappeport JM, Santos G, Gordon-Smith EC, Storb R (1979) A prospective study of androgens and bone marrow transplantation for treatment of severe aplastic anemia. Blood 53:504
4. Champlin R, Ho W, Gale RP (1983) Antithymocyte globulin treatment in patients with aplastic anemia. N Engl J Med 308:113
5. Coiffier B, Guyotat D, Vuvan H, Fiere D, Viala JJ (1984) Severe aplastic anemia: dose related effect of antitihymocyte globulins. Exp Hematol 12 [Suppl 15]:44
6. Fairhead SM, Chipping PM, Gordon-Smith EC (1983) Treatment of aplastic anaemia with antilymphocyte globulin (ALG). Br J Haematol 55:7
7. Griner PF (1980) A survey of the effectiveness of cyclophosphamide in patients with severe aplastic anemia. Am J Hematol 8:55
8. Jacobs P, Wood L, Martell RW (1985) Cyclosporin A in the treatment of severe acute aplastic anaemia. Br J Haematol, in press
9. Lafferty KJ, Borel JF, Hodgkin P (1983) Cyclosporine-A: models for the mechanism of action. Transplant Proc 15:2242
10. Lampacis A (1983) Complication of cyclosporine therapy – a comparison to azathioprine. Transplant Proc 15:2748
11. Miller WJ, Branda RF, Flynn PJ, Howe RB, Ramsay NKC, Condie RM, Jacob HS (1983) Antithymocyte globulin treatment of severe aplastic anaemia. Br J Haematol 55:17
12. Randall G, Jacobs P (1985) Cyclosporin A radioimmunoassay. A modified method for whole blood determination. Exp Hematol, in press
13. Skarberg KO, Engstedt L, Jameson A, Killander A, Lundh B, Pers B, Reizenstein P, Uden AM, Wadman B (1973) Oxymetholone treatment in hypoproliferative anaemia. Acta Haematol 49:321
14. Stryckmans PA, Dumont JP, Velu T, Debusscher L (1984) Cyclosporine in refractory severe aplastic anemia. N Engl J Med 310:655
15. Thomas ED, Storb R (1984) Perspective: acquired severe aplastic anemia: progress and perplexity. Blood 64:325
16. Young N (1981) Aplastic anemia: research themes and clinical issues. In: Brown EB (ed) Progress in hematology. Grune and Stratton, New York, p 227

Supported by the University of Cape Town Leukaemia Centre and Staff Research Fund, the Medical Research Council and the National Cancer Association; we thank Sandoz Laboratories for donation of the cyclosporin A, Institute Merrieux for the antilymphocyte serum, Jackie Davies for typing, and Dr H. Reeve Sanders for permission to publish.

Ciclosporin for Therapy of Severe Aplastic Anemia (SAA) and Pure Red Cell Aplasia (PRCA)

L. Debusscher and P. Stryckmans

Introduction

In severe aplastic anemia (SAA) there are several experimental and clinical observations which prompted us to test the efficacy of ciclosporin (CyA). Among them are laboratory observations which underline the autoimmune pathogenesis of SAA: (a) the prevention of CFU-GM suppressor T cells by in vitro preincubation with CyA of SAA T lymphocytes [5], and (b) the suppressive effect of CyA on the production of gamma interferon, a lymphokine recently designated as the in vivo soluble mediator of aplastic anemia [7, 8]. Clinically, in the field of bone marrow transplantation for SAA, a reduced occurrence of allograft failure with the use of CyA as prophylaxis of graft-versus-host disease was another important argument for the use of CyA [4].

A rationale for the treatment of pure red cell aplasia with immunosuppression is provided by the demonstration that many cases have an immune pathogenesis and that without therapeutic intervention most patients require life-long transfusion support [2].

Our preliminary experience with CyA in SAA and PRCA [3, 6] was encouraging and we report here the results obtained in more patients.

Patients and methods (Table 1)

We gave treatment to 5 patients with SAA and 2 patients with PRCA. Their age ranged between 14 and 82 (median 64). The SAA patients fulfilled the criteria of the International Aplastic Anemia Study Group [1]. The PRCA patients had reticulocytopenic anemia, with a normocellular marrow showing severe erythroblastopenia. The 2 cases appeared as primary PRCA.

Five patients had never been treated by immunosuppressive therapy whereas two SAA patients had been shown resistant to corticosteroids and antithymocyte globulin (ATG).

All the patients were off classical immunosuppressive drugs during CyA treatment. CyA was given orally, at an initial daily dose varying between 5 and 12 mg/kg body weight in two divided doses. The following doses were adjusted according to efficacy and toxicity.

The trough levels of plasma CyA, 12 hours after oral administration, were measured by radioimmunoassay using the RIA kit provided by Sandoz Ltd.

Results

In SAA 80, the drug was stopped after 67 days of total ineffectiveness.

In SAA 64, an incipient increase of granulocytes was noticeable on day 37, when CyA had to be interrupted because of severe but rapidly reversible renal failure.

In SAA 14, the partial remission obtained was questionable since a slow increase in granulocytes had already started before the CyA treatment.

In SAA 62, an excellent partial remission was clearly related to CyA. After a 13-month course, her granulocytopenia was moderate (mean 1480/mm^3) and her clinical status was quite critical with severe diffuse hemorrhages due to extreme thrombocytopenia unresponsive to massive platelet transfusions, despite several previous attempts at therapy (prednisolone,

Service de Médecine et Laboratoire d'Investigation Clinique H. J. Tagnon
Institut Jules Bordet, Centre des tumeurs de l'Université Libre de Bruxelles, Rue Héger Bordet 1, 1000 Brussels, Belgium

Table 1. Patient features prior to ciclosporin therapy

Diagnosis	Age	Sex	Days from diagnosis to start of CyA	Treatment attempts prior to CyA therapy
SAA	80	F	43	0
SAA	64	F	20	0
SAA	14	M	137	PDN, ATG+PDN
SAA	62	F	380	PDN, HD–PDN, ATG
SAA	20	F	24	0
PRCA	67	F	240	0
PRCA	82	M	390	Androgens

Table 2. Response to ciclosporin therapy

Diagnosis	Age	Range trough plasma levels ng/ml	Days to first signs of response	Response to 1st course of CyA	Outcome after decrease or withdrawal of CyA
SAA	80	310– 850	–	Failure	Death D14
SAA	64	175–1750	37	Minimal	No change
SAA	14	100–1470	–	Possible	No change D110
SAA	62	350– 850	14	Partial	Relapse D70
SAA	20	320–1370	30	Complete	Relapse D25
PRCA	67	60– 150	20	Complete	Relapse D160
PRCA	82	50– 270	10	Partial	–

high dose prednisolone, antithymocyte globulin). Fourteen days after the start of CyA, given at 10 mg/kg/day, a rise in the platelet count became evident, reaching 65,000/mm³ on day 47. The patient has been in excellent condition without any need for transfusion, with platelets around 35,000 per mm³ and Hb levels at 11 g/dl, during the 16 months of the CyA treatment. Maintenance doses resulted in rather low (100 ng/ml) trough plasma levels due to disphantoin administration. Seventy days after CyA interruption she relapsed, and required an RBC transfusion. At present, after resumption of the drug, a second response is becoming evident.

In SAA 20, CyA was started as the first treatment 24 days after diagnosis. A response was noticeable at day 30. The completely normalized blood parameters obtained after 5 months deteriorated when CyA doses were reduced, and returned to normal with drug re-increase.

PRCA 67 had required 36 units of packed red cells during an 8-month disease course. She showed a rise in the reticulocyte count 20 days after CyA initiation. A complete response obtained with low atoxic doses of CyA (4 mg/kg/day) lasted for the 4 months of CyA administration and another 4 months after CyA withdrawal. A second complete remission, obtained after CyA resumption, is still ongoing.

PRCA 82 had required 66 units of packed red cells during the 13-month course of his disease. He showed a rise in his reticulocyte count 10 days after CyA initiation at 5 mg/kg/day. Now, at day 100 of his treatment, he is in good partial remission with 10 gr hemoglobin per dl.

In the two PRCA cases, the low effective CyA doses resulting in trough plasma levels around 100 ng/ml did not cause any significant toxicity. Higher CyA levels (500 ng/ml), needed to reach optimal effect in SAA, led to severe toxicity in 2 cases (1 gingival hypertrophy and 1 renal failure). Both problems were rapidly reversible after drug withdrawal. In the other cases, tremor, hirsutism, paresthesias, weight gain, hyperuremia and hyperbilirubinemia were transient and acceptable.

Conclusions

CyA as a single agent, administered twice daily by mouth, induced partial or complete remission in SAA (2/5) and PRCA (2/2).

In 3 of the 4 responding patients, the role played by CyA was proven with certainty by the occurrence of relapse on withdrawal or reduction of the drug and the occurrence of a second response at resumption of the initial CyA therapy.

First signs of improvement became evident between 10 and 30 days in all responding patients.

SAA apparently required higher doses and higher trough levels of CyA than PRCA.

One SAA patient responded despite proven resistance to ATG and high-dose prednisolone.

Since relapse occurred in SAA and in PRCA after CyA withdrawal, maintenance therapy after normalisation of the blood picture seems warranted.

Severe but reversible toxicity sometimes required cessation of CyA therapy.

Acknowledgements

We wish to thank Drs. Otten J., Paridaens R., and Malarme M. for permitting us to evaluate their patients, and Mrs M. Cadière for her secretarial help.

References

1. Camitta BM, Storb R, Thomas ED (1982) Aplastic anemia (second of two parts). Pathogenis, diagnosis, treatment, and prognosis. N Engl J Med 306:712–718
2. Clark DA, Dessypris EN, Krantz SB (1984) Studies on pure red cell aplasia. XI. Results of immunosuppressive treatment of 37 patients. Blood 63:277–286
3. Debusscher L, Paridaens R, Stryckmans P, Delwiche F (1985) Cyclosporine for pure red cell aplasia. Blood 65:249
4. Hows JM, Palmer S, Gordon-Smith EC (1982) Use of cyclosporin A in allogeneic bone marrow transplantation for severe aplastic anemia. Transplantation 33:382–386
5. Podesta M, Bacigalupo A, Frassoni F, Raffo M, Piagigo G, Repetto M, van Lint M, Marmont A (1983) Generation of CFU-C suppressor T cells. VI. Effects of Cyclosporin A. Acta Haematol 70:163–169
6. Stryckmans PA, Dumont JP, Velu TH, Debusscher L (1984) Cyclosporine in refractory severe aplastic anemia. N Eng J Med 310:656–657
7. Zoumbos N, Djeu J, Young N (1984) Interferon is the suppressor of hematopoiesis generated by stimulated lymphocytes in vitro. J Immunol 133:769–774
8. Zoumbos NC, Gascon P, Djeu JY, Trost SR, Young NS (1985) Circulating activated suppressor T lymphocytes in aplastic anemia. N Engl J Med 312:257–264

Experience with Ciclosporin (CyA) in the Management of Pure Red-Cell Aplasia (PRCA) and Aplastic Anemia (AA)

T. H. Tötterman[1, 2], A. Killander[2], A. Kreuger[3], G. Gustafsson[3], J. Nisell[4] and N. Skage[5]

Summary

Six patients with therapy-resistant PRCA and 2 patients with AA were treated with CyA for 14–32 months. In most cases (6/8), CyA was added to previous prednisolone therapy. Complete remission or a definite response was obtained in 4/6 PRCA and 1/2 AA patients. No effect was seen in 2 children with PRCA, and there was only a partial response (reduced transfusion need) in a child with AA. Side effects were acceptable and included nephrotoxicity (6/8), hirsutism (5/8), gingival hyperplasia (4/8), gynecomastia (2/8) and tremor (1/8). It is concluded that CyA has a place in the management of PRCA and possibly also of AA.

Introduction

Pure red-cell aplasia (PRCA) and aplastic anemia (AA) are uncommon, serious disorders in which immune-mediated mechanisms are thought to cause a selective (PRCA) or broad (AA) suppression of marrow stem cell function; reviewed in [1].

Consequently, conventional immunosuppressive drugs and ALG may induce at least temporary remission in some 40% of the cases [2].

We have recently reported the successful treatment of severe PRCA with ciclosporin (CyA) alone or in combination with prednisolone [5]. Here we report the accumulated clinical experience with CyA of the Uppsala group in the management of 6 PRCA and 2 AA patients.

Patients

Pure red-cell aplasia. Four adult patients and 2 children with therapy-resistant PRCA were treated. Short case records are presented. *PRCA-1:* Male, 56 with acquired PRCA after thymectomy in 1971. Positive for autoantibodies to erythroblasts. Remission after prednisolone plus oxymetholone. Since 1975, 5 relapses treated with prednisolone plus cyclophosphamide/azathioprine, ALG (2 cycles), or plasmapheresis, with temporary effects only. *PRCA-2:* Male, 21 with Blackfan-Diamond syndrome since infancy. Declining hemoglobin (Hb) despite prednisolone 150 mg/week. *PRCA-3:* Male, 29 receiving prednisolone since 8 months of age for the Blackfan-Diamond syndrome. Unsatisfactory Hb with steroids (130 mg/week) only. *PRCA-4:* Female, with Coomb's positive PRCA at 8 years of age. Prednisolone plus azathioprine treatment. Temporarily higher Hb after thymectomy in 1971 and splenectomy in 1982. Cushingoid habitus contraindicated higher doses of steroids. *PRCA-5:* Girl, 2 years old with PRCA since birth. Treated without effect with RBC transfusions, prednisolone, anabolic steroids and ALG. *PRCA-6:* Boy, one year old with congenital erythroblastopenia treated with prednisolone plus transfusions.

Aplastic anemia. AA-1: Male, 69 following exposure to pesticides. Pancytopenia since 1983, treated with prednisolone without effect. *AA-2:* Boy, 5 years, with pancytopenia since 1982. Treated with oxymetholone, methylprednisolone (both low and high pulse doses) and ALG without effect, in addition to transfusions.

Clinical Immunology Section/The Blood Center[1] and Departments of Internal Medicine[2] and Pediatrics[3], University Hospital, Uppsala; Department of Internal Medicine, Mora Hospital[4]; Department of Internal Medicine, Fagersta Hospital[5], Sweden.

Correspondence: Dr. Thomas Tötterman, Clinical Immunology/The Blood Center, University Hospital, S-751 85 Uppsala, Sweden.

Results

Response rate and hematological effects of CyA treatment

Table 1 summarizes the drug doses and changes in hematological parameters and S-creatinine in the responder (6/8) patients. In two small children (PRCA-5 and 6) with congenital erythroblastopenia, no beneficial effects were observed during the 6 months of CyA (plus steroid) treatment (data not shown).

All four adult *PRCA cases* responded favourably, and a striking reticulocytosis (6–11%) was seen in 3 cases around day 10. CyA was added to previous (unchanged or reduced) steroid therapy in 3/4 patients. In case 3, CyA alone did not induce remission, but after addition of low dose prednisolone a definite response was seen. A temporary relapse occurred after a 50% reduction of steroids in case 2. In case 4, the CyA dosage was reduced due to nephrotoxicity, and this resulted in relapse. The patient received cyclophosphamide plus (increased dose) prednisolone in this situation, without effect. In case 1, a temporary relapse was noted after reduction of the CyA dose to only 3.5 mg/kg/d. This patient responded promptly to an increased CyA dose (no steroids). The PRCA patients have now been followed up for 14–32 months. *Fig-*

Table 1. Effect of CyA treatment on hematological variables and serum creatinine in patients with pure red-cell aplasia and aplastic anemia

Variable[a]	PRCA-1	PRCA-2	PRCA-3	PRCA-4	AA-1	AA-2
Before treatment						
Drug doses	0/100	0/30	0/0	0/15	0/20	0/5
Hb/Retics	70/0	37/0.7	69/0.8	72/0.4	73/2.8	72/0.2
WBC/TRC	6/122	5.1/308	2.8/330	14.7/726	2/10	0.2/11
Creat	83	64	80	67	127	32
CyA 2 months						
Drug doses	9.5/20	10/20	11/2	10/5	4.5/0	12.5/5
Hb/Retics	123/0.8	101/1.2	64/0.5	98/0.8	98/2.8	70/0.4
WBC/TRC	–	–	–	–	4.1/88	0.4/10
Creat	148	70	87	83	130	31
CyA 6 months						
Drug doses	8/0	4.5/20	11/8.5	7.5/7.5	4.5/0	25/5
Hb/Retics	127/0.7	87/0.4	93/1.2	85/3.1	100/0.4	64/6.2
WBC/TRC	–	–	–	–	2.5/89	3.1/15
Creat	144	68	87	136	145	68
CyA 12 months						
Drug doses	6.5/0	7.5/10	8/8.5	6/25	4.5/0	10/5
Hb/Retics	125/0.7	91/0.1	95/0.8	70/4.8	111/0.5	75/6.2
WBC/TRC	–	–	–	–	2.2/176	3.1/< 10
Creat	158	80	83	177	150	64
Latest follow-up[b]						
Drug doses	5/0	10/30	8/8.5	0/40[c]	4.5/0	10/5
Hb/Retics	128/0.9	62/1.3	97/4.2	66/1.6	110/1.8	57/3
WBC/TRC	4.8/159	2.6/256	2.6/248	5.7/399	2.6/110	1.3/< 10
Creat	114	109	96	120	159	60

[a] Drug doses as CyA (mg/kg/d)/Prednisolone (mg/d); Hb in g/l; Reticulocytes as %; WBC and TRC × 10/l; S-Creatinine in μmol/l.

[b] PRCA-1: 32 months, PRCA-2: 20 months, PRCA-3: 14 months, PRCA-4: 16 months, AA-1: 18 months, AA-2: 14 months.

[c] Switched to cyclophosphamide 50 mg × 3 daily.

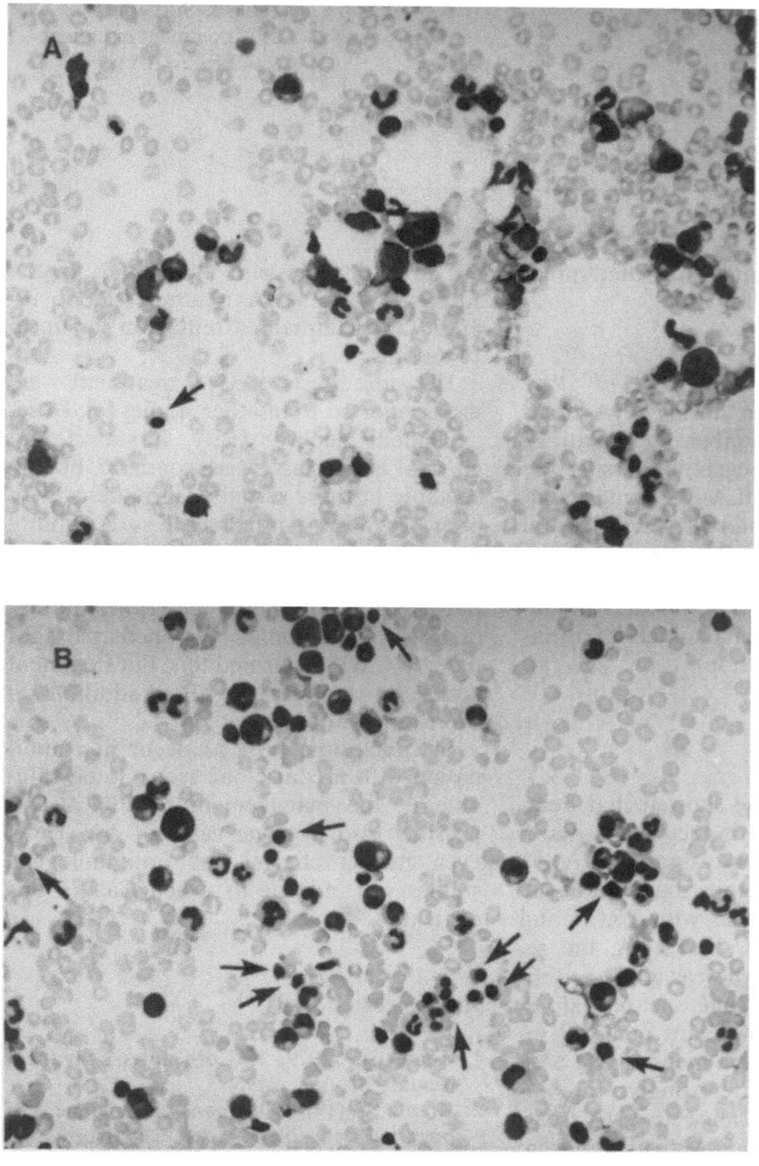

Fig. 1. Bone marrow morphology (May-Gruenwald-Giemsa stained aspirate smear) in PRCA patient 2 before (A) and after 6 months on CyA treatment (B). Note the increase in erythroid precursor cells (arrows)

ure 1 shows the changes in bone marrow morphology during CyA therapy in case 2.

Two *patients with AA* have to date been treated for 14–18 months with CyA (*Table 1*). In case 1, a very favourable effect on blood values has been noted with CyA alone. The child AA-2 received steroids plus relatively high doses of CyA, with moderate effects on the number of reticulocytes and polymorphs after 4–6 months. However, there was a drastic reduction in the demand of RBC and platelet transfusions in this case (not shown).

Side effects of CyA treatment

The types and incidence of adverse side effects of CyA treatment in our PRCA/AA patients are summarized in *Table 2*. The side effects seemed to be reversible and dose-dependent in every case. It is important to consider that in most cases CyA was

Table 2. Side effects of CyA treatment in patients with PRCA/AA (n=8)

1. Rise in S-creatinine	6/8
2. Increased hair growth	5/8
3. Gingival hyperplasia	4/8
4. Gynecomastia	2/8
5. Tremor	1/8
6. Increase in upper resp. viral inf. ??	2/8

combined with previously initiated prednisolone treatment (6/8 = 75%).

Immunomodulatory effects of CyA

There was a reduction during CyA treatment in the relative number of circulating/bone marrow lymphocytes expressing the activation markers HLA-DR, interferon-gamma and IL-2 receptor as well as natural killer (NK) cell markers. In particular, the number of HLA-DR positive suppressor T lymphocytes decreased in remission and reappeared in relapse (data subject of an independent communication).

Discussion

In an earlier report we showed that treatment with CyA could induce remission in four cases of therapy resistant PRCA [5]. The present paper extends these studies to include two further cases with PRCA and two patients with AA. In PRCA, the response rate was 75%, whereas in AA we observed one complete and one partial response. Recently, Stryckmans et al. [4] reported the successful treatment of one SAA patient with CyA. Interestingly, the patients with a poor response to CyA treatment in the present study were all children. A possible explanation could be that patients with PRCA/AA surviving to adult age on prednisolone/conventional cytostatic drugs represent a milder, immunologically mediated disease, whereas non-responders to such treatment may have an intrinsic stem cell defect [3]. In most of the cases presented here, CyA treatment had to be combined with prednisolone in order to be effective. This indicates that the two agents may act synergistically. In one PRCA patient, remission was initiated with this combination but has been maintained for up to 3 years with CyA alone. In the adult AA case, CyA treatment alone induced and maintained remission for up to 16 months.

The side effects of CyA treatment were those reported from other studies [6]. Dose-dependent nephrotoxicity, hirsutism and gingival hyperplasia were common, but acceptable in these seriously ill patients with poor prognosis. An increased susceptibility to upper respiratory infections was reported by 3 PRCA patients receiving CyA plus steroids. In one of these, the findings of bronchopneumonia and increased IgM titers to CMV confirmed this, but treatment could be maintained after addition of short-term antibiotics.

In conclusion, CyA alone or in combination with prednisolone seems to be valuable in the management of PRCA and possibly also in some cases of AA. However, further clinical and immunological studies will indicate its exact place in this context.

References

1. Geary CG (1979) Red cell aplasia. Baillière Tindall, London, p 195
2. Krantz SB (1976) Diagnosis and treatment of pure red cell aplasia. Med Clin North Am 60:945
3. Lacombe C, Casadevall N, Muller O, Varet B (1984) Erythroid progenitors in adult chronic pure red cell aplasia: Relationship of in vitro erythroid colonies to therapeutic response. Blood 64:71
4. Stryckmans PA, Dumont JP, Velu TH, Debusscher L (1984) Cyclosporine in refractory severe aplastic anemia. N Engl J Med 310:655
5. Tötterman TH, Nisell J, Illander A, Gahrton G, Lönnqvist B (1984) Successful treatment of pure red-cell aplasia with cyclosporin. Lancet II:693
6. White DJG (ed) (1982) Cyclosporin A. Elsevier Biomedical Press, Amsterdam

Ciclosporin in Idiopathic Thrombocytopenic Purpura and other "Auto-Immune" Cytopenias

B. Coiffier

We have tried ciclosporin (CyA) in 9 patients with auto-immune cytopenias: 5 with thrombopenia, 1 with pure red cell aplasia (PRCA), 1 with aplastic anemia (AA), 1 with neutropenia, and 1 with auto-immune hemolytic anemia (AIHA). We report here our preliminary results concerning the response of the cytopenia to this treatment, as well as the toxicity of CyA.

Methods

CyA was given per os at 5 mg/kg/day in two doses. Patient condition and blood count, blood pressure, creatinine and CyA dosage were surveyed once a week.

Results

1) Auto-immune thrombocytopenias.
Among the 5 patients, there were 3 with refractory idiopathic thrombocytopenic purpura (ITP), one with thrombopenia associated with scleroderma and one with sarcoidosis. In all cases, the thrombopenia was refractory to corticosteroids or corticodependent. In 2 of the ITP cases splenectomy had been done. The 3rd patient had a hepatic sequestration of Cr51-labelled platelets. All these patients were treated with CyA on the occasion of profound thrombopenia (less than 20 G/l) with hemorrhages.

Out of the 3 patients with an ITP, there were 2 partial responses (PR) (increase of platelets above 50 G/l) in less than 3 weeks. The 3rd patient had a complete response (CR) (platelets above 150 G/l). The patient with sarcoidosis also had a CR in 3 weeks. The patient with thrombopenia associated with scleroderma had a PR after 5 weeks. In all these patients, hemorrhages disappeared very soon after the commencement of CyA.

2) Pure red cell aplasia. This patient had a refractory PRCA of 8 years' standing, treated with corticosteroids, antithymocyte globulins (on two occasions), plasmapheresis, cyclophosphamide and azathioprine. After 2 weeks of therapy, transfusions were stopped and reticulocytes began to increase. At this time, after 11 weeks of CyA, there was an almost CR: hemoglobin more than 110 G/l, reticulocytes above 50 G/l, medullary erythroblasts at 10%.

3) Auto-immune hemolytic anemia. This patient had a history of a coeliac disease, one crisis of AIHA with IgG antibodies, and 3 crises of ITP responding to corticosteroids. He was rehospitalised with Evans' syndrome: hemoglobin at 30 G/l and platelets less than 100 G/l. Methylprednisolone (250 mg/m²), and plasmapheresis did not halt the hemolysis. CyA was begun iv at 5 mg/kg/day and within 8 days hemoglobin and platelets increased (Fig. 1). At this time, after 9 weeks of CyA therapy, hemoglobin was at 145 G/l and platelets at 324 G/l.

4) Aplastic anemia. This patient had moderate AA treated with norethandrolone for 15 months; initial results were good, but were followed by an aggravation of the cytopenias. CyA did not lead to an increase in hemoglobin, neutrophils or platelets after 8 weeks of therapy and was stopped. At present, this patient is responding to antithymocyte therapy.

5) Autoimmune neutropenia. This patient had an 8-year history of rheumatoid ar-

Service d'Hématologie, Hopital Edouard-Herriot, 69374 Lyon Cedex 8 France.

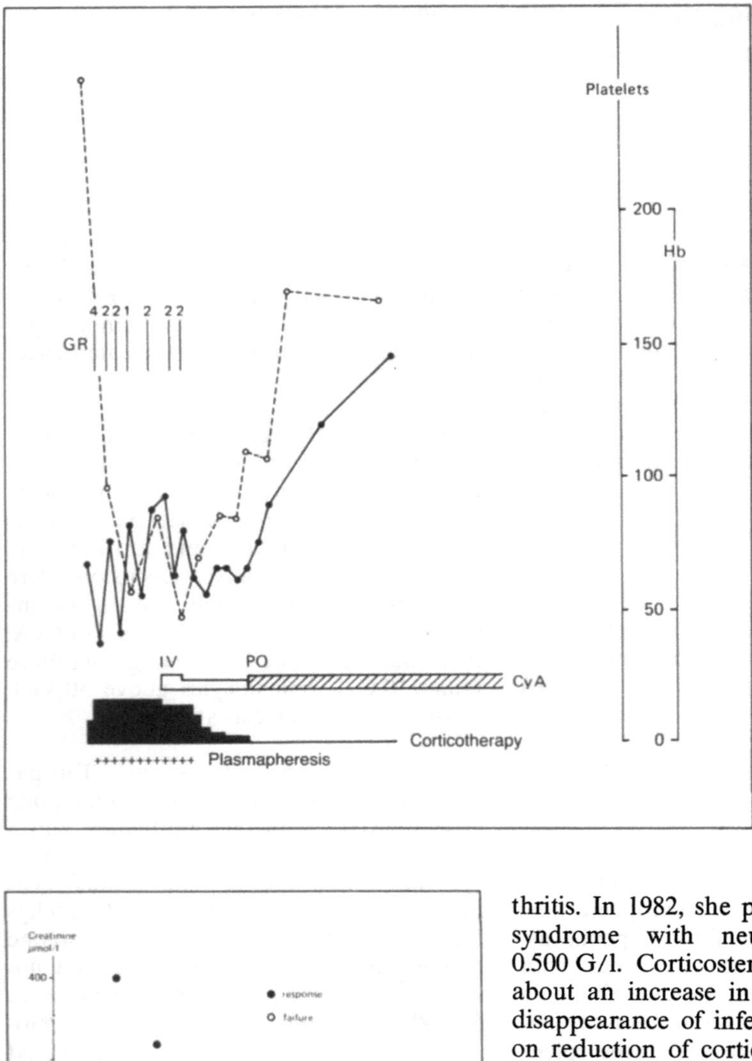

Fig. 1. Patient with autoimmune hemolytic anemia and thrombocytemia treated with CyA after failure of corticotherapy and plasmapheresis. Evolution of hemoglobin and platelets

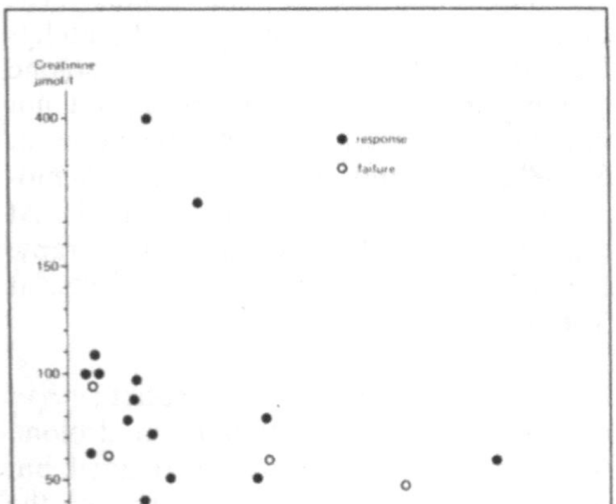

Fig. 2. Correlation of serum CyA level with toxicity (creatinine) and result of the treatment at the time of the determination

thritis. In 1982, she presented with Felty's syndrome with neutrophils less than 0.500 G/l. Corticosteroid therapy brought about an increase in neutrophils and the disappearance of infection. Unfortunately, on reduction of corticosteroid dosage, the neutropenia reappeared and persisted in spite of continuing corticotherapy. With CyA therapy, neutrophils increased from less than 0.200 G/l to more than 1000 G/l.

6) Toxicity. Renal: two patients had increased creatinine and urea levels after 8 weeks of therapy, although the serum level of CyA did not go above 200 µg/l. This abnormality is currently disappearing. None of the patients showed any increase in blood pressure. Two of the 6 female patients presented slight hirsutism (moustache). One patient showed a slight increase (less than 2 times the normal) in alkaline phosphatases without abnormali-

Table 1. Results of CyA therapy in 9 patients with "autoimmune" cytopenias

Type of cytopenia	Failure	Partial response	Complete response
Thrombocytopenia		3	2
Aplastic anemia	1		
Hemolytic anemia			1
Neutropenia		1	
PCRA			1
Total	1	4	4

ties of transaminases or gamma-GT. One patient had some problems with pre-existing gingivitis, which was aggravated. No other toxicity was identified.

The determination of CyA was carried out by RIA with the Sandoz Kit in blood and serum by 2 laboratories. The results were the same in all cases. However, this determination was of no value in the management of the patient because it did not correlate with efficacy (Fig. 2) or toxicity. The two patients with an increase in creatinine level had a normal CyA level (less than 200 μg/l).

7) Development. Three patients discontinued CyA therapy: one because of inefficacy, one because of toxicity, and one after 3 months of therapy. The 2 patients with some response stopped therapy for less than one month. The 6 other patients are at present at the end of the planned 3-month course of therapy. Thus, the effect of this treatment as determined in a long-term follow-up is not known.

Discussion

Our results (Table 1) are too premature to allow conclusions regarding the long-term efficacy of CyA in autoimmune cytopenias, but they are suggestive. Very few results have been published concerning this type of treatment: two PR in ITP [1], two CR and 4 PR in PRCY [1, 2, 5], 3 PR in AA [1, 3, 4]. If CyA has a therapeutic role in these diseases, we do not know either the therapeutic dosage or the appropriate duration of treatment.

Conclusion

In refractory autoimmune cytopenias, the use of ciclosporin results in the disappearance of clinical symptoms and an increase in the number of hemopoietic cells. Our results are too premature to indicate whether the response is likely to continue or if it is only temporary. Meanwhile, the results are encouraging and ciclosporin should be tried on a large scale in these autoimmune cytopenias.

References

1. Beris P, Miescher PA (1985) Hematologie. Med Hyg 43:121–126
2. Debusscher L, Paridaens R, Strychmans P, Delwiche F (1985) Cyclosporine for pure red cell aplasia. Blood 65:249
3. Finlay JL, Toretsky J, Hoffman R, Bruno E, Shahidi NT (1984) Cyclosporine in refractory aplastic anemia. Amer Soc Hematol, Miami 1984, abstr 326
4. Stryckmans PA, Dumont JP, Velu T, Debusscher L (1984) Cyclosporine in refractory severe aplastic anemia. N Engl J Med 310: 655–656
5. Totterman TH, Nisell J, Killander A, Gahrton G, Lonnquist B (1984) Successful treatment of pure red cell aplasia with cyclosporin. Lancet II:693

Ciclosporin (CyA) and Intravenous Immunoglobulin (i.v. IgG) in Chronic Immune Thrombocytopenic Purpura (ITP) in Childhood: A Clinical and Immunological Study (progress report)

P. Imbach [1], L. Luginbühl [1], P. Späth [2], A. Hirt [3], T. Huwyler [3], A. Morell [3], C. Mueller-Eckhardt [4], W. J. Pichler [5], H. P. Wagner [3, 1]

In our i.v. IgG (Sandoglobulin®) multicenter study for children with ITP unresponsive to previous treatment we observed some patients with an unsatisfactory long-term response to i.v. IgG [1]. They required more than one IgG infusion per month in order not to fall below 20×10^9/l platelets and/or not to show signs of hemorrhagic diathesis. Therefore, we proposed a trial combining i.v. IgG treatment and ciclosporin therapy for these children with such a severe form of chronic ITP.

The objectives of this trial were 1) to test the effects of the additional CyA treatment with respect to the platelet count and the frequency of the IgG infusions required; 2) to study the immunological profile prior to, during and after CyA and 3) to get to know the side effects of a 56- or 84-day treatment period with CyA.

The treatment plan and the laboratory investigations are shown in Table 1. When the thrombocyte count dropped below 10×10^9/l platelets we started a single i.v. IgG infusion of 0.4 g/kg bodyweight and the CyA treatment in a dosage of 10 mg/kg bodyweight per day. A further IgG infusion was only repeated, if the platelet count again dropped below 10×10^9/l platelets. Every 4 weeks we performed major immunological analyses (see Table 1). Further clinical and laboratory controls were scheduled weekly in order to note the side effects of the planned treatment.

As a pilot study we started the trial in two children. Patient A had previously had a long period of corticosteroid treatment with unsatisfactory response and was later pretreated with IgG infusions; i.v. IgG was given if the thrombocytes dropped below 10×10^9/l. She received an IgG infusion every 1 to 3 weeks for a period of 18 months. During and after a first period of additional ciclosporin medication lasting 56 days we saw that the intervals between IgG infusion became significantly longer while the platelet counts, measured 48 hours after every IgG infusion, were obviously higher. A second period of 84 days of CyA treatment showed a similar effect.

Patient B never showed a good response to corticosteroids or i.v. IgG and she was treated with courses of vincristine and prednisone at intervals of 3 to 6 weeks. After the beginning of ciclosporin treatment, this girl showed a continuous increase in her thrombocyte counts without any need for further IgG infusions. The thrombocyte count increased from a base line level of 15×10^9/l to over 200×10^9/l within the 84 days of CyA treatment.

The laboratory analyses in these two children also reflect the heterogeneity of ITP. In patient A we found an elevation of PAIg (platelet-associated antibodies) declining during the period of treatment with ciclosporin. Free antiplatelet antibodies (PBIg) were absent and the complement system normal. In contrast, patient B showed high values of PAIg and PBIg at the beginning of ciclosporin treatment, both of them declining during the treatment. Furthermore, this girl had a defect of her classical pathway complement system activation due to a marked decrease of C_2- and C_4-factors.

The analysis of the lymphocyte subsets of patient A during the first 56-day period with ciclosporin treatment revealed normal

---

1 Department of Pediatrics, University Hospital, Inselspital, Berne, Switzerland
2 Central Laboratory of the Swiss Red Cross Blood Transfusion Service, Berne, Switzerland
3 Institute for Clinical and Experimental Cancer Research, University of Berne, Switzerland
4 Institute of Clinical Immunology and Blood Transfusion, University of Gießen, Federal Republic of Germany
5 Institute of Clinical Immunology, University of Berne, Switzerland

Table 1. Treatment plan and laboratory investigations

	days 0	.	.	.	28	.	.	.	56	.	.	.	84	.	.	.	112
i. v. IgG (0.4 g/kg b.w.)	↓		↓***				↓***										
CyA (10 mg/kg b.w./d)	▭	▭	▭	▭	▭	▭	▭	▭	▭	▭	▭	▭	▭				
– Physical examination – Platelet counts** – Hemoglobin, reticulocyte count, WBC and differential – Creatine, BUN, Na, K, Ca, Mg, Ph, SGOT, SGPT, alk. Ph. – γ GT, bilirubin	×	×	×	×	×	×	×	×	×	×	×	×	×	×	×	×	×
CyA blood level			×	×													
Serum IgG*, IgA, IgM	×				×				×				×				×
PAIg, PBIg	×				×				×				×				×
Immune complexes and complement analysis (C10, C1–9, B, P, H, I ...., CI-INH, CH 50, APH 50)	×				×				×				×				×
T-, B-cells and subsets and functional analysis (lymphocyte stimulation, NK activity)	×				×				×				×				×

* Prior to each IgG infusion
** 24–48 hours after each IgG infusion
*** Only if platelet count again dropped below $10 \times 10^9/l$

values. T cells and T cell subsets slightly increased during ciclosporin therapy but B cells decreased under this immunosuppression. There was also a decrease in the T_4-/T_8-ratio (from 2.2 to 1.6).

Side effects under ciclosporin treatment were hypertrichosis, a slight decrease of serum magnesium in the otherwise unchanged laboratory analysis, and marked tiredness in patient B.

Certainly further periods of well-monitored ciclosporin medication in ITP have to be documented to allow general interpretations of these fascinating observations.

In conclusion we can say that 1) two children with severe chronic ITP and increased platelet-associated Ig showed different responses to ciclosporin treatment, reflecting the heterogeneity of ITP; 2) ciclosporin was more effective in ITP with positive platelet binding antibodies and a defective classic pathway of complement system activation; 3) no major side effects due to ciclosporin were observed.

The procedure employed seems to be feasible. We therefore wish to continue these fascinating investigations with international cooperation.

Acknowledgement

We thank Dr. M. P. Gianinazzi, Pediatrician, Lugano, and Dr. Voelckle, General Practitioner, Gersau, for their kind cooperation.

References

1. Imbach P, Gaedicke G, Joller P (1984) Interim evaluation of two cooperative studies assessing the effects of intravenous immunoglobulin (i.v. IgG) on childhood idiopathic thrombocytopenic purpura (ITP). Blut 48:357

Ciclosporin (CyA) in the Treatment of Autoimmune Blood Disorders

P. A. Miescher and P. Beris

This paper gives the case histories of four patients suffering from autoimmune blood disorders who were treated with ciclosporin (CyA) in combination with steroids. In all four patients, prior immunsuppressive treatment had been considered unsatisfactory either because it was not possible to control the disease activity even with intensive immunosuppression (cases 1 and 2), or because the patients found it unacceptable to take large doses of steroids (cases 3 and 4).

Case 1

The first case concerns a female patient born in 1951 who had suffered from pure red cell anemia since 1973 (Fig. 1). No thymoma could be detected. She was initially treated with transfusions. In the autumn of 1974 she was placed on immunosuppressive treatment (steroids plus azathioprine) which she continued until the beginning of 1977. In the summer of 1977, she developed abdominal pain diagnosed as salpingitis. At the same time, her hemoglobin dropped from 12.5 g% to 7.9 g%. Immunosuppressive therapy was resumed, initially with favourable results. In 1978, however, the hemoglobin dropped again to below 6 g% which made it necessary to give her weekly transfusions. In the spring of 1979, she was given an intensive course of anti-lymphocyte globulin. This treatment produced a favourable response of one year's duration despite severe side reactions in the form of serum sickness. She relapsed again in the spring of 1980. This time she received two courses of plasma exchange, 3 litres each time, associated with intensive i.v. immunosuppression (3×500 mg of cyclophosphamide plus 3×500 mg of methylprednisolone). Response to this treatment was only partial, necessitating blood transfusions to maintain a hemoglobin level between 4 and 6 g%. In July 1981, she was placed on a combined steroid/ciclosporin regimen with 600 mg of CyA daily (10 mg/kg). She responded after two weeks with a rise in her reticulocyte count. Water retention with ankle oedema and mild elevation of blood pressure (140/90 mm Hg) responded to chlortalidone. Furthermore, she developed quite severe hirsutism. The dosage was reduced to 400 mg daily after 5 months of treatment. In July 1982, the patient discontinued CyA. There was a prompt relapse of the pure red cell anemia necessitating blood transfusions in order to prevent a drop in hemoglobin to below 4 g%. CyA was resumed in September, and the hematological condition subsequently improved. In summer 1983, the patient gradually diminished the dose, and CyA was discontinued in September 1983. For the time being, the patient is maintaining a hemoglobin level between 9 and 10 g% without further treatment.

Case 2

The second case concerns a patient born in 1906 who developed aplastic anemia in late 1982 (Fig. 2). Pertinent family history concerns a sister of the patient who died in 1982 of a lupus-like disease. The patient was in good health until the end of 1982 when he developed pallor of the lips and increasing shortness of breath. On February 25, the following hematological data were obtained: red cell count 1.6 million/mm^3, WBC 2800/mm^3 with 30% neutrophils, platelets 18,000/mm^3. Bone mar-

Division of Hematology and Transfusion Centre, Geneva University Hospital

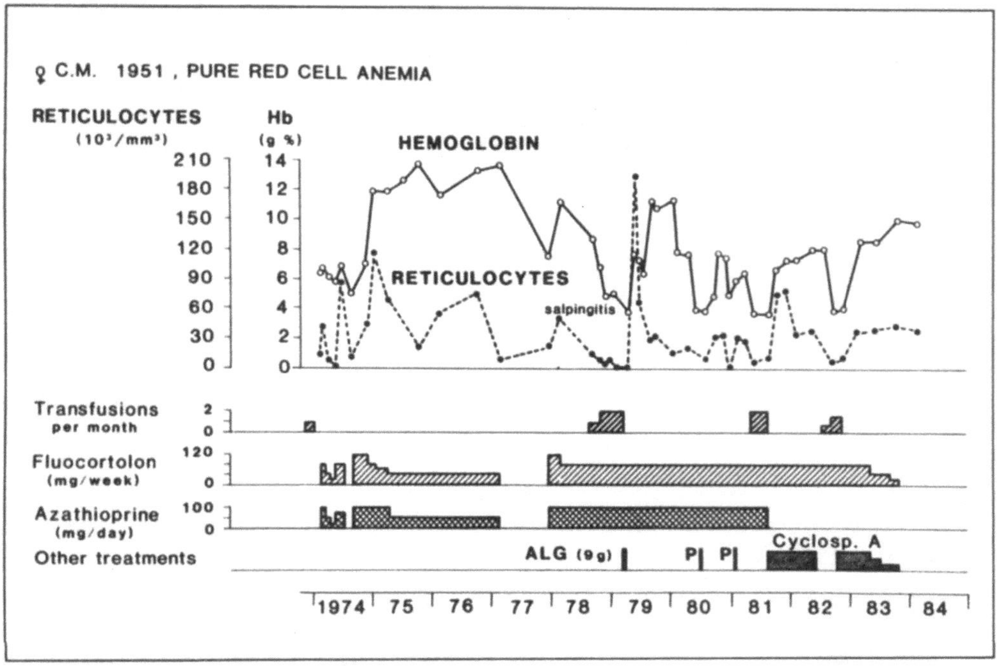

Fig. 1. Hematological course and treatment of case No. 1

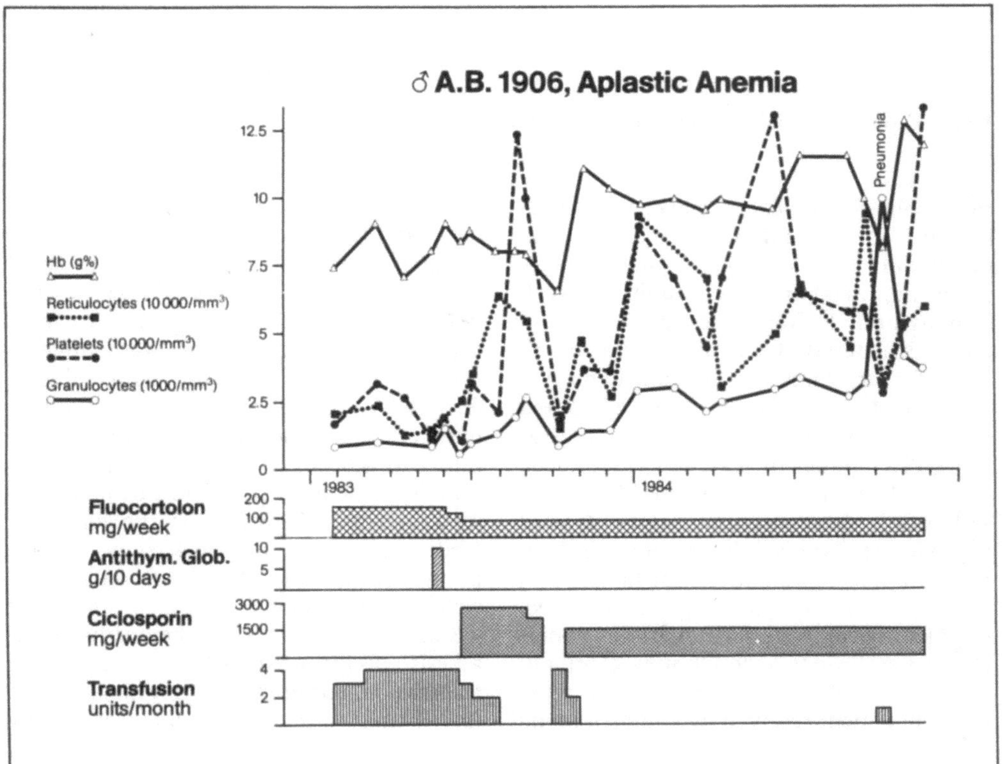

Fig. 2. Hematological course and treatment of case No. 2

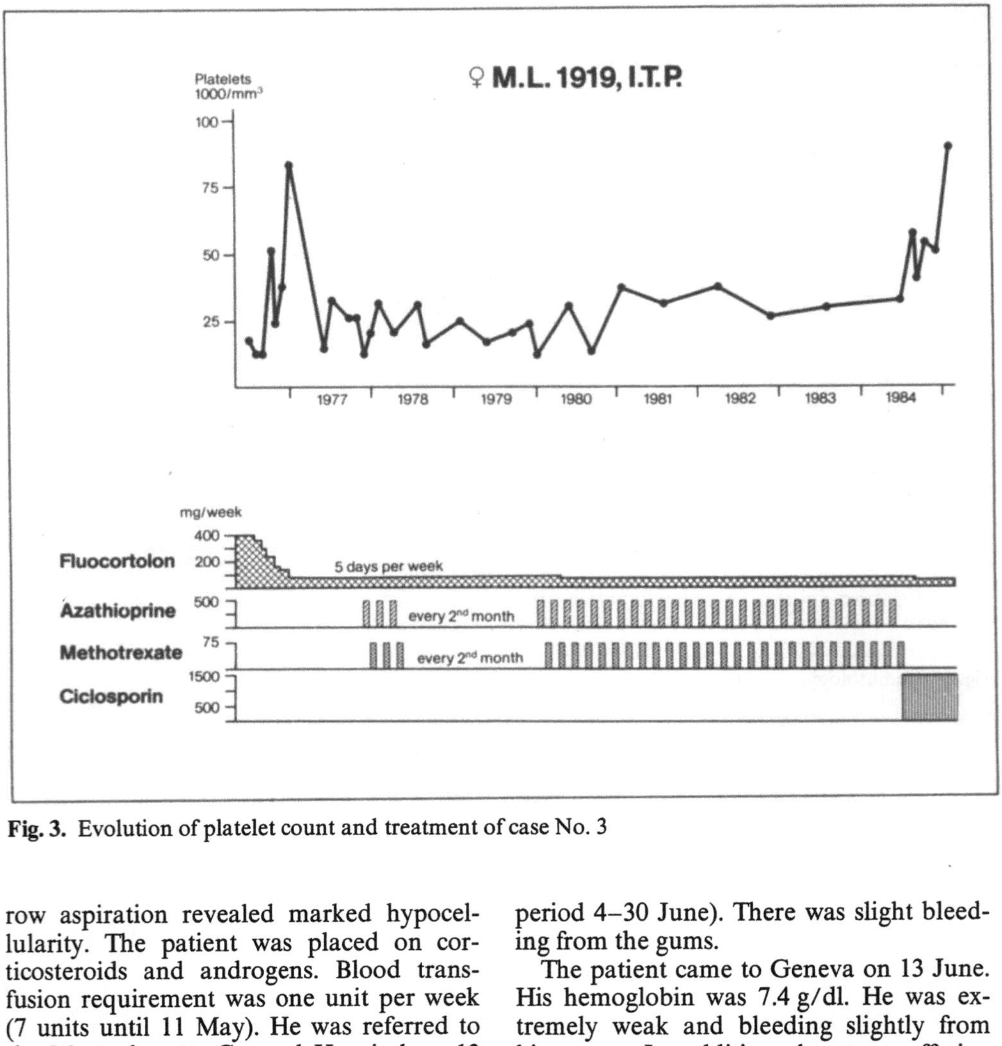

Fig. 3. Evolution of platelet count and treatment of case No. 3

row aspiration revealed marked hypocellularity. The patient was placed on corticosteroids and androgens. Blood transfusion requirement was one unit per week (7 units until 11 May). He was referred to the Massachusetts General Hospital on 13 May for treatment with anti-thymocyte globulin. On admission, the red blood count was 3 million/mm³ (after transfusion), the number of platelets was 10,000/mm³ and the number of white blood cells 2100/mm³. Bone marrow biopsy showed an extreme hypocellularity, the hematopoietic tissue representing less than 1% of what one would normally expect. No megakaryocytes were seen. A 10-day course of horse anti-thymocyte globulin (Upjohn) was given at a rate of 1 g per day. In addition, the patient received two units of blood and 10 units of platelets. Following this treatment, the patient continued to require one unit of blood per week (5 units in the period 4–30 June). There was slight bleeding from the gums.

The patient came to Geneva on 13 June. His hemoglobin was 7.4 g/dl. He was extremely weak and bleeding slightly from his gums. In addition, he was suffering from an enlarged prostate. With a blood ferritin level of 8250 ng/ml it was thought unwise to continue blood transfusions but rather to wait for a delayed therapeutic response to the antithymocyte treatment. On 25 June, he was placed on the following medication: CyA, 6.5 mg/kg/day, 6 days per week; fluocortolone, 20 mg, 4 times per week, oxymetholone, 50 mg, 3 times per week. After one week, his hemorrhagic diathesis disappeared. After three weeks, transfusion requirements dropped to less than 1 unit per month (2 units from 1 July to 12 October). CyA was discontinued in mid-September by the local physician because of gastric discomfort and a creatinine

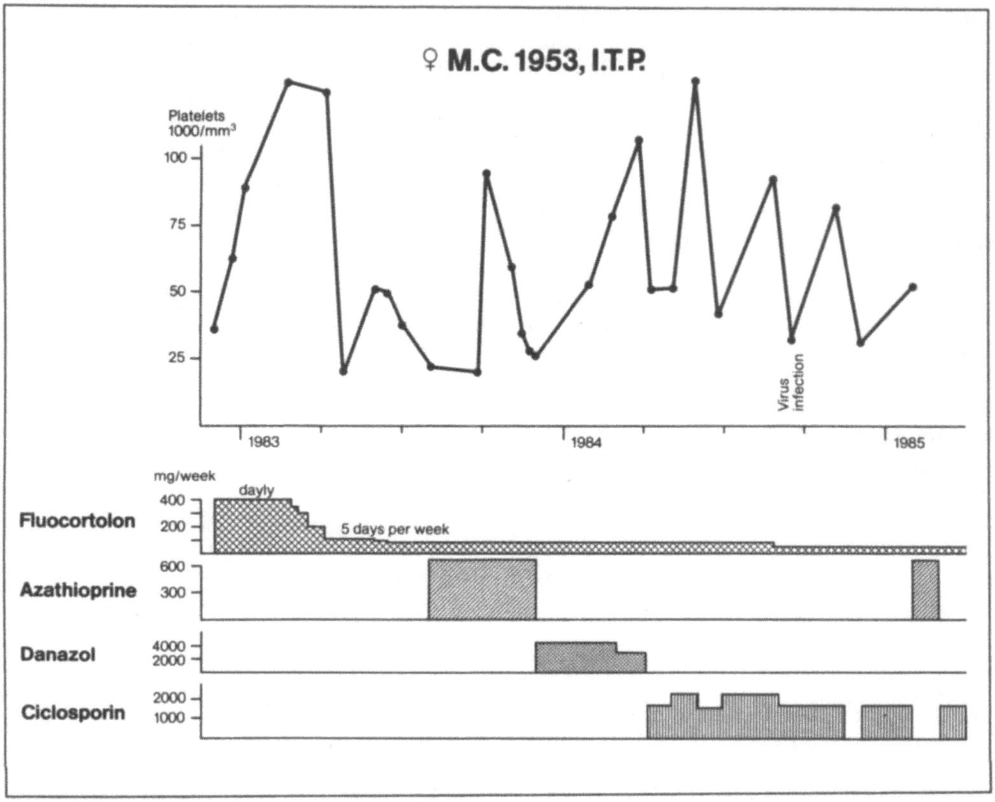

Fig. 4. Evolution of platelet count and treatment of case No. 4

level of 174 μmol/l. On 12 October, the red cell count dropped to 2.1 million/mm³. The patient received 5 units of blood between 12 October and 8 November when he entered our hospital for evaluation. CyA was resumed on 10 November. Meanwhile, hypertrophy of the prostate gland reached a level requiring transurethral resection which was performed on 24 November. The post-operative course was uneventful and the patient was discharged on 5 December with the following medication: CyA, 4 mg/kg, 6 day per week and fluocortolone, 20 mg, 4 times per week. On 13 January, blood creatinine was 150 μmol/l. The last transfusion was given on 3 December. Without further transfusions, the patient maintained a red cell count of 3 million/mm³, a white blood count varying between 3100/mm³ and 4900/mm³ and a platelet count between 56,000 and 90,000/mm³. In October 1984, a unit of blood was necessary during intercurrent bronchopneumonia.

CyA produced the following side effects in addition to an increased creatinine level: mild water retention, tremor and slight hirsutism.

The following two patients are suffering from chronic autoimmune thrombocytopenic purpura (ITP) (Figs. 3 and 4).

Case 3

This female patient born in 1919 has suffered from ITP since 1976 when she had a first episode of purpura and easy bruising. With an initial dose of 80 mg fluocortolone per day, 5 days per week, the platelet count rose to 82,000/mm³. However, when the steroid dose was adjusted to an acceptable maintenance level, the platelet number fell again to values between 15,000 and 30,000/

mm³. With the addition of azathioprine and methotrexate, the number was finally stabilized between 35,000 and 48,000/mm³. In June 1984, the antimetabolites were replaced by CyA (5 mg/kg/day). After one month, with a platelet count above 50,000/mm³, the fluocortolone dose was diminished from 70 to 60 mg per week. The last platelet count on 19 February 1985 was 88,000/mm³.

Case 4

This female patient born in 1953 is suffering from chronic ITP which was discovered in October 1982 at the end of the patient's second pregnancy. With 60 mg of fluocortolone per day, the number of platelets rose to 130,000/mm³. However, the patient suffered tremendously from the steroid side effects, developing a nervous state with a suicidal tendency. When the steroid dose was adjusted to an acceptable level, the number of platelets dropped to 22,000/mm³. The introduction of azathioprine was followed by a temporary rise in the number of platelets. When the platelet count fell again to 25,000/mm³, azathioprine was replaced by danazol at a dose of 600 mg per day. However, the side reactions to this drug were unacceptable with the development of acne and a feeling of puffiness of the face. After reaching 95,000/mm³, the number of platelets fell again to 50,000/mm³ upon reduction of the danazol dose. Danazol was finally replaced in April 1984 by CyA at an initial dose of 4 mg/kg/day. This dose was increased to 5 mg/kg/day after three weeks, followed by a rise in the platelet count to 130,000/mm³. The subsequent development of the platelet count appears erratic. However, there is a certain parallelism between the platelet count and the CyA dose. Reduction from 5 to 4 mg/kg/day was followed by a diminution in the number of platelets to 41,000/mm³ with a new rise to 93,000/mm³ after the dose was brought back to 5 mg/kg/day. However, a further reduction of platelets occurred after the dose was again diminished to 4 mg/kg (at the same time as the patient contracted an upper respiratory virus infection). Finally, a new drop occurred after the patient discontinued CyA medication. The patient is at present on a small dose of fluocortolone (30 mg per week) given with either azathioprine (100 mg, 6 days per week) or CyA (4 mg/kg, 5 days per week) on an alternate-month schedule. With this last regimen, she does not complain about side effects of the medication. Although the number of platelets is still diminished, the patient does not show any signs of hemorrhagic diathesis. The limiting side effect of CyA in this case was gingival hypertrophy which developed after only one week of therapy.

Discussion

The results obtained with the combined CyA/steroid treatment in the four patients suffering from autoimmune blood disorders justify the undertaking of large-scale studies on the usefulness of CyA in the treatment of this group of diseases.

In the three diseases the autoimmune mechanism is difficult to demonstrate in individual cases. There is still no reliable method which can be used in the routine laboratory for the demonstration of autoantibodies against platelets. However, careful investigations on the nature of chronic ITP permit the assumption that autoantibodies are responsible in the great majority of these cases.

With regard to pure red cell anemia, the situation is more difficult since even at the level of the research laboratory no suitable methods are available to demonstrate the autoimmune mechanism. It is mainly the results of immunosuppressive therapy that have led to the conclusion that most cases of chronic pure red cell anemia are due to autoimmunity.

Various mechanisms can lead to aplastic anemia. Once aplasia is present it is not possible, with today's methodology, to decide whether its origin is toxic or immunologic. In the toxic variety, bone marrow transplantation would seem to be the most logical therapeutic approach while there is no reason why immunosuppression should be effective. It is only in the autoimmune variety of aplastic anemia that immunosuppression is likely to be successful.

The patient described in this paper had a sister who suffered from SLE. With the genetic background of self-perpetuating diseases, it was logical to assume that the aplastic anemia was also the consequence of an autoimmune process, especially since there was no indication of exposure to toxic substances or radiation.

With regard to the evaluation of the effect of CyA in the four patients, the recurrence of the disease upon cessation of CyA medication in the first two cases appears important. Indeed, spontaneous remission can occur in pure red cell anemia and in aplastic anemia. Furthermore, antithymocyte globulin may produce a delayed remission. The fact that in both cases the disease recurred when the patients stopped taking CyA is a strong argument in favour of the efficacy of the drug in the two conditions. With regard to ITP, evaluation of treatment is difficult in view of the spontaneous variations of the platelet count which frequently occur in the course of this disease. However, it seems unlikely that the improvement in case 3 is purely coincidental after so many years of unsuccessful treatment. With regard to case 4, the evolution of the platelet count appears at first glance rather fortuitous. However, the result of the various attempts at therapy appears of sufficient relevance to us to report at a meeting where pilot studies are presented.

CyA induces too many side reactions for it to be accepted without reservation by patients. Hirsutism was severe in one patient, mild in two. Hypertension and water retension with the formation of ankle oedema occurred in case 1. Gingival hyperplasia was a serious problem in case 4. Finally, patient AB (case 2), who suffered from chronic cholecystitis, complained that CyA aggravated his gastrointestinal problems. These side reactions also explain the tendency of patients to discontinue CyA medication once an improvement has been achieved.

New solutions have to be found for long-term therapy in order to limit the extent of side reactions, including renal damage. We are at present alternating CyA with azathioprine on a monthly basis for maintenance therapy in the treatment of self-perpetuating autoimmune disease.

On the basis of our very limited experience with four cases of autoimmune blood disorders, CyA appears to be a promising new immunosuppressant which merits further investigation.

9. Rheumatoid Arthritis

Rheumatoid Arthritis

Øystein Førre

Rheumatoid arthritis is characterized by a chronic inflammatory synovitis in various joints. The cell infiltrates have the characteristics of a cell-mediated, or delayed type, immune reaction. The inflammatory cells produce various factors that can modulate the inflammatory reaction and cause the characteristic destructive features of the disease. All effective therapies modulate mononuclear cell function or influence the rate of production or elimination of these cells and/or cell products. Ciclosporin (CyA) represents a new and exciting way treating patients with rheumatoid arthritis.

Introduction

It has been estimated that 1% of all humans have rheumatoid arthritis. There is also general agreement that the current therapy for this disorder is very unsatisfactory. Rheumatoid arthritis is characterized by remissions and exacerbations which are unpredictable and which make therapeutic evaluations very difficult. The etiology of the disease is unknown, but genetic and immunological factors seems to play on important role in the pathogenesis. Thus rheumatoid arthritis is associated with the HLA-DR4 gene [5] and many immunological aberrations can be demonstrated in rheumatoid synovial tissues [24].

Characteristics of the rheumatoid synovial tissue

The normal synovial membrane is lined by a double layer of synovial lining cells which form a multilayer in the rheumatoid synovial membrane [3]. The synovial lining cells have previously been classified according to electron microscopic criteria as A and C cells, which have macrophage characteristics, and B cells which have fibroblast characteristics [9].

By means of immunohistological techniques and a panel of monoclonal antibodies it has been possible to confirm the macrophage and fibroblast nature of the synovial lining cells [9].

In addition, however, a new cell with dendritic appearance and abundant class II MHC antigens has been identified in the rheumatoid synovium [3, 8, 9].

In the rheumatoid tissues there are also large infiltrates of T lymphocytes which are activated and spontaneously produce various types of lymphokines [15] such as interleukin 2 [7]. A majority of these T cells express surface antigens associated with helper/inducer cell function, such as OKT4 and Leu 3A [10]. There are also observations which indicate that helper/inducer T cells are in close apposition to HLA DR bearing dendritic cells which have many accessory activities like antigen presentation and production of interleukin 1 [6, 8, 9]. These findings are strongly reminiscent of a cell-mediated immune hypersensitivity reaction, as similar findings can be seen in positive skin tuberculin tests [17] and in chronic lesions induced by persistent infectious agents [13].

In the rheumatoid synovial membrane there is also a spontaneous production of immunoglobulins, like self-associating IgG rheumatoid factors [14], which promote inflammation by means of deposition of immune complexes, followed by complement activation [14] (Table 1).

Recent observations indicate that mononuclear cells in the synovial tissue spontaneously generate mediators of fibroblast growth [15].

Oslo Sanitetsforenings Rheumatism Hospital, Akersbakken 27, Oslo 1

Table 1. Characteristics of the cell infiltrates in the synovial membrane in rheumatoid arthritis

Synovial cells
Macrophages (A and C type cells) (HLA-DR positive)
Fibroblasts (B type cell)
Dendritic cells (HLA-DR positive)
T lymphocytes
OKT4 > OKT8
HLA-DR positive T lymphocytes
Proliferating T lymphocytes
Spontaneous production of lymphokines (interleukin 2) (IL2)
Tac (IL2-receptor)-positive T lymphocytes
B lymphocytes
Spontaneous production of immunoglobulins (Self-associating IgG rheumatoid factors)

Table 2. Products of rheumatoid mononuclear cells which may contribute to inflammation and tissue destruction

Lymphocyte products
Monocyte chemotactic factor
Migration inhibition factor
Leukocyte migration inhibition factor
Lymphocyte mitogenic factor
Fibroblast-activating factor
Monocyte products
Interleukin 1
Mononuclear cell activator
Fibroblast activating factor
Synovial activator
Plasminogen activator
Collagenase
Prostaglandins
Lysosomal enzymes
Oxygen radicals
Dendritic cells
Interleukin 1

Thus cellular interactions are involved in the formation and function of the pannus which is composed of proliferating fibroblasts, numerous small blood vessels, collagen, and inflammatory cells [15]. Inflammatory cells mediate synovial proliferation, which produces the excessive levels of collagenase and prostaglandins [15, 21] that may in turn contribute to connective tissue destruction. Interleukin 1, which is produced both by macrophages [19] and dendritic cells [6] and has been demonstrated in the synovial fluid [23], can stimulate synovial cells to secrete increased levels of collagenase and prostaglandins [15]. Another monocyte product, synovial activator, stimulates plasminogen activator from synovial fibroblasts, resulting in the generation of plasmin which can degrade connective tissue constituents [15]. Monocytes/macrophages also secrete collagenase, prostaglandins and oxygen radicals, further augmenting tissue damage [15, 21] (Table 2).

Effects of antirheumatic drugs on rheumatoid inflammation

Nonsteroidal anti-inflammatory drugs. These drugs cause analgesia and are anti-inflammatory after repeated administration in high doses. They act rapidly and their effects decline promptly after termination of therapy. Nonsteroidal anti-inflammatory drugs do not prevent tissue destruction and probably cannot induce remission in rheumatoid arthritis.

These drugs act by inhibiting the enzyme cyclooxygenase which converts arachidonic acid to prostaglandins [21]. Some of these agents might also inhibit the formation of oxygen radicals [21].

Corticosteroids. These drugs act on many cell types. They inhibit monocyte chemotaxis. At high doses they cause a reversible monocytopenia and lymphocytopenia which is due to a redistribution of monocytes and lymphocytes from the circulation to the bone marrow [4]. These drugs also act on vessel walls leading to decreased vascular permeability and might thereby prevent extravasation of inflammatory mediators. Corticosteroids block the accumulation of polymorphonuclear leukocytes and monocytes at inflammatory sites. These drugs also inhibit the enzyme, phospholipase A2, which converts membrane phospholipids to arachidonic acid, thus leading to reduced formation of proinflammatory prostaglandins and leukotrienes [21]. It is possible that small doses of corticosteroids can prevent tissue destruction in rheumatoid arthritis.

Slowly acting drugs. These drugs include D-penicillamine, gold salts and antimalarial drugs. They have in common a slow onset of action. These drugs may induce remission and prevent the development of tissue destruction. D-penicillamine is able to inhibit lymphocyte proliferation and immunoglobulin production [12]. Gold salts may interfere with the functioning of macrophages as effector [20] and antigen-presenting cells [11]. This leads to diminished phagocytosis, reduced release of lysosomal enzymes and depressed lymphocyte responses to mitogens and antigens. Antimalarial drugs can inhibit lymphocyte functions, probably through inhibition of interleukin 1 [16] production by monocytes (synovial cells) and dendritic cells.

Cytostatic drugs. These drugs include the alkylating agents chlorambucil and cyclophosphamide, the purine analog azathioprine and the folic acid antagonist, methotrexate. They all inhibt DNA synthesis in proliferating cells and may thereby affect the proliferation of many kinds of cells in the rheumatoid synovium. Cytostatic drugs act very slowly and it can take weeks and months before they induce clinical remission [15].

Ciclosporin. The current treatment of rheumatoid arthritis with nonsteroidal anti-inflammatory drugs, slowly acting drugs and cytostatic agents is disappointing, as only marginal effects on tissue destruction can be achieved. Therefore rheumatologists are searching for new modalities which can represent a "breakthrough" in the treatment of rheumatoid arthritis. CyA may represent such a "breakthrough", alone or in combination with traditional antirheumatic drugs. CyA has greatly improved the graft survival rates in organ transplantation since it can effectively suppress the immune reactions which are responsible for graft rejection [2]. The drug is able to suppress various immune responses by inhibiting the production of various lymphokines like interleukin 2 [2] and by counteracting events induced by interleukin 1 [18]. The fact that cells from rheumatoid joint tissues produce various forms of lymphokines and monokines might indicate an important place for CyA in the future treatment of rheumatic diseases (Table 3). The beneficial effect of the drug on adjuvant arthritis in experimental animals [1] also indicates that CyA might be effective in rheumatoid arthritis.

In this workshop the present status of CyA treatment of rheumatoid arthritis is given. The results from these preliminary studies are promising but before the role of CyA treatment in rheumatoid arthritis can be defined, larger controlled studies have to be performed. These studies should give answers to the following questions: 1. Is CyA effective in rheumatoid arthritis? 2. How long should the treatment last? 3. What is the lowest effective dose of CyA 4. What are the beneficial and harmful drug combinations? 5. How can one avoid toxic effects of CyA treatment?

Table 3. Drug therapy in rheumatoid arthritis

Type of drug	Mode of action
Nonsteroidal anti-inflammatory drugs	Inhibition of cyclooxygenase Inhibition of oxygen radical release
Corticosteroids	Modulation of lymphocyte and macrophage function. Inhibition of interleukin 1 production. Redistribution of mono-/lymphocytes. Inhibition of phospholipase A2
Antimalarials	Inhibition of interleukin 1 production
D-penicillamine	Modulation of lymphocyte function
Gold salts	Modulation of lymphocyte and macrophage functions
Cytostatic drugs	Inhibition of DNA synthesis (cell proliferation)
Ciclosporin	Inhibition of lymphokine and monokine-production (Interleukin 2 and Interleukin 1)

References

1. Borel JF, Wiesinger D, Gubler HV (1978) Effects the antilymphocytic agent cyclosporin A in chronic inflammation. Eur J Rheum Inflam 1:237
2. Britton S, Palacios R (1982) Cyclosporin A. – Usefulnes, risks and mechanism of action. Immunol Rev 65:5
3. Burmeister GR, Locher P, Koch B, Winchester RJ, Dimitriu-Bona A, Kalden JR, Mohr W (1983) The tissue architecture of synovial membranes in inflammatory and non-inflammatory joint diseases. I. The localization of the major synovial cell populations as detected by monoclonal reagents directed towards Ia and monocyte/macrophage antigens. Rheumatol Int 3:173
4. Cupps TR, Fauci AS (1982) Corticosteroid-mediated immunoregulation in man. Immunol Rev 65:133
5. Doubloug JH, Førre Ø, Kåss E, Thorsby E (1980) HLA antigens and Rheumatoid arthritis. Association between HLA-DRw4 positivity of IgM-Rheumatoid Factor production. Arthritis Rheum 23:309
6. Duff GW, Førre Ø, Waalen K, Dickens E, Nuki G (1985) Rheumatoid synovial dendritic cells produce Interleukin 1-activity. Br J Rheumatol 24:108
7. Førre Ø, Egeland T, Waalen K, Mellbye OJ (1982) Interleukin 2 production by peripheral blood, synovial fluid and synovial tissue lymphocytes. Clin Rheumatol 1 (abstr)
8. Førre Ø, Waalen K, Pahle J (1984) Rheumatoid dendritic cells as accessory cells. Immunobiology 167:117
9. Førre Ø, Waalen K, Thoen J, Hovig T (1985) Macrophages and Dendritic cells in Rheumatic Diseases. In: Gupta S, Talal N (eds) Immunology of Rheumatic Disease. Plenum Publishing Corporation, New York, in press
10. Klareskog L, Forsum U, Wigren A, Wigzell H (1982) Relationships between HLA-DR-expressing cells and T cells of different subsets in rheumatoid arthritis synovial tissue. Scand J Immunol 15:501
11. Lipsky PE, Ziff M (1977) Inhibition of antigen- and mitogen-induced human lymphocyte proliferation by gold compounds. J Clin Invest 59:455
12. Lipsky PE, Ziff M (1980) Inhibition of human helper T cell function in vitro by D-penicillamine and $CuSO_4$. J Clin Invest 65:1069
13. Madlin RL, Gebhard JF, Taylor CR, Rea TH (1983) In situ characterization of T lymphocyte subsets in the reactional states of leprosy. Clin Exp Immunol 53:17
14. Munthe E, Natvig JB (1972) Complement-fixing intracellular complexes of IgG-Rheumatoid Factor in rheumatoid plasma cells. Scand J Immunol 1:217
15. NIH-Conference (1984) Rheumatoid Arthritis: Evolving Concepts of Pathogenesis and treatment. Ann Intern Med 101:810
16. Salmeron B, Lipsky PE (1983) Immunosuppressive potential of antimalarials. Ann J Med 75 [Suppl]: 19
17. Scheynius A, Klareskog L, Forsum U (1982) In situ identification of T lymphocyte subsets and HLA-DR expressing cells in the human skin tuberculin reaction. Clin Exp Immunol 49:325
18. Skjodt M, Gallagher JA, Beresford JN, Elford P, Gowen M, Poser JW, Wood DD, Russell RGG (1984) Modulation of Interleukin-1 effects on bone by Cyclosporine. Calcif Tissue Int 36 [Suppl 2]:50 (abstr)
19. Smith KA, Lachman LB, Oppenheim JJ, Fontana MF (1980) The functional relationship of interleukins. J Exp Med 151:155
20. Ugal K, Ziff M, Lipsky PE (1979) Gold-induced changes in the morphology and functional capabilities of human monocytes. Arthritis Rheum 22:352
21. Weissmann G (1982) The biochemistry of inflammation: Rheumatoid arthritis and anti-inflammatory drugs. Eur J Rheum Inflam 5:366
22. White DJG, Calne RY (1982) The use of cyclosporin A: Immunosuppression in organ grafting. Immunol Rev 65:115
23. Wood DD, Ihrie EJ, Dinarello CA, Cohen PL (1983) Isolation of an interleukin-1-like factor from human joint effusions. Arthritis Rheum 26:975
24. Zvaifler NJ (1973) The immunopathology of joint inflammation in rheumatoid arthritis. Adv Immunol 16:265

Ciclosporin in Rheumatoid Arthritis: Open Trials with Different Dosages

B. Amor, M. Dougados

We report on our experience of two pilot studies of ciclosporin (CyA) in the treatment of rheumatoid arthritis (RA), a disease in which functional T cell abnormalities have been clearly demonstrated [2].

Patients and Methods

Outpatients of both sexes who had given their informed consent after explanations about protocol were included in the trial. These patients were suffering from chronic RA in stage I to III according to criteria of the A.R.A. A patient was not included if he or she had been given slow-acting antirheumatic drugs in the 3 preceding months. Disease activity was judged by the presence of at least 3 of the following criteria: erythrocyte sedimentation rate ≧30 mms in the first hour; morning stiffness ≧60 minutes; Ritchie index [5] ≧10; Lee index [1]≧5 and at least 3 joints with effusion or synovitis. Corticosteroid and nonsteroidal anti-inflammatory drugs and/or analgesics were maintained and the doses during the trial were noted. The characteristics of the patients at the beginning of the trials are summarized in Table 1. Assessment criteria were as follows: 1 – morning stiffness (in minutes), 2 – grip strength (average in mmHg of 3 consecutive measurements on each side), 3 – proximal interphalangeal circumference (total of 10 joints), 4 – Ritchie index [5], 5 – Lee functional index [1], 6 – pain assessment (100 mm on visual analog scale), 7 – an assessment by the patient of his or her own state compared with that at the previous consultation (+3 = much better, +2 = better, +1 = a little better, 0 = identical, –1 = a little worse, –2 = worse, –3 = much worse), 8 – erythrocyte sedimentation rate measured by the Westergren method, 9 – Latex F2 agglutination test, 10 – Waaler Rose test.

Side effects were recorded either as spontaneous declarations by the patient but also as replies to an oral list of questions with special reference to hypertrichosis, gingivitis, tremor. Clinical tolerance assessment included blood pressure and biological tolerance liver enzymes, serum creatinine levels, blood count, and proteinuria determinations. All the patients were followed by the same physician two weeks after the beginning of the trial and then monthly. All patients received oral CyA twice daily (except 4 patients in the first trial). Initial dosage was 9 mg/kg/day in the first trial (6 patients) and only 5 mg/kg/day in the second (12 patients). The dosage of CyA was decreased if renal toxicity (creatinine plasma level increase more than 50% versus basal value) and/or hypertension occurred. CyA was discontinued if the side effect did not disappear one week after reduction of the dosage. After one month of therapy, the dosage was increased in case of clinical ineffectiveness and decreased after 4 months of therapy even in the absence of side effect.

Results

The changes in the clinical and the biological assessment criteria after 2 months of treatment in both trials and after 4 months in the trial using 5 mg/kg/day are summarized in Table 2. Furthermore, clinical improvement was observed at day 15 in the first trial, compared with only a slight improvement at day 30 in the second. The overall assessment by the patient of his or her own status was good in all cases after 2

Department of Rheumatology, Prof. B. Amor, Hôpital Cochin, 27 rue du Faubourg Saint-Jacques, 75014 Paris – France

Table 1. Characteristics of patients at the beginning of the trials

Characteristics*	CyA 9 mg/kg/day n=6	CyA 5 mg/kg/day n=12
Age (years)	59.2 (5.7)	50.1 (13.0)
Sex (F/M)	4/2	10/2
Duration of RA (years)	7.5 (4.2)	9.5 (4.8)
Rheumatoid factor +	6	11
Previous S.A.A.D**		
• Gold salts	6	11
• Penicillamine	5	10
• Levamisole	1	2
• Antimalarial drugs	4	7
• Chlorambucil	2	2
Morning stiffnes (minutes)	210 (117)	155 (138)
Pain (VAS)** mms	59.6 (22.8)	64.4 (18.3)
Grip strength (mm Hg)	191 (60)	198 (229)
PIP** circumference (mm)	633 (62)	623 (58)
Ritchie index	20.0 (3.4)	21.7 (9.8)
Prednisone consumption (mg/day)	15.5 (7.2)	5.2 (4.2)
Erythrocyte sedimentation rate (mm first hour)	66.1 (33.2)	69.4 (33.5)

* Number of patients or the mean (standard deviation)
** S.A.A.D.: slow-acting antirheumatic drug; V.A.S. = visual analog scale; P.I.P. = proximal interphalangeal joint.

Table 2. Changes in clinical and laboratory measurements after therapy

Measurements[a]	After 2 months		After 4 months
	CyA 9 mg/kg/day n=6	CyA 5 mg/kg/day n=11	CyA 5 mg/kg/day n=8
Morning stiffness (minutes)	– 133 (70)***	– 48.6 (56.5)**	– 103.8 (114.0)*
Pain (VAS) mm	– 24.6 (26.8)	– 15.6 (16.0)**	– 31.3 (5.8)****
Grip strength (mm Hg)	+ 157 (176)	+ 16 (78)	+ 101 (100)*
PIP circumference (mm)	+ 0.2 (9.6)	– 12.3 (10.1)**	– 15.9 (12.9)**
Ritchie index	– 16.3 (3.5)**	– 8.6 (8.9)*	– 12.2 (2.5)****
Lee index	– 5.3 (2.0)**	– 4.6 (2.5)**	– 5.9 (3.6)*
Prednisone consumption (mg/day)	– 6.0 (5.7)	– 0.3 (1.5)	– 1.1 (0.8)***
ESR (mm/1st hour)	– 4.6 (16.0)	– 7.9 (32.4)	+ 0.5 (28.8)
Latex F2 agglutination test	ND	ND	– 0.9 (2.6)
Waaler Rose	ND	ND	– 0.1 (2.7)
CyA posology (mg/kg/day)	7.7 (0.8)	5.7 (0.8)	6.5 (0.7)
CyA plasma level 12 hours after the last oral dose (ng/ml)	325 (179)	141 (156)	208 (178)

[a] Expressed in means (standard deviation); ND = not done, other terms as in Table 1. Statistical significance determined by Student's t-test: * $p<0.05$; ** $p<0.02$; *** $p<0.01$; **** $p<0.001$

Table 3. Reasons for dropout during the two trials

Side effect	CyA 9 mg/kg/day		CyA 5 mg/kg/day	
	No. of patients	Day of occurrence	No. of patients	Day of occurrence
Hypertension	2	80 – 120	1	60
Myocardial infarction	1	70		
Fatigue weight loss	1	60		
Thrombocytopenia	1	90	1	90
Renal toxicity			1	120
Skin rash			1	60
Dyspepsia			1	15
Total	5/6		5/12	

months therapy in the first trial; a minor benefit was observed in the second trial. Overall efficacy was considered good by all these patients after 4 months of therapy with, at this time, an increase in CyA dose from 5.7±0.8 mg/kg/day (day 60) to 6.5±0.7 mg/kg/day (day 120). This efficacy continued after 6 months (5 patients) while CyA dosage was slightly decreased (5.5±0.7 mg/kg/day). On the other hand, a flare-up of the disease occurred rapidly (2 to 10 weeks) after discontinuation of CyA because of side effect(s). Table 3 gives reasons for dropout in the two trials. Side effects were more frequent, severe and occurred sooner in the first trial using CyA 9 mg/kg/day. A patient with hypertension and corticosteroid therapy of long duration died from a myocardial infarction after 3 months of therapy. The autopsy revealed large atheromatous lesions of coronary vessels without any sign of vasculitis.

Previous hypertension was exacerbated in two patients, but no medication was given for this side effect and it disappeared in a few days after discontinuation of CyA. A patient with a good result of CyA treatment suddenly developed thrombocytopenia in the 3rd month of therapy without any clinical sign of haemorrhage (platelet count: 44,000 per mm^3). CyA therapy was immediately withdrawn. Myelogram revealed numerous megacaryocytes. Cytomegalovirus serology was positive and this virus was recovered from urine culture samples. Thrombocytopenia resolved spontaneously within 3 weeks. Because a viral aetiology was suspected and no previous case of thrombocytopenia with CyA had been reported, this patient was included in the second trial on recurrence of his disease. The drug was again effective, but in the 3rd month, thrombocytopenia recurred without any evident aetiology and the drug was definitively withdrawn.

Side effects were less frequent and less severe in the second trial. However, 5 patients had to discontinue CyA therapy: thrombocytopenia (1 case previously described); hypertension (1 case at day 60); dyspepsia (1 case at day 15); pruriginous skin rash with facial oedema (1 case at day 60) which disappeared in a few days after CyA withdrawal; increase in creatinine plasma level (1 case at day 120). It has to be noted that in this last patient cimetidine therapy was instituted two days after CyA withdrawal and the creatinine plasma level increased from 167 mmol/l (at the time CyA was discontinued) to 295 mmol/l one week later. Cimetidine therapy was stopped and the creatinine plasma level normalized within a week.

Other side effects occurred in this trial without necessitating CyA withdrawal: four other patients experienced an increase in plasma creatinine level (more than 50% versus basal value). In 3 of them, renal toxicity was associated with hypertension and in another patient with cimetidine therapy. Hypertension occured in 3 patients. In all these cases, previous hypertension was noted and was exacerbated after therapy. In 3 cases, hypertension was controlled with medication and/or reduction of CyA dose. Hypertrichosis (7 cases) was mild in 3 cases and moderate in 4, necessitating shaving twice a day in one male patient and monthly depilation in 3 female patients. Gingival hyperplasia (6 cases) was minor in 3 cases and associated with clinical functional signs in the other 3 cases. Local care (frequent tooth brushing, local antiseptic treatment) was able to cure gingivitis in all these cases. Transient paraesthesia of hands and feet (5 to 10 minutes, twice or three times a week) disappeared spontaneously within one month in 3 patients without change in CyA dosage. Only one patient developed moderate elevation of liver enzymes.

Discussion

These two trials suggest that CyA may be an effective treatment of RA. However, these open trials have to be confirmed by randomized double-blind controlled trials. The high frequency of good results observed and the benefit to the patients of this therapy, which is not devoid of side effects, suggest that the observed efficacy is not due to chance alone or to the attractiveness of a new drug. For us, the main problem of this treatment is the management of the patients. These two trials using two different dosages suggest that the onset and the strength of the drug's effect are dose related, as are the side effects. We therefore suggest that in the future it will be better to initiate the treatment with a dosage of 5 mg/kg twice a day (dyspepsia occurred more frequently when using CyA once a day and no advantage was observed when using CyA three times a day) and then to increase this dosage with regard to clinical efficacy. When a good result was obtained (in our experience after 4 months of therapy), it would be possible to decrease this dosage even in the absence of side effects and with a maintenance of the clinical efficacy.

All these precautions have to be taken because CyA is far from devoid of side effects. In these trials, we observed those previously reported in the literature [3, 4, 6]. Their occurrence and their severity were more frequent when using CyA 9 mg/kg/day, which led us to stop this trial. When using 5 mg/kg/day, we also observed many side effects necessitating discontinuation of the therapy in 5 cases. This frequency has to be discussed and calls for some precautions. In these trials, the frequency of the side effects might be overestimated because they were systematically sought in an oral list of questions at each consultation. Hypertension occurred only in patients with previous hypertension, suggesting that a history of hypertension, past or present, treated or untreated, might be a criterion against the institution of CyA treatment, even if controlled with therapy. Renal toxicity occurred in patients with hypertension and when cimetidine was associated with CyA, also suggesting that active peptic ulcer or the administration of an H2 antagonist might be an exclusion criterion. Moreover, to our knowledge, peripheral thrombocytopenia has never been previously reported in CyA treatments. Although this is a single case, we suggest that a platelet count has to be performed in the management of these patients. In our experience, some other side effects such as tremor and sometimes hypertrichosis were transient and did not necessitate discontinuation of the drug; gum hyperplasia is frequent but our experience suggests that oral hygiene might be a prophylactic therapy.

We know that the CyA plasma level is commonly determined in the management of these patients and we did so. We understand the interest of such a dosage when using CyA in transplantation. In these cases, the aetiology of a side effect such as hypertension or renal insufficiency is difficult to ascertain. In RA patients, management is easier so we suggest that this determination has to be performed in phase III therapeutic trials but that it should not constitute a criterion for changes in the CyA dosage. CyA dosage should be modified only with regard to clinical efficiency and/or occurrence of side effects.

In conclusion, CyA seems to be an effective treatment of RA. It will be interesting to conduct randomized controlled trials and long-term follow-up of the patients to confirm the observed efficacy and to determine the optimal dose of CyA.

References

1. Lee P, Jasani MK, Dick NC, Buchanan WW (1973) Evaluation of a functional index in rheumatoid arthritis. Scan J Rheumatol 2:71–77
2. NIH Conference; Moderator: Decker JL (1984) Rheumatoid arthritis: evolving concepts or pathogenesis and treatment. Ann Intern Med 101:810–824
3. Palestine AG, Nussenblatt RB, Chanc C (1984) Side effects of systemic cyclosporine in patients not undergoing transplantation. Am J Med 77:652–656
4. Powles RL, Clinck HM, Spence D, et al. (1980) Cyclosporin A to prevent graft-versus host disease in man after allogeneic bone marrow transplantation. Lancet I:327–329
5. Ritchie DM, Boyle JA, Mc Innes JM, Grieveson P, Buchanan NN (1968) Clinical studies with an articular index for the assessment of joint tenderness in patients with rheumatoid arthritis. J Med 7:393–406
6. Starzl TE, Iwatsuki S, Bahnson HB (1982) Cyclosporin A and steroids for liver and heart transplantation. In: White DJG (ed) Cyclosporine A. Elsevier Biomedical Press, Amsterdam, p 431–436

A Pilot Study of CyA in Patients with Rheumatoid Arthritis (RA)

C. Bombardier, P. Tugwell, M. Gent, W. Buchanan, D. Ludwin, C. Stiller

A before-and-after pilot study is currently in progress to obtain preliminary evidence on the role of ciclosporin (CyA) as a third line agent in RA. Twenty patients with definite or classical RA who have failed NSAID, gold and penicillamine therapy will be maintained on CyA for six months and observed for an additional six months. Currently fourteen patients have been entered into the study. Patients were initially started on 10 mg/kg/day of CyA in two doses, and monitored closely for the first five weeks; dosage was adjusted to achieve a trough level of 50 to 200 ng/ml of CyA. Initial dosage is currently reduced to 5 mg/kg/day to minimize side effects. When a stable CyA level is achieved, patients are followed every three weeks for side effects and every six weeks for efficacy. Efficacy assessments include: Joint count, morning stiffness, grip strength, 50-foot walk time, global assessment of efficacy and a functional assessment. Four patients were withdrawn because of side effects: three patients had renal toxicity and one had liver toxicity. All side effects improved after discontinuing the drug. It is too early to comment on drug efficacy, but the lower dosage (5 mg/kg/day) appears to be reasonably well tolerated by patients.

McMaster University and University of Toronto, Canada.

Low Dose Ciclosporin (CyA) and Prednisone – a Step in the Direction of Selective Immunosuppression in Rheumatoid Arthritis Refractory to Treatment (6-Month Follow-Up)

Ch. Herzog, D. Gross

Summary

In our study 15 patients with severe rheumatoid arthritis refractory to treatment were treated with low dose CyA (max. 5 mg/kg body weight/day) in combination with prednisone (6-month follow-up at end of February 1985). 12 patients exhibited a surprising clinical improvement after an average of 7.5 weeks (6–11 weeks). In 3 patients the result was only partly satisfactory. In the course of the 6 months, we did not observe any serious nephrotoxicity such as has been described in other studies with a dosage of 10 mg/kg/day [18]. We believe that individual adjustment of the dose during the first 90 days is of decisive importance. An improvement was seen in various parameters of the disease, such as morning stiffness, number of swollen joints, etc. Little correlation was seen between the clinical improvement and the humoral and cellular laboratory parameters. All virus titres tested were negative throughout the six months. The increased incidence of side effects in HLA-DR4 positive patients (in 8 of 15 patients) is interesting. The slight side effects seem to be dose-dependent and exhibit little correlation with the ciclosporin A levels.

Introduction

The conventional treatment of severe forms of rheumatoid arthritis with gold, cyclophosphamide, penicillamine etc. is largely unsatisfactory, partly because of side effects and also because of a non-selective mechanism of action [25, 29]. Severe complications have also been seen with attempts at total lymph-node irradiation (TLI) (4 deaths in 12 patients) [33].

Preliminary experiments using CyA (monotherapy) in rheumatoid arthritis by Müller and Hermann in 1979 [18] resulted in considerable renal side effects with clinical efficacy in about one-third of the patients at most (dosage approx. 10 mg/kg/day). CyA is currently used for short- or long-term therapy in various dosages for a number of autoimmune diseases. It appears, however, that nephrotoxicity is a limiting factor with all high-dose monotherapy [19]. For this reason cautious combined therapy with max. 5 mg/kg bodyweight/day of CyA and low-dose prednisone has been used. We did not observe any nephrotoxicity in 9 patients. A 1- to 2-week treatment-free interval had to be intercalated on account of a deterioration of creatinine clearance in 6 patients.

Patients and methods

15 patients – 9 men, 6 women – with active rheumatoid arthritis that had proved refractory to previous therapy (Table 1) were admitted to our study. 6 of them were in stage II and 9 in stage III (ARA criteria) and 14 of them had had a 3-month treatment-free interval before the start of CyA therapy. Average age was 61 years (36–72 years). Average duration of the disease: 6 years (½–12 years). Entry into the study was optional. Informed consent was given by all patients.

Plan of treatment

CyA was given in a gradually increasing dosage (maximum 5 mg/kg body weight/day) in combination with low-dose prednisone (initially max. 10 mg/kg/day with

---

Rheumatology and Rehabilitation Clinic, Triemli City Hospital, Zürich

Table 1. Previous basic therapy

Case	Stage	Previous basic therapy	NSAID	Pause of 3 months prior to beginning of therapy
1	II	Prednisone	+ + +	Yes
2	III	Gold, cyclophosphamide, holoxan, TP-5, prednisone	+ + +	Yes
3	II	Resochin, azathioprine, prednisone	+ + +	Yes
4	III	Gold, cyclophosphamide, prednisone	+ + +	No
5	II	Methotrexate, prednisone, radiotherapy	+ + +	Yes
6	III	Gold, cyclophosphamide, azathioprine, prednisone	+ + +	Yes
7	III	Endoxan, azathioprine, prednisone	+ +	Yes
8	II	Gold, prednisone	+ + +	Yes
9	III	Gold, cyclophosphamide, prednisone	+ + +	Yes
10	III	Gold, prednisone	+ +	Yes
11	II	Prednisone	+ + +	Yes
12	III	Gold, prednisone	+ +	Yes
13	III	Gold, cyclophosphamide, prednisone	+ + +	Yes
14	III	Gold, penicillamine, cyclophosphamide, azathioprine, prednisone	+ + +	Yes
15	II	Gold, resoquine	+ +	Yes

NSAID = nonsteroidal anti-inflammatory drug, + = small dose, + + = moderate dose, + + + = high dose

graduated reduction below adrenal dose), with adjustment to the individual gastrointestinal and renal side effects. A 1- to 2-week treatment-free interval was intercalated for patients with signs of nephrotoxicity (increase in serum creatinine above approx. 20%). The dose was always adjusted in accordance with clinical criteria. In the course of the first 90 days we were able to distiuguish two groups of patients with regard to ciclosporin toxicity, these being largely associated with the HLA-DR4 heterozygote status. Two schedules of therapy were developed in this observation period of 90 days, and were used from the 3rd to the 6th month.

Treatment schedule A: High-risk = HLA-DR4 (heterozygote)-positive patients: 3 weeks of therapy/7-day treatment-free interval.

Treatment schedule B: Low-risk = HLA-DR4-negative patients: 4 weeks of therapy/14-day treatment-free interval.

Dosages: CyA: max. 5 mg/kg body weight/day (one patient needed 6.2 mg/kg body weight). Maintenance dose generally defined after 3 months (min. 2–3 mg/kg body weight). Prednisone: initially max. 10 mg/day. After 3 months 2.5–5 mg/kg on average.

Special investigations

Immunoglobulins, immunoelectrophoresis, kappa/lambda coefficient, rheumatoid factors, C3, C4, $C3_B$, immune complexes, ANA, EBV, CMV at start of therapy and after 6 months. T subtypes, Ia expression at weeks 0 and 12. HLA typing (especially DR loci), hydroxylator/acetylator status at start of therapy.

Investigation of joint aspirate (if aspiration possible): T subtypes, Ia expression, interleukins.

Results

Most of the patients exhibited a substantial improvement in the course of the 6 months of therapy (Fig. 1). At the clinical evaluation after 6 months, 12 patients were virtu-

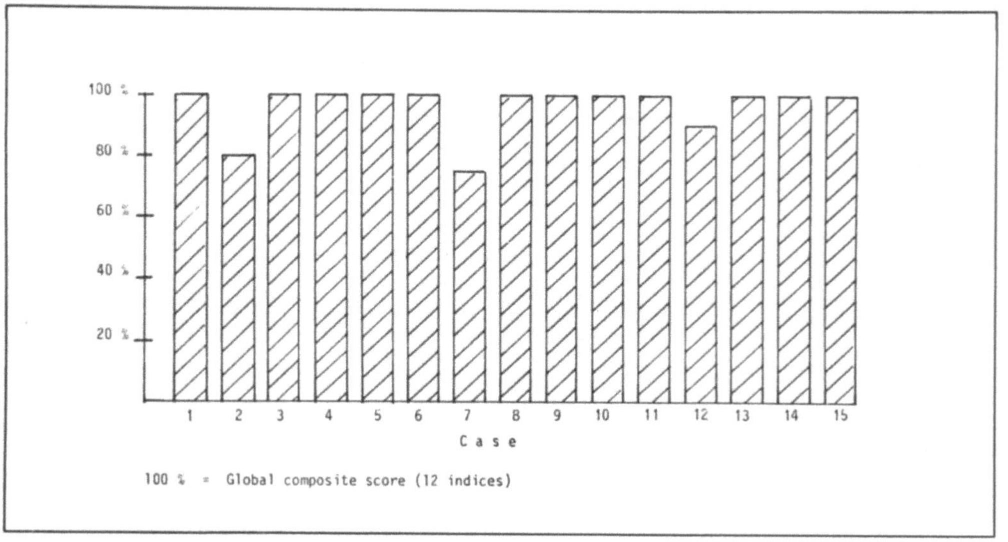

Fig. 1. Changes in clinical variables in patients completing 24 weeks of therapy (%)

ally free of symptoms. Two patients showed no satisfactory response. The treatment had to be interrupted in one patient because of hypertension. On average the onset of action occurred after 4 weeks, the maximal clinical effect being reached after 7.5 weeks. The tolerability of the combined therapy was generally good. In isolated cases we observed slight tremor (3 patients), hypertrichosis (3 patients), slight nausea at the start of therapy (3 patients) and slight diarrhoea for 3 days (1 patient). No infections, in particular EBV, CMV and lymphoma, were seen.

Side effects

We did not observe any serious nephrotoxicity during the period of the study. As already mentioned, a 1- to 2-week treatment-free interval had to be intercalated for each of 6 patients with increased creatinine. Fig. 2 shows the clinical course in a typical case, patient 9. Treatment was stopped in the 5th week because of an increase in creatinine (161 μmol/l). The value became normal during this 14-day interval. Surprisingly enough we did not observe any activation of the inflammatory process

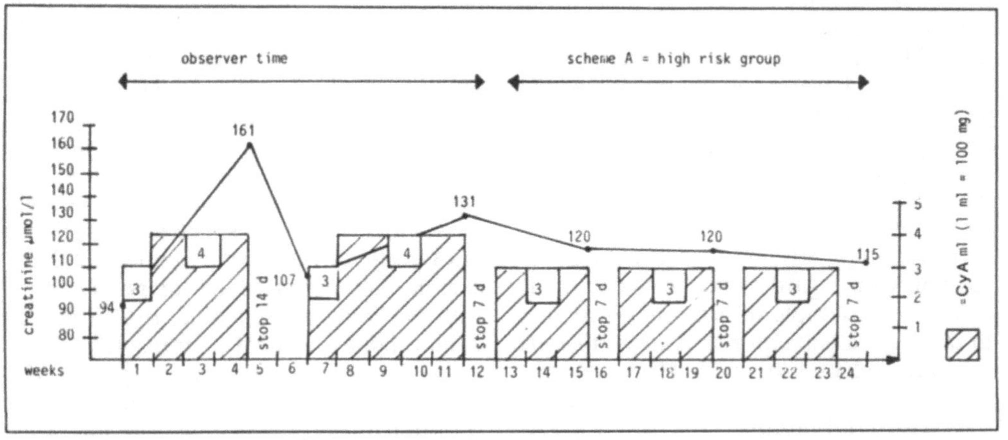

Fig. 2. Clinical course in a 'high-risk' patient

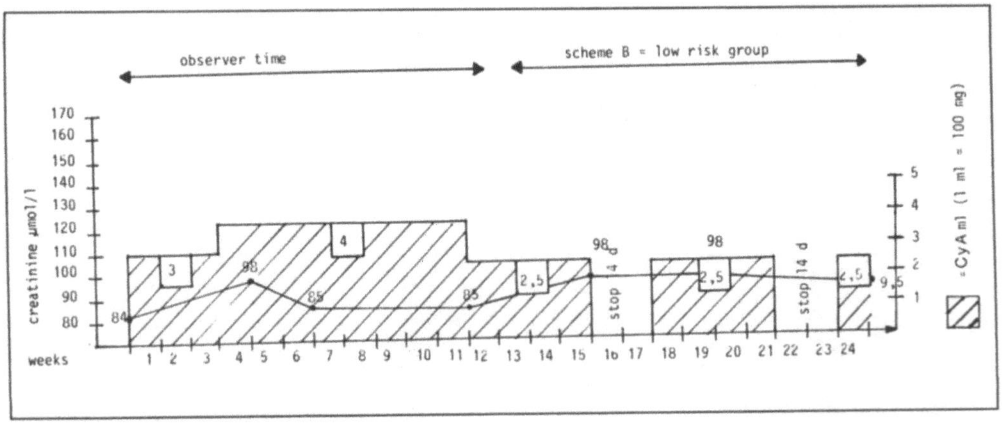

Fig. 3. Clinical course in an unproblematic 'low-risk' patient

at this time. A cautious increase in dosage was tried again: in the 7th week 300 mg/day (=3.3 mg/kg BW) in combination with low-dose prednisone. Week 8–11, 400 mg/day (=4.4 mg/kg BW). Because of a renewed increase in the creatinine value to 131 µmol/l, a second treatment-free interval of 7 days was intercalated. A schedule of 3 weeks of treatment/7 day interval was observed from the 13th week. The creatinine was subsequently reduced to 115 µmol/l and stabilised. Maintenance dose: 300 mg/day (=3.3 mg/kg BW).

In contrast to this so-called high-risk patient, the following is a description of the course of the disease in a unproblematic case. Figure 3, patient 13: initial dose 300 mg/day (=3.6 mg/kg BW). From weeks 4–12, 400 mg/day (=4.8 mg/kg BW). Maximum creatinine value in the 4th week 98 µmol/l. Schedule of therapy from 13th week: 4 weeks of treatment/14 day treatment-free interval. Maintenance dose: 250 mg/day (=3.0 mg/kg BW). There was a striking absence of nephrotoxicity despite the relatively high CyA level (754 ng/ml) in the 4th week.

In our study we observed two forms of reaction with regard to nephrotoxicity. Patient 9 is a example of extreme sensitivity. In these so-called high-risk patients there is a certain relationship with HLA-DR4. In the less sensitive group only one patient was HLA-DR4-positive. The seven HLA-DR4-negative patients were characterised by an unproblematic course during the first 90 days, particularly as regards any nephrotoxicity. These observations undoubtedly still have to be confirmed in a larger number of patients. Regular urinalysis did not reveal any pathological findings in any of the patients. Because of risk/benefit considerations we have not so far carried out renal biopsies to obtain a precise assessment of proximal tubule and glomerular damage.

Hypertension: One patient exhibited a rise in blood pressure values to 190/110 mm Hg in the 7th week. The values were normalised by means of enalapril. During the 3-week treatment-free interval, however, there was slight recurrence of the inflammatory symptoms. A cautious increase in dosage was tried again from the 10th week, with a satisfactory therapeutic result in the 15th week. Schedule of therapy from the 16th week: 3 weeks of therapy/7 day treatment-free interval. Maintenance dose: 250 mg/day (=3.9 mg/kg BW). In this patient there was also little correlation between the ciclosporin A level and side effects. Interestingly this patient was HLA-DR4-positive. The other 14 patients did not exhibit any raised blood pressure values with our low-dose schedule. In contrast to kidney/bone marrow transplantations, where hypertension is seen in up 70% [39], this side effect was very infrequent (6.6%) with our low-dose schedule. The following are currently under discussion as possible causes of the hypertension which develops under CyA: activation of the renin-angiotensin system, increase in sympathetic tone through the CNS, inhibition of prostacyclin [36].

Four other side effects of CyA – nausea, tremor, hypertrichosis, gingival hyperplasia – were recorded weekly on a semi-quantitative scale (+ = slight, + + = moderate, + + + = severe). Three patients had a + score for nausea, tremor and hypertrichosis (in one 24-year old SLE patient, outside the protocol, severe arthralgia went into complete remission after 6 weeks of treatment. There was no nephrotoxicity but therapy was discontinued on account of hypertrichosis). Gingival hyperplasia and hepatotoxicity were not seen in any of the patients.

Laboratory parameters

The Hb, leucocytes, thrombocytes, erythrocytes, SGOT, SGPT, alkaline phosphatase and potassium did not exhibit any significant changes. There was an average reduction of 14% in the ESR after 6 months.

Immunological parameters

Humoral: There was no significant change in the immunglobulins, immunoelectrophoresis, kappa/lambda coefficient, rheumatoid factors, C3/C4, C3B. There was an increase in immune complexes (3 patients) and ANA (2 patients) during treatment.

Cellular: The T-helper/suppressor quotient before therapy was 3.13 on average (normal = 1.5 to 2.5); under therapy: 2.23, i.e. a reduction of 29%. Interleukin-2 could not be demonstrated with certainty in the joint aspirate of any of the patients.

HLA typing: Seven out of 15 patients were HLA-DR4-negative, and a strikingly low CyA toxicity was seen in this group.

CyA levels: There was generally little correlation between these and nephrotoxicity, and no correlation between onset of action/immunosuppression.

Discussion

Patients with rheumatoid arthritis present signs of disturbed immune regulation. Until a recognised pathogenic mechanism can be determined specific forms of pharmacologic immunosuppression are being tried in an attempt to increase the efficacy and reduce the side effects of current therapy.

It was recently shown in hybridisation experiments that, at the mRNA transcription level, CyA selectively inhibits the synthesis of interleukin-2 and gamma-interferon, but not the interleukin-2 receptors at the cell surface [17, 40]. It is believed that with prednisone, macrophages and other interleukin-1-producing cells are blocked [1, 2]. For this reason we used a combined treatment. Our good clinical results, in particular the absence of gingival hyperplasia, may be seen as confirmation of this assumption [1]. Interleukin-1 is probably a decisive mediator in the fibrous, collagenic proliferation of gingival hyperplasia. [4, 46].

We tried to include these theoretical considerations in our plan of treatment. The good clinical results and only slight nephrotoxicity are a clear indication that in future monotherapy will generally be abandoned. Using a treatment protocol which permitted individual dosage in the first 90 days and a classification into high-/low-risk patients, we were able to define two schedules of therapy. In the more sensitive group of patients (essentially HLA DR_4 positive) we kept to a schedule of 3 weeks of therapy/7 day treatment-free interval from the 3rd month and in the less sensitive group (HLA DR_4 negative) a schedule of 4 weeks of therapy/14 day treatment-free interval. Treatment-free intervals were routinely intercalated from the 3rd to the 6th month, on the basis of the observations of the first 90 days.

In 4 patients who were treated beyond the duration of the study, we have even demonstrated a lasting clinical effect with a further reduction in the maintenance dose. From the example of a patient with concomitant diabetes mellitus, we have indications that after the saturation phase treatment-free intervals of up to 4 weeks can be intercalated with no loss of clinical effect.

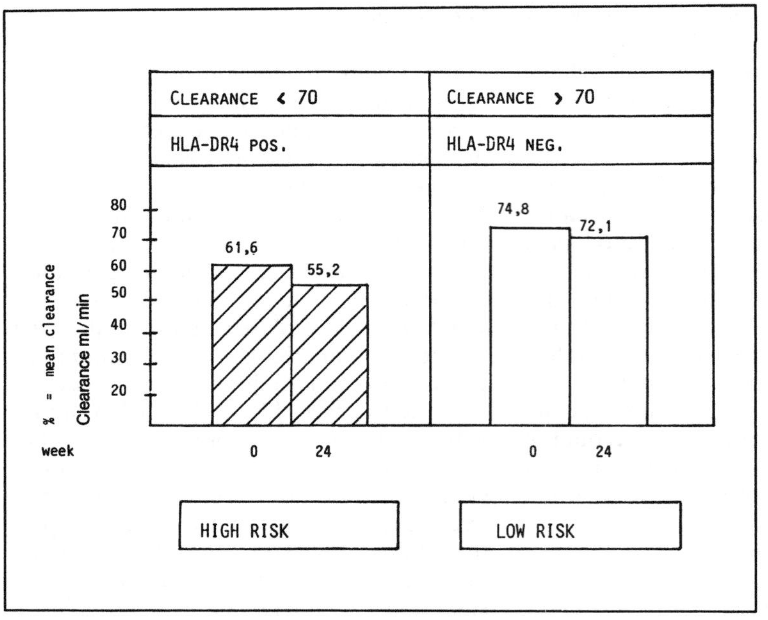

Fig. 4. High/low risk patients

The attempt to carry out more differentiated therapy with the use of the latest immunological markers and hydroxylator/acetylator status, did not proceed in accordance with our expectations [12]. High age was not a risk factor (in contrast to other studies). Only the HLA typing and creatinine clearance below 70 ml/min showed extensive correlation with the more sensitive group of patients (Fig. 4). The CyA level similarly permitted few predictions as to nephrotoxicity. We had patients in the low-risk group with excessive levels and with no signs of toxicity. The humoral investigations also resulted in surprising findings, i.e. 2 patients with a raised ANA, 3 patients with a raised IC, with otherwise unaltered findings. At the present time the question of the extent to which the humoral factors are of diagnostic and pathogenetic significance needs to be answered [29–32]. The clinical results might be additionally supported by the findings of the T-subset investigations (T4/T8-ratio, fall from 3.13 to 2.23), but in rheumatoid arthritis there is little correlation between these peripheral phenotype changes and the immunological status of the synovia [44], as we were also able to confirm. At a constant dosage, there are also considerable variations in the ciclosporin levels depending on the compartment [39]: low in CSF and muscle, moderate in the kidneys, high in the pancreas and liver. This fact will have to be taken into account in clinical investigations.

To sum up, the risk/benefit criteria were fulfilled in our 15 patients with extremely severe forms of the disease. Long-term investigations will show to what extent minimal dosage (2–3 mg/kg CyA/low-dose prednisone) will still exhibit clinical efficacy without appreciable tubular and glomerular damage.

References

1. Bendtzen K (1985) Ciclosporin in polymyositis In: Schindler R (ed) Ciclosporin in Autoimmune Diseases. 1st International Symposium, Basle, March 18–20, Springer, Berlin Heidelberg New York Tokyo p. 110
2. Carpenter CB et al. (1984) Immunosuppressive Therapy for Renal Transplantation. Springer Semin Immunopathol 7/1:43–57
3. Cohen IR et al. (1982) Immunology 128 (3):1450–1457
4. Gery I et al. (1984) Interleukin-1: Uniqueness of Its Production and Spectrum of Activities. Lymphokines 9:109–125

5. Goding JW et al. (1982) Biological Effects of Antibodies to Lymphocyte Surface Receptors. Springer Semin Immunopathol 5/4:463–477
6. Hess A et al. (1982) Effect of Cyclosporin A on human lymphocyte responses in vitro: III. CSA inhibits the production of T lymphocyte growth factors in secondary mixed lymphocyte responses, but does not inhibit the response of primed lymphocytes to TCGF. J Immunol 128:355–359
7. International Workshop on Ciclosporin in Autoimmune Diseases, ed Schindler R, Basle, March 18–20, 1985, Springer, Berlin Heidelberg New York Tokyo
8. Janeway CA et al. (1984) Quantitative variation in Ia antiregulation. Immunology Today 5/4:99–104
9. Janossy G, Panayi G, Goldstein G et al. (1981) Rheumatoid arthritis, a disease of T-lymphocyte/macrophage immunoregulation. Lancet 2:839–842
10. Kappler IW et al. (1981) B cell helper factors. I. Requirement for both Interleukin 2 and another 40,000 mol. wt. factor. J Exp Med 154:1681–1693
11. Keown PA, Stiller CR et al. (1981) Mechanism of Immunosuppression by Cyclosporin. Transplant Proc 13:386–389
12. Küpfer A, Preisig R et al. (1983/84) Pharmakogenetik in der täglichen Praxis. Arzneimittelkompendium der Schweiz, Band 2, S. 1542–1550
13. Kunkel HG et al. (1984) T cell factors regulating B cell activation and differentiation. Current Topics Microbiology and Immunology, vol 113. Springer, Berlin Heidelberg, pp 77–85
14. Melchers F (1984) Introduction. BII: Annual Report (1–12) 1983/Mechanism in B-cell neoplasia. Immunology Today 5/8:213–217
15. Melchers F (1984) Multiple Steps in the Transformation of Normal B cells Towards Neoplasia. Current Topics in Microbiology and Immunology, vol 113. Springer, Berlin Heidelberg, pp 56–61
16. Mingari MC et al. (1982) Surface Markers of Resting and Activated Human T cells. Functional Implications and Experimental Limits, Springer Semin Immunopathol 5/4:477–488
17. Mizel SB et al. (1984) Induction of Interleukin 2 Messenger RNA Inhibited by Cyclosporin A. Science 226:1439
18. Müller W, Hermann B (1979) Die Therapie der chronischen Polyarthritis mit Cyclosporin A, einem neuen Immunsuppressivum. Act Rheumatol 4:173–186
19. Myers B et al. (1984) N Engl J Med 311:699–705
20. Neckers LM et al. (1984) Transferrin Receptors Regulate Proliferation of Normal and Malignant B Cells. Current Topics in Microbiology and Immunology, vol 113. Springer, Berlin Heidelberg, pp 63–68
21. Nussenblatt RB et al. (1982) Modulation of Experimental Autoimmune Uveitis with Cyclosporin A. Arch Ophthalmol 100:1146–1149
22. Palacios R (1982) Production of lymphokines by circulating human T lymphocytes with and without receptors for interleukin-2. BII: Annual Report, p 54
23. Palacios R et al. (1982) Mechanism of T cell activation: role of functional relationship of HLA-DR antigens and interleukins. Immunol Rev 63:73
24. Palacios R, Britton S et al. (1982) Cyclosporin A – Usefulness, Risks and Mechanism of Action. Immunol Rev 65:5–23
25. Panayi GS et al. (1982) Scientific Basis of Rheumatology. Churchill Livingstone, Edinburgh, London, Melbourne, New York, pp 1–71, 114–130
26. Robb IM et al. (1984) Interleukin 2: the molecule and its function. Immunology Today 5/7:203–209
27. Roitt IM et al. (1984) Prevailing Theories in Autoimmune Disorders. Triangle 23, 3/4:67–76
28. Rolink T: BII. Personal communication
29. Schlossman SF, Personal communication
30. Schlossman SF et al. (1980) Regulation of B cell immunoglobulin secretion by functional subsets of T lymphocytes in man. Eur J Immunol 10:570
31. Schlossman SF et al. (1982) Communicative interactions between subpopulations of human T lymphocytes required for generation of suppressor effector function in a primary antibody response. J Immunol 128:1645
32. Schlossman SF et al. (1984) Human T-cell Subsets in Health and Disease. Springer Semin Immunopathol 7/1:9–18
33. Schlossman SF et al. (1984) Total lymphoid irradiation therapy in refractory rheumatoid arthritis. Arthritis Rheum 27/5: 481–488
34. Schreier M (1984) Interleukin-2 and its Role in the Immune Response. Triangle, vol 23, No 3/4:141–152
35. Shevach EM et al. (1978) The Guinea Pig I-Region. A Functional Analysis of Ia-Ir Associations. Springer Semin Immunopathol 1/2:207–234
36. Siegel H, Ryffel B et al. (1982) Effect of Cyclosporin on renin angiotensin aldosterone system. Lancet 2:1274
37. Steinberg AD et al. (1984) Autoimmunity and Increased c-myb Transcription. Science 226:1087–1089

38. Steinberg AD et al. (1984) The basis of autoimmunity in MRL/lpr mice: a role for self Ia-reactive T cells. Immunology Today 5/3:64
39. Stiller CR et al. (1984) Cyclosporine therapy in perspective. In: Morris, P.J., Tilney. N. (Eds) "Progress in Transplantation". vol 1, Churchill Livingstone, Edinburgh, London, Melbourne, New York, pp 11–45
40. Stobo J et al. (1984) The requirement for two stimuli for the coordinate production of interleukin-2 and gamma-interferon reflects evebts occurring at a pretranslational level. Arthritis Rheum 27/4:41
41. Talal N, et al. (1978) Autoimmunity and the immunogenetic network. Arthritis Rheum 21:853–861
42. Talal N et al. (1983) A clinician and a scientist look at AIDS. Immunology Today 4/7:180–183
43. Taniguchi N et al. (1983) Kinetics of Expression of T-cell "Activation" Antigens on In Vivo- and In Vitro-Stimulated T Cells. Diagnostic Immunology 1/3:104–111
44. Veys EM et al. (1982) T lymphocytes in blood and Synovial fluid in rheumatoid arthritis. Lancet i:225–226
45. Waldmann TA et al. (1984) Interleukin-2 Receptors on Activated Malignant and Normal B-cells. Current Topics in Microbiology and Immunopathology, vol 113. Springer, Berlin Heidelberg, pp 96–101
46. Wood DD et al. (1983) In "The Reticuloendothelial System", vol 6, Plenum, New York

Ciclosporin in Rheumatoid Arthritis – Preliminary Results

R. Madhok, H. A. Capell

Introduction

There is a relatively limited choice of second line ("slow acting", "disease modifying") drugs for the treatment of rheumatoid arthritis. These drugs have considerable toxicity and need to be used over a period of 3–6 months before clinical and laboratory monitoring of inflammation may be expected to improve. Most patients who discontinue therapy do so because of side effects. Agents with second line properties include gold, penicillamine and sulphasalazine, in addition to cytotoxic agents such as azathioprine, cyclophosphamide and chlorambucil. Rheumatologists are constantly searching for effective, less toxic preparations and the relatively benign effect of ciclosporin in terms of bone marrow toxicity suggested that it would be worthy of study.

Patients and methods

Twenty patients with progressive classical or definite rheumatoid arthritis were enrolled in an open study. No patient was receiving steroid therapy during the study and none had received a second line drug in the 3 months prior to study. All continued their non-steroidal anti-inflammatory drugs throughout.

Patients were started on 5 mg/kg/day and the dose was increased by 2.5 mg/kg/day every 4 weeks until 10 mg/kg/day was reached or the occurrence of toxicity meant that the dose had to be adjusted. Assessments of toxicity were done fortnightly when urea and electrolytes, liver function tests and drug levels were checked. Clinical efficacy was monitored by a clinical metrologist: pain and function were measured on a 10 cm visual analogue score, morning stiffness was recorded in minutes and the Ritchie articular index was performed. In addition the erythrocyte sedimentation rate and rheumatoid factor were checked every 6 weeks.

In view of the uncertain long-term effects of this drug the study was at this stage restricted to patients older than 45 years. No patient, however, had had the disease for longer than 7 years at the time of study.

Centre for Rheumatic Diseases, Glasgow Royal Infirmary, Glasgow, Scotland

Results

Of the 20 patients studied 8 were male and 12 were female. The median duration of the disease was 3 years, range 1–7. The dosage used and initial median and range for urea, creatinine, bilirubin, articular index, morning stiffness, pain score, functional index, ESR and rheumatoid factor are shown in the accompanying table, along with the changes over the 24 weeks. At the time of writing all patients had reached 6 weeks, 16 patients 12 weeks, 14 patients 18 weeks and 12 patients 24 weeks; clearly, further analysis will be necessary at a later stage.

Toxicity

As can be seen from the table there was a tendency for urea and creatinine to increase over the period of study, (significant; Wilcoxon) and bilirubin showed a slight rise (not significant). Dose-related changes in renal function were seen in 13 patients and a dose-related hyperbilirubinaemia in one. Hypertrichosis occurred in 2 patients, tremor in one and mild gingival hyperplasia in one; none of these events led to cessation of therapy. One patient stopped treatment at 6 weeks because of an unrelated medical problem.

Table 1. Medians and ranges for changes in laboratory and clinical values over 24 weeks

Week	0	6	12	18	24
n	20	20	16	14	12
Urea mmol/l	6.8 (3.9–103)	10.0 (3.2–129)	8.9 (2.6–15.8)	9.9 (3.9–17.7)	8.6 (4.7–14.4)
Creat µmol/l	83 (45–120)	102 (70–180)	100 (50–150)	109 (30–160)	100 (60–140)
Bilirubin	8 (5–12)	10 6–21	10 (4–22)	9 (4–15)	11 (5–23)
AI (Articular Index)	13 (4–26)	9 (1–24)	10 (0–24)	8 (0–21)	11 (0–26)
AMS (Morning Stiffness – minutes)	68 (15–1440)	29 (0–1440)	21 (5–1440)	16 (0–120)	33 (0–120)
Pain	60 (20–95)	31 (0–80)	28 (0–64)	12 (0–50)	25 (0–77)
Function	83 (10–100)	40 (2–95)	25 (0–93)	12 (0–70)	21 (1–85)
ESR mm/hr	66 (16–128)	61 (9–105)	57 (16–87)	48 (12–84)	47 (8–83)
RF	533 (64–1024)	496 (64–1024)			

Efficacy

Over the period of study the articular index tended to fall as did pain score, and the degree of functional incapacity also improved. Morning stiffness decreased and the ESR and rheumatoid factor titre tended to fall. In the majority of instances these results achieved statistical significance (Wilcoxon) but not much weight can be placed on the statistics at this time, since not all patients have completed the 24 week follow-up period.

Discussion

There seems little doubt that ciclosporin is producing a 'second line effect' in the patients studied. It is true that there is no control placebo group and that patients who have rheumatoid arthritis may show subjective improvement over a short spell. However, without an active second line drug it is most unusual for patients with this disease severity to show a sustained fall in ESR. The results are much like those which might be expected with gold or penicillamine. Nevertheless there is anxiety about long-term cumulative toxicity with ciclosporin and with its prolonged use in a non-fatal disease such as rheumatoid arthritis, this aspect will be very important. Thus, before embarking on larger controlled studies of ciclosporin in RA it would seem desirable to have available as much information as possible about the effects of the drug when used over many years.

Ciclosporin Treatment in Rheumatoid Arthritis: A Preliminary Report of a Multicentre Placebo-Controlled Double-Blind Study

A. W. A. M. van Rijthoven [1], B. A. C. Dijkmans [2], H. S. Goei The [3], Z. L. B. M. Montnor-Beckers [1], P. J. C. Jacobs [3], A. Cats [2]

The efficacy, safety, and tolerance of ciclosporin (CyA) was assessed in a multicentre placebo-controlled double-blind study in patients with rheumatoid arthritis (RA).

The patients admitted to the study were persons with active and erosive, definite or classical RA according to the ARA criteria who had previously been treated with antimalarials and gold salts or d-penicillamine. Further inclusion criteria were anatomical and functional stage II or III, while corticosteroids had to have been stopped at least 6 months before the start of the study. Patients were excluded if they showed abnormal liver and/or renal function or extra-articular manifestations of RA, or if they had undergone joint surgery within the previous 3 months.

After informed consent had been obtained the patients were assigned at random to either CyA or placebo, in accordance with a separate randomization list for each centre. The initial dosage of the test medication was 10 mg/kg in one dose per day for 2 months. If a satisfactory therapeutic response was obtained, the dosage of the test medication was reduced to 7.5 mg/kg (month 3 and 4) and to 5 mg/kg (month 5 and 6). The dosage was adjusted according to the clinical response and side effects. In addition, patients were monitored by means of CyA trough blood levels; if these exceeded 1000 ng/ml the dosage was adjusted. After 6 months the test medication was stopped. Nonsteroidal anti-inflammatory drugs were prescribed according to individual needs. The efficacy of medication was evaluated monthly by clinical and laboratory parameters (Table 3). Safety and tolerance were assessed by physical examination (body weight, blood pressure and pulse rate) and laboratory tests (serum creatinine, liver enzymes, serum potassium).

Preliminary results

A total of 36 patients (28 females and 8 males, mean age 54.9 years ± 11.2, range 24–69) were admitted to the study. The CyA group consisted of 17 patients, and the placebo group 19 patients; the demographic characteristics of the patients and the disease are shown in Table 1, indicating an equal distribution over the groups. A considerable number of dropouts occurred in both groups (Table 2). There was (severe) nausea in almost all CyA patients, four of whom had to stop the drug as a result. In the CyA group there was a significant ($p < 0.005$) rise in serum creatinine in comparison with the pre-treatment values, mean values of serum creatinine being 98.7 (S.D. 31.4) and 72.6 (18.2) µmol/l, respectively. In the placebo group the initial serum creatinine was the same as in the CyA group (mean value 71.5 ± 13.5 µmol/l); during test medication the mean serum creatinine was 72 ± 10.8 µmol/l. The test was interrupted in the placebo group in 4 patients for reasons of inefficacy (Table 2). The clinical and laboratory efficacy parameters are given in Table 3. The patients in the CyA group showed an improvement in comparison with those in the placebo group as measured by the number of swollen joints, Ritchie articular index, pain at rest, and active movement. A statistical analysis to assess the significance in these differences has not yet been performed.

Departments of Rheumatology, Deaconess Hospital Eindhoven [1], University Hospital Leiden [2], Hospital "De Wever" Heerlen [3], The Netherlands.

Table 1. Characteristics of the patients with rheumatoid arthritis

Parameter	CyA group (n=17)	Placebo group (n=19)
Sex	13F/4M	15F/4M
Age (y)	54.5 (13.2)*	55.3 (9.7)
Duration of illness (y)	11.8 (6.2)	14.5 (11.3)
Functional stage (I–IV)	12 pts.=II 5 pts.=III	10 pts.=II 9 pts.=III
Anatomical stage (I–IV)	6 pts.=II 11 pts.=III	8 pts.=II 11 pts.=III

* mean (S.D.)

Table 2. Reasons for discontinuations

	CyA group	Placebo group
Inefficacy	1	4
Nausea	4	0
Duodenal ulcer	0	1
Rise in serum creatinine	2	0
Hyperkalemia	1	0
Arthroplasty	0	1
Non-compliance	1	0
Total number of patients	8	6

Table 3. Clinical and laboratory parameters of efficacy

Parameter	CyA group		Placebo group	
	At 0 months	At 6 months	At 0 months	At 6 months
Morning stiffness (min)	68.5 (43.2)*(n=17)** 57.8 (32.2) (n=9)***	56.3 (77.6) (n=8)	68.3 (56.0) (n=18) 51.5 (42.7) (n=13)	47.3 (42.8) (n=13)
Number of swollen joints	10.5 (2.8) (n=17) 10.3 (2.5) (n= 9)	3.8 (4.8) (n=9)	9.1 (3.3) (n=19) 8.3 (3.0) (n=13)	6.1 (2.7) (n=13)
Ritchie index	22.2 (8.1) (n=17) 23.6 (8.1) (n= 9)	11.1 (5.8) (n=9)	22.9 (8.0) (n=19) 21.3 (6.9) (n=13)	18.3 (6.5) (n=13)
Pain on active movement (score range 0–3)	2.4 (0.6) (n=17) 2.4 (0.7) (n= 9)	1.6 (1.0) (n=9)	2.2 (0.7) (n=19) 2.0 (0.6) (n=13)	2.2 (0.7) (n=13)
Pain at rest (score range 0–3)	1.5 (1.2) (n=17) 1.3 (1.3) (n= 9)	0.6 (0.9) (n=9)	1.1 (0.9) (n=19) 0.9 (0.8) (n=13)	1.1 (1.0) (n=13)
ESR (mm/hr)	59.0 (40.0) (n=16) 65.0 (42.0) (n= 8)	50.0 (24.0) (n=9)	58.0 (31.0) (n=19) 44.0 (23.0) (n=13)	58.0 (25.0) (n=13)

* Mean (S.D.)
** Number of patients
*** Number of patients assessed up to 6 months

Conclusions

In the present study there were many discontinuations in both groups; the discontinuations in the CyA group were mainly due to gastrointestinal intolerance and to an elevation of serum creatinine. The main preliminary conclusion with regard to efficacy is that the CyA-treated group showed an improvement, when compared with the placebo group, in the scores for pain, joint tenderness and joint swelling.

Acknowledgement

The authors are greatly indebted to Dr. J. D. Macfarlane for correcting the English and to Gerda J. C. van den Hout for typing the manuscript.

Ciclosporin versus Azathioprine in Rheumatoid Arthritis

O. Førre, F. Bjerkhoel, H. E. Rugstad, K. J. Berg and E. Kåss

Summary

Ciclosporin (CyA) and azathioprine were compared with respect to efficacy, safety and tolerance in rheumatoid arthritis. Twelve patients were treated with ciclosporin 10 mg/kg/day and 12 patients with azathioprine 2.5–3 mg/kg/day for 26 weeks in an open, controlled and randomized study. All patients received prednisolone 5 mg/day as basic therapy. Both groups demonstrated an improvement in the majority of clinical parameters. There was a tendency towards more improvement in the ciclosporin group than in the azathioprine group. At the end of the study the patients on ciclosporin used a lower prednisolone dose than those on azathioprine. Reduction in the C-reactive protein (CRP) levels was seen in both groups, while the sedimentation rate was augmented in the ciclosporin group and reduced in the azathioprine group compared to baseline levels.

Four of the patients on azathioprine and 2 of the patients on ciclosporin had to discontinue the treatment due to side effects and one of the patients on azathioprine had to discontinue due to an unacceptable increase in disease activity.

An increase in serum creatinine and potassium as well as in systolic and diastolic blood pressure compared with baseline values was observed in the ciclosporin group but not in the azathioprine group. These parameters returned to normal after termination of treatment, except for an irreversible augmentation in serum creatinine in one patient who had signs of renal dysfunction prior to therapy.

Introduction

Immune reactions are involved in the pathogenesis of rheumatoid arthritis [13, 19]. The rheumatoid inflammation resembles a delayed hypersensitivity reaction which is mediated by various monokines and lymphokines [13]. Thus rheumatoid synovial lymphocytes spontaneously produce various lymphokines like interleukin 2 [6] that may be important both for B [11] and T cell responses [17], both of which promote inflammation in the synovial tissues. Rheumatoid synovial monocytes/ macrophages and dendritic cells produce interleukin 1 [18], which is essential for immune responses [17] and also mediates tissue destruction in rheumatic disorders [13].

Ciclosporin has been reported to suppress various immune responses by inhibiting the production of interleukin 1 [16] and interleukin 2 [4, 7]. This, together with the fact that CyA has been shown to prevent the development of adjuvant arthritis in experimental animals [2], prompted us to perform the pilot study now reported on.

Results and discussion

Twenty-four patients with classical or definite rheumatoid arthritis [15] were studied for 26 weeks. Twelve patients were treated with CyA 10 mg/kg/day and 12 patients were treated with azathioprine 2.5–3 mg/ kg/day in an open, controlled and randomized study. All the patients received prednisolone 5 mg/day as a basic therapy. The characteristics of the patients are given in Table 1.

Oslo Sanitetsforenings Rheumatism Hospital, Department for Clinical Pharmacology and Medical Department B; Renal Section, Riksshospitalet, The National Hospital, Rikshospitalet, Oslo, Norway

Table 1. Patient characteristics

Characteristics	Ciclosporin group	Azathioprine group
Number of patients	12	12
Age (years)	52.8±12.3*	55.8±10.3
Range	(34–69)	(42–73)
Sex		
F: Female; M: Male	7 F/5 M	8 F/4 M
Anatomical stage	6 (II), 6 (III)	6 (II), 6 (III)
Functional class	1 (I), 9 (II), 2 (III)	11 (II), 1 (III)
Duration of disease (years)	4.5±4.1	8.8±6.0
Range	(1–15)	(1–18)

* Standard deviation: SD

Table 2. Discontinuations during the trial

Patient group	Unacceptable increase in disease activity	Side effects	Treatment week of discont.
Ciclosporin	0	2 – Angina pectoris	5
		– Dyspepsia, fever	18
Azathioprine	1	4 – Liver toxicity	5
		– Nausea	1
		– Allergic exanthema	1.5
		– Liver toxicity, nausea	8

Table 3. Effect of ciclosporin and azathioprine treatment on various clinical parameters in patients with rheumatoid arthritis

Parameters		Before start	After 10 weeks		After 26 weeks	
Time to walk	CyA	13.1± 4.1	9.6± 3.0	(−27%)	9.5± 1.9	(−27%)
50 feet (sec)	Aza	13.1± 3.4	11.8± 3.0	(−10%)	11.2± 2.8	(−15%)
Grip strength	CyA	103 ±39	166 ±79	(+61%)	137 ±59	(+33%)
(mean both hands) (mmHg)	Aza	120 ±66	147 ±83	(+23%)	157 ±86	(+31%)
Assessment of	CyA	9.7± 2.7	8.5± 3.2	(−12%)	8.8± 1.9	(− 9%)
patient (cm VAS)	Aza	7.4± 2.2	7.6± 2.5	(+ 3%)	7.5± 2.1	(+ 1.5%)
Ritchie joint	CyA	14.6± 5.8	5.5± 5.2	(−62%)	6.2± 6.5	(−58%)
index	Aza	11.9± 7.4	7.1± 4.3	(−40%)	7.7± 4.6	(−35%)
PIP joints total (mm)	CyA	457 ±43	445 ±37	(−3%)	437 ±38	(− 4%)
	Aza	460 ±49	451 ±48	(−2%)	448 ±53	(− 3%)

CyA: Ciclosporin A; Aza: Azathioprine
In brackets: % increase/decrease.

Two of the patients on CyA and 5 of the patients on azathioprine had to discontinue the treatment due to various intolerable side effects (Table 2). For the various clinical parameters tested an improvement was seen in both patient groups (Table 3). The improvement obtained with CyA was greater than with azathioprine as regards grip strength and global assessment of patients (Table 3).

After 26 weeks of treatment the patients in the CyA group were on a mean prednisolone dose of 2.9 ± 1.1 mg/day, while the patients treated with azathioprine were on 4.7 ± 1.7 mg/day, corresponding to a reduction of 42% and 6%, respectively. The mean CyA dose after 26 weeks was 6.4 ± 1.7 mg/kg/day while the mean azathioprine dose was 156 ± 1.7 mg/kg/day.

There was a comparable decrease in both C-reactive protein (CRP) and Waaler reaction titers after 26 weeks of treatment in both groups. A reduction in platelets of 20% was seen in the CyA group while the reduction in the azathioprine group after 26 weeks was 7%. Conversely an augmentation in the sedimentation rate of 14% was seen in the CyA group while a reduction of 35% was seen in the azathioprine group after 26 weeks of treatment.

Almost all patients on CyA showed an increase in serum creatinine during the treatment (Fig. 1). This was reversible in all cases except for one patient (patient no. 11) who had a reduced creatinine clearance prior to therapy and also had the highest serum creatinine before the start of the treatment (Fig. 1). The creatinine values in the azathioprine group were unchanged throughout the study. In parallel with the increase in serum creatinine an augmentation in systolic and diastolic blood pressure from 142.3 ± 23.2 mm Hg to 160.9 ± 29.5 mm Hg and from 84.1 ± 4.9 mm Hg to 92.3 ± 14.0 mm Hg respectively was seen in the CyA group, while the blood pressure values in the azathio-

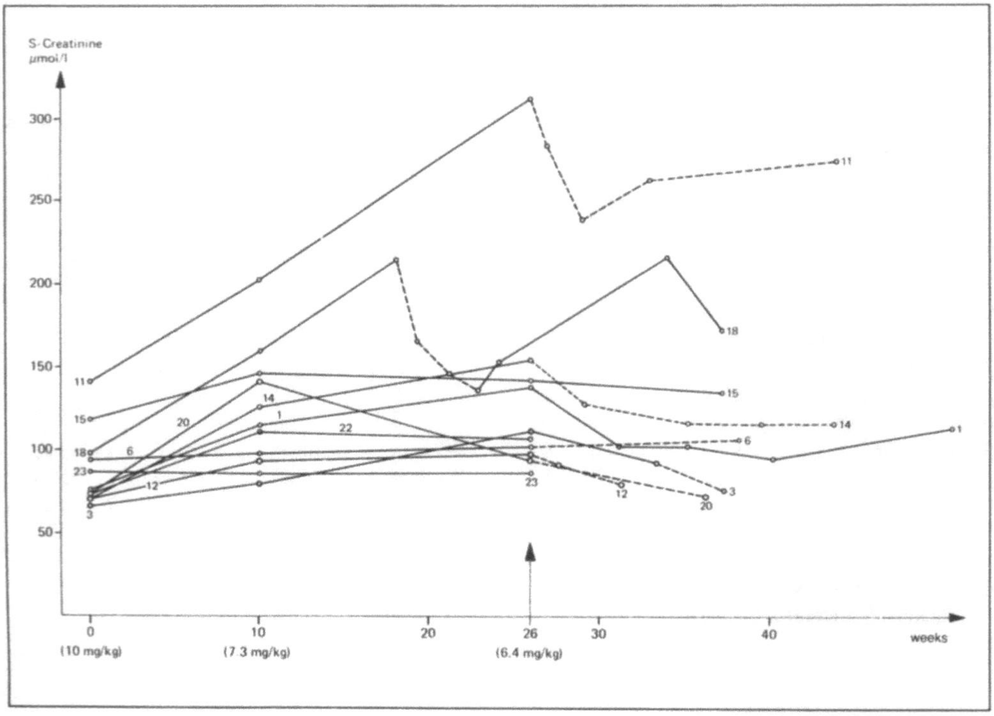

Fig. 1. This figure shows serum creatinine for each patient during the study. Broken lines represent the creatinine values after termination of treatment at 26 weeks. In brackets: mean blood concentration of ciclosporin at different periods of treatment

prine group were unchanged during the study. Serum potassium in the CyA group increased from 4.1±0.3. mmol/l prior to treatment to 4.6±0.2 mmol/l after treatment for 26 weeks. The values of serum creatinine were unchanged during the study in the patients treated with azathioprine.

The present results with a favourable effect of CyA treatment are in accordance with a previous report dealing with a small number of rheumatoid patients [8].

Renal toxicity, detected by a significant increase in serum creatinine, was the most common and serious toxic reaction seen in our patients. Renal toxicity of CyA has previously been reported in both transplanted patients [5, 12] and patients with autoimmune uveitis [14]. One of our patients developed an irreversible increase in serum creatinine, while the creatinine in all the others returned to normal values after the CyA treatment was stopped. This indicates that rheumatoid patients with signs of renal derangements should not be subjected to CyA therapy. Our rheumatoid patients on CyA also showed a rise in blood pressure and in serum potassium which is in agreement with observations in transplanted patients [1, 9]. The majority of our patients were on nonsteroidal anti-inflammatory drugs (NSAIDs), which could account for some of the nephrotoxicity, hypertension and increase in serum potassium seen by Brater et al. [3]. However, our patients treated with azathioprine also received NSAIDs without developing signs of renal toxicity or hypertension. An unfavourable interaction between NSAIDs and CyA may occur and should be looked for in future studies.

Many subjective side effects caused by CyA were noted in our patients. Most of these side effects have been described previously [10, 14]. The majority of our patients had paraesthesias and increased hot/warm sensation as well as a fine tremor most pronounced just after start of therapy. These side effects ceased in time and with dose reduction. Hypertrichosis was also observed in a majority of the patients and was a major problem for the females. This side effect might represent a considerable problem in connection with CyA therapy of autoimmune disorders as such diseases are much more frequent in women than in men.

However, most side effects and toxic phenomena seen due to CyA could be controlled by dose reduction. The mean trough blood levels were between 470 and 570 ng/ml throughout the present study. To reduce side effects and toxic reactions we therefore propose blood concentrations of CyA below 400 ng/ml in individual patients in future studies.

The results of the present pilot study are promising and have prompted us to plan a Scandinavian Multicenter Study which will start soon. In that study, which has a double-blind type of design, ciclosporin will be compared with placebo to further mark out a future place for ciclosporin treatment in rheumatoid arthritis.

References

1. Adu D, Turney J, Michael J, McMaster P (1983) Hyperkalaemia in cyclosporin-treated renal allograft recipients. Lancet II:370
2. Borel JF, Wiesinger D, Gubler HV (1978) Effects of the antilymphocytic agent cyclosporin A in chronic inflammation. Eur J Rheum Inflam 1:237
3. Brater G, Anderson S, Baird B, Campbell W (1985) Effects of ibuprofen, aproxen and sulidac on prostaglandins in men. Kidney Int 27:66
4. Britton S, Palacios R (1982) Cyclosporin A. – Usefulness, risks and mechanism of action. Immunol Rev 65:5
5. Flechner SM, van Buren CT, Kahan BD (1983) Nephrotoxicity in renal recipients. Transplant Proc 15:2689
6. Førre Ø, Egeland T, Waalen K, Mellbye OJ (1982) Interleukin 2 production by peripheral blood, synovial fluid and synovial tissue lymphocytes. Clin Rheumat 1 (abstr)
7. Granelli-Piperno A, Inoba K, Steinman RM (1984) Stimulation of lymphokine release from T lymphoblasts. Requirement for mRNA synthesis and inhibition by Cyclosporin A. J Exp Med 160:1792
8. Herrman B, Muller W (1979) Die Therapie der chronischen Polyarthritis mit Cyclosporin A, einem neuen Immunosuppressivum. Akt Rheumatol 4:173
9. Joss DV, Barrett AJ, Kendra JR (1982) Hypertension and convulsions in children receiving cyclosporin A. Lancet II:906

10. Laupacis A (1983) Complications of cyclosporine therapy – a comparison to azathioprine. Transplant Proc 15:2748
11. Mingari MC, Gerasa F, Carra G, Accolla RS, Moretta A, Zubler RH, Waldman TA, Moretta L (1984) Human Interleukin 2 promotes proliferation of activated B cells via surface receptors similar to those of activated T cells. Nature 312:641
12. Myers BD, Ross J, Neveton L, Leutcher J, Perlroth M (1984) Cyclosporine-associated chronic nephropathy. N Engl J Med 319:699
13. NIH Conference (1984) Rheumatoid Arthritis: Evolving concepts of pathogenesis and treatment. Ann Intern Med 101:810
14. Palestine AG, Nussenblatt RB, Chan CC (1984) Side effects of systemic cyclosporine in patients not undergoing transplantation. J Med 77:652
15. Ropes MW, Bennet GA, Cobb S, Jacox R, Jessar RA (1958) 1958 revision of diagnostic criteria for rheumatoid arthritis. Bull Rheum Dis 9:175
16. Skjodt M, Gallagher JA, Beresford JN, Elford P, Gowen M, Poser JW, Wood DD, Russell RGG (1984) Modulation of Interleukin-1-effects on bone by cyclosporine. Calcif Tissue Int 36 [Suppl 2]:50 (Abstr)
17. Smith KA, Lachman LB, Oppenheim JJ, Fontana MF (1980) The functional relationship of interleukins. J Exp Med 151:1551
18. Wood DD, Ihrie EJ, Dinarello CA, Cohen PL (1983) Isolation of an Interleukin-1-like factor from human joint effusions. Arthritis Rheum 26:975
19. Zvaifler NJ (1973) The Immunopathology of joint inflammation in rheumatoid arthritis. Adv Immunol 16:265

Preliminary Observations from a Comparison of Ciclosporin and Azathioprine in Rheumatoid Arthritis

H. A. Bird

Ciclosporin (CyA) may have a beneficial effect in the treatment of rheumatoid arthritis. If so, in view of its immunosuppressive action, it is likely to behave as a "second- line" or disease-remitting agent. It was therefore decided to compare ciclosporin with azathioprine in a six-month study of patients with rheumatoid arthritis of sufficient disease severity to merit the use of second-line drugs. Although the drug may act by immunological means, it was decided to include standard biochemical assessments that have been validated in the detection of second-line activity in previous studies from this Unit in addition to standard immunological assessments of the sort routinely performed in rheumatoid arthritis.

Patients and methods

All patients will have definite or classical rheumatoid arthritis (ARA criteria) with at least 3 of the following:

a) tenderness of more than 6 joints
b) swelling of more than 3 joints
c) morning stiffness longer than 45 minutes
d) Ritchie articular index greater than 20
e) ESR greater than 28 mm/hr.

Of the 40 patients, 20 will be allocated to azathioprine in a dose of 1.5 mg/kg/day rounded up or down to the nearest 50 mg increment and given in divided doses, and 20 will receive CyA. The dosage scheme for CyA is very flexible but it is envisaged that all patients will start at 5 mg/kg/day, having the option of increasing to 7.5 mg/kg/day at 4 weeks and 10 mg/kg/day at 8 weeks. There is an option to reduce dose if side-effects occur or if impending toxicity is found, judged by renal function or trough blood levels of the drug.

Patients will not be allowed other second-line agents and no patient will be receiving steroid therapy. The back-up non-steroidal anti-inflammatory therapy will be restricted to a single agent either (a) enteric-coated aspirin or (b) naproxen or (c) diclofenac. A single analgesic will also be allowed as back-up therapy, this being either (a) paracetamol or (b) dextropropoxyphene.

Clinical assessments performed at −2, 0, 2, 4, 8, 12, 16, 20 and 24 weeks will comprise: pain score (1–5 scale), change score (20 cm visual analogue scale), early morning stiffness (minutes), Ritchie articular index, grip strength (sphygmomanometer cuff), functional grade (1–5 scale), analgesic/non-steroidal anti-inflammatory drug usage. In addition x-rays will be taken at 0 and 24 weeks. Laboratory assessments of disease activity performed at each of the special clinic visits will comprise: rheumatoid factor (latex fixation and SCAT methods), IgG, IgA, IgM, C3 and C4. In addition ESR, plasma viscosity, serum histidine, total serum sulphhydryl, C-reactive protein and haptoglobin will all be recorded. Safety parameters recorded at each clinic visit include blood pressure, pulse, body weight, full blood count and platelet count, liver function tests and renal function tests comprising urine testing, electrolytes and urea and creatinine. Levels of CyA (radioimmunoassay method) will be measured before the next dose.

Dr. H. A. Bird, M.D., M.R.C.P. Senior Lecturer in Rheumatology, University of Leeds and Honorary Consultant Rheumatologist, General Infirmary at Leeds and Royal Bath Hospital, Harrogate.
Clinical Pharmacology Unit,
Royal Bath Hospital
Cornwall Road,
Harrogate,
N. Yorks., HG1 2PS.

Results

At the time of preparation of this paper (7th March 1985), 13 patients had been recruited to the study. Seven have been allocated to azathioprine and 6 to ciclosporin by the randomisation code. The maximum duration of treatment for any single patient is 4 months.

It was felt inappropriate to analyse any clincial or biochemical parameters at this early stage. Such results might produce a misleading impression at an early stage of the study and would certainly have no statistical usefulness in view of the small number of patients recruited. However, the study is being conducted using blind assessors (clinical metrologists) with a physician supervising the dosage levels in the light of side effects occurring. It was felt ethical and possibly of value to other investigators to present data on the side effects noticed to date.

In the azathioprine group, 7 out of 7 patients continue on treatment. One has reported loss of appetite and one has described dyspepsia but the remaining five have complained of no side effects.

In the CyA group, 4 out of 6 patients continue on the drug but 2 out of 6 patients have temporarily discontinued dosing. All patients commenced at 5 mg/kg/day and 3 out of 6 patients increased to 7.5 mg/kg/day at 4 weeks of treatment. The others declined an increase in dose in view of side effects. To date no patient has climbed to 10 mg/kg/day. Of the 3 patients who climbed to 7.5 mg/kg/day, one reduced immediately to 5 mg/kg/day because of vomiting, one produced raised CyA levels (greater than 200 μg/ml; plasma) after increasing the dose, so has temporarily discontinued, and one continues with no side effects. One patient receiving 5 mg/kg/day developed a raised creatinine (greater than 130 μg/l) after seven weeks of therapy and according to the protocol temporarily discontinued treatment. Side effects noticed in the others include loss of appetite (1 patient), burning of the hands (1 patient), flushing of the extremities (1 patient) and tingling of the hands (1 patient). Only one of the six patients on CyA has been free of side effects.

Recruitment to the study continues and it is hoped that results will be available for statistical analysis in about one year's time.

10. Glomerulonephritis and Systemic Lupus Erythematosus

Ciclosporin in Glomerulonephritis – A Pilot Study

D. C. Cattran, J. Dossetor, P. F. Halloran, C. Cardella, C. Stiller, P. Keown, W. F. Clark

Introduction and objectives

The nephrotoxic potential of ciclosporin (CyA) was first established in the area of renal transplantation [1, 3] but has since been recognized as a risk in non renal related organ transplants such as liver and heart [2, 4]. Our study was designed to determine if there was any unexpected nephrotoxicity of this agent in patients with glomerulonephritis by observing the drug's effect on the prime markers of glomerular function, namely the glomerular filtration rate determined by monitoring the creatinine clearance and abnormal permeability determined by assessing quantitative proteinuria. Careful documentation of other side effects was also determined. A tertiary objective was to assess the information and attempt to determine the direction of future controlled studies using CyA in the treatment of glomerular diseases.

Material and method

All patients had biopsy proven glomerulonephritis. Total patients studied were 28 and included IgA-IgG nephropathy (2), membranous glomerulonephritis (MGN) (7), diffuse proliferative glomerulonephritis (DP) (3), focal segmental glomerulosclerosis (FSGS) (10), and membranoproliferative glomerulonephritis (MPGN) (4). Two patients had systemic lupus erythematosis (SLE) but with no systemic dysfunction except rapidly deteriorating renal function unresponsive to conventional steroid therapy.

At study entry the patient's plasma creatinine must have been between 150 and 500 μmol/l and all patients had to have a documented decline in creatinine clearance ≧10% in the 12 months preceding trial entry. Patients with MGN or FSGS must have had proteinuria in excess of 3 gm/day as well as the above criteria. There was to be no evidence of any systemic disease with the exception of the patients with documented SLE. The project was approved by the university ethics committees and informed consent was obtained from all patients prior to trial entry.

Exclusion criteria included age less than 16 years, immunosuppressive agents, corticosteroid therapy or plasmapheresis within 4 months of trial entry (with the exception of the 2 lupus nephritis patients), pregnancy and treatment with any nonsteroidal, anti-inflammatory agent within 2 months of initiating the study.

All patients were to receive CyA therapy for 4 months unless one of the following stop points was reached.

1) Decrease in creatinine clearance ≧50% of the initial entry value.
2) Persistent increase in liver enzyme values despite a reduction in CyA dose
3) Life-threatening infection.
4) The development of any neoplasia.

CyA was given on a twice-a-day schedule. Started at 4 to 6 mg/kg with 12-hour trough plasma levels to be maintained between 50–200 ng/ml. Twenty-eight patients were entered into the study. Twenty-five of these patients fulfilled all the entrance criteria. Three children, 2 with FSGS and 1 with MPGN, were entered after obtaining special permission because all other medication had failed to influence their severe proteinuria. These patients are included in the

University of Toronto, University of Western Ontario, University of Alberta, Edmonton, Alberta
Toronto General Hospital, CW 3-217, 101 College Street, Toronto, Ontario, M5G 1L7
Study Support: Kidney Foundation of Canada (Ontaria Branch)

proteinuric response numbers but because of their normal initial creatinine clearances are not included in the results relating to changes in clearance. The sex distribution was 20 males and 8 females. Age range excluding the 3 children was from 16 to 66 with a mean age of 32 years.

Results

Figure 1 shows the slope of the creatinine clearance in the 25 patients in the 2 years preceding the introduction of the ciclosporin therapy. All patients have been zeroed at the start time in order to study the mean changes in slopes utilizing multiple linear regression analysis. The actual initial trial entry creatinine clearance varied from 0.3 to 1.3 mls/sec. There was an overall reduction in corrected clearance in the group of 0.75 mls/sec in the 2 years prior to trial entry, i.e. the mean monthly decline was 0.03 mls/sec.

Figure 2 illustrates the change in the corrected creatinine clearance during the 4 months of drug therapy. In 1 case therapy was repeated for a second 4-month period and this is the reason for the single points beyond the 4-month time frame. The over-

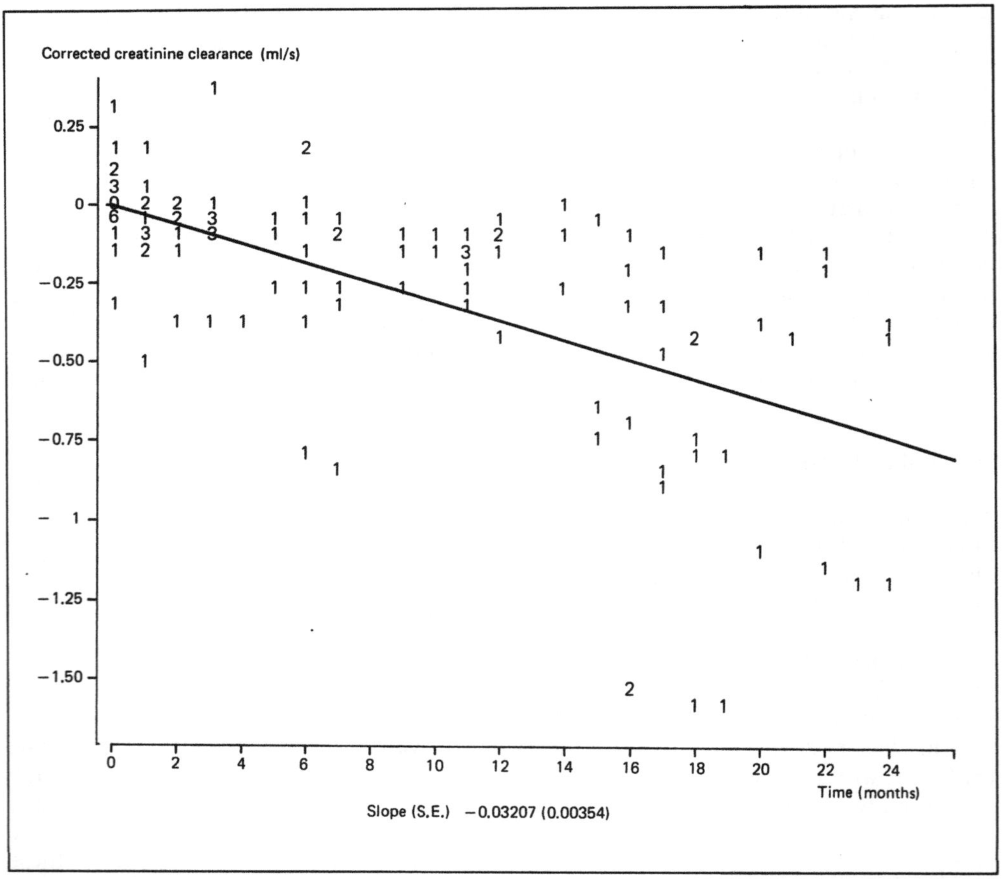

Fig. 1. This represents the change in renal function as measured by variations in the corrected creatinine clearances in the 25 patients in the 2 years prior to trial entry. The regression line indicated is the mean regression of all the individual patients. All patients had their initial clearance zeroed for the sake of clarity of presentation. The numbers on the graft represent the number of patients with similar clearances at that point in time. The letters occur starting at 10 points (i.e. A = 10, B = 11, C = 12, etc.). The mean slope of the creatinine clearance is negative (−0.03 ml/sec/month)

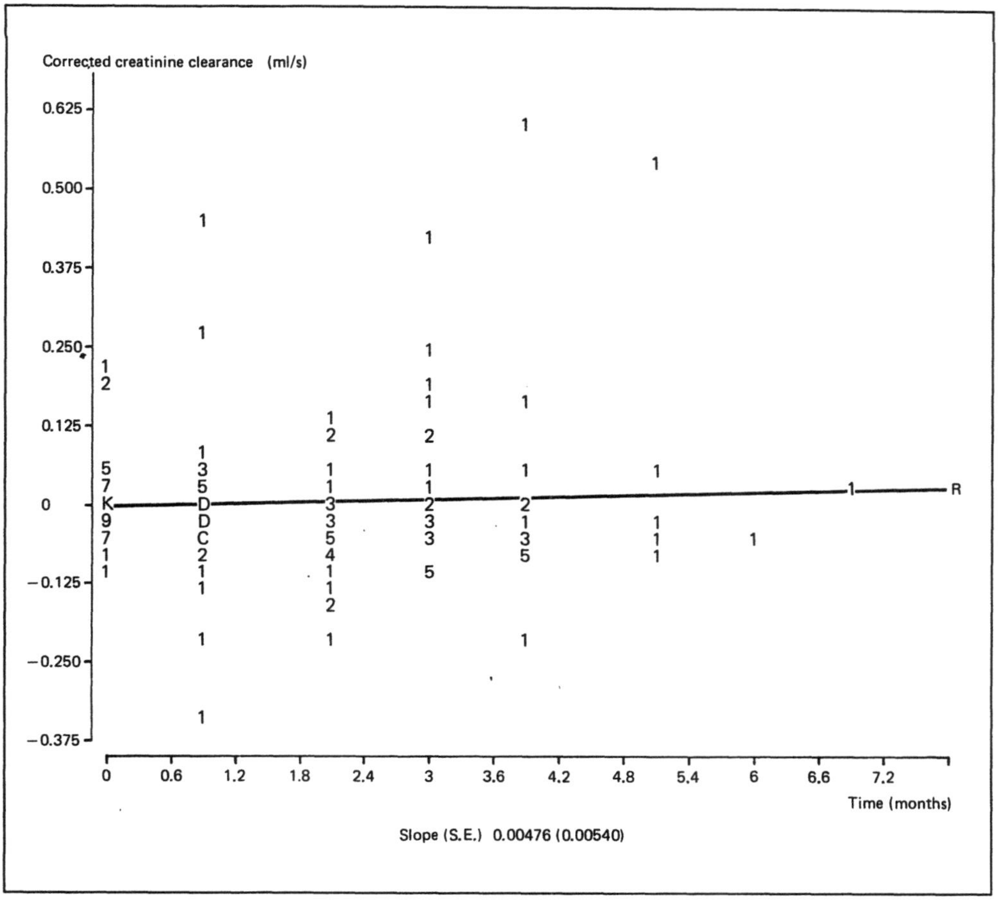

Fig. 2. This figure represents the change in function during the drug period. The overall regression line is positive with the change in creatinine clearance equal to 0.004 ml/sec/month). The number of points at each time is represented in the same fashion as in Fig. 1

all slope during this alteration of the period was positive, 0.005, i.e. a mean increase in creatinine clearance of 0.04 mls/sec over the 8 months of observation.

Figure 3 illustrates the change in slope in the 10 months of follow-up although only 4 of the 25 patients have been followed longer than 6 months. The regression line becomes negative again with a slope of 0.007. This translates to a decline in clearance of 0.07 ml/sec over the 10 months observation post treatment.

The changes in proteinuria are more difficult to assess. Some of the patients did not complete the urine protein assessments and others have not finished the post drug study period. However none of the patients had an increase in proteinuria during the drug period. Seven patients had declined in proteinuria and reached 50% of their initial value, although none reached the normal range. Seven others had reductions of 25 to 50% of their initial values and the rest showed no change in the severity of their proteinuria. One MGN patient was particularly instructive in that the introduction of a second course of CyA, after a marked relapse in proteinuria following the initial stoppage of the drug, produced another dramatic reduction from 14 gm/day to 1 gm/day. There appears to be some rebound effect post treatment in some of these patients but this observation period is still short.

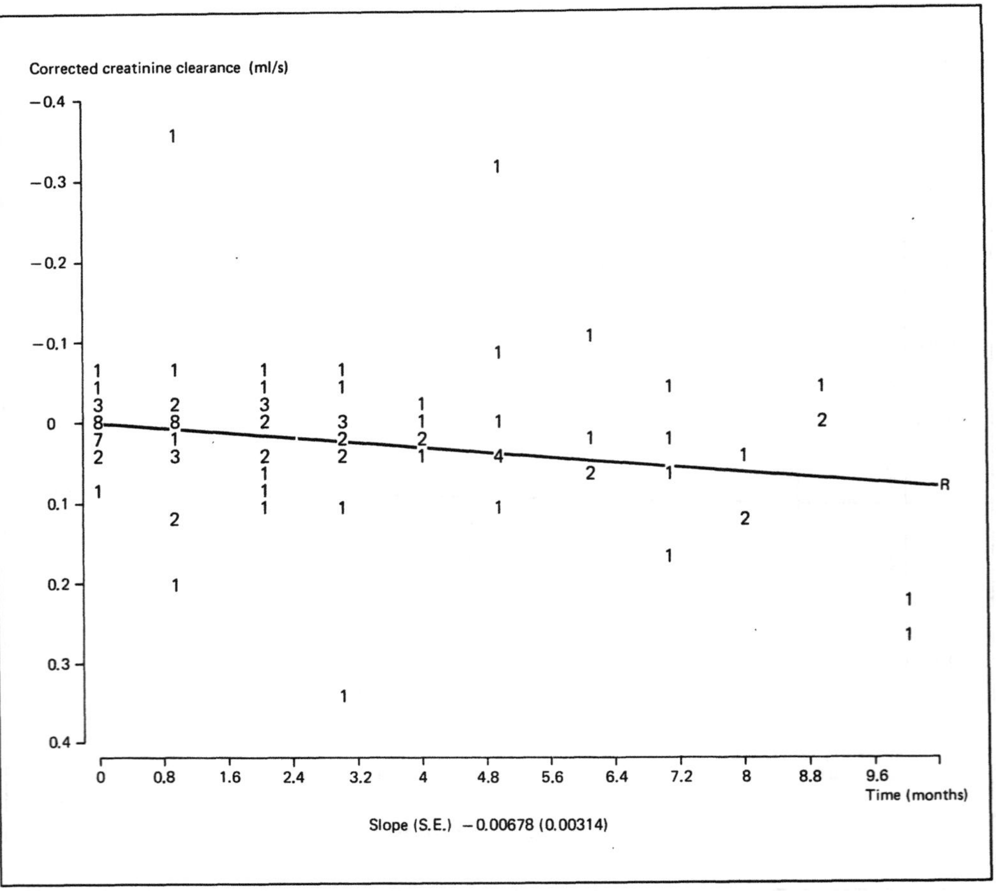

Fig. 3. The regression line in this figure represents the mean change in creatinine clearance in the 10 months post drug period and has again become negative (−0.007 ml/sec/month). The number of points at each time is represented in the same fashion as Fig. 1

Side effects were numerous but minor. Six patients had significant nausea and 1 patient had to have the drug completely withdrawn. This particular patient also developed the clinical syndrome of gout while on the drug. Three patients developed mild gum hypertrophy which was not apparent to the patient but was to the clinician. Two patients had a substantial increase in headaches and 2 developed a noticeable tremor on the medication. All these effects resolved with drug dose reduction. Four patients noticed mild hirsutism. Two patients had an increase in blood pressure as documented by an increased requirement of blood pressure medication despite either no change or an improvement in plasma creatinine values. Four intercurrent infections were documented. All were mild. Two were viral in nature, two bacterial, including one skin infection, and one pneumonia. This latter patient had significant uremia prior to trial entry. One patient developed acute pulmonary edema within two weeks of initiating therapy. This was in the absence of known cardiovascular disease and in the absence of a significant change in clearance. The patient responded to diuretic therapy and the edema did not recur following the reintroduction of the drug.

Conclusions

No patients had a significant decline in creatinine clearance following the introduction of the ciclosporin therapy. In 5 cases there was a minor increase in plasma creatinine values in the first 2 to 4 weeks following initiation of therapy but this plateaued or subsequently improved in the following 3 months of observation. We can conclude that CyA can be used without any unexpected nephrotoxicity for short periods of time in patients with glomerulonephritis.

Other side effects of the drug in these patients were similar in severity and percentage to other studies utilizing this medication. The one possible exception was the severity and frequency of the gastrointestinal side effects. This may relate to a combination of uremia and the preservation of the taste sensation not commonly preserved in the renal transplant patient where preceding dialysis therapy seems to alter taste perception.

These preliminary observations also suggest that there may be a role for CyA in a variety of types of glomerulonephritis. This is substantiated by the apparent stabilization of the glomerular filtration rate in these patients with previous well documented declining creatinine clearances and supported in several patients by remarkable reductions in proteinuria not associated with declines in glomerular filtration rate. These studies should form the foundation for the construction of prospective properly controlled drug trials in patients with glomerulonephritis.

References

1. Hamilton DV, Evan DB, Henderson RG, et al. (1981) "Nephrotoxicity" and metabolic acidosis in transplant patients on cyclosporine A. Proc Eur Dial Transplant Assoc 18:400–409
2. Klintmalm GBG, Iwatsuki S, Starzl TE (1981) Nephrotoxicity of cyclosporine A in liver and kidney transplant patients. Lancet I:470–471
3. Merior RM, White DFG, Thiru S, et al. (1984) Cyclosporine: Five years experience in cadaveric renal transplants. N Engl J Med 310:148–154
4. Myers BD, Ross J, Newton L, et al. (1984) Cyclosporine-associated chronic nephropathy. N Engl J Med 311:699–705

Use of Ciclosporin in Idiopathic Corticoresistant or Corticodependent Nephrotic Syndrome (Minimal Change Glomerulopathy and Focal-Segmental Hyalinosis)

A. Meyrier MD [1], P. Simon MD [2], G. Perret MD, P. D., M. Sc. [3] and M.-C. Condamin-Meyrier MD

Conduct of the study

This was an open study. The patients were selected among adult (> 15 years of age) nephrotics with a corticoresistant or corticodependent nephrotic syndrome (NS) or short-term relapsing disease with more than 3 relapses in the preceding year or with unacceptable risks from conventional therapy by biopsy. In all cases any systemic cause of NS was ruled out. The diagnosis of MCLN (minimal change glomerulopathy or "lipid nephrosis") or FSH (focal-segmental hyalinosis) rested on at least one renal biopsy, comprising a minimum of 10 glomeruli and studied by light microscopy and IF (immunofluorescence). The histological diagnosis (Table 1) was in accordance with established criteria [6]. Any systemic cause of NS was excluded. Corticoresistance and corticodependence are defined in Table 1. Any ongoing treatment of the NS was interrupted: cytotoxic agents 4 months and corticosteroids 10 days before the beginning of the trial. During the first 2 weeks, the patient started to take a placebo. Proteinuria was determined twice a week. The patient was then hospitalized for 18 days. On the first 3 days he was kept on placebo, and proteinuria was measured each day. After having checked that NS was still present (i.e. excluding spontaneous remission) ciclosporin (CyA) was given at an initial dosage of 5 mg/kg/24 h. Whole blood CyA levels were measured thrice weekly before the morning dose and drug dosage was adjusted to obtain whole blood trough levels between 100 and 400 ng/ml. After 6 weeks, blood levels were monitored once a week. In 2 patients urinary CyA was assayed while they were still proteinuric, and we have verified that unmetabolised CyA was undetectable in urine by our method. After discharge from hospital the patients were examined twice a week and blood and 24-h urine samples were collected for the following determinations: creatinine clearance, 24-h protein and sodium excretion, serum protein electrophoresis, liver tests, fibrin degradation products in blood and urine, complete blood count. No other "specific" medication was allowed during the first three months of the study, such as corticosteroids, cytotoxic agents or nonsteroidal anti-inflammatory drugs. Informed consent was obtained in each case.

Case reports

Case 1. This Black african female (H.D.) was 21 years old when she became nephrotic in the 6th month of her 2nd pregnancy, in July, 1980. Blood pressure was normal. She gave birth to a normal baby at 9 months. The NS persisted. Surgical renal biopsy yielded 200 glomeruli. Light microscopy and IF revealed no lesion. Treatment was initiated with 2 mg/kg/24 h of prednisone. Complete remission was obtained within 3 months. Treatment was tapered to a stop after 7 months. The NS recurred 4 months later. She again went into remission within 1 month with 2 mg/kg/24 h of prednisone. The NS recurred when the dosage was 10 mg/24 h and remitted within 2 weeks when it was increased to 1 mg/kg/24 h. A 2nd renal biopsy ruled out FSH. Steroid dosage was tapered to 10 mg/24 h. The NS recurred and persisted despite treatment with 2 mg/kg/24 h of

---

1 Nephrology and Hemodialysis Unit, Hôpital Avicenne, 125 route de Stalingrad, 93000 Bobigny
2 Nephrology and Hemodialysis Units, Hôpital La Beauchée, 22000 Saint-Brieuc
3 Hôpital Avicenne, 125 route de Stalingrad, 93000 Bobigny

Table 1. Definitions and abbreviations

1. *Nephrotic syndrome (NS):* a condition in which 24-hour urinary protein excretion is superior or equal to 3 grams and serum albumin concentration is less than 31 grams/liter.
2. *Recurrence:* a period of at least 3 days during which proteinuria is superior to 0.50 gram/24 hours.
3. *Complete remission:* a period equal to at least 2 weeks during which proteinuria is nil, with a regression of hypoalbuminemia (and of edema in a patient not treated with diuretics).
4. *Partial remission:* a period during which proteinuria has not totally disappeared, but is low enough to allow a rise of serum albumin and normalization of sodium balance with spontaneous loss of edema.
5. *Corticoresistant:* no remission after 6 weeks of corticosteroid therapy at a dosage of 1 mg of prednisone/kg/24 h.
6. *Corticodependent:* relapses occurring within 2 weeks, each time the dosage is reduced to 15 mg prednisone/24 h or less.
7. *Lipoid nephrosis (LN):* NS in which a renal biopsy comprising a minimum of 8 glomeruli is considered as normal or as "minimal change" on light microscopy and in which immunofluorescence (IF) is negative.
8. *Minimal change (MCLN):* a mild mesangial proliferation shown by light microscopy, without capillary wall changes, no capsular adhesion, and negative IF.
9. *Focal-segmental hyalinosis (FSH):* a glomerular lesion with varying degrees of severity. The minimum consists of capsular adhesion(s); the typical lesion is one of sclerosis occurring predominantly at the periphery of the tuft, caused by a combination of vascular collapse and of excess matrix. The "hyalin" material is homogeneous, PAS positive and silver negative. It is often associated with mesangial hypercellularity. A typical feature is the frequent positive fluorescence of the sclerotic lesion with anti-IgM and anti-C3 antisera. Such a lesion found in 1 glomerulus is considered as diagnostic, even if the sample comprises less than 8 glomeruli.

prednisone. She was started on cyclophosphamide plus prednisone and went into remission within 2½ months. This remission lasted 10 months. The NS recurred in March, 1984. Remission was obtained with four boli of methylprednisolone. She was maintained on 2 mg/kg/24 h prednisone. She was still being treated with 25 mg/24 h in Dec., 1984 when the NS recurred and persisted.

CyA treatment was begun on Jan., 4, 1985. On Jan., 12, she was admitted for severe sepsis and diarrhea. Blood cultures yielded pneumococci. CyA treatment was interrupted. She made a rapid recovery with antibiotics. After a 14-day lag, CyA was reintroduced. On day 15 of this second course she is still proteinuric (6 g/24 h) but has no edema and excretes sodium normally.

Case 2. This 59-year-old female (R.M., Figs. 1a and b) became nephrotic in June, 1982. Renal biopsy showed normal glomeruli by light microscopy and IF. Proteinuria disappeared after 29 days of prednisone (1 mg/kg/24 h). The NS recurred 3 days after steroids were stopped, at 8½ months. Remission was slowly obtained with ½ mg/kg/24 h, but the NS recurred twice when the dosage was reduced and she finally developed steroid resistant NS in Dec., 1984 and showed cushingoid features. CyA treatment began on Jan., 4, 1985. Progressive natriuresis was noted from day 20. Proteinuria started to decline from day 24 onwards, persisted between 1 and 2 g/24 h and subsided on day 45. She has been in complete remission since.

Case 3. This 27-year-old female (P.R., Figs. 2a and b) became nephrotic in Aug., 1981. Renal biopsy showed MCLN. She was totally corticoresistant from the beginning. After she had completed an unsuccessful 8 month course of treatment with prednisone (1 mg/kg/24 h) she had a spontaneous 2-month remission, then a recurrence, and was therafter corticoresistant. A 2nd renal biopsy disclosed severe FSH and tubulo-interstitial lesions. Systematic oral anticoagulation treatment was begun.

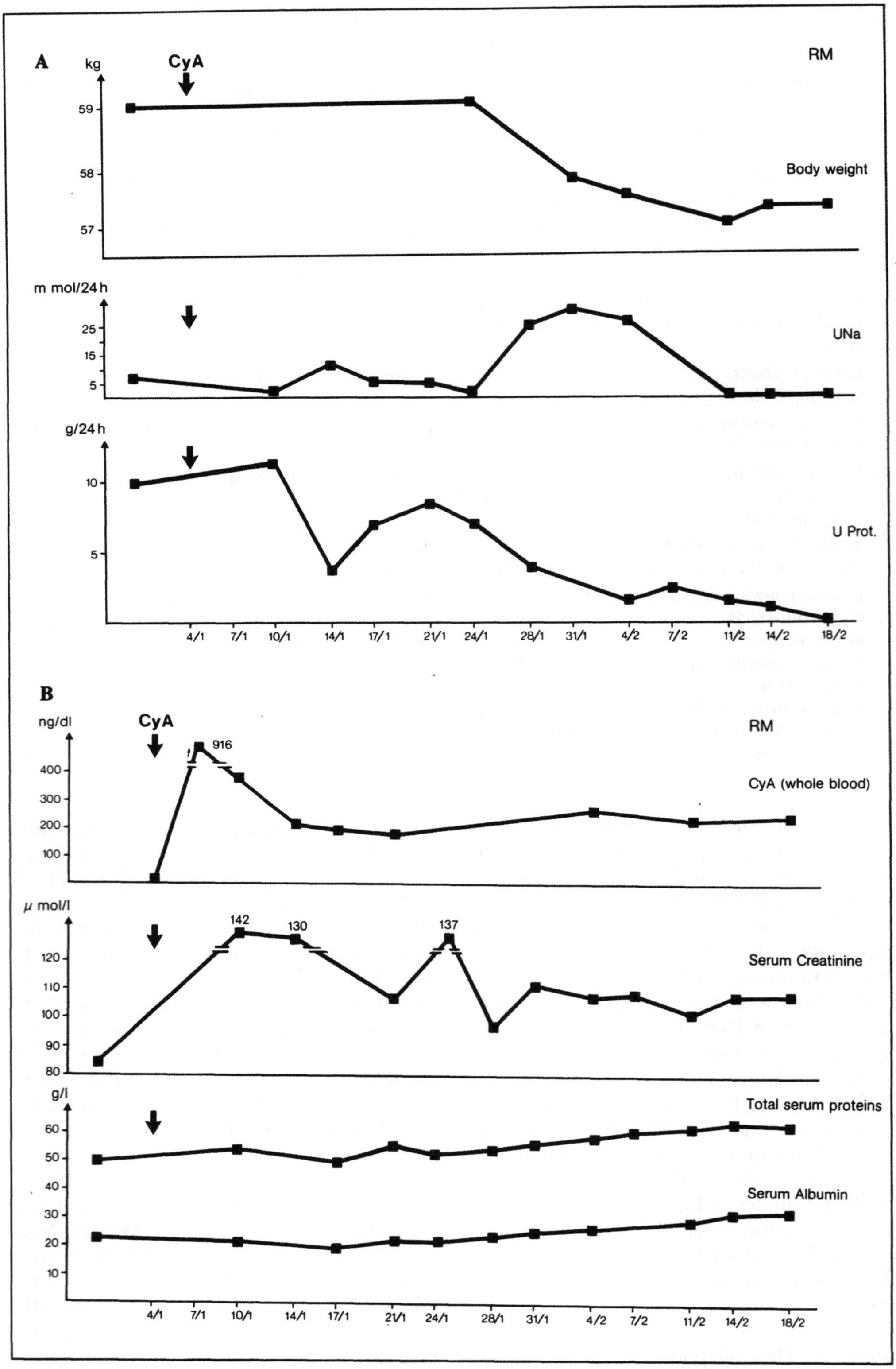

Fig. 1. Case 2 – Evolution of corticoresistant nephrotic syndrome in a patient with MCLN. 1 A: Remission appeared on day 20 and was complete on day 40. After disappearance of edema the patient continued to follow a sodium-free diet and low urinary Na excretion reflects normal renal response to dietary restriction. 1 B: Initial 5 mg/kg CyA dosage had to be rapidly reduced to 3.75 mg/kg, and this low dose was sufficient to maintain therapeutic blood levels. Renal tolerance was good, but serum creatinine closely paralleled CyA blood levels, and it was felt that care should be taken to keep 12 h post-dose trough levels below 300 ng/ml

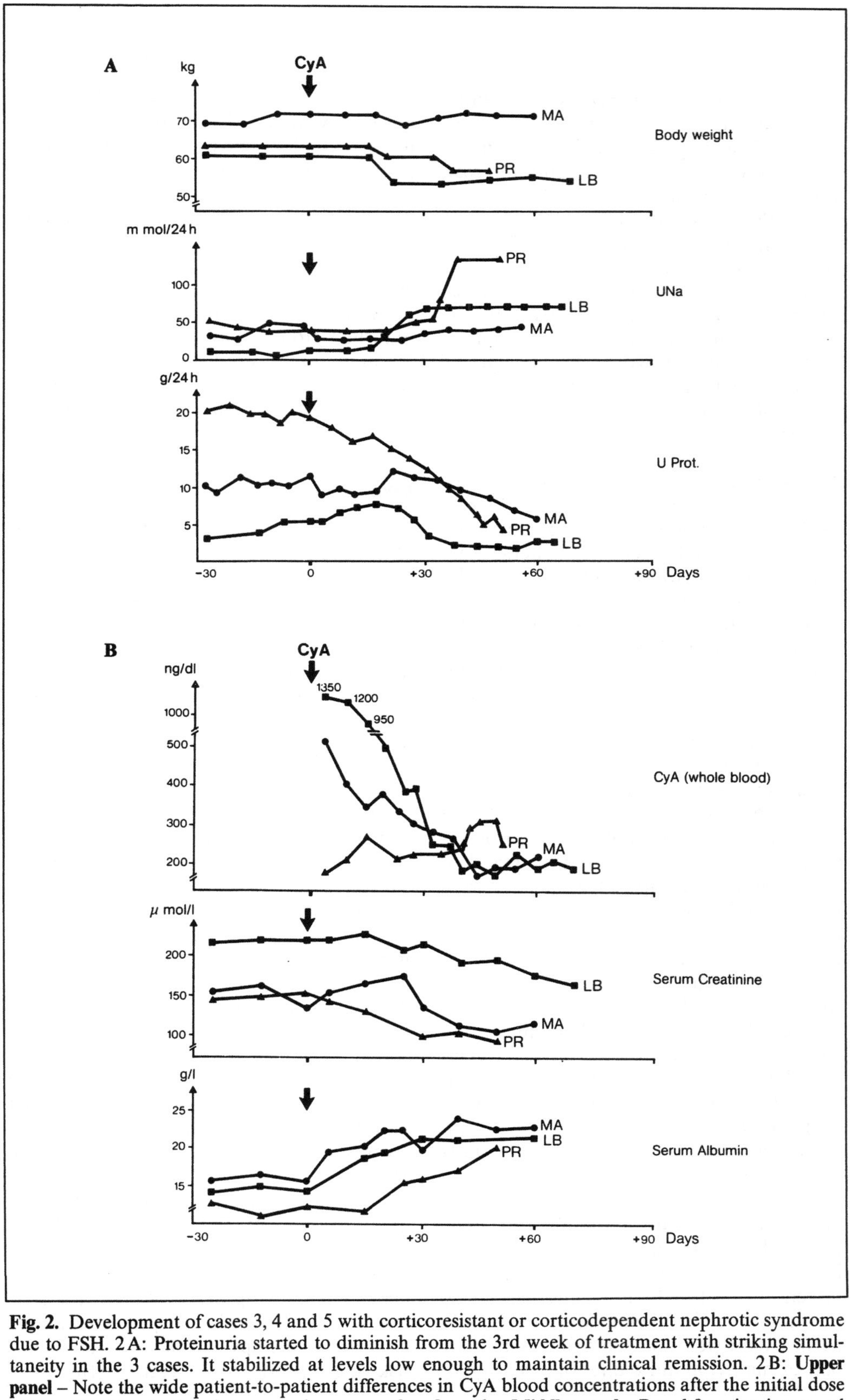

Fig. 2. Development of cases 3, 4 and 5 with corticoresistant or corticodependent nephrotic syndrome due to FSH. 2 A: Proteinuria started to diminish from the 3rd week of treatment with striking simultaneity in the 3 cases. It stabilized at levels low enough to maintain clinical remission. 2 B: **Upper panel** – Note the wide patient-to-patient differences in CyA blood concentrations after the initial dose of 5 mg/kg. The final maintenance dosage was 3 to 5 mg/kg. **Middle panel** – Renal function improved as serum albumin rose, presumably due to amelioration of functional renal insufficiency

On Dec., 18, 1984, CyA treatment was initiated. From day 25 natriuresis was noted and she lost 4 kg. 24 h urine protein regressed from 24 to 4 g. Serum albumin rose from 1.7 to 2 g/dl. This partial remission was stable on day 50 when she complained of angina pectoris and died suddenly of cardio-respiratory arrest. This patient was a heavy smoker and several members of her family had had coronary disease. The diagnosis retained was that of myocardial infarction, possibly provoked by the state of hypercoagulability of the NS and by the rapid volume contraction induced by the remission.

Case 4. This 56-year-old male (L.B.. Figs. 2a and b) became nephrotic in March, 1979. Serum creatinine was 555 μmol per liter and he had microscopic hematuria. Renal biopsy disclosed severe FSH. The discovery of an active duodenal ulcer precluded corticosteroid therapy and he was treated with cyclophosphamide alone for 4 months. He remained nephrotic but renal function improved (serum creatinine 150 μmol per liter). After healing of the ulcer he was started on prednisolone and went into remission in 55 days. Corticosteroids were tapered to a stop at 10 months and the NS recurred 3 months later. A 2nd course of cyclophosphamide had to be interrupted because of severe skin reaction. Chlorambucil and plasma exchanges were unsuccessful. A course of prednisolone induced remission, but the patient was corticodependent. Serum creatinine rose to 250 μmol per liter A 2nd renal biopsy again showed severe FSH. CyA treatment began on Dec., 8, 1984. 25 days later increasing natriuresis was noted with a 6 kg weight loss. Urine protein fell and stabilized at 3 g/24 h. Serum albumin rose from 1.6 to 3.4 g/dl. Renal function improved (serum creatinine 125 μmol per liter). Follow-up is now 95 days.

Case 5. This 20-year-old male (M.A., Figs. 2a and b) became nephrotic in Jan., 1979. He had microscopic hematuria and hypertension (150/100 mm Hg). Renal biopsy cast doubt on the likelihood of FSH. Only partial remission was obtained with four boli of methylprednisolone followed by an 18-month course of prednisone. A 2nd renal biopsy disclosed typical FSH and tubulointerstitial lesions. One month after cessation of corticosteroid therapy the NS recurred and was thereafter corticodependent and finally corticoresistant, with no effect from cyclophosphamide. CyA treatment began on Jan., 9, 1985. An increase of natriuresis was noted from day 21 onwards. Edema regressed, proteinuria diminished from 12 to 4 g/24 h and serum albumin rose from 1.5 to 2.5 g/dl. Renal function improved (serum creatinine 95 μmol per liter). This partial remission is stable at day 65.

Comments

In the spectrum of the nephrotic syndrome (NS), two clinico-pathologic entities represent an indication for corticosteriod therapy: minimal change glomerulopathy (MCLN or "lipoid nephrosis") and focal-segmental hyalinosis (FSH) [1, 6, 15, 16]. The nosology of these conditions is still a matter of debate, and there is no definite argument in the present state of our knowledge to decide whether they are two aspects of the same underlying disorder, or if they represent separate entities.

That an immunological derangement is responsible for the increased glomerular permeability of these two forms of NS was suggested 30 years ago by the favorable effect of corticosteroids on proteinuria. This was substantiated when it was shown that immunosuppressive therapy can be successful in cases resistant to steroids [3]. Among many immunological studies devoted to the pathophysiology of these two conditions there are arguments to support a T_h/T_s imbalance [4, 13, 14, 16], and some data suggest that the T lymphocytes of such patients secrete a lymphokine which increases vascular permeability [4, 8, 12, 15, 16].

Corticosteroids remain the keystone of treatment. Nevertheless, many patients are multi-relapsers, some are totally corticoresistant, and the rest are corticodependent [10]. In such a case, the control of the NS requires permanent corticosteroid therapy, with the attendant risk of long-term complications. Immunosuppressive therapy entails risks of opportunistic infections, of later development of malignancy and of sterility in the male. In the case of total corticoresistance, the chronic development of persistent NS is a debilitating condition, dangerous infections can supervene and the progression of the disease can lead to terminal renal insufficiency [1]. These possibilities undoubtedly justify a therapeutic trial of any new immunosuppressive agent, even if its side effects include some degree of nephrotoxicity. The mode of action of CyA is compatible with an expected favorable effect on the immunological derangement(s) which lead to nephrosis ([2, 7, 11], see also part 1 of this symposium).

At present there is no published experience of this drug in idiopathic NS. We therefore undertook a feasibility study of CyA treatment of selected cases of MCLN and FSH in which failure or unacceptable risks of corticosteroids and/or of immunosuppressive therapy represented a therapeutic dead-end.

Of 5 patients with corticoresistant or corticodependent NS, one with MCLN was in complete remission after 46 days of CyA treatment, 3 with FSH were in partial remission (still proteinuric but no longer nephrotic) after 25 to 32 days of the same regimen, and one met a temporary stop point when pneumococcal septicemia supervened at a time when the NS still persisted. A 5th patient with FSH was in partial remission when she died suddenly of a cardio-vascular event. This ongoing trial gives the opportunity to discuss the feasibility, the therapeutic effects and the tolerance of CyA in adult idiopathic NS resisting conventional therapy. Some of these very preliminary results also open the door to theoretical considerations on the nosology and the physiopathology of idiopathic NS, and on conceivable further therapeutic strategies comprising CyA associated with steroids and/or other immunosuppressive agents. The following discussion should of course be considered as speculative, as further studies could yield entirely different results.

Efficacy. In 4 patients remission started between the 3rd and the 4th week of treatment. This simultaneity is an argument for rejecting the hypothesis of spontaneous remission and, if verified on a larger series, could represent a clue to the disappearance rate of the hypothetical factor(s) which increase(s) glomerular permeability in idiopathic NS. In 3 patients with FSH, remission was incomplete. Does the persistence of proteinuria mean that the effect of CyA was only partial? In fact these patients had glomerular lesions, and one can accept the idea that CyA suppressed a factor of generalized glomerular hyperpermeability and left unchanged the lesional component of proteinuria.

In all cases we noticed that the control of edema became extremely easy after 3 weeks of treatment. There is no reason to think that CyA induced tubular lesions with an associated tendency to salt loss. It is now established that an intrarenal mechanism of sodium retention is at work in NS [5, 9]. Did CyA exert an effect on this component of nephrotic derangement of sodium excretion?

Tolerance. Case 1 had pneumococcal septicemia. This is a classical complication of NS. Conversely, CyA is rarely responsible for opportunistic bacterial infections. We therefore consider that sepsis was probably coincidental. It remains to be established whether CyA enhances or diminishes the incidence of sepsis in nephrotics and the figures have to be compared with conventional treatments. Case 3 died of a cardiovascular accident. A computer search (Sandoz, data on file) indicated that in transplant patients CyA treatment is only exceptionally complicated by thrombotic events. This may not be the case in NS, so that systematic anticoagulation is possibly justified in this specific indication.

Renal tolerance in this short-term trial was excellent. In fact, renal function improved in the 3 cases with FSH, probably due to the improvement of functional renal insufficiency. Nevertheless, we do not know what will be the long-term renal effects of CyA. The same applies to hepatic and hematological tolerance.

Future developments. This trial indicates that CyA treatment of MCLN and FSH is feasible and possibly effective even when every other treatment has failed. This represents a great hope in one of the most vexing therapeutic issues of nephrology. If our initial impressions are confirmed, a host of questions will call for answers: How long will remissions last? When should we stop the treatment and for what reasons? What will be the long-term renal tolerance? Should we combine CyA with corticosteroids and/or immunosuppressive agents in the case of resistance?

There is clearly an urgent need for launching a large-scale multi-center study of CyA in idiopathic NS.

Note added in proof: in case 1 remission of the NS was obtained on day 35 of the second treatment course

References

1. Brown CB, Cameron JS, Turner DR, et al. (1978) Focal segmental glomerulosclerosis with rapid decline in renal function ("malignant FSGS"). Clin Nephrol 10:51
2. Bunjes D, Hardt C, Rollinghoff M, Wagner H (1981) Cyclosporine A mediates immunosuppression of primary cytotoxic T-cell responses by impairing the release of interleukin-1 and interleukin-2. Eur J Immunol 11:657
3. Editorial (1976) Immunosuppression in the Nephrotic Syndrome. Lancet II:1121
4. Fillit HM, Zabriskie JB (1982) Cellular Immunity in Glomerulonephritis. Am J Pathol 109:227
5. Geers AB, Koomans HA, Roos JC, Boer P, Dorhout-Mees EJ (1984) Functional relationships in the nephrotic syndrome. Kidney Int 26:324
6. Heptinstall RH (ed) (1983) The nephrotic syndrome. In: Pathology of the kidney, 3rd edn Little Brown and Co, Boston, vol II: pp 637–740
7. Hess AD, Tutschka PJ, Santos GW (1982) Effect of cyclosporine A on human lymphocyte responses in vitro. III. CyA inhibitis the production of T lymphocyte growth factors in secondary mixed lymphocyte responses but does not inhibit the response of primed lymphocytes to TCGF. J Immunol 128:355
8. Hoyer JR, Raij L, Vernier RL, et al. (1972) Recurrence of idiopathic nephrotic syndrome after renal transplantation. Lancet II:343
9. Ichikawa I, Rennke HG, Hoyer JR, et al. (1983) Role for intrarenal mechanisms in the impaired salt excretion of experimental nephrotic syndrome. J Clin Invest 71:91
10. International study of kidney disease in children (1979). Nephrotic syndrome in children: a randomized trial comparing two prednisone regimens in steroid-responsive patients who relapse early. J Pediatr 95:239
11. Kalman VK, Klimpel GR (1983) Cyclosporine A inhibits the production of gammainterferon but does not inhibit production of virus-induced alpha/beta interferon. Cell Immunol 78:122
12. Lagrue G, Xheneumont S, Branellec A, Hirbec G, Weil B (1975) Lymphokines and nephrotic syndrome. Lancet I:271
13. Shaloub RJ (1974) Pathogenesis of lipoid nephrosis: a disorder of T-Cell function. Lancet II:556
14. Wu MJ, Moorthy AV (1981) Enhanced suppressor cell activity in minimal change nephrotic syndrome. 8th Int. Congr. Nephrol., Athens 1981, p 134
15. Zimmerman SW (1984) Increased urinary protein excretion in the rat produced by serum from a patient with recurrent focal glomerular sclerosis after renal transplantation. Clin Nephrol 22:32
16. Zucchelli P, Cagnoli L, Casanova S (1983) Minimal change glomerulopathy in humans. In: Bertani T, Remuzzi G (eds) Glomerular Injury 300 Years after Morgagni: Wichtig Publ., Milano, p 179

Ciclosporin (CyA) in Steroid-Insensitive Nephrotic Syndrome in Durban, South Africa

M. Adhikari, M. D., F. C. P. (Paed.) (SA)

The nephrotic syndrome (NS) among African children in South Africa has many features which make it quite distinct from the disease among children in most other parts of the world [1]. In some respects, especially the relationship with quartan malaria, the syndrome among black South Africans is different even from that in tropical Africa [4]. The commonest histological category among these patients is membranous nephropathy which appears to be causally linked to HB_sAg [2]. The nature of the Hb_s infection is invariably the carrier state. The outcome in these children is not entirely clear as follow-up studies are exceedingly difficult in the third world. However, about one third go into remission, a third have persistent proteinuria and the

Department of Paediatrics and Child Health, Faculty of Medicine, University of Natal, PO Box 17039, Congella 4013 Durban, South Africa.

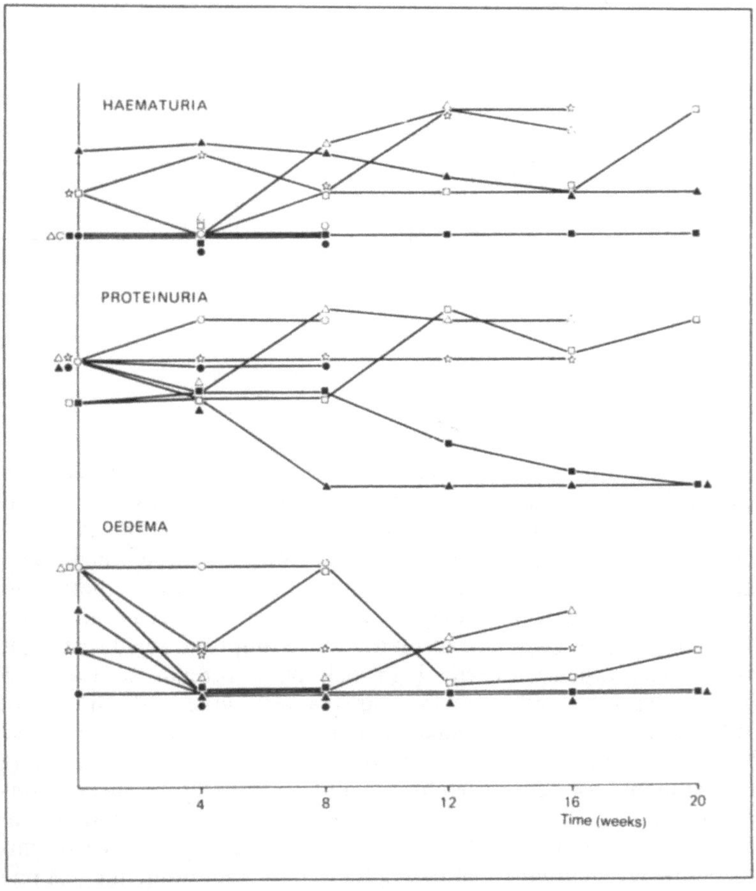

Fig. 1. Clinical Features

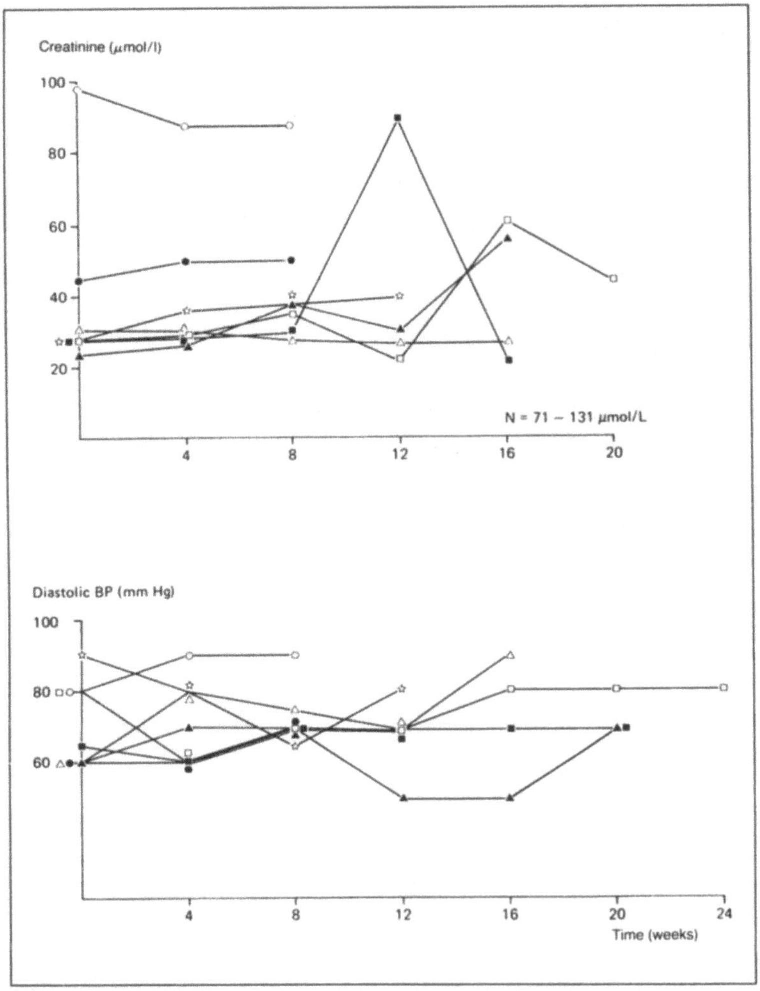

Fig. 2. Renal function

remainder have severe proteinuria with oedema. Morbidity is significant in the last-mentioned group with repeated hospital admissions for severe oedema. Management is quite unsatisfactory and nothing remotely like the success of steroids or cytotoxics in minimal change has been achieved. A high protein diet (expensive and often unattainable among black patients), diuretics and intravenous 20% salt-free albumen have been the mainstay of therapy. Accordingly treatment for this condition has to be innovative.

Indian South Africans have a fairly typical disease with a predominance of minimal change which is, as expected, steroid-responsive. The major clinical problem, as in most similar situations, is focal glomerulosclerosis (FGS) [1]. This is an exceedingly dangerous condition which often leads to renal failure. At present, there is no adequate therapy for this disease and even transplantation is unpromising because of the high risk of recurrence of the FGS in the transplanted kidney [5]. Nine % of Indian nephrotics have FGS. Their course is a protracted one with 50% remaining nephrotic and eventually requiring consideration for dialysis and transplantation. CyA is known to have major effects on immunoregulation by inhibiting the expression of T helper cell function [3]. These ef-

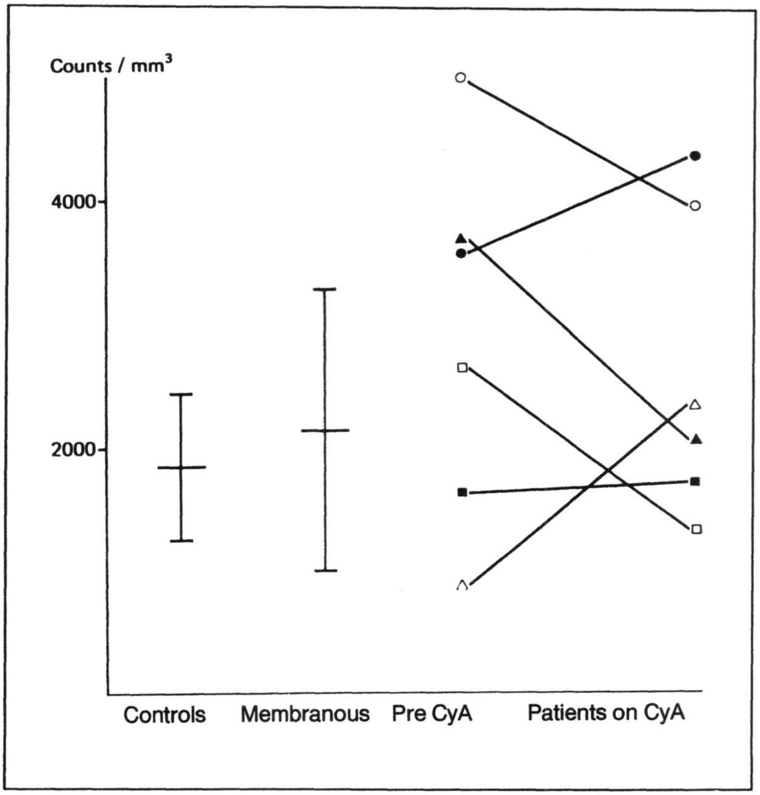

Fig. 3. Changes in OKT3

fects have been adequately discussed. The nephrotic syndrome is associated with abnormalities in these immunoregulatory cells and therefore it was appropriate to try this drug in this condition. A pilot study was designed to establish the dosage and side effects of this drug.

Patients

The inclusion criteria are shown in Table 1. Nine patients, 8 Africans and 1 Indian aged 3½ to 14 years, of whom 5 were males, were entered into the study. One child was withdrawn from the study by the parents, a second was withdrawn when he developed massive haematuria. 4 patients have membranous nephropathy all HB_sAg positive, 2 patients have focal glomerulosclerosis and 1 is unclassified.

Table 1. Inclusion criteria

1.	Oedema
2.	Hypoalbuminaemia
3.	Proteinuria
4.	Histological diagnosis: membranous, FGS
5.	African/Indian (FGS)

Dosage of ciclosporin and monitoring of patients

It was decided to commence at the lowest dosage of 2.5 mg/kg/day in 2 doses for a month and the dose was increased by 2.5 mg/kg/day if the trough blood levels were not adequate, an adequate level being 250–1000 ng/ml. The blood level was tested weekly. Once an adequate level was achieved the patient was maintained at that dosage. Six patients achieved adequate levels at a dosage of 10–15 mg/kg/day and 1 at 7.5 mg/kg/day.

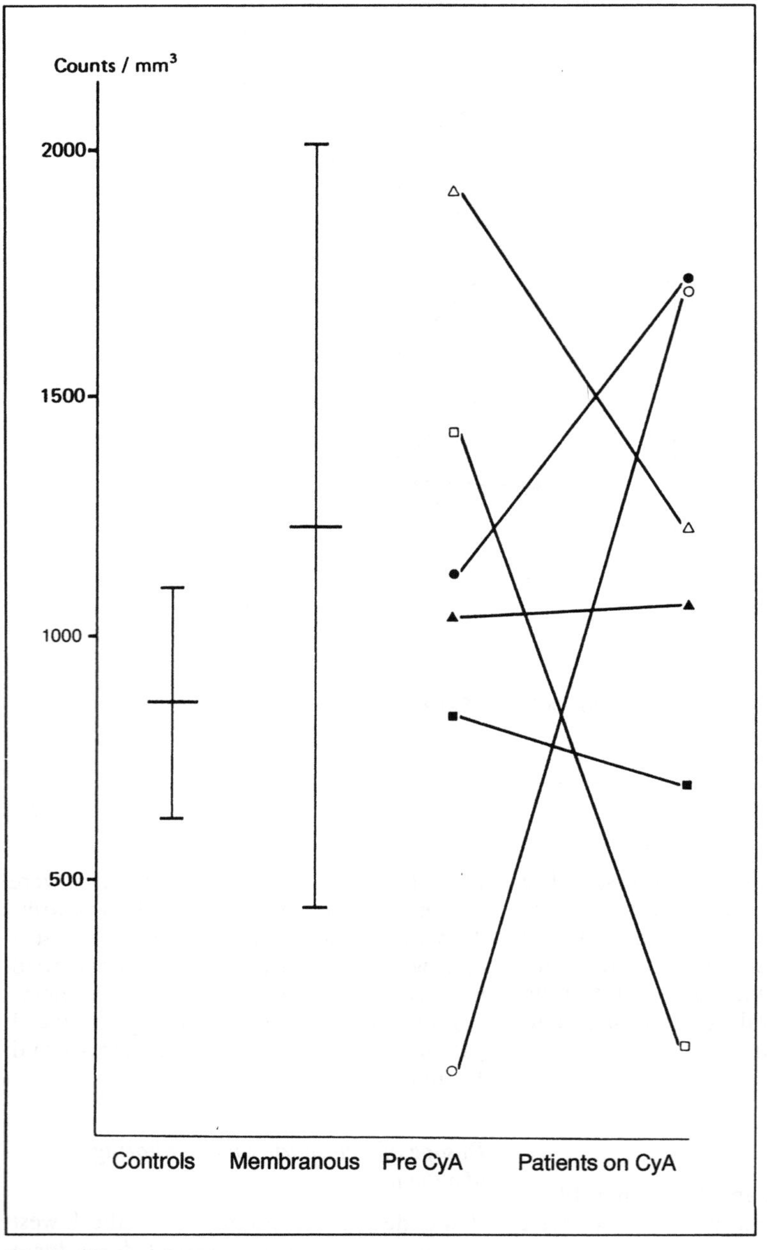

Fig. 4. Changes in OKT4

A careful clinical examination was performed before the drug was commenced. Initially a weekly, then 2-weekly and monthly recordings were made of the clinical and biochemical status of the patient. Careful attention was paid to the development of hypertension, evidence of hepatic, renal, nervous system disturbances, hirsutism, the development of infections and the urinary findings.

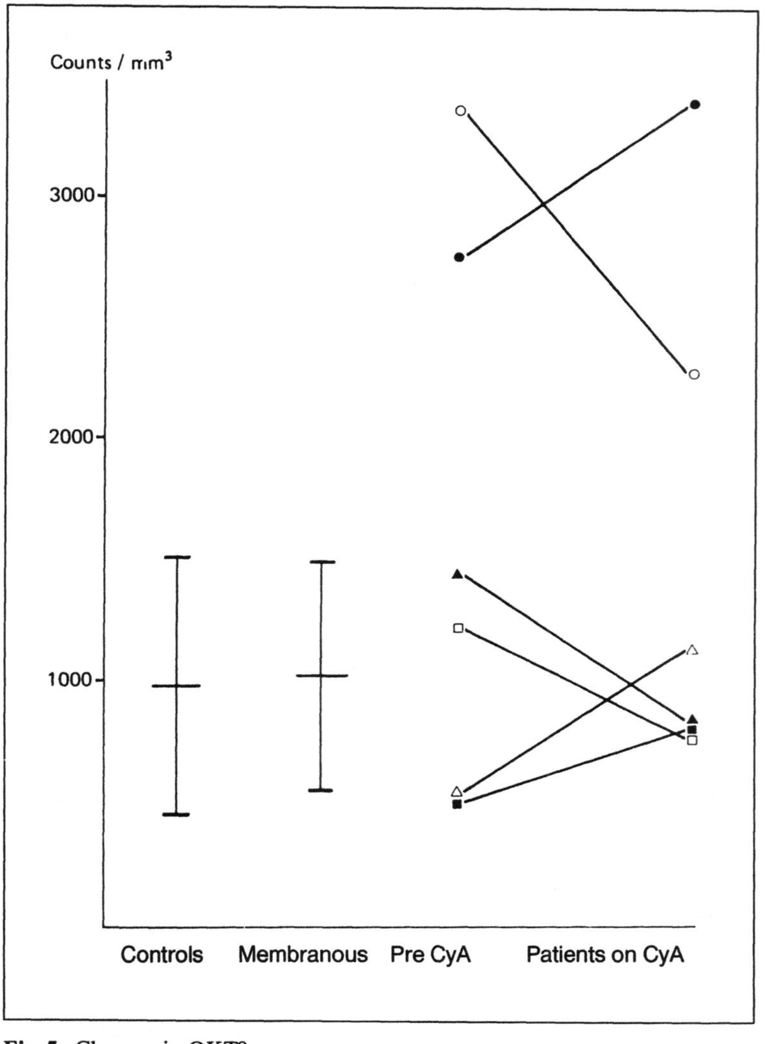

Fig. 5. Changes in OKT8

Clinical outcome

Of the 7 patients, 2 have remitted on an inadequate dosage of CyA. Both these are cases of membranous nephropathy and may well have remitted spontaneously, 5 have remained proteinuric or nephrotic (Fig. 1). The serum creatinines and blood pressures have remained within normal limits for all patients (Fig. 2).

The patient who was withdrawn from the study because of massive haematuria was found on investigation to have a normal blood picture, coagulation screen and ultrasonography of the urinary tract, and phase contrast microscopy revealed normal red cells, suggesting that the bladder was the site of bleeding. The haematuria subsided rapidly over 3–4 days.

Immunological changes

These are given in Figures 3–6. Results are available for 6 patients. It can be seen that there is a tendency for the numbers of total T cells (T3), helper T cells (T4) and suppressor T cells (T8) to regress towards the mean of the controls and patients.

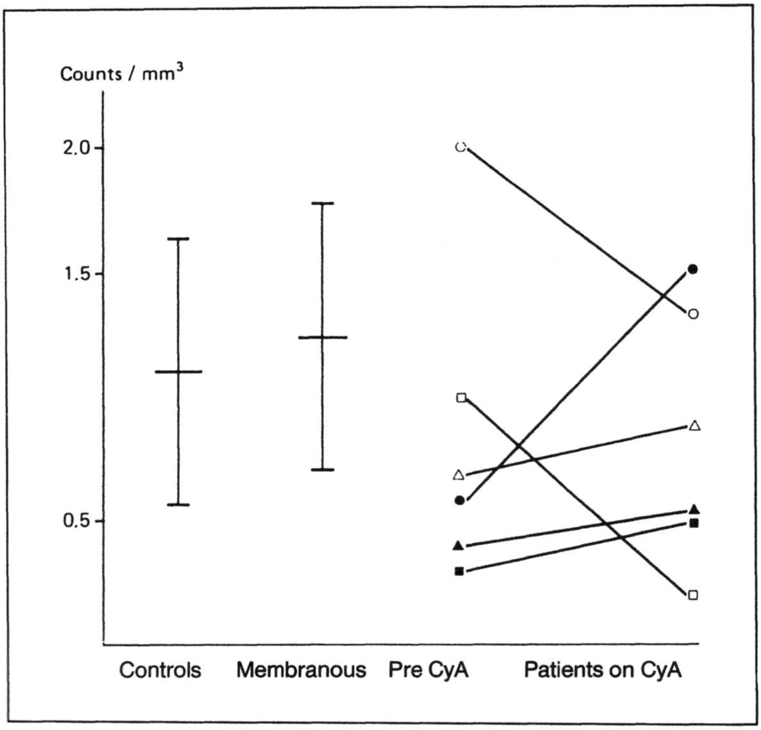

Fig. 6. Changes in OKT4/OKT8 ratio

From this study, although a small number of patients have been studied, the dosage of CyA has been established as ranging between 7.5–15 mg/kg/day with no side effects to date, good compliance and an indefinite clinical outcome in NS at present. A double-blind controlled study is planned to commence shortly.

References

1. Adhikari M (1981) Nephrotic Syndrome in African and Indian children in South Africa. M. D. Thesis, University of Natal
2. Adhikari M, Coovadia HM, Chrystal V (1983) Extramembranous nephropathy in Black South African children. Ann Trop Paed 3: 17–24
3. Borel JF, Lafferty KJ (1983) Basic Science Summation in Cyclosporin, Volume 1, Biological Activity and Clinical Applications. Editors Kalian BD, Grune and Stratton, New York
4. Hendrickse RG, Adeniyi A, Edington GM, Glasgow EF, White RHR, Houba V (1972) Quartan malariae nephrotic syndrome, collaborative clinicopathological study in Nigerian children. Lancet 1:1143–1149
5. Tejani A, Nicastri AD, Sen D, Chek CK, Phadke K, Adamson O, Butt KM (1983) Long-term evaluation of children with nephrotic syndrome and focal segmental glomerulosclerosis. Nephron 35:225–231

Ciclosporin Treatment of Idiopathic Nephrotic Syndrome in Children (Minimal Change Disease and Focal Segmental Glomerulosclerosis)

J. Brodehl, P. F. Hoyer

Ciclosporin has been used in our center for kidney and liver transplantation in children since September 1982 [3, 5]. The first not transplanted, but *nephrotic* child was tentatively started on ciclosporin in January 1984, when her glomerular filtration rate revealed a definitive downhill course and when it became evident that she presumably would go into renal failure in the near future [6] and would in any case receive ciclosporin for kidney transplantation. Since then we have treated three more cases, i.e. a total of 4 children with nephrotic syndrome. Two of them suffered from the steroid-responsive type with minimal change disease, the other two from steroid-resistant focal segmental glomerulosclerosis. We shall present the 4 cases and then briefly report on the recommendations we have issued in the "Arbeitsgemeinschaft für Paediatrische Nephrologie (APN)" for a pilot study of ciclosporin treatment in a specified group of nephrotic children.

Case reports

Case 1 (Fig. 1, H. Sch. male, born 6. 8. 1973) had suffered from nephrotic syndrome since 1974. He was treated with prednisone in a standard APN regimen [2], i.e. 60 mg/m²/day for 4 weeks followed by alternate-day prednisone (40 mg/m²/48 h) for another 4 weeks. He responded to prednisone, but relapsed frequently and became steroid-dependent (for definition see Arbeitsgemeinschaft Paediatrische Nephrologie [1]). Renal biopsy revealed minimal change disease. He was therefore treated with cytotoxic drugs and received two courses of chlorambucil (cumulative dose 7 mg/kg and 10.5 mg/kg, respectively) and one course of cyclophosphamide (cumulative dose 115 mg/kg). After the second course with chlorambucil, he remained in remission for almost 6 years. Thereafter, he again relapsed and had to be treated with prednisone in a standard manner. After the third successive relapse it became evident, that again he was steroid-dependent. At this point we started treatment with ciclosporin. The daily dose was 100 mg (i.e. 100 mg/m² body surface area) which was increased stepwise to 180 mg/day. The trough blood level of ciclosporin was estimated by radioimmunoassay [4]. It remained in the range of < 100 to 366 ng/ml. Ciclosporin treatment was combined with alternate-day prednisone in the first three months in analogy to our treatment schedule with cyclophosphamide (Arbeitsgemeinschaft für Paediatrische Nephrologie [1]), in order to avoid an early relapse. Despite this a relapse occurred after 4 weeks of treatment with ciclosporin plus alternate-day prednisone, but responded promptly to an increase in prednisone dose. After 3 months prednisone was withdrawn completely and ciclosporin continued for another 3 months. Thus, the treatment with ciclosporin lasted for a total of 6 months. No further relapse took place during this period, but relapse did occur 10 weeks after complete cessation of therapy. The patient responded to standard prednisone. It is intended to observe him for the next months, in order to establish whether he again relapses and becomes steroid-dependent.

Case 2 (Fig. 2, M.E. male, 2. 7. 1973) had suffered from idiopathic steroid-responsive nephrotic syndrome since 1977. He became steroid-dependent and was treated with cyclophosphamide (cumulative dose 140 mg/kg), but relapsed quickly after the

Professor Dr. med. Johannes Brodehl, Dept. Paediatric Nephrology and Metabolic Diseases, Children's Hospital, Medical School Hannover, D-3000 Hannover 61, Fed. Rep. Germany

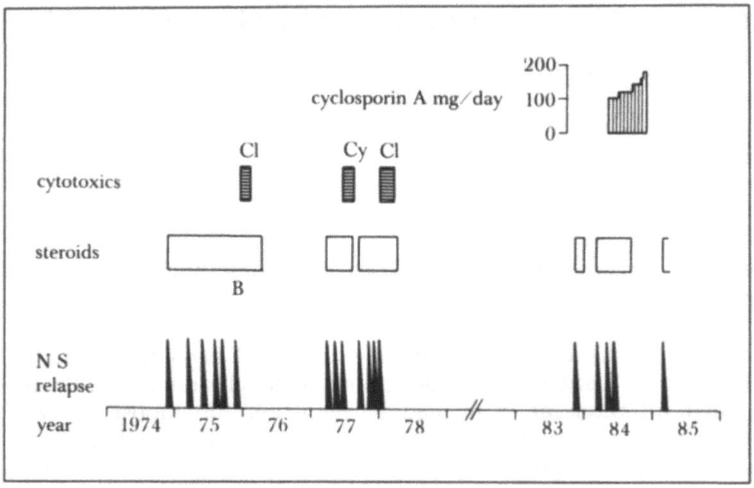

Fig. 1. H. Sch. 6. 8. 73 m. Steroid-dependent MCNS (see text); Cl = chlorambucil, Cy = cyclophosphamide, B = renal biopsy

end of cytotoxic treatment. Renal biopsy revealed minimal change disease. From mid 1983 he was continuously treated with prednisone by titrating his daily requirement, but nevertheless showed several relapses. Therefore, in July 1984 treatment with ciclosporin was started with a daily dose of 120 mg (i.e. 100 mg/m²), which was increased stepwise to 200 mg/day. Blood levels of ciclosporin were in the range of 100–260 ng/ml. Prednisone was administered on alternate days for 3 months, and then discontinued. The patient has now been off ciclosporin for 6 weeks, and off prednisone for 4½ months. So far, no relapse has occurred. Kidney function and plasma proteins are completely normal.

Case 3 (Fig. 3, U.H. female, 8. 7. 1969) had suffered from nephrotic syndrome since 1979. Initial steroid treatment for 8 weeks revealed primary steroid resistance. She then was referred to our hospital. Her renal function was normal apart from the severe proteinuria. The renal biopsy revealed mesangial proliferative glomerulonephritis with focal segmental sclerosis. Only symptomatic therapy with diuretics was therefore instituted. During the following years proteinuria was variably high and serum protein and albumin remained in the nephrotic range. At the end of 1983 serum creatinine rose above 200 μmol/l, and it was anticipated that she now would rapidly go into renal failure. It therefore

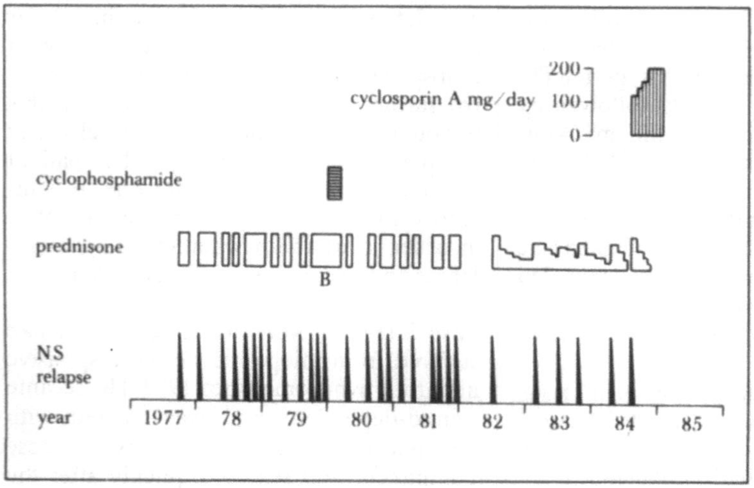

Fig. 2. M. E. 2. 4. 73 m. Steroid-dependent MCNS (for abbreviations see Fig. 1)

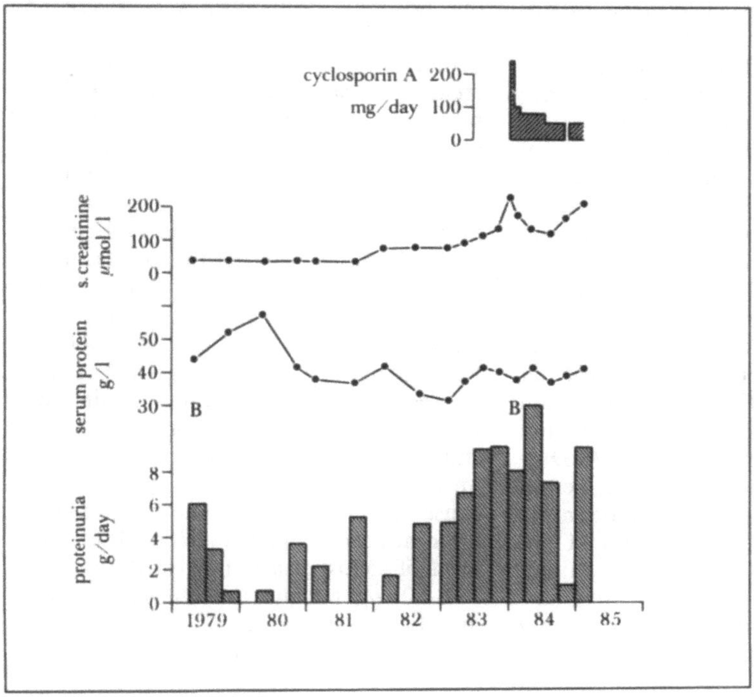

Fig. 3. U. H. 8. 7. 69 f. Foc.-seg. Glomerulosclerosis

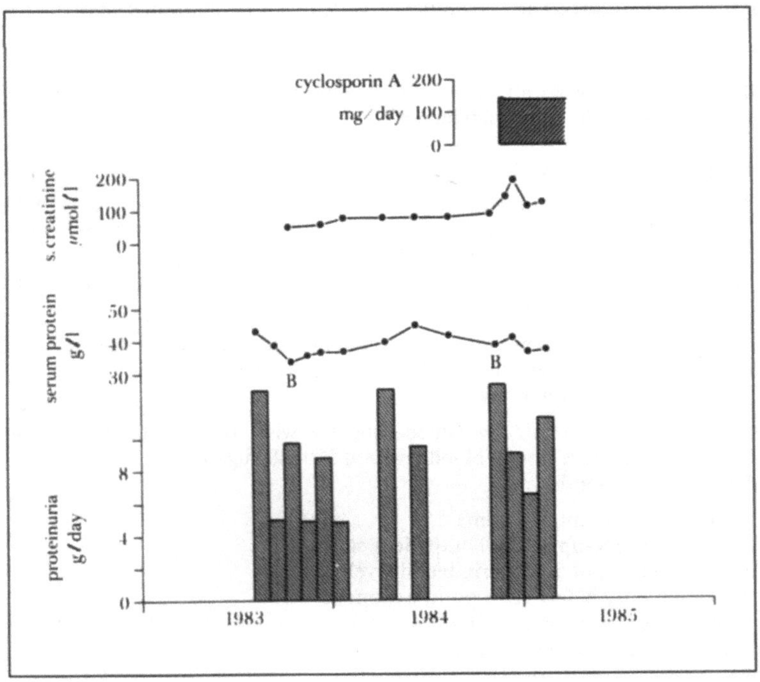

Fig. 4. C. I. 30. 4. 70 m. Foc.-seg. Glomerulosclerosis

seemed justified to try ciclosporin as immunosuppressive treatment. The second renal biopsy revealed severe changes of focal segmental glomerulosclerosis. Since this was the first case a dose of 240 mg/day ciclosporin was administered, i.e. half of the initial CyA dose used in renal transplantation (500 mg/m²). This, however, led to high ciclosporin blood levels (maximum 1002 ng/ml). Therefore ciclosporin dosage was reduced to 50–70 mg/day. Under this regimen blood levels remained between 167 and 661 ng/ml. The patient responded favourably to ciclosporin and in particular her well-being improved markedly. Serum creatinine did not increase further, but dropped to a minimum of 101 µmol/l. During the last few months, however, serum creatinine has increased again. Proteinuria and hypoproteinemia have remained unchanged. Ciclosporin treatment was initially scheduled for one year, but it has now been decided to continue and see whether the deterioration of renal function can be halted further.

Case 4 (Fig. 4, C.L. male, 30. 4. 1970) had suffered from nephrotic syndrome since June 1983. He was treated with standard prednisone regimen for 8 weeks but did not respond to it. He was therefore referred to our hospital. Proteinuria was severe and hypoproteinemia (34 g/l) and hypoalbuminemia (11 g/l) were marked, but serum creatinine was normal (55 µmol/l). Renal biopsy revealed focal segmental glomerulosclerosis. The patient was treated symptomatically with diuretics, co-trimoxazole and antihypertensive drugs, and his proteinuria persisted. At the end of 1984 serum creatinine started to rise, reaching a maximum of 130 µmol/l. The patient was therefore started on ciclosporin after a second renal biopsy. Dosage of ciclosporin was 140 ng/day (i.e. 100 mg/m²). During the second week the serum creatinine level rose to 178 µmol/l. The patient who was still on co-trimoxazole to prevent peritonitis, was changed over to penicillin because co-trimoxazole is known to increase CyA-induced nephrotoxicity. The blood level of ciclosporin is now in the range of 117–501 ng/ml and the last serum creatinine level was 112 µmol/l. Proteinuria and hypoproteinemia remained unchanged.

Summary and conclusions

The preliminary analysis of our ciclosporin trial in 4 children with nephrotic syndrome seems to reveal some evidence that ciclo-

Table 1. Protocol of a pilot study on ciclosporin treatment of children with idiopathic nephrotic syndrom (Arbeitsgemeinschaft für Pädiatrische Nephrologie, APN)

Patients:	Children 2–16 years with 1. Frequently relapsing and steroid-dependent nephrotic syndrome with minimal glomerular lesions, who have already received cytotoxic treatment but have relapsed again. 2. Steroid-resistant focal and segmental glomerulosclerosis with impairment of GFR (not below 40 ml/min/1.73 m²)
Aim:	re 1. prevention of relapses and prolongation of steroid-free remissions, re 2. slowing of progression of glomerular impairment, reduction of proteinuria
Ciclosporin	Dosage: 100 mg/m²/day, increasing stepwise by 10–20 mg/day to achieve trough blood levels of 200–400 ng/ml Duration: 6 months
Preconditions:	1. Informed consent of parents 2. Regular check-up in renal outpatient clinic 3. Measurement of ciclosporin blood levels 4. Renal biopsy before ciclosporin treatment 5. Strict observation of contraindications and early cessation of CyA medication if side effects arise.

sporin could have a favourable influence on the course of the disease. In the steroid-responsive and -dependent minimal change nephrotic syndrome, ciclosporin treatment may prevent relapses, at least for as long as it is administered. We have no data as to whether it could be effective as a sole drug, since we have combined it with prednisone. In the steroid-resistant nephrotic syndrome with focal segmental glomerular sclerosis ciclosporin could possibly interfere with the progression of the glomerular insufficiency. Whether it will stop the progressive decline of renal function in this condition is questionable but, if it did, this alone would justify further treatment. Ciclosporin treatment with blood level monitoring is a fairly safe treatment, since no severe side effects have been observed in our cases. It is noticeable that all patients tolerated the treatment very well and experienced a marked improvement of their well-being.

The Arbeitsgemeinschaft für Paediatrische Nephrologie (APN) has therefore issued a protocol for a pilot study to collect more cases (see Table) before the initiation of a controlled trial on ciclosporin treatment in children can be considered. According to this protocol, two disease entities should be treated with ciclosporin: 1. Children with frequently relapsing and steroid-dependent nephrotic syndrome with minimal changes (MCNS), who have already undergone at least one course of cytotoxic drug treatment and subsequently relapsed again. 2. Children who have steroid-resistant focal segmental glomerulosclerosis (FSGS) and already show marked impairment of glomerular filtration rate, which, however should not be below 40 ml/min/1.73 m^2.

Preconditions for the pilot study are: 1. informed consent of the parents, 2. regular check-ups in the renal outpatient clinic, 3. measurement of the blood level of ciclosporin, 4. renal biopsy before start of ciclosporin treatment.

The starting dosage of ciclosporin is 100 mg/m^2/day in two doses. It should be increased stepwise by 10–20 mg/day in order to avoid nephrotoxicity and to achieve a trough blood level of 200–400 ng/ml. The scheduled duration of ciclosporin treatment is 6 months.

Patients with steroid-dependent nephrotic syndrome should first be brought into remission by standard prednisone relapse therapy [1], and then started on ciclosporin. In order to avoid an early relapse, they additionally should receive prednisone on alternate-day regimen for 8 weeks (40 mg/m^2/48 h for 6 weeks, 20 mg/m^2/48 h in 7th week and 10 mg/m^2/48 h in 8th week).

The laboratory and clinical data are to be collected, and the results evaluated every six months, by the pilot study center in Hanover.

The principal criterion for the effectiveness of ciclosporin treatment is the recurrence of relapses and the duration of the steroid-free interval in steroid-dependent MCNS and the development (progression or nonprogression) of renal insufficiency and the degree of proteinuria and hypoproteinemia in steroid-resistant FSGS. Only if the pilot study shows promising results will a controlled study of ciclosporin treatment be considered by the APN.

References

1. Arbeitsgemeinschaft für Paediatrische Nephrologie (1982) Effect of cytotoxic drugs in frequently relapsing nephrotic syndrome with and without steroid dependence. N Engl J Med 306:451
2. Brodehl J, Krohn HP, Ehrich JHH (1982) The treatment of minimal change nephrotic syndrome in children: cooperative studies of the Arbeitsgemeinschaft für Paediatrische Nephrologie (APN). Klin Paediatr 194:162
3. Brodehl J, Offner G, Hoyer PF, Schirg E, Pichlmayr R, Wonigeit K (1985) Normal growth rates of children with kidney transplantation treated with cyclosporin A (submitted for publication)
4. Donatsch P, Abisch E, Homberger M, Traber R, Trapp M, Voges RA (1981) Radioimmunoassay to measure cyclosporin A in plasma and serum samples. J Immunoassay 2:19
5. Hoyer PF, Offner G, Wonigeit K, Brodehl J, Pichlmayr R (1984) Dosage of cyclosporin A in children with renal transplants. Clin Nephrol 22:68
6. Tejani A, Nicastri AD, Sen D, Chen CK, Phadke K, Adamson O, Butt KMH (1983) Long-term evaluation of children with nephrotic syndrome and focal segmental glomerular sclerosis. Nephron 35:225

What Can the NZB/W Mice Teach us about the Treatment of SLE with Ciclosporin?

H. C. Gunn, B. Ryffel, P. C. Hiestand and J. F. Borel

Female NZB/W hybrid mice spontaneously develop a disease that resembles human systemic lupus erythematosus (SLE) [1]. Briefly, by 4 months of age these mice develop anti-DNA antibodies; by 10 months of age they develop anti-red-blood cell (RBC) antibodies and a systemic immune complex (IC) disease with glomerulonephritis (GN) and proteinuria, and by 12 months of age they have a predictable course to chronic renal failure with about 50% mortality.

Preclinical Research, Sandoz Ltd, Basel, Switzerland

The drug ciclosporin (CyA) is a powerful inhibitor of lymphocyte functions in vitro and a highly specific immunosuppressive agent in vivo [2].

In this study we have used CyA to ask 2 questions which may possibly be applicable to human autoimmune disease: (i) can CyA suppress a strong on-going autoimmune response? and (ii) is CyA beneficial to the pathology which results from the disease?

Effect on autoantibody production

CyA was given 5 times a week for 12 weeks at a daily oral dose of 100 mg/kg to old

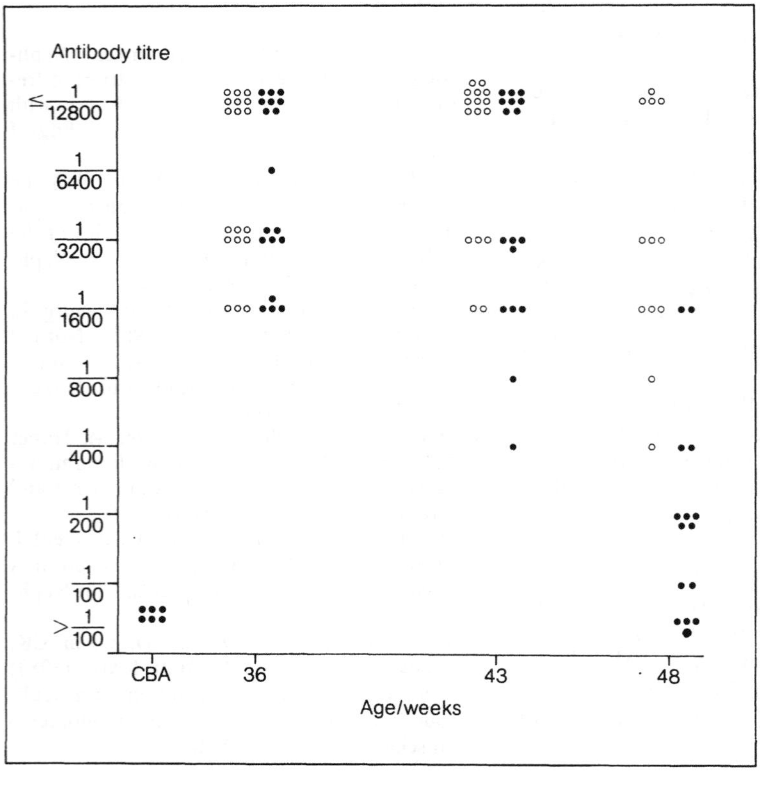

Fig. 1. Effect of ciclosporin on anti-DNA autoantibodies in old NZB/W mice. (○) – animals given olive oil, (●) – animals given ciclosporin

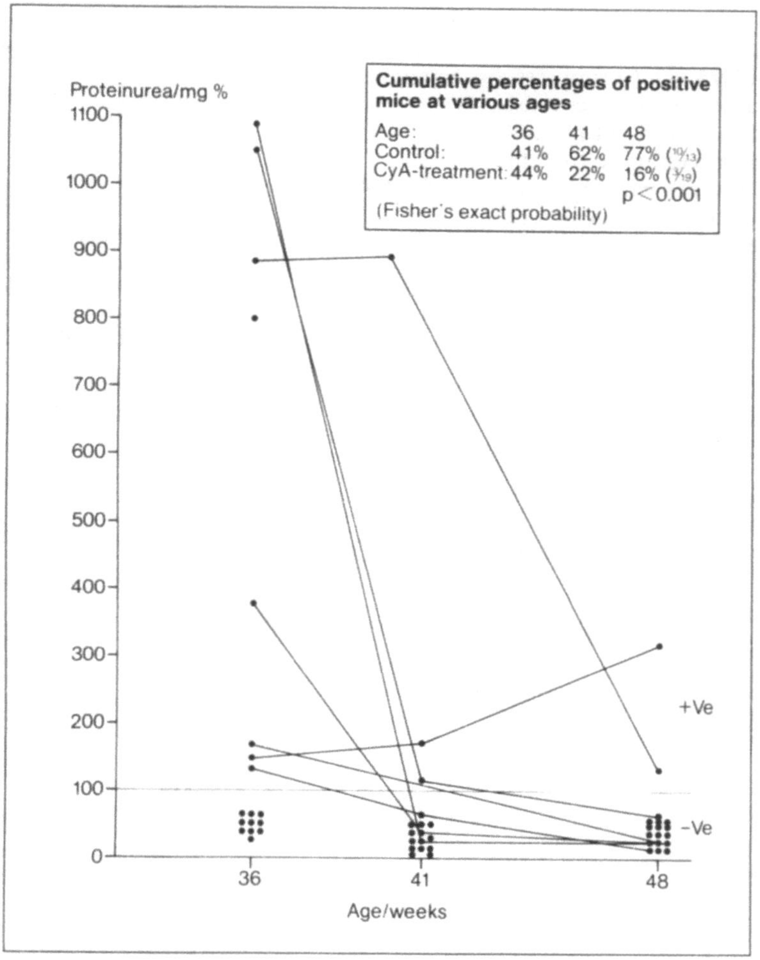

Fig. 2. Proteinurea of old NZB/W mice treated with ciclosporin

NZB/W mice which already had high titres of anti-DNA antibodies. Figure 1 shows that after several weeks of treatment the autoantibody levels were lowered ($p<0.05$ by an unpaired Student's test). The antibodies were assayed by the enzyme-linked-immunosorbant assay. Identical results were obtained for another set of autoantibodies against autologous RBC (data not shown). The latter set of autoantibodies was assayed by a direct agglutination Coombs' test.

Effect on proteinurea

A simple method for the estimation of glomerular damage caused by IC deposition in the NZB/W mouse is the measurement of the degree of proteinurea. This was estimated by staining urine spots on filter paper with bromophenol blue. A thin-layer chromotography scanner connected to an integrating computer was then used to quantify the intensity of the stained urine spots to a serial dilution of bovine serum albumin. Figure 2 shows that CyA reduced the proteinurea in 6 out of 7 mice. 1 mouse died before the end of the 12-week experiment. However, none of the 10 mice which were proteinurea negative (< 100 mg%) became positive. This is in contrast to an olive-oil-fed control group where 41% of the mice were positive at 36 weeks and this percentage increased to 77% (no mouse remitted to negative proteinurea) by the end of the experiment at 48 weeks.

Conclusions

We have shown that CyA can (i) suppress a strong, on-going autoimmune response, and (ii) reverse proteinurea in old NZB/W mice. However, it was necessary to treat the animals for about 12 weeks with this compound before the autoantibody levels were reduced to non-detectable levels. This may be clinically relevant, since patients may show little sign of a drop in autoantibody levels in the first few weeks of treatment. We have reported elsewhere that the reduction of proteinurea is probably due to the reduction of glomerulonephritis [3, 4]. The above observations support the possibility that CyA might be effective in the treatment of certain autoimmune diseases in man.

References

1. Andrews BS, Eisenberg RA, Theofilopoulos AN, Izui S, Wilson CB, McConahey PJ, Murphy ED, Roth JB, Dixon FJ (1978) J exp Med 148: 1198
2. Borel JF, Feurer C, Gubler HU et al. (1976) Agents Actions 6:468
3. Borel JF (1984) Triangle 23: No 3/4, 153
4. Gunn HC, Ryffel B (in press) Clin Nephrology

Combined Ciclosporin-Steroid Treatment of Systemic Lupus Erythematosus

P. A. Miescher and A. Miescher

Introduction

Systemic lupus erythematosus (SLE) is a complex autoimmune disorder for which there is multigenic predisposition, which varies from patient to patient. Its clinical expression depends on a multitude of exogenous factors which again vary tremendously from patient to patient as well as during the course of the disease. It is therefore understandable that a precise evaluation of any treatment in biological terms had to be and will be a difficult task.

Among the various drugs which have been applied in the treatment of SLE, corticosteroids have been found by all clinicians to represent the most efficient single therapeutic agent, unequalled by any non-steroidal agent. Immunosuppressive drugs such as cytotoxic agents help in the management of SLE patients by permitting a reduction, but not usually the replacement, of steroid medication [3].

While the treatment of mild cases of SLE has become possible with minimum side effects, severe cases still pose many problems. In particular, the daily use of steroids is limited by the disabling long-term side effects.

Ciclosporin (CyA) is a non-steroidal immunosuppressive agent whose mode of action is different from that of cytotoxic agents. It acts primarily on helper T cells with reduction of the various lymphokines they produce [1]. Since T cells are instrumental in the regulation of B cell activity, it was hoped that CyA might be beneficial in the treatment of diseases presenting pathological B cell activation.

In the present study, CyA was given in combination with steroids to 20 SLE patients. In view of the not inconsiderable toxicity of CyA [5], for an initial assessment of this treatment in the management of SLE we selected 4 patients with skin involvement resistant to steroids, cytotoxic agents and hydroxychloroquine, but with an otherwise benign course of SLE. The short-term results were sufficiently encouraging for us to investigate the steroid-CyA association in 16 more severe cases of SLE that had not responded well to conventional treatment. In view of the negative effect of CyA on glomerular function [4], we excluded any cases with persistantly elevated creatinine values. In all patients, cytotoxic agents were replaced by CyA at a dose of 5 mg/kg/day. For basic steroid medication we selected fluocortolone, a derivative of cortisone which does not produce sodium retention and which has a higher Cushing threshold than prednisone [3].

Table 1 summarizes the clinical data of patients included in this study.

Results

Of the four patients suffering from therapy-resistant skin involvement, one patient did not respond at all after an 8-week trial (case 1); in two patients, the skin eruption diminished in intensity but recurred upon discontinuation of the drug (cases 2 and 3). In the fourth patient, who was also suffering from arthralgia, skin lesions were mostly localised on the hands and in particular on the terminal phalanges of the fingers at the site of the nailbed. In this last patient, the skin lesions and arthralgia disappeared on replacing cytotoxic agents with CyA (case 4). This patient is still on CyA, which, after 20 months of continuous treatment, is now given on an alternate-month schedule with azathioprine, and remains well controlled with this combination. The evolution of corresponding laboratory parameters is shown in Table 2 (cases 1–4).

Table 1. Clinical data of 20 SLE patients

Patient, Initials, sex birthdate	Year of onset of disease	Main disease manifestations	Duration of immunosuppression before addition of CyA (years)	Duration of CyA medication (months)*
1) A.A. F 18.10.59	1977	Skin involvement, adenopathy, kidney involvement, convulsions	3	2
2) M.A. F 25.07.55	1974	Fever, skin, joint, heart and kidney involvement (diffuse proliferative glomerulonephritis)	3	3
3) N.L. F 04.07.46	1975	Skin and joint involvement, pleural and G.I. involvement, arthralgia, psoriasis	6	5
4) R.M. F 04.05.31	1964	Skin and joint involvement, renal calculi (creat. cl. 68 ml/min).	2	23+
5) B.G. F 01.09.50	1972	Skin, joint and heart involvement, kidney involvement (diffuse proliferative glomerulonephritis, arterial occlusions)	9	2+
6) C.P. F 24.08.63	1980	Joint involvement, pleurisy, kidney involvement (diffuse proliferative glomerulonephritis)	3	2+
7) F.V. M 13.09.67	1981	Fever, joint and liver involvement, pericarditis, kidney involvement (diffuse proliferative glomerulonephritis, creatinine clearance 40 ml/min, CNS involvement)	0.6	4+
8) G.S. F 12.11.68	1963	Fever, joint and heart involvement, kidney involvement, chorea	4	28+
9) K.S. F 18.11.54	1969	Skin and joint involvement, hemolytic anemia, thrombocytopenia, pericarditis, lung involvement, phlebitis, renal involvement (focal proliferative glomerulonephritis)	13	10+
10) M.M. F 11.08.43	1981	Fever, skin and joint involvement, tooth infections	3	4
11) M.S. F 08.06.68	1981	Heart, CNS and kidney involvement (membrano-proliferative glomerulonephritis)	2	3+
12) M.C. F 13.10.68	1980	Joint involvement, phlebitis, nephrotic syndrome, renal insufficiency (membrano-proliferative glomerulonephritis), interstitial cystitis	6	5
13) P.G. F 13.07.40	1958	Joint, lung, heart and kidney involvement (creatinine clearance 48 ml/min.), CNS involvement, autoimmune hemolytic anemia	0.75	8+
14) P.E. F 21.06.65	1975	Skin and joint involvement, splenomegaly, CNS involvement, kidney inv. (creatinine cl. 70 ml/min.)	6	9+

* + = still under CyA medication

Table 1. (Continued)

Patient, Initials, sex birthdate	Year of onset of disease	Main disease manifestations	Duration of immunosuppression before addition of CyA (years)	Duration of CyA medication (months)*
15) R.C. F 21.04.70	1978	Skin and joint involvement, pleurisy, nephrotic syndrome	3	6+
16) R.S. F 19.12.73	1982	Skin and heart involvement, kidney involvement (nephrotic syndrome)	1	3
17) R.D. F 12.06.59	1974	Joint and pleural involvement, kidney involvement (membranoproliferative glomerulonephritis)	8	3+
18) S.D. F 20.05.39	1981	Skin, joint, heart and kidney involvement	2	6+
19) S.M. F 06.11.48	1984	Fever, joint involvement, kidney involvement (membranoproliferative glomerulonephritis, creatinine clearance: 58 ml/min.)	0.5	2+
20) S. G.P. M 17.08.56	1976	Joint, heart and kidney involvement	4	6+

The results of CyA-steroid treatment in the 16 more severe cases are listed in Table 2 (cases 5–20). In two patients (cases 5 and 11), no improvement occurred during the first three months of treatment. In six patients, improvement was mild to moderate (cases 7, 10, 12, 16, 18, 19). In all of them, CyA medication could be evaluated only after a three-month course.

Eight patients showed a marked improvement in clinical as well as in laboratory terms (cases 6, 8, 9, 13, 14, 15, 17, 20): antibody titers to ssDNA diminished in 6 patients and dsDNA antibody titres in 5, while there were improvements in blood and urinary protein levels in seven of the eight patients.

Three case histories are given in detail in Figures 1–3. Case 17 (Fig. 1) is a patient with long-standing proteinuria. An increase in the fluocortolone dose led to a temporary decrease in proteinuria. This girl now has only traces of proteinuria after replacement of antimetabolites with CyA.

The following two cases represent severe forms of SLE not responding well to conventional therapy. In case 8 (Fig. 2), replacement of antimetabolites with CyA allowed reduction of steroid medication with resultant resumption of linear growth. After 20 months of continuous CyA medication, this drug was then administered on an alternate-month schedule with azathioprine.

Case 13 (Fig. 3) concerns a patient who developed a most severe course of SLE, with hemolytic anemia, thrombocytopenia, kidney involvement, pleural effusion, arthralgia and retinal involvement, not responding to treatment with massive doses of steroids and cyclophosphamide. This lady responded to a short i.v. course of methylprednisolone followed by a combined steroid-CyA medication. The steroid medication before introduction of CyA was 100 mg of methylprednisolone daily; after introduction of CyA, she received 300 mg of fluocortolone per week (60 mg daily, 5 days per week).

The following side reactions attributable to CyA medication were observed: hirsutism in eight patients, water retention in six, tremor in two, abdominal discomfort in four, and elevation of diastolic blood pres-

Table 2. Laboratory data before and 3 and 6 months after replacement of cytotoxic immunosuppressants with CyA

Case No.	Months treatment CyA	Creatinine	Serum protein	Urinary protein	ESR	Antibody activity to ssDNA	Antibody activity to dsDNA	CH50	C_3d
		μm/l	g/l	g/l	mm/h	Δ% fix.	Δ% fix.	%	%
1	0	68	68	0	18	19.8	2.7	62	4
	3	72	70	0	28	10.3	4.6	81	5.6
2	0	84	72	0.3	18	9	1	98	5
	3	83	77	0.3	23	12.9	0	103	5
3	0	68	74	0	8	33	2.4	52	18.5
	3	107	67	0	25	44.8	3.5	51	0
4	0	82	78	0	6	20.7	1.1	83	1
	3	125	70	0	15	18.3	1.0	54	0
	6	106	71	0	12	21.7	1.4	62	2
5	0	83	67	1	37	1	0	75	11
	3	89	63	1.0					
6	0	79	58	5	24	0	0	88	6
	3	124	66	0.3	19				
7	0	121	69	1	58	55.4	28.5	54	22
	3	124	65	0.3	35	22	13	61	5
8	0	63	57	5	61	43	11.1	47	16.4
	3	52	61	0.3	61	16.4	0	51	8
	6	54	56	0	40	8	0	68	3
9	0	71	70	1	75	27	14	44	0
	3	75	71	0.3	40	3	2.4	40	0
	6	71	76	0.3	31	14	1	50	0
10	0	81	68	0.3	73	61.6	43.6		
	3	98	72	0	64	55.5	23.1	59	17
11	0	85	49	6	55	0	0	67	16
	3	124	45	10	106	17.3	1.6	49	9
12	0	62	60	5	40	43.9	2.7	57	7
	3	90	64	0.5					
13	0	114	54	6	22	7.7	0	83	12
	3	123	77	0.3	25	0	0	84	9
14	0	83	67	0	32	52	7	26	5
	3	141	68	0					
	6	98	69	0.3	15	30	1.5	52	0
15	0	54	45	6	56	44.2	2.7	42	12
	3	59	45	2	52	9.4	0.2	78	2
	6	72	65	0.4					
16	0	47	72	5	58	0	0	80	0
	3	80	75	1	32				
17	0	79	55	5	35	4.8	0	83	15
	3	80	57	1	22	6.8	0	62	3
18	0	92	48	1	23	29.4	22.8	24	13
	6	100	64	0	16	18.0	1.6	77	0
19	0	83	56	5	35	1.3	0	122	2
	3	150	63	2.37	25	0	0	115	0
20	0	74	60	5	48	71.2	72.9	65	4
	3	107	63	1	27	0	0.3	112	0

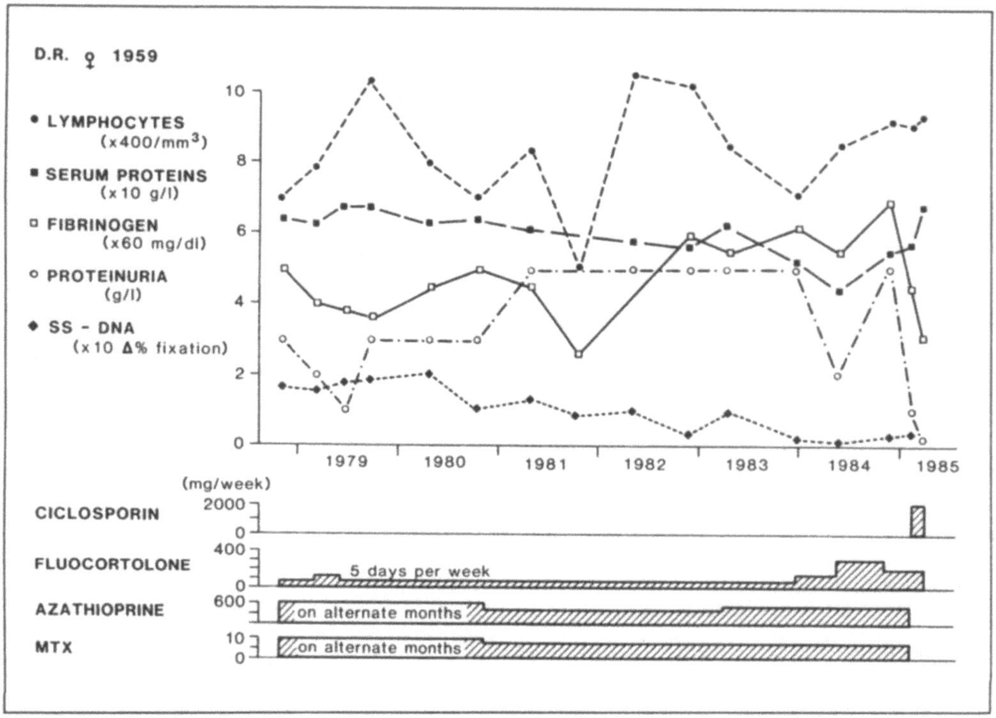

Fig. 1. Summary of laboratory data of case 17. This female patient born in 1959 has suffered from SLE since the age of 15 years, when she developed fever, arthralgia and proteinuria. The family history includes one case of rheumatoid arthritis (mother's sister). Her initial treatment consisted of intermittent daily prednisone medication and cyclophosphamide. She came to Geneva in November, 1977 after developing Cushing's syndrome with the clinical and laboratory findings of a nephrotic syndrome. With the introduction of two days per week without steroids and the replacement of prednisone with fluocortolone, the Cushing symptoms were attenuated. In the first year there was a marked improvement of the nephrotic syndrome, but in subsequent years urinary protein again increased. In March 1983, urinary protein rose to 8 g/l and the patient developed ankle oedema. A kidney biopsy permitted histological evaluation of 20 glomeruli which showed the picture of membranoproliferative glomerulonephritis. In addition, the interstitial tissue was characterized by periglomerular and periarteriolar lympho-monocytic cell infiltration. Immunofluorescence showed massive finegranular deposition of IgG and complement throughout all glomeruli. Increase of the steroid dose brought only a temporary improvement of the nephrotic syndrome. Upon replacement of antimetabolites with CyA, proteinuria diminished for the first time to levels below 1 g/l

Table 3. Serum creatinine levels in 20 SLE patients before and after CyA treatment

	Serum creatinine (μmol/l)	% of initial level
Before CyA	89.3±23.2	100%
After CyA		
2– 4 mo.	104.7±30.9 (p<0.005)	116.3±22.4
5– 7 mo.	88.4±24.1	109.6±15.6
8–10 mo.	80.2±22.0	102.2±14.2
11–13 mo.	98 ±32.1	97.5±16.8

sure of >10 mm Hg in four patients. Creatinine levels were influenced in most patients, with a significant increase in the first 4-month period (Table 3). The increase was particularly marked in patients with reduced kidney function (cases 4, 6, 11, 14, 19).

Discussion

In a disease as complex as SLE, it is necessary to try a new drug first in a pilot study.

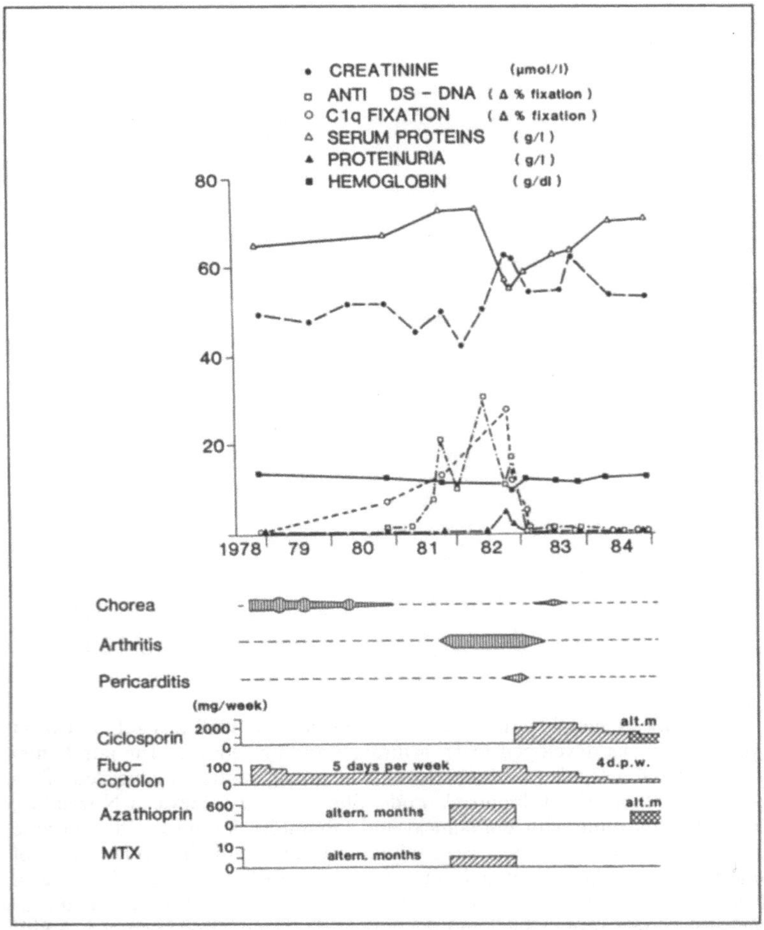

Fig. 2. Summary of laboratory and clinical data of case 8. In this female patient, the first manifestations of SLE appeared in July 1977 at the age of 11, with fever, convulsions, chorea and hemolytic anemia. Large doses of steroids were necessary to control disease activity. Prednisone was given on a daily basis at a dosage of 15–25 mg. At that time, the patient measured 120 cm and weighed 25 kg. In December 1978, an extremely severe Cushing syndrome developed. The girl weighed 33 kg but had gained only 1 cm in height. Prednisone was replaced by fluocortolone, and two steroid-free days were gradually introduced. The weekly amount of fluocortolone was slowly diminished from 100 mg to 50 mg. In addition, azathioprine was given, alternating with methotrexate on a monthly basis. At the end of 1979, the Cushing syndrome had completely disappeared. In one year, the patient had gained 7 cm in height. In 1980, the clinical condition improved further with the disappearance of chorea. In the autumn of 1981, the girl started to suffer from arthralgia which responded well to piroxicam. In the autumn of 1982, the patient developed mild fever. The biological parameters became more prominent. Furthermore, proteinuria of 5 g/l together with cylindruria reflected kidney involvement. Increase of fluocortolone was insufficient to prevent further exacerbation of disease in the form of severe pericarditis. After a 5-day course of i.v. methylprednisolone (500 mg per day), the antimetabolites azathioprine and methotrexate were replaced by ciclosporin at an initial dose of 350 mg daily which was increased to 400 mg (10 mg/kg). The clinical and biological condition improved in a few weeks. A third steroid-free day was introduced in January 1983. CyA was gradually reduced to the present dose of 1200 mg per week (5 mg/kg). During 1983 and 1984, there was a 17.5 cm increase in height (from 136 to 153.5 cm). Since September 1984, CyA has been alternated on a monthly schedule with azathioprine. This patient is at present free of symptoms

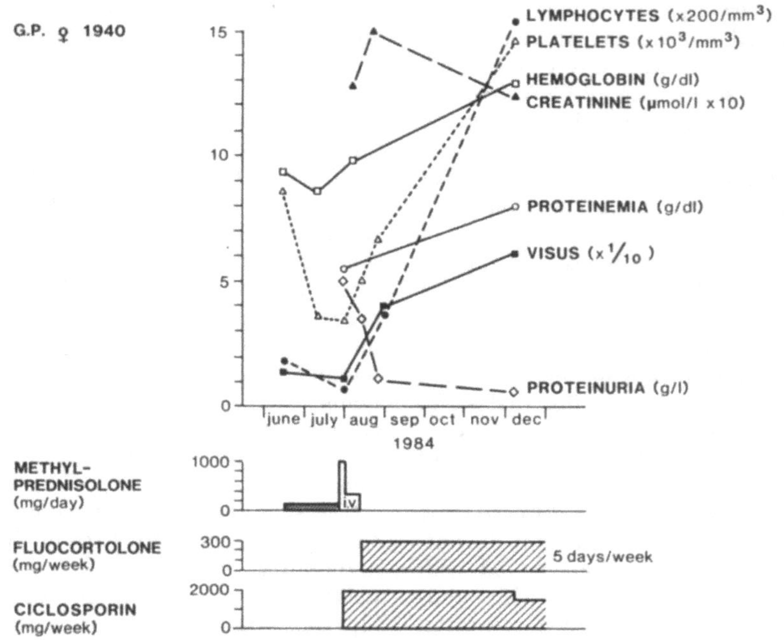

Fig. 3. Evolution of laboratory data of case 13. This female patient born in 1940 has a sister who suffers from rheumatoid arthritis. In 1981, she also developed a similar articular condition involving initially her knees and subsequently her hands, elbows, and finally ankles. Rheumatoid arthritis was diagnosed. In January 1984, she contracted typhoid fever which responded well to chloramphenicol and tetracycline. However, clinical recovery was delayed. In March, she suffered from a slow exacerbation of her arthritis. In May, she became subfebrile and her vision deteriorated rapidly. She was hospitalized in Cagliari, where the diagnosis was made of active SLE with Coombs'+ hemolytic anemia, thrombocytopenia, pleural effusions, severe kidney involvement with elevation of serum creatinine to 224 μmol/l and 6 g/l urinary protein. Following ophthalmologic examination, occlusive microangiopathic exudative retinitis was diagnosed. She was given methylprednisone, initially 40 mg per day, gradually increasing to 100 mg per day. Her condition did not respond to this treatment. Her vision dropped to less than 1/10, and her blood pressure rose to 200/230 mm Hg. Creatinine clearance was reduced to 48 ml/min. Methylprednisolone pulse therapy was started in the last week of July, a few days before her transfer to the Geneva University Hospital (August 1, 1984). I.v. steroids were continued, together with CyA, 5 mg/kg/day. Intercurrent bronchopneumonia was treated with i.v. amoxycillin. The patient improved rapidly with this treatment and could be discharged from hospital three weeks later

While the results thus obtained must be considered as preliminary, they are important as a first assessment.

For the evaluation of combined CyA-steroid medication, 20 patients were selected according to their previous insufficient response to conventional therapy. Some patients were seriously ill. Four had impaired kidney function (cases 7, 13, 14 and 19), but no patient with chronic kidney failure was included. The fact of not including desperate cases has certainly influenced the patients' overall response to this treatment. Indeed, no treatment will have an effect on kidneys which have been damaged beyond repair.

The overall treatment strategy is to achieve maximum benefit in terms of disease control with minimum side reactions. According to this principle, it appeared unjustifiable to try CyA on its own since this would have taken away the proven steroid benefit for patients with severe SLE. Furthermore, the side effects of CyA are such that it does not seem advisable to increase its dosage to a level of marked subjectively and objectively assessible side effects. For these reasons, in all patients we combined CyA with fluocortolone, a derivative of cortisone which produces less sodium retention and less Cushing side effects than prednisone but which has an otherwise comparable mg/mg activity.

The overall results with the combined steroid/CyA medication in this first series of 20 patients are summarized in Table 2. In the majority of patients, the course of the disease was favourably influenced by this treatment. In 17 of the 20 cases, the therapeutic results appeared more favourable when steroids were associated with CyA than when associated with antimetabolites. In the remaining three cases, three months of CyA medication may have been too short a period to ascertain a benefit to the patient.

The effect of CyA-steroid treatment on proteinuria and proteinemia in patients not responding to steroids associated with antimetabolites appeared particularly favourable. The failure of case 11 to respond is interesting to analyse in more detail. After the first two months of CyA-steroid medication, blood protein increased from 49 to 59 g/l with urinary protein diminishing from 6 to 1 g/l. This patient then contracted acute pharyngitis with rapid deterioration of her nephrotic syndrome, her urinary protein increasing to 15 g/l and her blood protein decreasing to 36 g/l. Subsequently there was a slight improvement, but the 3-month urinary protein value is still above the pre-CyA value. This result shows the importance of incidental environmental factors in the clinical course of SLE.

Among the immunological parameters, the antibody titer to native DNA and increase of C3d are good indicators of SLE activity, while the antibody titer to ssDNA appears to reflect the degree of non-specific B cell activation. In 16 patients, immunologic data are available after CyA treatment. In eight patients, there was a marked drop in antibody activity against ds-DNA, and in ten patients the level of C3d decreased. In one case with no demonstrable antibody titer to dsDNA before CyA medication, a low titer activity was detected three months later. With regard to antibodies to ssDNA, eleven patients had a decrease and four an increase, while the titer remained variable in one (case 4). The same trend is reflected in lymphocyte cultures (improvement of Con-A induced suppressor function, diminution of spontaneous in vitro IgG formation). Erythrocyte sedimentation rates diminished in most patients. The overall tendency of patients receiving CyA medication was thus towards an attenuation of inflammatory and immune parameters.

The side effects of CyA were in no case sufficiently intense to warrant discontinuation of CyA medication. In no case did we observe an angioedema-like complication [2]. Those patients in whom we replaced a continuous CyA medication with an alternate-month regimen experienced in general fewer side reactions. Two patients reported a feeling of heaviness in the legs during the CyA months, probably the result of water retention.

Since idiopathic SLE is a self-perpetuating disease frequently requiring many years of treatment, caution must be exercised regarding long-term toxicity of drugs. In the case of steroids, daily medication produces the worst side effects. With two steroid-free days per week, long-term treatment has become possible with minimal side reactions, the main complication remaining cataract formation. We also hope to reduce steroid toxicity with the introduction of CyA since it appears that the steroid-sparing effect of CyA is superior to that of antimetabolites. With regard to CyA, the development of renal interstitial fibrosis in certain patients who received large doses of CyA for more than one year represents a serious warning [4]. We hope to reduce long-term CyA toxicity by alternating this drug on a monthly basis with azathioprine.

Acknowledgements

This work has been supported by the Dr Henri Dubois-Ferrière/Dinu Lipatti Foundation. The authors would like to thank Dr. B. von Graffenried for his continuous stimulation, D. Grossiord for performing computer analysis of laboratory data, and Jean Ringrose and Ruth Preston for help in preparation of the manuscript.

References

1. Borel JF (1985) Mechanism of action of CyA and rationale for use in autoimmune disease. In: Schindler R (ed) Ciclosporin in Autoimmune Diseases. 1st International Symposium, Basle, March 18–20, 1985. Springer Berlin Heidelberg New York Tokyo
2. Isenberg DA, Snaith ML, Morrow WJW, et al. (1981) Cyclosporin A for the treatment of systemic lupus erythematosus. Int J Immunopharmacol 3:163–169
3. Miescher PA, Beris Ph (1984) Immunosuppressive therapy in the treatment of autoimmune diseases. Springer Semin Immunopathol 7:69–90
4. Mihatsch JM, Ryffel B (1985) Effects of CyA on the kidney – animal and human data. In: Schindler R (ed) 1st International Symposium, Basle, March 18–20, 1985. Springer, Berlin Heidelberg New York Tokyo
5. van Graffenried B (1985) Side effects and safety of CyA in patients with autoimmune disease. In: Schindler R (ed) Ciclosporin in Autoimmune Diseases. 1st International Symposium, Basle, March 18–20, 1985.

Ciclosporin (CyA) and Therapeutic Plasma Exchange in Steroid-resistant SLE

R. Bambauer [1], G. A. Jutzler [1], H. Pees [2], H. Daus [2], H. J. Schoenenberger [3], G. Biro [3], H. E. Keller [4]

Introduction

Systemic lupus erythematosus (SLE) may give rise to an extremely variable symptomatology with different clinical pictures ranging from an acute attack with high fever, anaemia, leucocytopenia and thrombocytopenia, arthritis, exanthema and polyserositis to the isolated involvement of organs including the kidneys, bone marrow or joints. Over recent years, aggressive therapy has ensured a continual increase of survival rates. The 5- and 10-year survival rates have been given as 75% and 60% for SLE with nephrotic syndrome and as 88% and 79% for other forms of SLE [9]. In addition to immunosuppressive therapy with cyclophosphamide, azathioprine and steroids [4], more recently the prognosis has been improved by administering high doses of prednisone and by combining therapeutic plasma exchange (TPE) with immunosuppression.

Over the last 2–3 years CyA has been successfully used to treat SLE [1, 7]. We report on 7 female patients with rapidly progressive SLE who, after combination therapy consisting of therapeutic plasma exchange and immunosuppression, were also treated with CyA.

Method and patients

The patients had been suffering from progressive SLE on average for 5.4 years (2–9 years). The diagnoses were made on the basis of clinical symptomatology and results of serological examinations. SLE in all patients was progressive despite highly dosed immunosuppressive therapy with methylprednisolone, azathioprine and/or cyclophosphamide in the last years. Besides immunosuppression the patients were also treated with TPE before CyA therapy. Following a series of 7–15 TPE treatments at 2- to 3-day intervals, additional plasmapheresis treatment was carried out, depending on symptomatology, every 7, 14 or 21 days. Membrane plasma separations were carried out with the Cobe unit or the system developed by us [2]. The first plasmapheresis treatment phase was usually effected using the single needle technique over a large bore catheter [3] placed in the superior vena cava. Periodical treatment was effected via peripheral vascular access points using the double needle technique. The amount exchanged corresponded to 3–4% body weight. The substitution solution consisted of a 3–5% human albumin electrolyte solution and/or 5% plasma protein fraction. Anticoagulation of the extracorporeal circulation was achieved with heparin (2000–6000 U/TPE).

The criteria applied for including a patient in the CyA pilot study and the concomitant disorders observed are shown in Table 1.

All patients were informed of the effects and side effects of CyA and gave their written consent to their inclusion in the pilot study.

The patients undergoing the therapy were administered CyA at 2.5 mg/kg body weight/day (2.0–3.1 mg/kg/day). On the basis of weekly determinations of the CyA plasma concentrations, doses were chosen to obtain a plasma concentration of 150–200 ng/ml. The patients were initially examined once a week, and later examined

1 Abteilung für Nephrologie
2 Bereich Innere Medizin I
3 Bereich Innere Medizin II
4 Klinisch-Chemische Laboratorien: Med. Univ.-Klinik und Poliklinik, D-6650 Homburg/Saar

Rolf Bambauer, MD, Abt. für Nephrologie, Med. Universitätsklinik und Poliklinik, Universität des Saarlandes, D-6650 Homburg/Saar, FRG

1. Progressive SLE	(n=7)
2. Steroid resistance and/or severe side effects	(n=7)
3. Proliferative glomerulonephritis (renal biopsy) Nephrotic syndrome	(n=2) (n=5)
4. Arthritis without deformity of most peripheral joints	(n=7)
5. Central nervous involvement: headache, edema	(n=2) (n=2)
6. Hypertension	(n=5)
7. Liver involvement	(n=5)
8. Pleural effusion	(n=1)
9. Facial erythema	(n=7)
10. M. Cushing	(n=7)
11. Blood sedimentation rate ↑	(n=7)
12. DNA-Ab ↑	(n=7)
13. Circulating immune complexes ↑	(n=5)
14. Antinuclear antibodies ↑	(n=5)

Table 1. Inclusion criteria (1, 2) and concomitant disorders of the pilot study of CyA in systemic lupus erythematosus (n=7 female patients)

I. Laboratory tests once a week	
– Hb, RBC, WBC, platelets	(Coulter counter)
– WBC with differential counts	
– Serum electrolytes	
– Serum creatinine, urea	(Hitachi 705)
– Bilirubin, SGOT, SGPT, gamma-GT, AP	
– *Urine:* 24-h proteinuria, sediment glucose, bacteriology	
II. Immunological tests once a week	
– DNA-Ab	(Radioimmunoassay)
– Circulating immune complexes	(Raji + cell + assay)
– CyA plasma level	(Ciclosporin Ria Kit)

Table 2. Investigations of the pilot study of CyA in systemic lupus erythematosus

as outpatients every two weeks. The following laboratory parameters which were analysed are shown in Table 2 and Table 3.

Initially CyA was administered in addition to conventional therapy. On starting CyA therapy 2 patients were not treated with further plasma exchanges, while the other 5 patients had to be given plasmapheresis treatment at irregular intervals (3–12 TPE).

Immunological markers

Mononuclear cells were isolated from peripheral blood on Ficoll-Hypaque and washed in PBS. For enumeration of T-cells, 10^6 cells were incubated in 200 µl with monoclonal antibodies (OKT4, OKT8, OKT11; Ortho) for 40 min on ice. After additional washings, cells were stained for 40 min with goat anti-mouse antibody FITC-labelled (Coulter).

For enumeration of B-cells, direct immunofluorescence was used with a polyclonal anti-immunoglobulin reagent (Behring) for 30 min.

Cytocentrifuge spreads were made and covered with glycerol containing 25 mg/ml 1.4-diazabicyclo-(2,2,2)-octane. The cells were counted with a Zeiss photomicroscope II with a 40 objective and epifluorescence condenser equipped with selection filters for FITC.

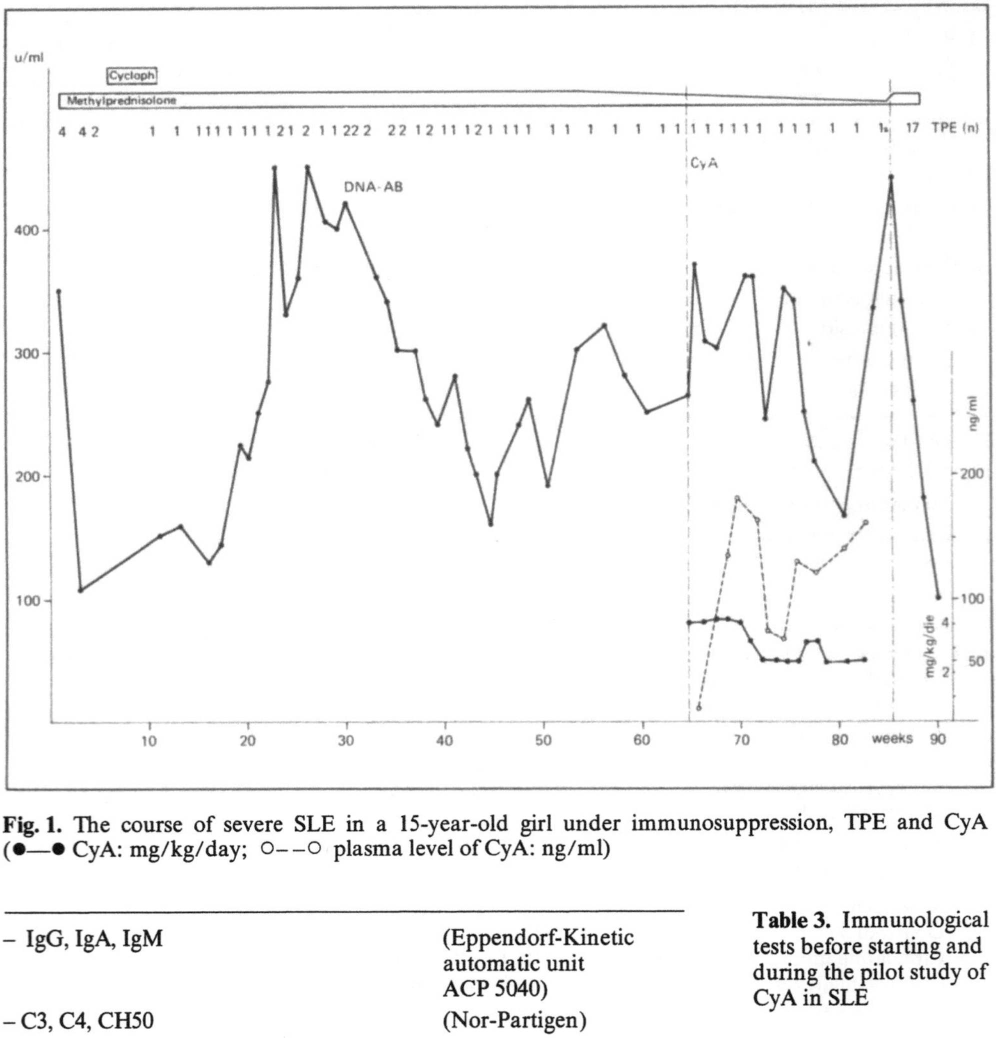

Fig. 1. The course of severe SLE in a 15-year-old girl under immunosuppression, TPE and CyA (●—● CyA: mg/kg/day; ○--○ plasma level of CyA: ng/ml)

Table 3. Immunological tests before starting and during the pilot study of CyA in SLE

– IgG, IgA, IgM	(Eppendorf-Kinetic automatic unit ACP 5040)
– C3, C4, CH50	(Nor-Partigen)
– Antinuclear antibodies	(Immunofluorescence)
– Coombs' test	
– Rheumatoid factor	(Latex, Rose Waaler)
– B-lymphocyte level	(Membrane immunoglobulin)
– T-lymphocyte level	(OKT_3 + population))
T-helper cells	(OKT_4 + cells)
T-cytotoxic and -suppressor cells	(OKT_8 + cells)

Results

The previous therapy of all SLE patients, who had a mean age of 26.6 years (15–37 years) is shown in Table 4. CyA was on average administered over 24.6 weeks (13–52 weeks) to all patients. In 5 of the 7 cases a sufficiently high plasma concentration of 150–200 ng/ml was achieved by administering appropriate doses. In two patients (Nos 4 and 5) no sufficiently high serum concentration could be detected de-

Table 4. Symptoms, therapy and course for the beginning of CyA therapy for 7 patients with SLE

	Pat. 1 30 years	Pat. 2 27 y.	Pat. 3 15 y.	Pat. 4 23 y.	Pat. 5 30 y.	Pat. 6 37 y.	Pat. 7 24 y.
SLE since:	1980	1976*	1980	1981	1976	1983	1981
Symptoms							
– Rapid progression	+	+	+	+	+	+	+
– Renal involvement	○	+	+	+	+	○	+
Nephrotic syndrome	○	○	+	+	+	○	+
– Arthralgia	+	+	+	+	+	+	+
– Cerebral involvement	+	○	+	+	○	+	○
– Hypertension	○	+	+	○	+	+	+
– Recurring pleural effusions	○	○	○	○	○	+	○
– Hepatic involvement	○	+	+	+	+	+	○
– Facial erythema	+	+	+	+	+	+	+
– M. Cushing	+	+	+	+	+	+	+
Previous therapy	Massages	Me	Me, Cy, Az	Me, Cy, Az	Me, Cy, Az	Me, Az	Me, Az
Combination therapy							
TPE	56 (4/83–2/84)	58 (2/81–10/82)	55 (2/83–4/84)	37 (5/84–11/84)	29 (9/82–9/84)	4 (11/84)	17 (7/84–11/84)
HD	–	–	–	–	36	–	–
Methylprednisolone (Me)	+	+	+	+		+	+
Cyclophosphamide (Cy)	+	+	+	+		○	+
Azathioprine (Az)	+ stopped due to leucopenia	+ stopped 1981 due to tox. hepatosis	+ stopped due to leucopenia	+		+	+

[a] Incorrectly diagnosed as chronic aggressive hepatitis, SLE diagnosis since 1981
TPE: Therapeutic Plasma; HD: Hemodialyses

Table 5. Laboratory data in 7 female patients with SLE under CyA and TPE

		Patient 1	Patient 2	Patient 3	Patient 4	Patient 5	Patient 6	Patient 7
CyA therapy (weeks)		52	45	24	12	13	13	12
CyA (mg/kg/day)		3.3± 0.95	2.8± 0.7	3.2± 0.7	4.7± 1.5	4.8±1.3	2.6	2.4± 0.4
	(n)	39	36	23	18	13	13	12
CyA plasma level (ng/ml)		194.4±127	157.6±102	118.7±61.4	35.6	111.2	211.3±121.6	257.9±125.5
	(n)	39	31	14	16	13	8	7
TPE	(n)	12	–	29	8	11	–	2
HD	(n)	–	–	27	–	–	–	–
Methylprednisolone	(mg/day)	17 ± 7.2	20.1± 11	11.1± 2.6	43.4±10.7	32.7	8 ± 2.6	6.8± 4.3
Azathioprine	(mg/day)	–	–	–	108.7±36	–	115 ± 33.8	83.3± 25.8
Laboratory tests:								
Hb	(g/dl)	10.8±1.3	11.8±0.6	10.5±0.6	10.1±0.9	10.1±0.8	11.2±33.8	12.9±0.8
WBC	(/ul)	5168±1505	8600±1672	4524±1080	8100±2315	6781±1515	6710±1987	7320±1905
DNA-Ab	(U/ml)	147.3±35.9	84.5±21.7	321.8±87.1	35.6±3.2	23.6±14.1	18.9±2.4	40.5±1.9
24-h proteinuria	(g)	0.42±0.12	–	4.0±2.3	0.3±0.17	9.2±3.9	–	2.0±1.3

Table 6. Immunoglobulins, complement factors, B-lymphocyte and T-lymphocyte levels in 7 female patients with SLE under TPE and CyA therapy

		Normal range	Patient		Patient 2		Patient 3		Patient 4		Patient 5	
			a	b: 39w	a	b: 22w	a	b: 15w	a	b: 15w	a	b: 13w
IgG	(g/l)	9 – 18	2.5	9.08	9.6	12.5	7.6	4.6	8.55	13.1	3.32	3.32
IgA	(g/l)	1.2 – 3.6	0.7	1.18	1.18	2.1	2.3	1.44	1.53	1.9	0.7	0.7
IgM	(g/l)	0.8 – 2.2	0.63	1.92	1.84	2.08	0.6	0.32	0.43	0.54	0.65	0.32
CH50	(%)	80 – 120	45	50.5	24	48.5	22	–	119.1	167.9	138	141.7
T-helper cells:												
OKT4+cells	(%)	29 ± 8	38	36	24	13	28	42	47	15	15	6
T-cytotoxic and suppressor cells:												
OKT8+cells	(%)	21 ± 7	23	16	27	13	24	28	29	16	18	20
OKT11+cells	(%)	50 ± 10	50	46	–	56	–	–	42	21	35	15
B-lymphocyte level (membrane immunoglobulin)	(%)	5 – 15	18	8	24	7	–	–	8	8	8	20

a: before CyA therapy
b: after CyA weeks

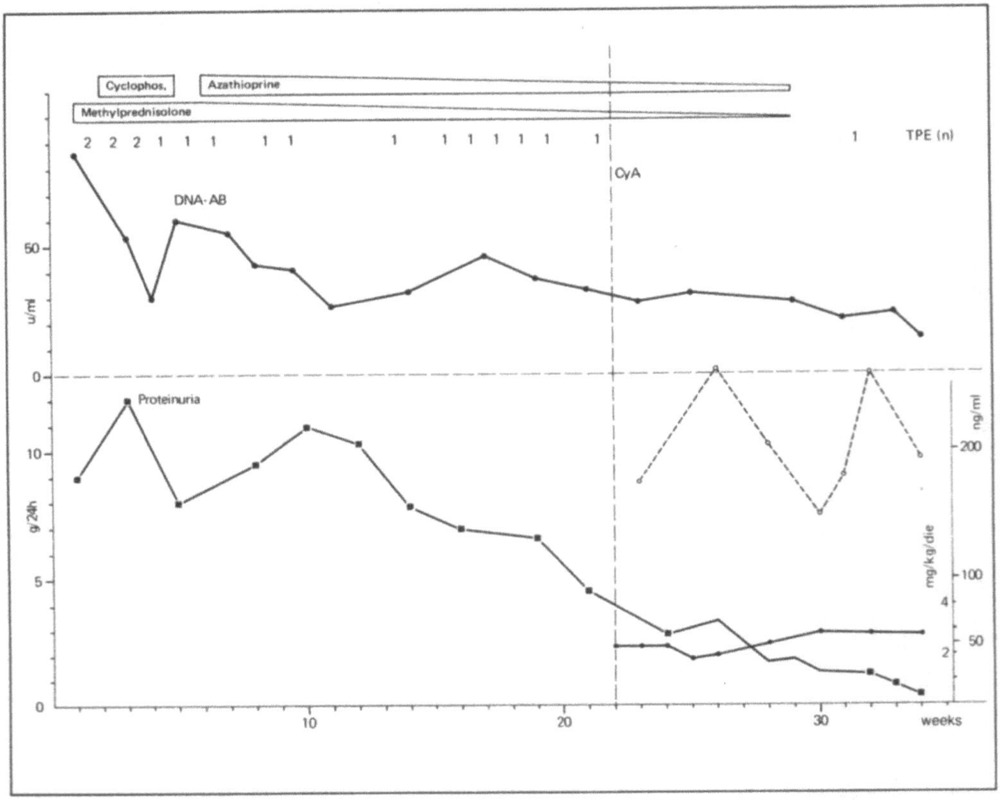

Fig. 2. Immunosuppression, TPE and CyA in 24-year-old female patient with SLE, proliferative glomerulonephritis and nephrotic syndrome (●—● CyA: mg/kg/day; ○--○ plasma level of CyA: ng/ml)

spite their taking CyA twice daily (Table 5). Nonetheless, the SLE symptomatology improved and the administration of methylprednisolone and/or azathioprine could also be reduced.

The 15-year-old patient who had been suffering from rapidly progressive SLE over a period of 4 years, with numerous intermittent manifestations of the disease, died of massive cerebral hemorrhage 24 weeks after CyA therapy was started. In a moribund state she was treated with TPE for the first time in February 1983 during a severe attack of SLE involving sepsis, thrombopenia, leucopenia and sudoriparous abscess. Once the sepsis had been brought under control and a clinical improvement was observed, she was also treated with methylprednisolone and cylcophosphamide. Following this combination therapy the patient could be discharged in a good general condition, free of pain. In September 1983, she again suffered a SLE attack which was once more overcome with plasma exchange.

This patient was given CyA for the first time on 11. 4. 84. Despite regular TPE (12 TPE during the CyA therapy), methylprednisolone and CyA therapy, five months later she had another attack of SLE with increased DNA antibodies, cerebral spasms and rapidly progressive renal insufficiency. Despite intensive therapy including TPE and hemodialysis (HD) treatments the patient died as a result of severe cerebral hemorrhage 23 days after CyA had been discontinued. An autopsy was refused (Fig. 1).

No conclusive statement can be made regarding this patient who, despite initial improvement on TPE, methylprednisolone, and CyA, suffered from renewed SLE at-

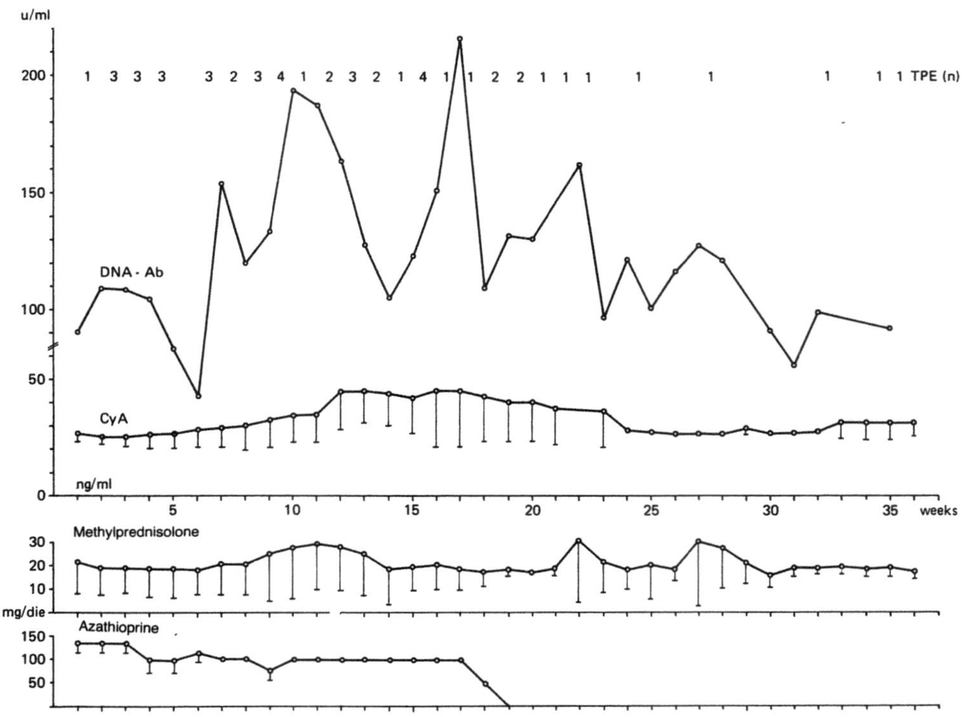

Fig. 3. DNA antibodies, plasma levels of CyA, TPE and immunosuppressive drugs in 7 female patients with SLE

tacks and died following massive cerebral hemorrhage.

During treatment with CyA the methylprednisolone dose could be reduced for 5 of 7 patients by an average of 26–40%. In 2 of the 3 patients who were also receiving azathioprine, this drug was reduced as much as 62%. The 24-year-old patient was able to do without azathioprine and methylprednisolone 7 weeks after CyA therapy was started. Proteinuria, which was between 3–4 g/24 h before therapy was started, improved visibly and was below 0.5 g/24 h 8 weeks later. The other symptoms improved correspondingly (Fig. 2).

The fluctuations of the DNA antibodies and complement factors under CyA therapy were too large to enable any correlation to be established with the therapy (Fig. 3). During treatment the immunoglobulins tended to increase while both T-

Table 7. Side effects during CyA and TPE therapy in 7 female patients with SLE

	Other immunosuppressive drugs (n)	CyA (n)
Bronchitis	2	–
Cystitis	2	–
Acute renal insufficiency	–	1
Leucopenia	2	–
Headache	1	–
SGOT, SGPT ↑	4	1
LDH ↑	1	–
	12	2

and B-cell antigens clearly decreased (Table 6). In 2 cases an increase in the circulating immunocomplexes parallel to the IgG increases was recorded.

The following side effects were registered during CyA therapy: 4 patients suffered from infections with fever, namely cystitis in two cases and bronchitis in another two. These infections improved with the administration of antibiotics. The 30-year-old patient suffered twice from leucopenia and 4 other patients from intermittent increases of transaminases, improvement occurring spontaneously. Only once was it necessary to reduce the dose of CyA. Ciclosporin had to be reduced temporarily for patient No. 2 because of renal insufficiency. The increased LDH and intermittent headaches suffered by 2 patients were related to the primary disease (Table 7).

Discussion

The cyclic polypeptide CyA, composed of 11 amino acids, had a distinct immunosuppressive but not cytostatic effect. Its immunosuppressive action obviously depends on a selective inhibition of T-cell activation, possibly at a very early stage [5]. The main target cell in this process appears to be the helper T-cell, while the influence on suppressor T-cells is still a controversial matter. CyA inhibits in vitro the release of interleukins. In addition, it also blocks the T-cell dependent release of interleukin by macrophages. Potentially reactive T-cells do not therefore mature to cytotoxic cells.

In addition to a large number of autoantibodies detectable in the serum of patients with SLE, a defective cellular immunoreactivity, namely a defective suppressor T-cell function, is also to be found [6]. Whether this defect represents a primary malfunction of the T-cell system or arises as a secondary effect due to cytotoxic antibodies specific for lymphocyte subpopulations is at present undecided because cytotoxic antibodies specific to suppressor T-lymphocytes have also been detected [8]. Multiplication of the immunoglobulin secretory B-lymphocytes in circulating blood has also been demonstrated [6]. Whether this hyperactivity of the B-cell system is caused by the suppressor T-cell defect already described, or whether polyclonal B-cell stimulation is ultimately due to an unknown cause, also remains an open question.

It must be assumed that the selective immunosuppressive effect of CyA is the inhibition of T-cell activation, essentially of the helper T-cells. This is supported by the fact that during CyA treatment we measured a clear decrease in T-cell and B-cell antigens. This was also observed by White in kidney transplant patients [10]. At present we are not able to make any conclusive statement, because neither the type of intracellular antigens nor its clinical significance for SLE is yet defined.

Summing up, the following can be said:

1. An acute attack of SLE can be well controlled by TPE.
2. Intermittent TPE treatment of chronic or sub-acute SLE does not appear to improve with conventional therapy.
3. 6 out of 7 patients did not suffer from renewed SLE attacks during the complementary therapy (CyA 24.6 weeks [$\bar{X}$]).
4. The frequency of TPE could be considerably reduced.
5. The previously required doses of methylprednisolone could be reduced by 26–40% in 5 patients and those of azathioprine by 62% in 2 patients.
6. After only 7 weeks one patient required only CyA.
7. DNA antibodies and complement factors fluctuated widely and showed no correlation to therapy.
8. Immunoglobulins increased during CyA treatment; the circulating immunocomplexes increased in proportion to IgG.
9. T-cell and B-cell antigens decreased during CyA therapy.
10. No conclusive statement can be made on CyA therapy for chronic cases of SLE.

References

1. Bach JF (1983) Present and perspectives of T-cell manipulation in the treatment of autoimmune disease. In: Weimer W, Marquet RL, Bijnen AB, Ploeg RJ (eds) Proceed-

ings, “Modern Trends in Clinical Immunosuppression”. A. C. V. Erasmus University, Rotterdam, pp 53–58

2. Bambauer R, Jutzler GA, Mauch H, Keller HE, Zaun H (1981) Ein vereinfachtes Plasmapherese-Behandlungsverfahren, Technik und erste klinische Ergebnisse. Nieren- und Hochdruckkrankheiten 10:126–134
3. Bambauer R, Jutzler GA (1982) Transcutaneous Insertion of the Shaldon Catheter Through the Internal Jugular Vein as Access for Acute Hemodialysis. Dial Transpl 11:766–773
4. Borsch G, Neumann R, Ricken D (1983) Therapie des systemischen Lupus erythematodes. Dtsch Med Wochenschr 108:792–794
5. Graf N, Marbet U, Müller W, Thiel G (1981) Cyclosporin-A-Wirkungen und Nebenwirkungen bei der Behandlung der chron. Polyarthritis und der Psoriasisarthritis. Immun Infekt 9:20–28
6. Kelly WN, Harris ED, Ruddy S (1981) Textbook of Rheumatology, vol II. Saunders, Philadelphiy London Toronto
7. Le Francois N, Deteix P, Laville M, Zech P, Fraeger J (1984) Treatment of Systemic lupus with cyclosporin A: 1 patient with a 1-year follow-up. Kidney Int 26:225
8. Sagawa A, Abdou NJ (1979) Suppressor-cell antibody in systemic lupus erythematosus. J Clin Invest 63:536–539
9. Wallace DJ, Podell T, Weiner J, Klinenberg JR, Forouzesh S, Dubois EL (1981) Systemic lupus erythematodes-survival patterns: Experience with 609 patients. JAMA 245:934–938
10. White JG (1982) Cyclosporin A clinical Pharmacology and Therapeutic Potential. Drugs 24:322–334

Possible Beneficial Effect of Ciclosporin in Some Cases of Severe Systemic Lupus Erythematosus

P. F. Halloran, E. H. Cole, A. A. Bookman, M. B. Urowitz, and W. T. W. Clarke

Introduction

The success of ciclosporin (CyA) in organ transplantation naturally raises the question of its usefulness in treating collagen diseases such as systemic lupus erythematosus (SLE). Isenberg et al [1, 2] reported five cases of SLE which were treated with CyA with relatively little effect, and with angioedema as a significant side effect. We recently performed a pilot study in which seven cases of severe and potentially fatal SLE were treated with CyA, without angioedema or other serious toxic effects. In 5 of these cases no beneficial effect was observed, and 4 of these patients died. However, two patients seemed to show a response and one had a relapse when CyA was withdrawn. The results suggest that, although CyA in the doses used here may not benefit the average patient with severe SLE, occasional patients may respond and further studies are warranted.

Materials and methods

This pilot study was approved by the Ethics Committee of the University of Toronto. Patients in the Toronto General or Wellesley Hospitals whose disease (diagnosed by the ARA criteria) was considered refractory to high doses of prednisone, and who were in danger of dying on their current therapy from either SLE or infection, were eligible for entry after informed consent had been obtained. Ciclosporin was administered every 12 hours in doses – usually about 8 mg/kg/d – adjusted to keep the 12-hour trough plasma level (monitored by RIA) at 100–150 ng/ml. The level was deliberately kept low to minimize toxicity during this pilot study.

Seven patients were entered into the trial (Table 1). Six of the seven were either very prednisone-dependent (case 3) or were refractory to high-dose prednisone (cases 2, 4, 5, 6, 7). The exception was case 1, in which severe cutaneous herpes from previous high-dose prednisone and cyclophosphamide were considered a contraindication to high-dose prednisone. Five had cerebritis; 5 had nephritis; all were seropositive at some time, although one (case 1) was seronegative immediately prior to ciclosporin therapy. In each case the current steroid dose was initially maintained, then an attempt was made to reduce the steroid dose.

Results

Five patients showed no benefit from the therapy, and 4 died within one year of starting CyA therapy (Table 2). In one case (case 6) the duration of CyA therapy was short (2 weeks) due to emergence of fatal systemic aspergillosis which may, in retrospect, have predated CyA therapy. In case 5 death from sepsis followed 6 months after discontinuation of CyA therapy. In cases 3 and 6, CyA was being administered when a fatal infection was diagnosed.

In 2 cases, some evidence of a beneficial effect of CyA was observed, and these cases are described in detail below.

Case 1 (Fig. 1): This obese female whose mother and sister both had SLE, presented in 1973 at age 24 with arthralgias, nephritis, and positive SLE serology. A renal biopsy confirmed the diagnosis of SLE – diffuse

Mount Sinai and Toronto General Hospitals,
Mount Sinai Hospital
Suite 435, 600 University Ave.,
Toronto, Ontario,
Canada
M5G 1X5

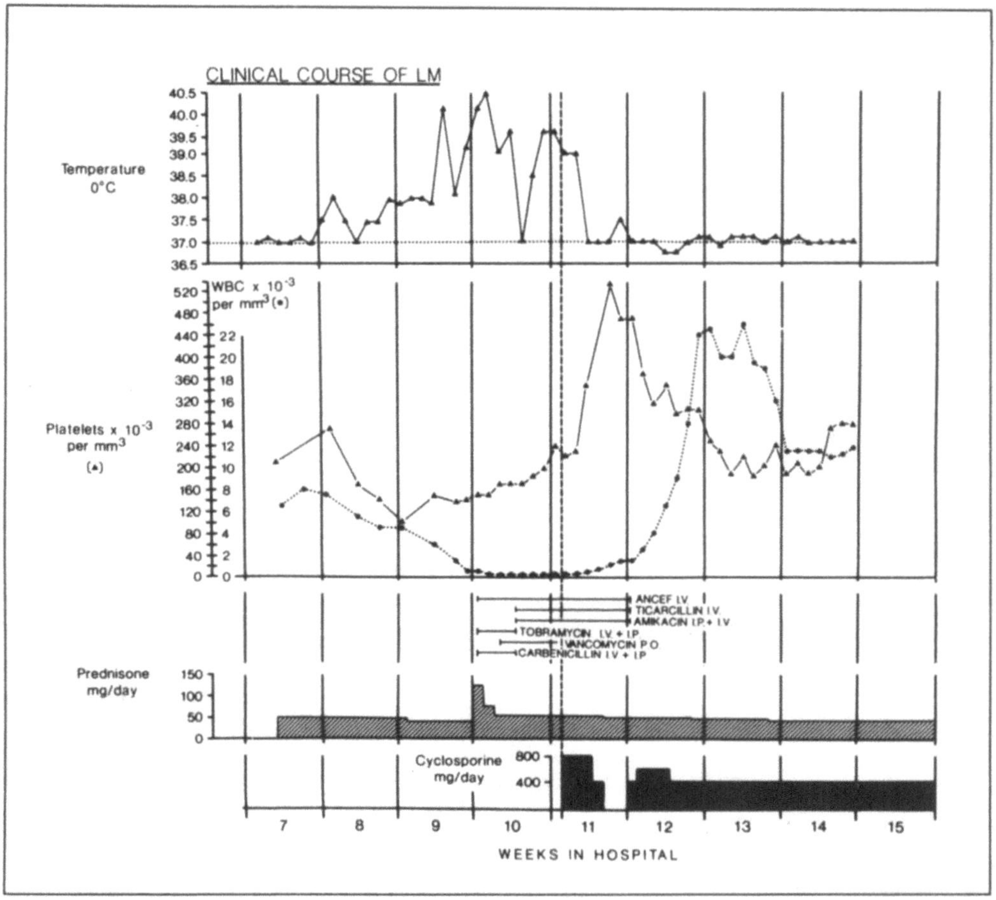

Fig. 1. Clinical course of case No. 1

Table 1. SLE patient data

#	Sex/Age	Duration of SLE	Previous prednisone	Other immuno-suppressives	Serology
1	F 32	10 yr.	++	Cyclophosphamide	+/–
2	F 20	3 mo.	++++	–	+
3	M 64	4 yr.	++++	Azathioprine	+
4	F 37	12 yr.	+++	Azathioprine	+
5	F 31	15 yr.	++++	Azathioprine	+
6	F 48	2 mo.	++++	–	+
7	M	1 yr.	+++	–	+

proliferative type. Over the next 9 years, she developed progressive renal failure and hypertension despite prednisone, azathioprine, and latterly a course of cyclophosphamide, and began peritoneal dialysis. After 3 weeks in hospital her cyclophosphamide was withdrawn and her prednisone was reduced because of large gluteal and perineal herpetic ulcerations. In the eighth week in hospital she developed fever, leukopenia, and thrombocytopenia which persisted despite trials of various

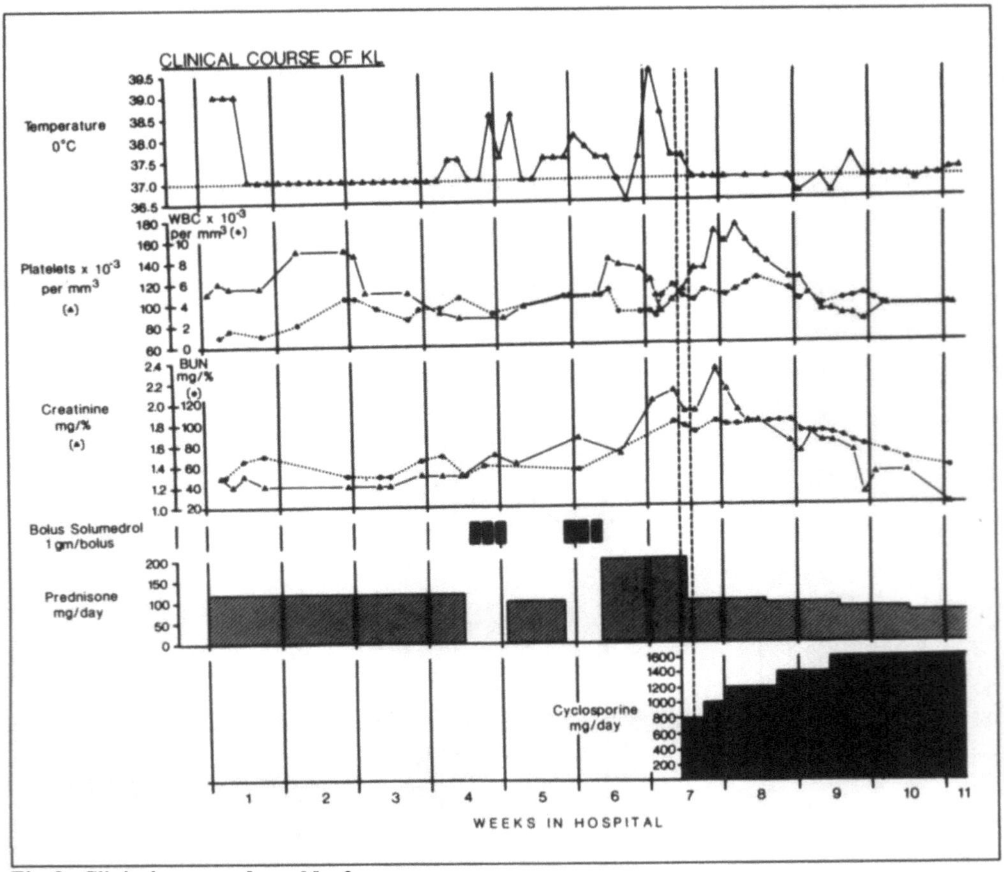

Fig. 2. Clinical course of case No. 2

Table 2. SLE patient data (2)

#	Principal manifestation	Duration of CyA	Outcome	Improved after starting CyA
1	Renal failure; fever, leukopenia	1.5 yr	Acute resolution of fever, leukopenia	?
2	Nephrosis, arthritis, retinitis	2.0 yr	Slow resolution, relapse of withdrawal	?
3	Arthrits; steroid-dependent	1 mo.	Death–sepsis	No
4	CNS, skin, cytopenia	2 mo.	Perforated ulcer	No
5	Nephritis, skin, CNS	2 mo.	Death–pneumonia	No
6	CNS, cardiac, etc	0.5 mo.	Death–aspergillosis	No
7	Nephrotic	6 mo.	Still nephrotic	No

antibiotics until week 11. Blood and urine cultures and viral studies (including EBV and CMV) were and remained negative, with the exception of one urine culture which grew a significant growth of gram negative bacilli sensitive to her antibiotics. The SLE serology was negative, but SLE flare-up was diagnosed as the likely cause of her illness. Because of her severe herpes, additional high dose prednisone and cytotoxic drugs were considered to be relatively contraindicated.

Accordingly, after being febrile for 19 of 21 days she was started on CyA. The fever disappeared and the leukocyte count and platelet count rose. Her herpetic ulcers continued to heal slowly and she remains well on dialysis, awaiting renal transplantation. She was continued on CyA for 18 months, then withdrawn without recurrence. She is currently maintained on low-dose prednisone.

Case 2 (Fig. 2): This 20 year old female developed multiple SLE symptoms in August and September of 1982 and deteriorated rapidly with multi-system involvement, including cerebritis, retinitis, nephritis with nephrotic syndrome, pancytopenia, typical skin lesions, arthritis, polyserositis, and positive serology. Despite 13 g of prednisone or methylprednisolone over a 2-month period her SLE was deemed to be still "active" clinically and serologically in December, 1982. She was started on CyA therapy and required very high doses (25 mg/kg) to obtain blood levels of 100–150 ng/ml. Her daily prednisone was steadily decreased and her clinical, hematologic, biochemical and serologic abnormalities improved. She was discharged and her prednisone was reduced to 15 mg/d. In September, 1983 after 9 months of CyA therapy, her CyA therapy was reduced and discontinued. In October, 1983 she developed fever, abdominal pain, severe leukopenia, elevated liver enzymes, and a recurrence of positive serology. She was hospitalized, treated with high-dose prednisone, and re-started on CyA. She improved in all respects and was discharged. She is currently well in remission with weakly positive serology, on prednisone 15 mg/d and CyA. It is worth noting that her renal function and proteinuria improved on CyA (Fig. 2) and remain stable after 2 years of CyA therapy, with serum creatinine of 120 μM/l (January, 1985) and a trough plasma CyA level of 50 ng/ml or less. She requires antihypertensive therapy, however.

Discussion

There are many ways to interpret this pilot study, and no definite conclusions. This group of seriously ill patients, believed to be at high risk of dying from SLE, represents a severe challenge for the modest doses of ciclosporin used in the present protocol. The fact that infection developed during CyA therapy in two cases raises a note of concern: perhaps CyA can contribute to the susceptibility to infection even when it is not clinically effective in suppressing SLE manifestations. We must point out that the risk of fatal infection was considered to be high without CyA in these patients and we consider that these infections may be unrelated to CyA. Thus our report in general confirms previous experience with CyA therapy for SLE – namely, that the average patient may not expect much benefit.

Nevertheless cases 1 and 2 suggest that certain patients with SLE may be improved by CyA therapy even if the majority are not. Even in these cases, however, the possibility that the observed improvement was unrelated to CyA therapy cannot be excluded.

Establishing a rationale for the use of CyA in SLE is complicated by the lack of understanding of the fundamental abnormalities in SLE, despite the enormous amount of descriptive information available. One possibility which would fit the present observations is that the basic process of SLE is not responsive to CyA, but that certain aggravating factors may be susceptible to CyA therapy. For example, some patients with SLE have elevated gamma interferon levels [4], and interferons are known to aggravate lupus-like autoimmune diseases in mice [3, 6]. CyA is known to inhibit gamma interferon release [5]. Thus we may find that CyA is capable of helping certain patients by inhibiting the release of gamma interferon or other lymphocyte mediators, which may play an ancillary role in some SLE patients, even though the basic disorder in SLE (whatever that may be) is not affected by CyA.

The failure of CyA to help 5 of the 7 patients in the present study does not rule out the possibility that higher doses of CyA alone or combinations of CyA and other immunosuppressive agents such as azathioprine, may be of value in SLE. Finally, even if CyA fails as a remission-inducing agent, the relapse of Case 2 on CyA withdrawal suggests that the use of CyA as a remission-maintaining agent should still be evaluated.

Our conclusions, based on this pilot study of moderate doses of CyA in severe SLE, are as follows: (1) most patients (5/7) derived no apparent benefit from CyA; (2) occasional patients (2/7) may have benefited, however; (3) the drug is well enough tolerated to justify continued studies, perhaps in patients with less severe and refractory illnesses, in order to define circumstances in which a response to ciclosporin is likely.

References

1. Isenberg DA, Snaith ML, Al-Khader AA, Cohen SL, Fisher C, Morrow WJ, Mowbray J (1980) Cyclosporin relieves arthralgia, causes angioedema. N Engl J Med 303:754
2. Isenberg DA, Snaith ML, Morrow WJ, Al-Khader AA, Cohen SL, Fisher C, Mombray J (1981) Cyclosporin A for the treatment of systemic lupus erythematosis. Int J Immunopharmacol 3:163–169
3. Heremans H, Billiau A, Colombatti A, Hilgers J, DeSomer P (1978) Interferon treatment of NZB mice: accelerated progression of autoimmune disease. Infect Immun 21:925–930
4. Hooks JJ, Moutsopoulos HM, Geis SA, Stahl NI, Decker JL, Notkins Al (1979) Immune interferon in the circulation of patients with autoimmune disease. N Engl J Med 301:5–8
5. Reem GH, Cook LA, Vilcek J (1983) Gamma interferon synthesis by human thymocytes and T lymphocytes inhibited by cyclosporine A. Science 221:63–65
6. Rosenberg YJ, Steinberg AD, Santoro TJ (1984) The basis of autoimmunity in MRL-lpr/lpr mice: a role for self Ia-reactive T cells. Immunol Today 5:64–67

Open Therapeutic Trial of Ciclosporin in Systemic Lupus Erythematosus. Preliminary Results in 4 Patients

P. Deteix, N. Lefrançois, M. Laville, S. Colon, P. Zech, J. Traeger

Steroids alone or in association with immunosuppressive drugs have until now been the mainstay of therapy for severe forms of systemic lupus erythematosus (SLE) [2]. Some patients have numerous relapses and severe steroid-related side effects. Ciclosporin (CyA) prolongs the life span of NZB/NZW F1 mice, reducing the level of anti-DNA antibodies and glomerular injury [6]. CyA is known to reduce antibody production against T cell dependent antigens, abolishing interleukin-2 (IL2) production with preservation of suppressor cell activation [4, 5, 7]. For all these reasons we tested CyA effects in patients with highly steroid-dependent SLE to see if CyA had a place in the therapy of SLE poorly controlled by steroids.

Patients and methods

Preliminary results concern 4 women with chronic active SLE, all of them having nephritis. The trial in which 10 patients will be included is an open trial without control group. All our patients were more than ten years old, gave informed consent (parents for children) and had severe steroid side effects without stable control of SLE with less than 0.5 mg/kg/d of prednisone. Exclusion criteria were: uncontrolled hypertension, pregnancy or risk of pregnancy, patients with very severe SLE and bad short term prognosis, non cooperative patients and patients with well-controlled SLE with low dose of prednisone and absence of important steroid side effects. Control of the disease means no clinical sign, no anti-DNA antibodies (negative Farr assay) normal C3 and C4 complement fractions.

CyA was given every 12 hours with an initial oral dose of 9 mg/kg/d, then tapered to maintain 12-hour trough levels of 80 to 150 ng/ml (plasma levels followed by radio-immunoassay). No drug having toxic interference with CyA was prescribed during the trial. All patients received steroids, patient 2 was on chloroquine (300 mg/d) and patient 3 underwent plasma exchanges during the first five months.

Evaluation was based on efficacy and side effects. Efficacy was defined as the possibility of tapering steroid dosage with a decrease of steroid-related side effects without clinical and biological relapses of SLE. Anti-DNA antibodies were measured by immunoflurescence and Farr radioimmunoassay. Other antinuclear antibodies were detected by immunofluorescence, anti-histone by enzyme linked immunosorbent assay, anti-extractable nuclear antigens (ENA) by immunodiffusion, C3 and C4 with specific antibodies and nephelometry. Renal function was checked by blood creatinine and 24-hour urine protein determinations. Side effects of CyA were checked by clinical examination, measure-

Table 1. Case histories before CyA therapy

Patient No.	1	2	3	4
Age at disease onset	26	13	16	13
Lupus duration (years)	7	5	6	4
Therapeutic regimens				
Prednisone	+	+	+	+
Azathioprine	+		+	
Chloroquine	+	+		
Thalidomide	+			
Levamisole	+			
Plasma exchanges	+	+	+	+
Relapses	5	2	3	2
Blood creatinine (μmol/l)	87	66	86	CRF[1)]

[1)] Chronic renal failure

Clinique de Néphrologie, Hôpital E. Herriot, 69374 Lyon cedex 8, France

Table 2. CyA range dose and plasma levels during trial

Patient No.	1	2	3	4
Follow-up (months)	26	14	9	8
Ciclosporin (mg/kg/d)	5 – 7	9 – 10	8 – 9	5 – 6
Ciclosporin trough plasma levels				
(ng/ml) mean (SE)	126 (59)	75 (27)	116 (58)	101 (44)
(ng/ml) median (range)	115 (50 – 285)	75 (40 – 120)	95 (35 – 225)	95 (45 – 210)

ment of bilirubin, transaminases, alkaline phosphatases, gamma-glutamyl transferases, red and white blood count. Heterogeneity of immunoglobulin was determined by isoelectric focusing on thin layer with pH gradient.

Biological studies were performed weekly in the first month, every two weeks till the third month, monthly till the sixth month, then four times per year. Case histories before CyA therapy are shown in Table 1. Blood creatinine was normal in three patients, and one had chronic renal failure with dialysis.

Results

In February 1985 the patients' follow-up period was respectively 26, 14, 9 and 8 months for patients 1, 2, 3 and 4. The CyA dose range and plasma levels during the study are shown in Table 2. Reduction of steroid dose was achieved for the four patients with clinical control of SLE. Patient 1 had SLE relapse after two years, patients 3 and 4 had biological exacerbations after six months. The cushingoid appearance regressed dramatically in patients 1 and 2. At the end of the follow-up period the four pa-

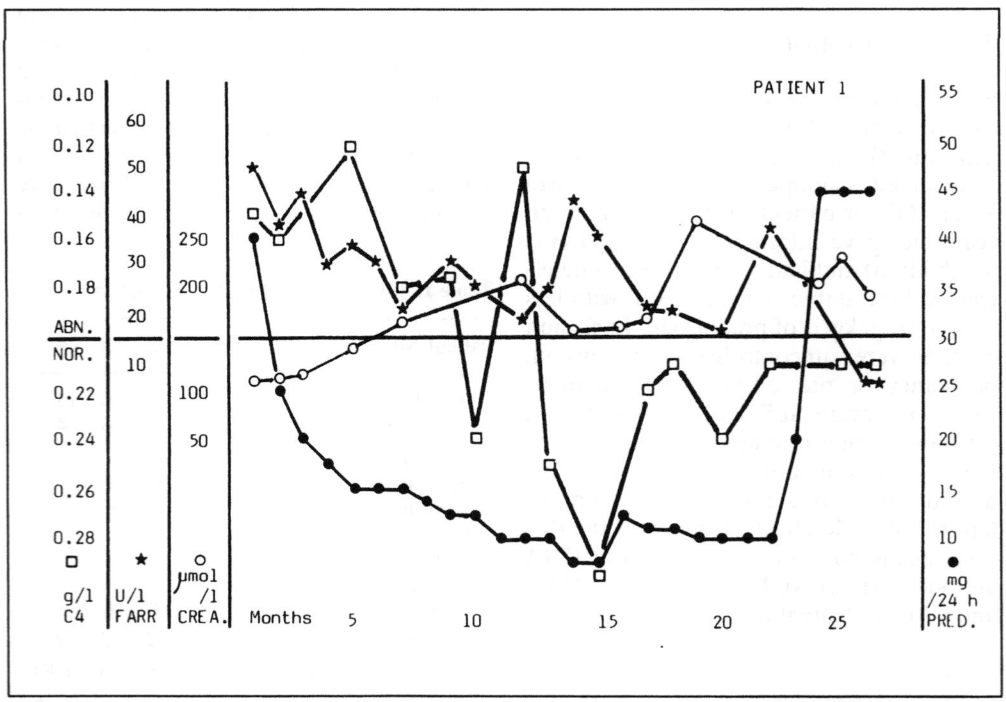

Fig. 1. Biological development and prednisone dose, patient 1

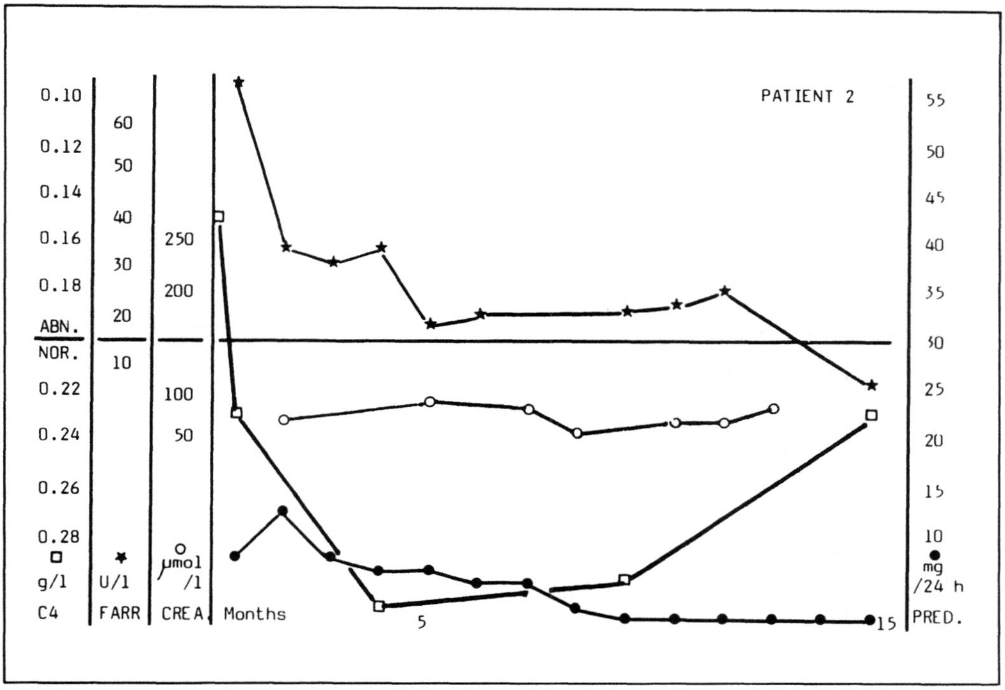

Fig. 2. Biological development and prednisone dose, patient 2

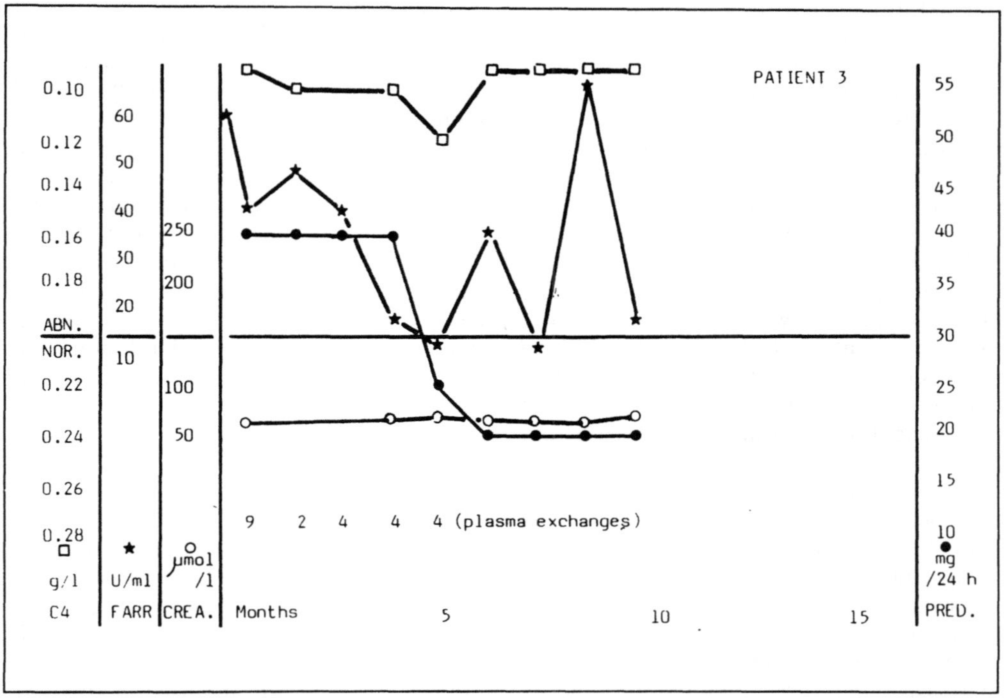

Fig. 3. Biological development and prednisone dose, patient 3

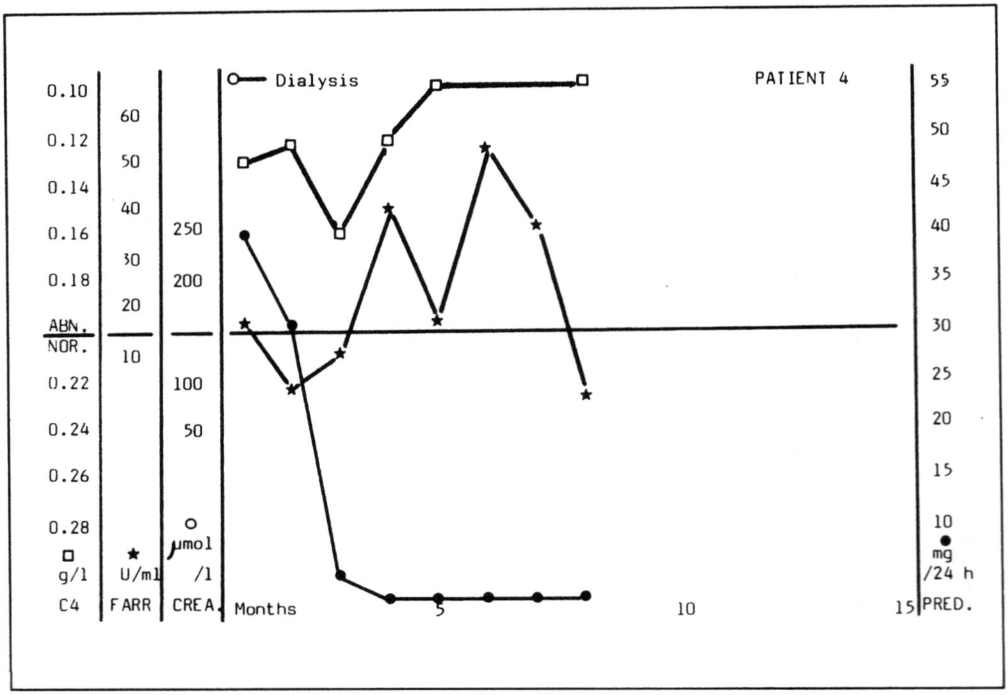

Fig. 4. Biological development and prednisone dose, patient 4

tients had no anti-DNA antibodies. C4 was normal in patients 1 and 2, low in patients 3 and 4. C3 followed the same tendencies. Proteinuria remained absent in patients 2 and 4, and low in patient 1 (0.77 g/d). Blood creatinine remained normal for patients 2 and 3 and went steadily up in patient 1 to reach 180 µmol/l at the end of the follow-up period. Biological development during trial (blood creatinine, Farr assay, C4) is illustrated in Figures 1–4. It was possible to taper the steroid dose to very low levels in patient 1 with a good clinical and biological control of SLE from the 13th to the 23 rd month when relapse occurred, and in patient 2 from the 5th month to the end of follow-up 10 months later. For patients 3 and 4 clinical control was achieved but C4 remained low, steroids for patient 3 still being prescribed at high dose at the end of the follow-up period.

Specific CyA-related side effects were present. All four patients developed hypertrichosis with increased hair growth on limbs and face. Patient 2 had gingival hyperplasia after three months, and biopsy showed plasma-cell infiltration without monoclonality. High blood pressure which was difficult to control and progressive renal failure were observed in patient 1. A repeat renal biopsy was performed after 24 months on CyA. Histologic study showed more severe tubular lesions than in the previous biopsy before CyA therapy. Proximal convoluted tubular epithelial cells were particularly damaged with cellular swelling, hydropic degeneration, micro-vacuolization along the brush border and apical vacuolization. Glomerular and interstitial lesions were more pronounced than on the first biopsy, as were vascular lesions. No other specific CyA-related side effect was observed.

Discussion

Our trial is a first approach to the therapy of SLE with CyA. Experience of past years has shown the difficulty of proving the efficacy in SLE of a drug other than steroids [2]. Our results are preliminary and longer follow-up periods are required to compare the period before CyA introduction with the period of CyA administration for each patient. Randomized trials will also be required. Results of treatment in these four patients with severe SLE suggest that CyA could be an advance in the treatment of SLE as in other autoimmune diseases [10, 11]. Particularly for patients 1 and 2 good results were achieved, with control of SLE and a decrease of morphologic steroid side effects.

Nephrotoxicity probably occurred in patient 1. Tubular lesions seen on repeat kidney biopsy with vacuolization can be compared to experimental and clinical lesions already reported [1, 8, 12]. SLE itself can be responsible for progression of glomerular lesions to sclerosis, and both CyA and SLE nephropathy can be responsible for high blood pressure and progression of vascular lesions. Clinical renal toxicity was not evident (stable blood creatinine) in patients 2 and 3, even if mean CyA plasma levels were the same as for patient 1, but the follow-up period was much shorter.

Mechanisms of action of CyA in SLE have to be specified. A defect in production of and responsiveness to IL2 by OKT4+ cells was recently reported in animals [3] and in patients [9] with SLE, irrespective of the degree of SLE activity. CyA, which by itself reduces IL2 production and possibly the responsiveness of T cells to IL2, could act in another way in SLE. More experimental and clinical information is needed to gain greater knowledge of the therapeutic action of CyA in SLE. This calls for prolongation of the present trial and the development of trials to test which stage of the disease and which combination of drugs, as in transplantation (azathioprin), seems suitable. One must bear in mind the difficulty of measuring drug efficacy in SLE, which is a complex disease with its own development besides the therapeutic effect.

Conclusion

With CyA it has been possible, in cases of severe steroid dependent SLE, to taper the steroid dose without an increase of disease activity in three cases and with one easily overcome relapse of the disease in one case. Renal tubular injury with renal failure in one case was the main side effect. More patients are now needed in order to consolidate these preliminary findings.

References

1. Devineni R, McKenzie N, Duplan J, Keown P, Stiller C, Wallace AC (1983) Renal effects of cyclosporine: clinical and experimental observations. Transplant Proc XV [Suppl 1]:2695
2. Felson DT, Anderson J (1984) Evidence for the superiority of immunosuppressive drugs and prednisone over prednisone alone in lupus nephritis. N Engl J Med 311:1528
3. Fischbach M, Talal N (1983) Effect of cyclosporine on antigen presentation: relationship to lupus. Transplant Proc XV [Suppl 1]:2899
4. Hess AD, Tutschka PJ, Santos JW (1983) Effect of cyclosporine on the induction of cytotoxic T lymphocytes: role of interleukine-1 and interleukine-2. Transplant Proc XV [Suppl 1]:2248
5. Hess AD (1985) Effect of interleukin 2 on the immunosuppressive action of cyclosporine. Transplantation 39:62
6. Jones MG, Harris G, Cowing G (1983) Response of murine autoimmune disease to cyclosporine and thiols. Transplant Proc XV [Suppl 1]:2904
7. Kupiec-Weglinski JW, Filho MA, Strom TB, Tilney NL (1984) Sparing of suppressor cells: a critical action of cyclosporine. Transplantation 38:97
8. Mihatsch MJ, Thiel G, Spichtin HP, Oberholzer M, Brunner FP, Harder F, Olivieri V, Bremer R, Ryffel B, Stöcklin E, Torhorst J, Gudat F, Zollinger HU, Loertscher R (1983) Morphological findings in kidney transplants after treatment with cyclosporine. Transplant Proc XV [Suppl 1]:2821
9. Murakawa Y, Takada S, Ueda Y, Suzuki N, Hoshino T, Sakane T (1985) Characterization of T lymphocyte subpopulations responsible for deficient interleukin 2 activity in patients with systemic lupus erythematosus. J Immunol 134:187
10. Vladutiu AO (1983) Effect of cyclosporine on experimental autoimmune thyroiditis in mice. Transplantation 35:518
11. Weetman AP, Ludgate M, Mills PV, McGregor AM, Beck L, Lazarus JH (1983) Cyclosporin improves Graves' ophtalmopathy. Lancet II:486
12. Whiting PH, Simpson JG, Thompson AW (1983) Nephrotoxicity of cyclosporine in combination with aminoglycoside and cephalosporin antibiotics. Transplant Proc XV [Suppl 1]:2702

The Effects of Ciclosporin in Twelve Patients with Severe Systemic Lupus

G. Feutren, S. Querin, L. Chatenoud, L. H. Noel, G. Beaurain, F. Tron, Ph. Lesavre and J. F. Bach

The treatment of severe forms of systemic lupus resistant to steroid therapy is still unsatisfactory. The risks of the life-threatening manifestations of the disease are not abrogated and chronically administered high doses of corticosteroids generate major side effects. The efficacy of other immunosuppressive drugs (azathioprine, cyclophosphamide) is not clearly established.

Ciclosporin (CyA) is a potent immunosuppressive drug that has been shown to improve the life span of (NZB × NZW) F_1 female mice with lupus [2, 3] and to decrease anti-DNA antibody production in male mice of the same strain. It is also active in a number of other autoimmune diseases. These data have prompted us to initiate an open trial of ciclosporin in steroid-resistant or steroid-dependent forms of lupus.

Patients and treatment

Twelve patients with systemic lupus erythematosus (fulfilling 4 or more of the A.R.A. criteria) were studied in this open trial. All of them had a severe form of lupus, as defined either by steroid resistance (dosage ≧1 mg/kg/d prednisone) or by steroid dependence (dosage≧0.5 mg/kg/d prednisone) for more than 6 months. All these patients showed severe side effects of steroid therapy. The main clinical features of individual patients appear on Table 1.

Ciclosporin was given orally once daily at an initial dosage of 5 to 10 mg/kg/d in 5 cases and only 5 mg/kg/d in 7 cases because of the poor tolerance of higher doses observed in the first 5 patients. The treatment was continued for 6 months at full dosage and thereafter tapered with a 20% decrease every month. Additionally, the dosage was decreased in the case of side-effects or when the ciclosporin blood trough level (Sandoz RIA kit) was above 750 ng/ml. Steroid therapy was maintained with the aim of decreasing their dosage. Prednisone dosage was plateaued after it had reached 0.2 mg/kg/d, a dose known not to induce major chronic side effects.

Immunological methods

Antinuclear antibodies were determined by indirect immunofluorescence on mouse liver frozen sections. Anti-DNA antibodies were assessed by a ^{14}C-DNA binding assay (Farr test). Complement fractions were measured by nephelometry (C3, C4) or rocket immunoelectrophoresis (C1 INH). Hemolytic activity of the serum and C1 INH activity were evaluated by functional assays. Serum immunoglobulins were determined by nephelometry. Anti-erythrocyte antibodies were absent in all patients. There was a false positive syphilis test in one. No circulating anticoagulant was detected.

Blood T lymphocyte subsets were enumerated using the OKT series of monoclonal antibodies. IL-2 production was determined after a 2-day stimulation of E^+ rosetting-lymphocytes by 0.4 µg/ml PHA. Supernatants were tested on a CTLL-2 IL-2 sensitive cell line.

Kidney biopsies were performed before and after 6 months of ciclosporin treatment in patients presenting a proteinuria exceeding 0.5 g/d except for one who had minor coagulation abnormalities and a history of perirenal hematomas at 2 previous needle kidney biopsies.

Service d'Immunologie Clinique and INSERM U 25, – Hôpital Necker, 161, rue de Sèvres, 75743 Paris CEDEX 15, France

Table 1. Clinical features of patients with systemic lupus treated with ciclosporin

Patient #	Sex	Age (years)	Duration of lupus (years)	Clinical manifestations (duration, response to steroids)
1	F	28	15	Right hemiparesis (6 months, CS[1] resistant) aphasia
2	F	32	7	Cerebral vasculitis (2 months, CS resistant)
3	F	19	2	Brain stem vasculitis (3 months, CS resistant) Cranial nerve palsies
4	F	22	1	Diffuse proliferative GN[a] (6 months, CS resistant)
5	F	26	6	Diffuse proliferative GN (6 months, CS resistant) + side effects of chronic steroid therapy.
6	M	36	2.5	Focal proliferative GN (6 months, CS resistant)
7	F	41	15	Diffuse proliferative GN (6 months, CS resistant)
8	F	27	17	Pulmonary hypertension (pulmonary vasculitis) (4 months, CS resistant)
9	F	55	5	Pulmonary interstitial fibrosis (8 months, CS resistant)
10	F	58	6	Pleuropericarditis, arthritis and skin vasculitis (2 years, CS dependent)
11	F	22	8	Pleuropericarditis (2 years, CS dependent) (+ nephrotic syndrome)
12	M	47	5	Arthritis, tenolysis, skin vasculitis (3 years, CS dependent) (+ membranous GN).

[a] Glomerulonephritis [1] Corticosteroid

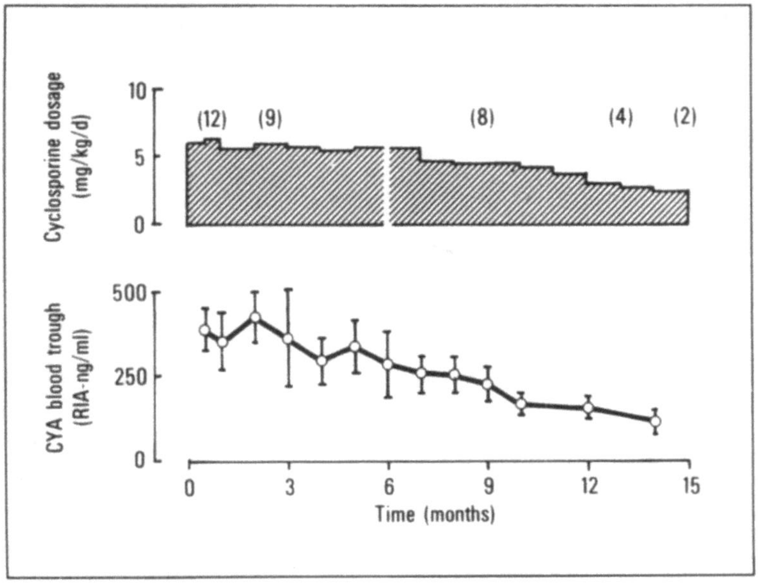

Fig. 1. Mean daily ciclosporin dosage and corresponding mean whole-blood ciclosporin trough level (Sandoz RIA kit) in patients with lupus. Results are expressed as the mean ± SEM. In parentheses: number of patients

Results

Clinical data

The treatment could be administered at full dosage for 6 months in only 8 patients. Mean ciclosporin dosage, duration of treatment and ciclosporin blood trough levels are shown in Figure 1. All but one (# 6) of the eight patients who were treated with ciclosporin for 6 months were clinically improved. Two young females with severe central neurological manifestations recovered completely with a return to normal life. A vespertilio that had resisted steroids and anti-malarial drugs for one year completely disappeared within a week of ciclosporin therapy. One patient with pulmonary hypertension due to pulmonary vasculitis suffering from a severe exertional dyspnea was clearly improved, as was the patient with severe arthritis and skin vasculitis. These favorable results were substantiated by the decrease in the steroid doses (Fig. 2). One patient with lupus-related pulmonary interstitial fibrosis has to date received ciclosporin for 3 months and is improving.

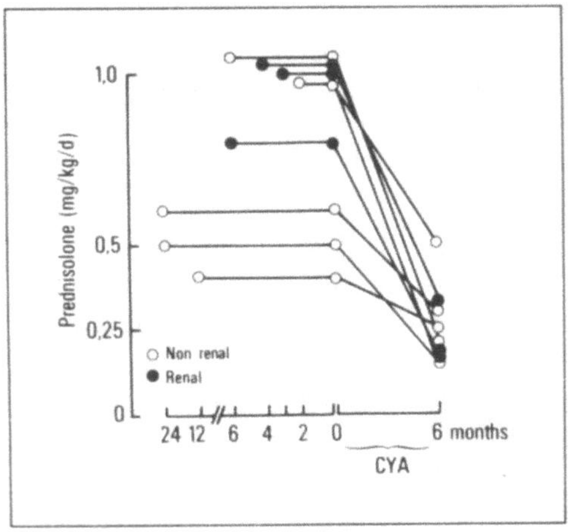

Fig. 2. Time-course of steroid requirement of patients (expressed as mg/kg/d prednisolone) in the preceeding two years without ciclosporin and after 6 months of ciclosporin treatment

In patients with nephritis, biological signs (proteinuria, hematuria) regressed (Fig. 3). Iterative kidney biopsies were performed in 4 cases: 3 had proliferative glomerulonephritis; activity of the disease (as defined by an activity index described elsewhere [4]) clearly declined in 2 patients but was unchanged in one. The fibrosis index remained unchanged in 3 patients (includ-

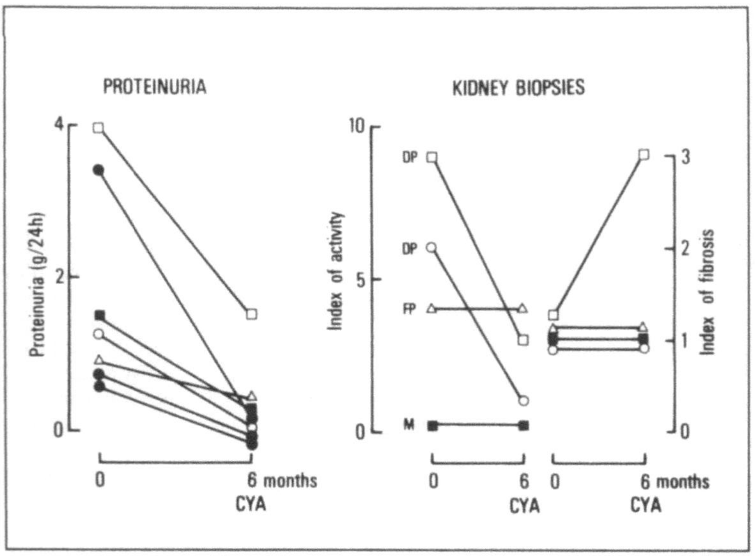

Fig. 3. Proteinuria and kidney biopsies before and after 6 months of ciclosporin. Results of biopsies ar expressed as activity and fibrosis indexes of lupus nephritis. DP: diffuse proliferative, FP: focal proliferative and M: membranous glomerulonephritis. The same symbol is assigned to each patient in the three panels

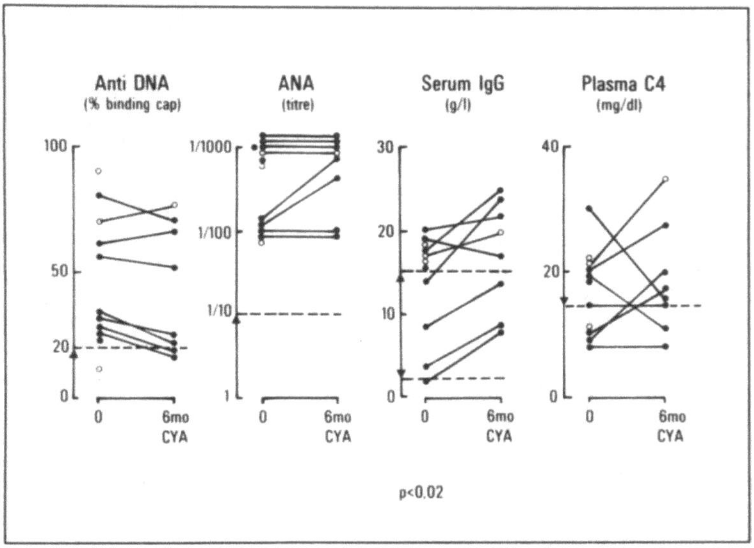

Fig. 4. Immunological parameters (anti ds-DNA, antinuclear antibodies, C4 plasma level and serum IgG level) before and after 6 months of ciclosporin

ing a case with membranous nephritis) and worsened in one (Fig. 3). No vascular lesions were noted.

In 2 patients, ciclosporin was rapidly stopped because of adverse effects: after 15 days in the first patient because of abdominal discomfort and weakness and after one day in the other patient because of facial edema and erythema. In one case, a 2-month pregnancy was diagnosed and ciclosporin was stopped after 15 days.

Limited data are available on the disease course after 6 months when the dosage of ciclosporin is tapered. It is important to note, however, that mild signs of lupus (fever, arthritis, skin rash) recurred in 3 patients after respectively 9, 14 and 16 months, when the ciclosporin dosage became lower than 2.5–3.0 mg/kg/d.

Immunological tests

Contrasting with the clinical improvement observed in most cases, anti-DNA antibody titers remained unchanged; the titers of antinuclear antibodies (detected by im-

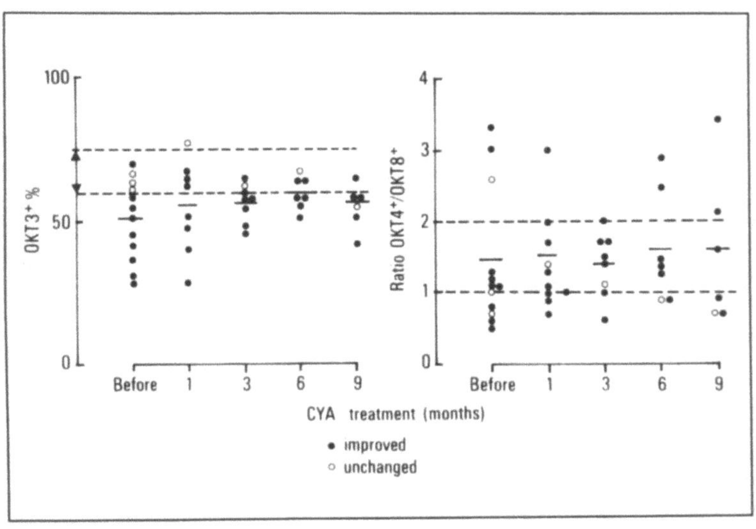

Fig. 5. Time-course of blood T lymphocyte subsets of patients with lupus during ciclosporin treatment ($OKT3^+$: total T lymphocytes; $OKT4^+$ helper/inducer subset; $OKT8^+$: cytotoxic/suppressor subset). Dotted lines and arrows: normal values

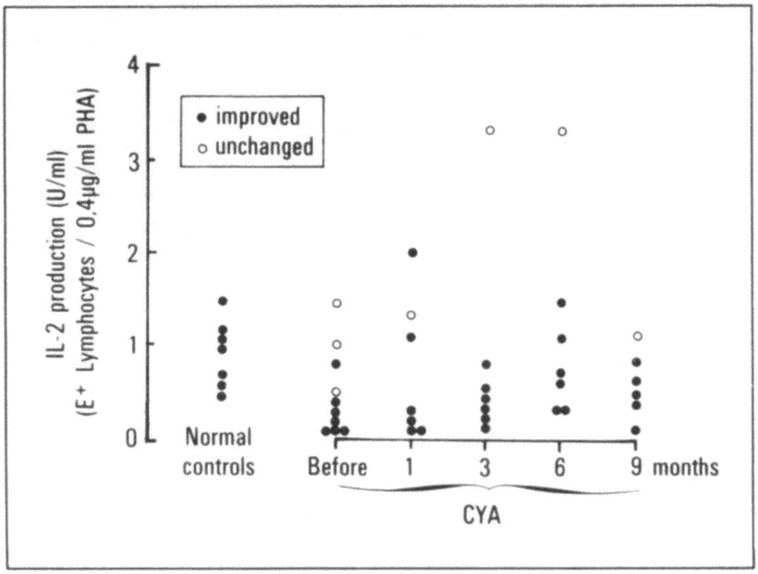

Fig. 6. Time course of IL-2 production by purified blood T lymphocytes of patients with lupus during ciclosporin treatment in comparison with normal controls

-munofluorescence) also remained unaltered. The false-positive syphilis test remained positive in the patient in whom it was initially present. Similar resistance to ciclosporin was noted for the abnormalities of the complement fractions, especially decreased C4 level (Fig. 4). Interestingly, IgG plasma levels were significantly increased at 6 months, an effect probably linked to the decrease in steroid dosage allowed by the clinical improvement.

The initially low percentage of $OKT3^+$ lymphocytes progressively increased with time on ciclosporin. The helper/suppressor ratio, which was initially in the normal range, was not significantly modified (Fig. 5). In vitro production of IL-2 was low before ciclosporin treatment although not significantly. No clear changes in IL-2 production were noted during ciclosporin treatment (Fig. 6). Finally, none of the immunological tests performed was clearly correlated with the clinical evolution. It can be noted that IL-2 production was higher in patients unchanged on ciclosporin than in those who were improved.

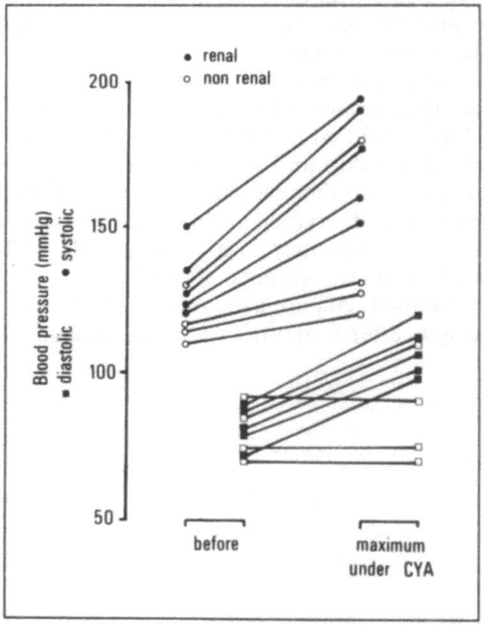

Fig. 7. Maximum increase in blood creatinine observed during ciclosporin treatment and at last determination (after reduction or interruption of ciclosporin therapy) in comparison with pre-ciclosporin levels (HT: vascular hypertension)

Side effects

A transient and moderate nephrotoxicity was observed in 6 patients (Fig. 7). In all cases, plasma creatinine did not exceed a

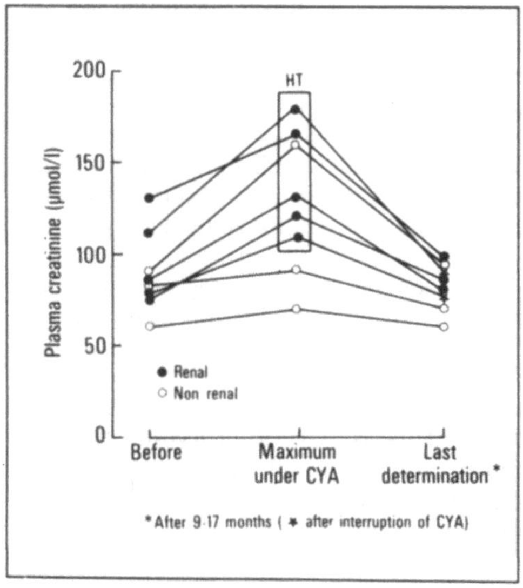

Fig. 8. Maximal rise in systolic (○, ●) and diastolic (□, ■) blood pressure during ciclosporin treatment (before antihypertensive therapy), in comparison with pre-ciclosporin values

two-fold increase from the pre-ciclosporin level (remaining lower than 180 μmole/l). Blood creatinine returned to normal in all cases after the ciclosporin dose was decreased or treatment was interrupted. An increase in blood creatinine was frequently observed when the ciclosporin dosage exceeded 5 mg/kg/d even when the ciclosporin trough level remained in the accepted range. The occurrence of nephrotoxicity did not strictly correlate with the presence of lupus nephritis.

Systemic hypertension was the most frequent side effect (Fig. 8). It was observed in 7 out of 12 patients; 5 of these had never had hypertension before ciclosporin was started. It was completely controlled with antihypertensive therapy and disappeared after the end of ciclosporin treatment. Hypertension was particularly frequent in patients showing nephrotoxicity but was also seen in patients with normal blood creatinine levels.

Other side effects are summarized in Table 2. No significant changes were noted in the levels of hemoglobin (11.8 ± 9.5 g/dl before vs 11.5 ± 0.5 after 6 months of ciclosporin), bilirubin, alkaline phosphatases and transaminases. No modification of the plasma C1 inhibitor (determined serially by antibody and functional tests) was observed, even in the female patient who developed facial oedema after one day of ciclosporin treatment.

Discussion

Data obtained in this limited series of patients indicate that ciclosporin is beneficial in a majority of steroid-resistant or steroid-dependent systemic lupus patients, allowing a significant reduction in the steroid dosage. The heterogeneity of the patients studied does not allow general conclusions

Table 2. Side effects (and their mean time of occurrence) in lupus patients treated with ciclosporin

Adverse effects	n	Occurrence
Nephrotoxicity (reversible in all)	6	1 month
Hypertension	6	15 – 30 days
Weight gain (mild, reversible)	7	2 – 5 months
Hypertrichosis (women) mild	5	2 months
severe	1	
Paresthesias	4	1 day
Symptomatic gingival hyperplasia	2	4 – 6 months
Weakness	1	3 days
Facial oedema + erythema	1	1 day
Epileptic fit	1	20 days
Infection skin pityriasis	2	
warts	1	
sepsis	1	

to be drawn. In most cases, the improvement was assessed on a clinical basis. In 2 out of the 3 subjects with proliferative glomerulonephritis the improvement was substantiated by the clear decrease of activity indexes in iterative kidney biopsies.

Adverse effects were frequently observed. These included mainly nephrotoxicity, which remained moderate and reversible in all cases, and especially hypertension. Nephrotoxicity was observed with doses exceeding 5–6 mg/kg/d, suggesting that higher doses should be avoided in systemic lupus. In contrast to data recently reported in heart transplant recipients treated with high dose ciclosporin, no chronic nephrotoxicity was observed in our patients, as confirmed in 4 cases by biopsies [5]. Hypertension always responded to antihypertensive drugs and never justified a premature interruption of ciclosporin. In contrast to the study of Isenberg et al. [1], no modifications of C1 INH were observed.

At variance with the favorable clinical effect, immunological abnormalities were not corrected: anti-DNA and antinuclear antibodies as well as complement decrease remained unchanged, while the IgG level even increased, probably due to a decrease in steroid dosage.

This contrasting effect of ciclosporin on clinical activity and immunological parameters is at variance with data observed with steroids, which usually induce simultaneously a clinical improvement and a decrease in anti-DNA antibody titer. This does not mean that ciclosporin will not depress anti-DNA antibodies in other cases of lupus, as it can do at high doses in (NZB×NZW) F_1 mice, since the cases studied here represent a particular subpopulation selected for its resistance to steroids. In any case, the fact remains that patients were clinically improved in spite of the persistence of high antibody titers. This discrepancy may be explained in several ways: 1) pathogenic antibodies or immune complexes are not detected by the tests that are currently used: decreased production of such antibodies or complexes could have been missed; 2) ciclosporin acts on immune-complex induced inflammation that could involve a ciclosporin-sensitive T cell contribution and 3) cell-mediated immunity could play a direct (although still unknown) role in the pathogenesis of systemic lupus.

From the practical viewpoint, our data call for a further investigation of the drug's effect in the disease. Our globally favorable result could prompt studies in a wider range of indications in patients with less advanced disease. Ciclosporin could thus be tried in cases of initial steroid dependence where the disease recurs as soon as steroid dosage is lowered.

Acknowledgments

We wish to thank Pr. J. Dormont, Pr. P. Godeau and Pr. M. F. Kahn for clinical cooperation.

References

1. Isenberg DA, Snaith ML, Al-Khader AA, Cohen SL, Fisher C, Morrow WJW, Mowbray J (1980) Cyclosporin relieves arthralgia, causes angioedema. N Engl J Med 303:754
2. Israel-Biet D, Noel LH, Bach MA, Dardenne M, Bach JF (1983) Marked reduction of DNA antibody production and glomerulopathy in thymulin (FTS-Zn) or cyclosporin A treated (NZB×NZW) F1 mice. Clin Exp Immunol 54:359
3. Jones MG, Harris G, Cowing G (1983) Response of murine autoimmune disease to cyclosporine and thiols. Transplant Proc 15 [Suppl 1]:2904
4. Morel-Maroger L, Mery JPH, Droz D, Godin M, Verroust P, Kourilsky O, Richet G (1976) The course of lupus nephritis. Contribution of serial renal biopsies. Adv Nephrol 6:79
5. Myers BD, Ross J, Newton L, Luetscher J, Perlroth M (1984) Cyclosporine-associated chronic nephropathy. N Engl J Med 311:699

Ciclosporin and Autoimmune Disease – an Overview

C. R. Stiller, London/CAN

We have been treated this week to a tantalizing smorgasbord of acute and chronic inflammatory diseases (generally grouped under 'suspected autoimmune diseases') which, with one exception, has been a very selective and anecdotal sampling from a very large menu. Some of these anecdotal studies have impressed on us that we have seen an effect of ciclosporin, and encourage us to go back for more. And to complete the analogy, I have to tell you that some of them have only left a bad taste in our mouths! Overall however, the scientists looking at autoimmune diseases in the human would like to ask the question: "Does ciclosporin cause a significant change in the immune response relevant to the disease?" (Fig. 1). But, as we have seen, in most of these disorders we have a 'black box phenomenon' – that is, we are studying diseases in which the primary clinical measurements are those of effects of inflammation, but for which in the majority of cases we do not know the relevant immune responses or have no reliable in vitro measurements of them. These papers also tell us that we probably know less about the relevant immune responses than we thought we knew prior to these studies. For example, most of us believe systemic lupus erythematosus is an antigen-antibody mediated disease, that the T cell has little role in the process, and that the agent ciclosporin really shouldn't have any impact on the disease. Yet CyA alters the disease process, at least in the mouse, and possibly in the human. Because we don't know the relevant immune response in most of these

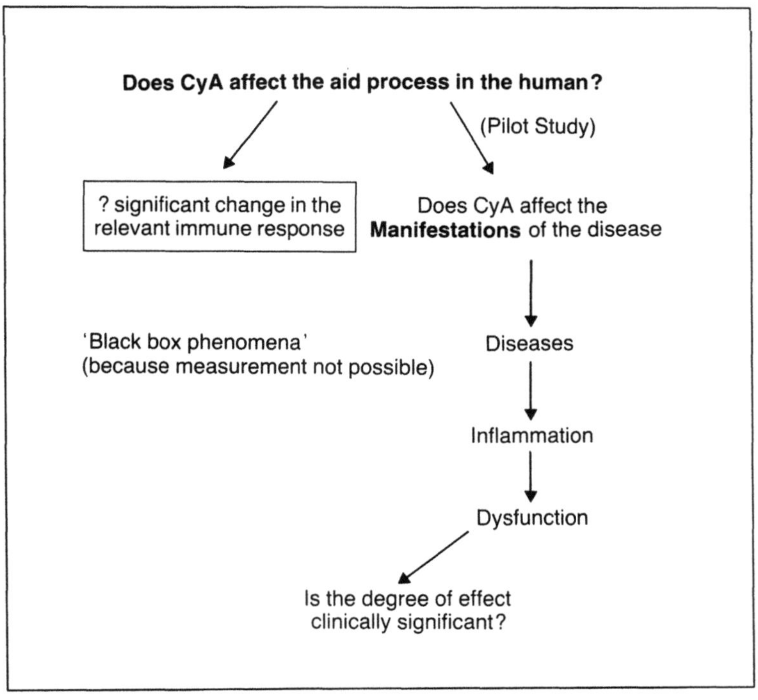

Fig. 1. Does CyA affect the autoimmune disease process in the human?

diseases we have to ask a more primitive question: "Does ciclosporin affect the manifestations of the disease in the patient?" And I should underscore the fact that we are talking about clinical *effect*. We are not talking about benefit! There have been no studies presented which talk about benefit, except in the short term. On the basis of the study presented by Masuda I can say, with confidence, that ciclosporin affects the uveitis of Behçet's disease. That was clear from the studies presented, but nobody would claim to know whether it benefits the patient in the long term because that study hasn't been done. I would caution all of the investigators that we should not rush into studies that ask the question of benefits, even though our colleagues want to know that answer, and certainly the regulatory agencies and fund-granting bodies are anxious to address that problem. But until we know whether the agent *affects* manifestations of the disease it is not possible for us to go on and design *benefit* trials: the clinical and laboratory measurements may be different, the number of requirements is usually different, and the length of study, particularly in these diseases, is significantly different.

If our pilot studies suggest that ciclosporin has affected the manifestation of disease then, as clinical scientists, we have to ask the hard question: "Is the degree of effect seen clinically significant?" and be very honest with ourselves in this regard. This whole process would, of course, be different if we had the ability to measure a significant change in the relevant immune response, but so often that eludes us and so we are left at the level of testing a clinically significant effect. With acute disease it is not such a problem. If a patient is dying of myasthenia gravis and ciclosporin is administered and in a small trial they get dramatically well – then we have a definite immediate risk/benefit ratio that can be quantified. But it is very different in the primary diseases that we have largely studied up to this point with ciclosporin (Fig. 2). These diseases take their toll in life over a long period, and because we don't know the long-term risk of ciclosporin therapy we are calculating the risk of therapy versus risk of disease in the short term (really a risk/risk ratio, not a risk/benefit ratio). But we are dealing largely with chronic diseases in these studies, and the decremental deterioration as a result of the disease is in general a slow one. On the other side of the ledger, it has been proposed by Myers that the risk of the therapy is also a slow one. So this is the toughest

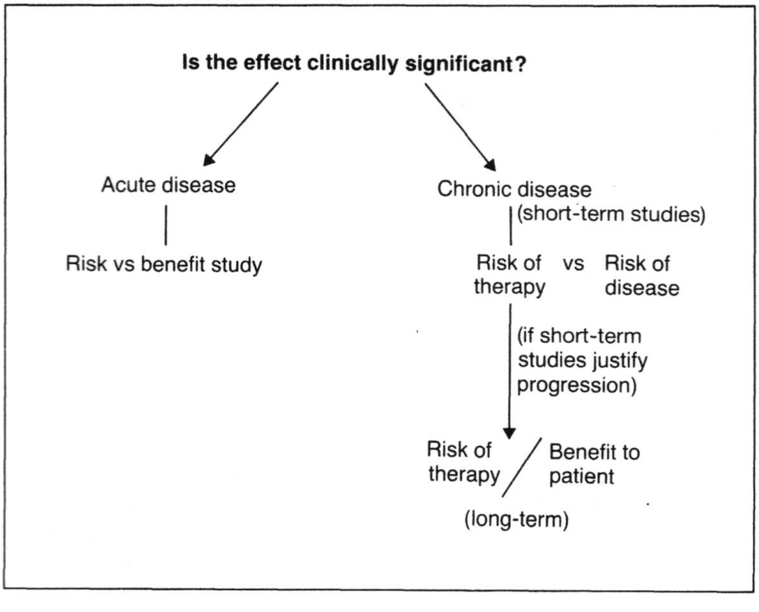

Fig. 2. Is the degree of effect clinically significant?

measure of the therapy: "Is there a significant improvement in the risk/benefit ratio in the long term?"

Site of action of ciclosporin

The classical, or generally understood, concept of how ciclosporin effects its action is at the level of the T helper cell. This is based on fundamental work carried out by Borel and others to demonstrate that the T helper cell is shifted to a resting phase in the presence of ciclosporin. The implication of this in the transplant situation is that ciclosporin is of benefit in preventing and arresting T helper cell dependent responses in their initiation. Although it is now generally appreciated that ciclosporin terminates T helper cell dependent reactions by inhibiting interleukin 2 production on the one hand and B cell growth factors on the other, it also inhibits and terminates the production of all lymphokines. The rationale for using ciclosporin in autoimmune disease was to choose those diseases that were clearly cell-mediated, and for which ciclosporin would probably have an effect similar to that in transplanation. What wasn't generally appreciated, (although it had been clearly pointed out by Borel in earlier work) and which is evident in these clinical papers, is that ciclosporin is a very important anti-inflammatory agent (Fig. 3). This lymphokine-dependent inflammation is 'down stream' from the T helper cell, and the effects seen clinically may be abrupt, or may have a certain lag-time before becoming apparent. We have seen in these papers dramatic evidence of cessation of active inflammation, but few observations that would suggest a fundamental change in the immune response – that is, immunosuppression. That is not to say that it hasn't occurred – it is just that most of the measurements reported are reflections of inflammation and disease rather than measurements of immune function.

On cessation of ciclosporin therapy it would appear that the immune response 'picks up where it left off'. As someone noted, almost as if the network had had an opportunity to clear itself, and the immune response has been held in suspended animation, the inflammation evidences itself within a very short period of time after discontinuation of ciclosporin. In an odd sort of way, the proof of the effect of ciclosporin on these diseases was that, on removal of the drug, the inflammatory response oc-

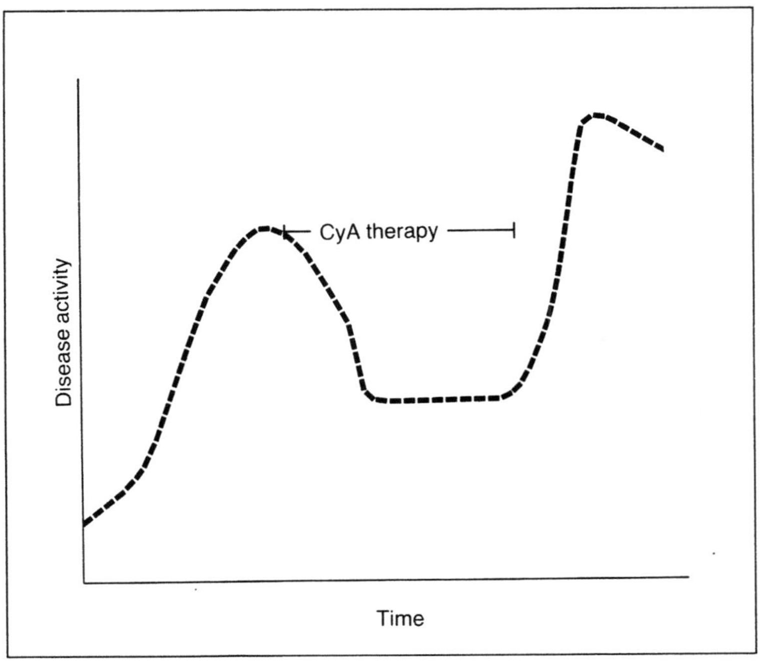

Fig. 3. Recurrence of inflammation after discontinuation of CyA

curred in an accelerated way. This appeared to be true in both the diabetes and uveitis story, for example.

Natural history of disease and immunosuppressive therapy

To reiterate, in these studies the primary measurement of activity of the disease is inflammation, not measured immune responses. Diseases that have been examined here are diseases which have had inflammation present intermittently or continuously for months to years, with which there is an increasing disability. Figure 4 demonstrates that with each wave of inflammation there is a progressive and irreversible disability. In the measurement of the effects of an anti-inflammatory or immunosuppressive agent, we are interested in the ability both to reverse inflammation and to maintain quiescence. In an individual with a small amount of background disability (in say a joint, or the kidney, or in the islets of the pancreas), the fluctuation in function that occurs with inflammation is easily seen. However, with time, the background disability increases and the ability to demonstrate reversibility or effect becomes more and more difficult. These studies represented here are studies that have largely been conducted at the terminal part of a chronic disorder in which the degree of disability is very great. With the residual function so small, it would be virtually impossible to have demonstrated a therapeutic *benefit,* and even to demonstrate an *effect* where the 'background noise' is so high is very difficult. A prime example of this was the study on the SLE and rheumatoid arthritic patients. Should we in lupus, for example, be examining a phase where the background noise is not so great and where the degree of residual function is such that, in fact, we can ultimately determine benefit? I think that is the approach that must be taken. The only consideration that would preclude it is if the therapy is too risky.

How risky is the treatment? (Fig. 5). In terms of *host defence,* I think we have all been pleasantly surprised that ciclosporin is not that risky. The Canadian Study showed that in transplantation the incidence of infections in the transplant recipients treated with ciclosporin was less frequent than in

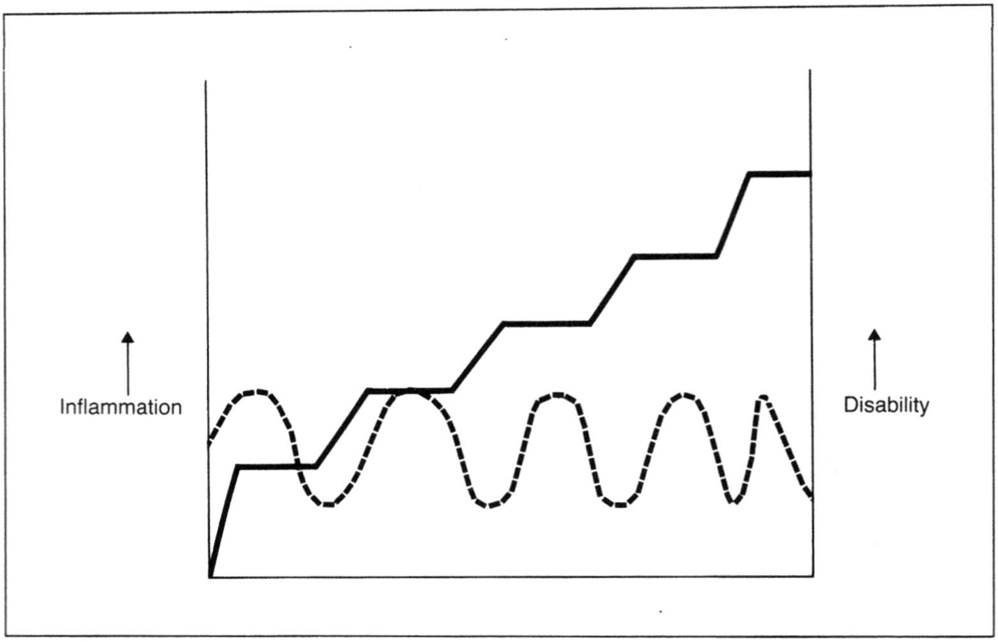

Fig. 4. Progression of disability with recurrent episodes of inflammation in chronic inflammatory disease

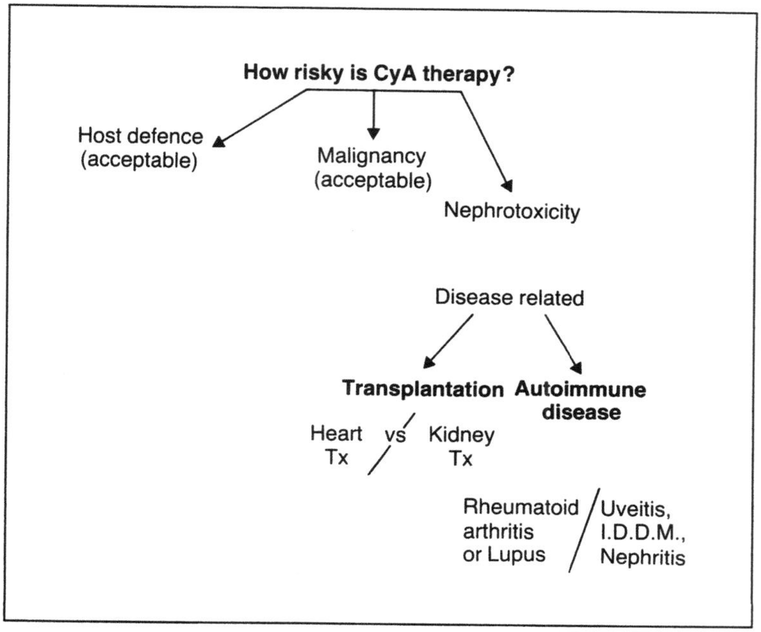

Fig. 5. Assessment of risk with CyA therapy

those treated with azathioprine or prednisone, and much less than in those treated with ALG. The studies in autoimmune disease have been surprisingly free of complicating infections, and indeed in the diabetes study, children went through varicella and herpes zoster infections without difficulty. In terms of *malignancy,* it is recognized that over-immunosuppression will result in an increased incidence of malignancy. But the use of ciclosporin is more judicious than it once was, and in patients not treated with multiple immunosupressive therapy, lymphoma and other cancers have not been a problem, to date. It would be wrong for us to believe that malignancy will not occur at some time but I suspect this will occur in individuals who are on ciclosporin (possibly with reasonable measured ciclosporin levels) but who are over-immunosuppressed if the degree of immunosuppression is measured. The primary risk, of course, is *nephrotoxicity* and this remains with us as a problem in both the short and the long term. These autoimmune studies have demonstrated that the observations made with regard to nephrotoxicity in the transplants probably hold here as well. That is, certain risk factors increase the likelihood of drug toxicity and nephrotoxicity. In the transplant it is preexisting renal ischemia. In heart and liver transplants, ciclosporin is more toxic than in kidney transplants. We now know, in terms of some of the reports contained here, that ciclosporin is more toxic in rheumatoid arthritis than other disorders, probably because of the use of non-steroidal anti-inflammatory drugs (NSAID), but I would caution that this is not definitely known. Rat models would suggest it, and until further evidence to the contrary is presented, NSAID and ciclosporin shouldn't be mixed. There also appears to be some increased manifestation of toxicity in certain disease states such as the presentation in lupus. The reports of the side effects were not in keeping with the ones seen in the uveitis or diabetes mellitus studies. I don't know why that is. Perhaps it is because the primary toxicity of ciclosporin is at the level of the endothelium and any disease process which, in fact, has a primary vascular phenomenon as part of its pathogenesis is a 'set-up' for its toxic effect. En passant, I would point out that ciclosporin has not been shown to promote fibrosis but, rather, indirectly to cause fibrosis. There is an important difference. What ciclosporin does is to have an effect on vascular supply leading to ischemia and, in the kidney, nephron drop-out and interstitial fibrosis. Fibrosis is probably relative to the ischemia so I think we need to be very careful in studying disorders where there is a vascular component. In those situations ciclosporin should be used with care, and in the absence of additional risk factors. The suprising thing, and I think the most exciting report contained in these studies, is the effect of ciclosporin on glomerulonephritis – an area where we didn't think the difference between the potential risk and the benefit would be great enough for us to pursue studies. In fact, CyA seems to have a demonstrable short-term effect on the renal disease and if any study should be aggressively pursued in a properly designed trial, it should be this one.

Pattern of autoimmune disease

In studying these autoimmune diseases it is important to understand the natural history or 'pattern' of the disease. I think it is important for us to classify the disease we are studying with respect to its clinical pattern, for purposes of discussion, with no claim that this is anything but a classification to facilitate the designing of immunosuppressive therapy. I would do this on the basis of three patterns.

Pattern I (Fig. 6) would be those diseases in which there is an explosive onset with a great deal of inflammation, and a rapid loss in most cases of end organ functions, with little chance of recovery over the shorter period. The time interval would vary according to the disease, the age of the patient, and the genetic background. We are considering here interventional immunosuppressive therapy and if the disease is of this pattern then the approach to immunosuppresive therapy is not dissimilar to the approach to the induction of immunosuppression that you use in graft rejection. In this situation you have a relatively short time in which to 'make your move'.

The second pattern of autoimmune disease (Fig. 7) is one in which, over a long period, there is a chronic inflammatory disorder in which there is a slow loss of function. One may take issue with my as-

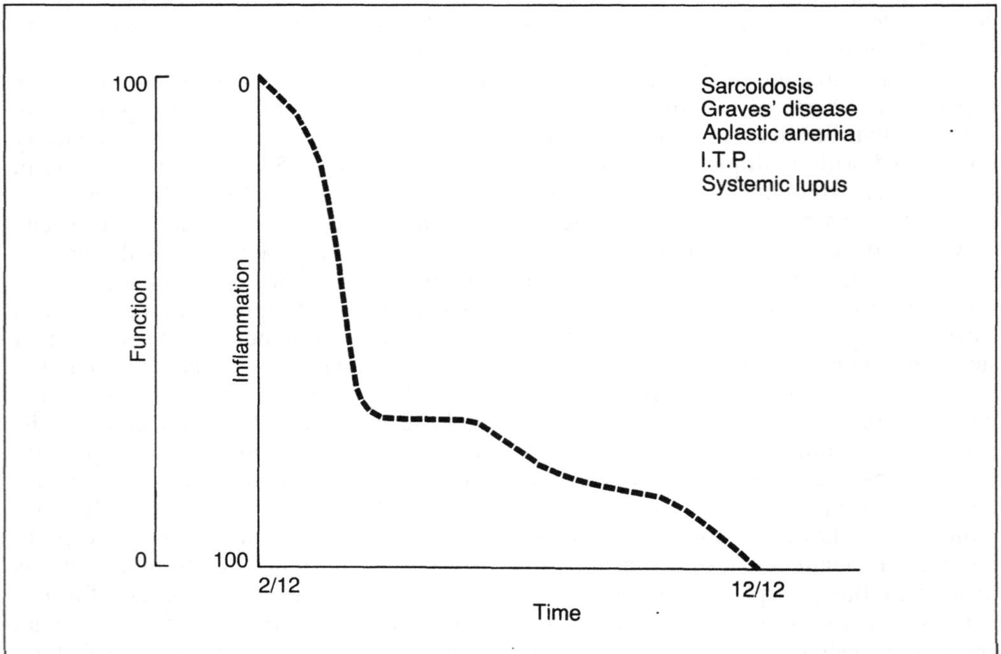

Fig. 6. Pattern I autoimmune disease

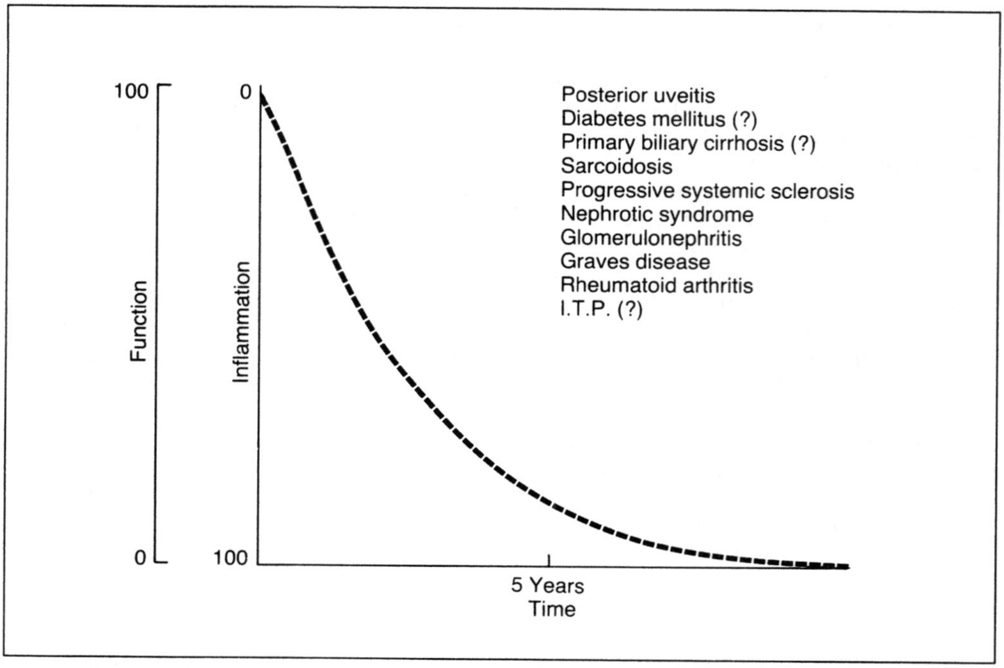

Fig. 7. Pattern II autoimmune disease

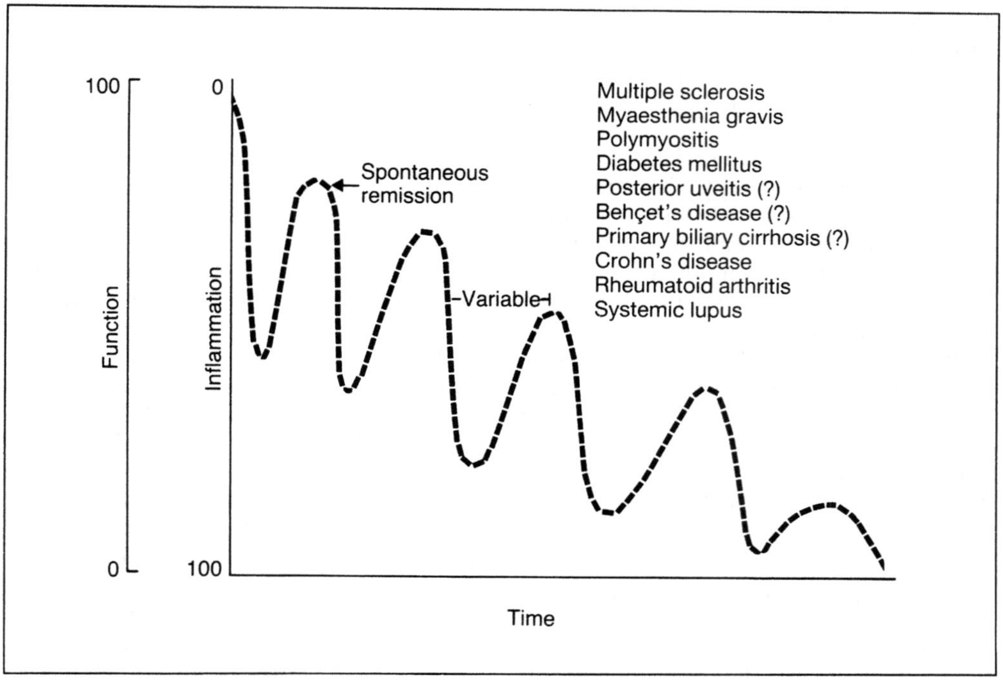

Fig. 8. Pattern III autoimmune disease

signment of certain diseases to these different patterns. For example Eisenbarth would put IDDM in Pattern II. I happen to think it is not, but would be more typical of Pattern III. The approach to designing immunosuppressive intervention in this kind of disease is different from that for Pattern I. In this pattern, one doesn't have to reach therapeutic levels of immunosuppression by ciclosporin in the first few days. One doesn't have to run the risk of 'over-shooting' therapeutic levels into toxic ranges and end up with toxic manifestations of the drug. One must think in terms of the chronicity of the disease, and measure the effect on the disease on the basis of preserved function and, secondarily, on evidence of reduced chronic inflammation.

Pattern III (Fig. 8) is a pattern of relapsing/remitting disease which may, on the surface, look like the same course as Pattern II but is in fact one of remission and recrudescence. If the target organ is a surface tissue in which pain and inflammation can be seen, as in rheumatoid arthritis, then the relapsing/remitting undulations of the disease can been seen. If, on the other hand, it is 'black box disease' like multiple sclerosis or diabetes mellitus, then it may look like a chronic loss, as in Pattern II, when in fact there are spontaneous remissions occurring. This Pattern III suggests that there is alternating autoimmunity/autoregulation etc. If this is the case, then one must bear in mind, in designing the interventional therapy, that autoregulation does occur spontaneously and is the state that we, in fact, want to capture. We want to prevent autoimmunity and we want to preserve autoregulation. I happen to think that diabetes mellitus is in this category and that interventional therapy is associated with a fairly large degree of potential recovery. Depending upon the periodicity, it may be necessary to use an induction type of immunosuppression regimen, converting to a maintenance type of therapy once remission is obtained.

Designing immunosuppressive strategies

In considering these different patterns of autoimmune disease there are fundamental differences in the strategic approach to a) induction immunosuppressive therapy, b) maintenance immunosuppression, and c) promotion of autoregulation. Can one induce immunosuppression in these disorders? In an acute phase disorder, the risk of the immunosuppressive therapy is not one's primary concern, because high-dose or multiple therapy is going to be used for only a short period during the induction phase. But what about maintenance? Can we develop a strategy in which the doses are low enough for the 'Achilles heel' of ciclosporin, nephrotoxicity, to be avoided? Is the right approach to the maintenance program one of drug holiday, or triple therapy (azathioprine, ciclosporin and prednisone) with low doses of ciclosporin, or is interval therapy reasonable? All of these questions are, to some extent, not answerable until a fundamental challenge to basic science is met in these diseases. Our first requirement is to find a method in animals or humans by which we can move from an induction or maintenance immunosuppressive regimen into one that allows the state of autoregulation to re-express itself, and that doesn't lead to the accelerated re-activation of the disease, such as we have seen in some of these reports.

Future directions

The time of anecdotal experience with ciclosporin and autoimmune disease should largely be over. We now have to enter a phase of study in which, where possible, the following four criteria should be met: First of all, the disease should be studied in the phase in which benefit can be detected. To study when chronic disability is established, and then to try to measure clinically the anti-inflammatory effect, is to doom oneself to frustration, if not failure. Secondly, it is imperative that assays that measure the relevant immune response to the disease under study be developed. It could be an extraordinary contribution if our studies included not only the monitoring of drug levels to monitor compliance and toxicity, but also assays from which we could know with certainty that we were affecting the relevant immune response. Thirdly, clinical study protocols must be

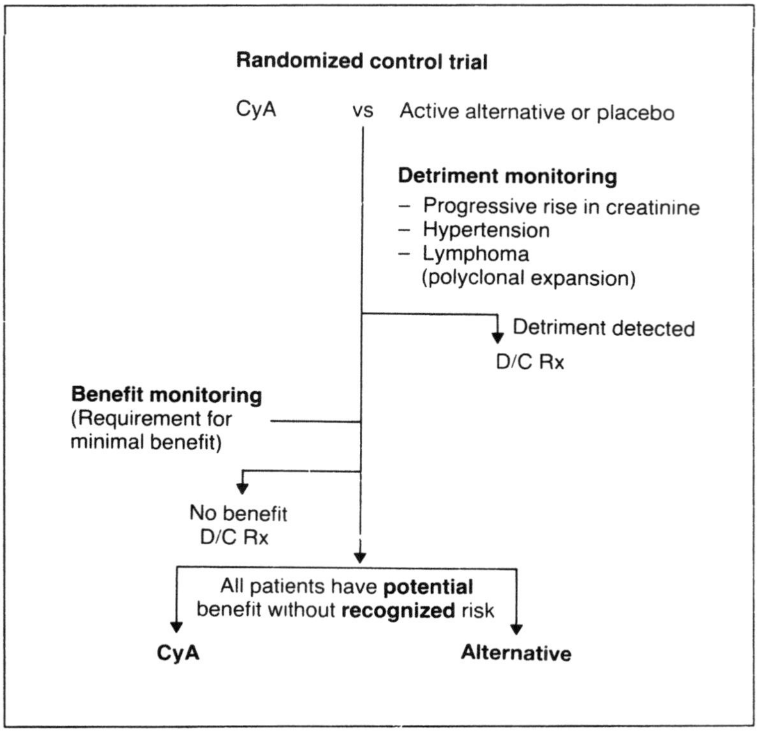

Fig. 9. General protocol for selection of lowest-risk patients in CyA clinical trials

developed that include frequent assessment, and elimination of those patients who have a potential for, or have demonstrated, risks of therapy, but do not have potential benefit. Figure 9 demonstrates such a general protocol. The diabetes studies are designed in this way and I believe the rheumatoid arthritis studies must also be of this design. Lastly, randomized controlled trials are necessary in all of these disorders! In terms of the design, where possible, ciclosporin should be tested against either an active alternative therapy or placebo, but with this agent 'detriment monitoring' should be included so that any progressive rise in creatinine, hypertension or polyclonal B cell expansion results in the patient's being withdrawn from therapy. At the end, one is left only with patients who have potential benefit without demonstrated risk. This is, after all, the way we practice medicine, and it is in this context that we should study the effects of ciclosporin.

In the multiplicity of anecdotal studies that we are of necessity dependent on for our opinions at this time, we are in danger of 'losing sight of the forest because of the trees' and dismissing ciclosporin as offering too little benefit for the risk involved. Standing back and looking at this from a little distance, I have no doubt that ciclosporin, or its derivatives, will have an important effect in autoimmune diseases. It has already demonstrated to us that diseases we thought were not likely to be amenable to immunosuppresive therapy may have exciting potential. We have been shown that the 'suspended animation' in which the immune response is held by ciclosporin in chronic inflammatory diseases is probably very *effective* (although that is different from benefical), and that to demonstrate it to be beneficial in the long term, chronic immunosuppressive therapy will be necessary. More importantly, we have seen that our only way to arrive at the truth in this area will be through objectivity, and studies that demand that of us will be the 'bench-mark' against which all future studies of ciclosporin will be measured.

Concluding Impressions

J. R. Batchelor

As I have, not surprisingly, come to very much the same conclusions as mentioned by Dr. Stiller, I shall deal with them briefly.

The first question that arises is: which diseases are likely to benefit from treatment with ciclosporin? It is my view that these should be the diseases in which there is cogent evidence that an abnormality of self-regulation of the immune response is present. For example, we have heard of some very appropriate animal examples, like the rat model of thyroid autoimmunity mentioned by McGregor. From this we can learn two things. The first is that only with early treatment of the autoimmune thyroiditis is permanent benefit obtained. The second is that only short-term treatment seems to be needed in these circumstances. Once down-regulation of the immune system is established, this usually remains unchanged. So we should be attempting to achieve the same effect in human diseases.

Which of the human diseases that we've heard about over the last few days would fit into that kind of category?

Insulin-dependent diabetes would seem to fit, but there are, of course, special problems. Clearly, so much damage to islets occurs before we ever see our patients that immunosuppressive therapy at that late stage presents very great difficulties.

In the case of Behçet's disease and uveitis, it seems to me very likely the anti-inflammatory effects of ciclosporin may be responsible for the effects seen. This perhaps explains why there is a strong rebound phenomenon when patients are taken off ciclosporin. It has not been possible, really, to establish the desired down-regulation of the immune response as a whole.

Department of Immunology, Royal Postgraduate Medical School, London, UK

In the case of SLE, it appears from the animal models that there are several different genetic abnormalities that are responsible for susceptibility to the disease. For example, it seems that the genetic defect in MRL mice is totally different from that in the NZB mouse and the BXSB. Whether any of these are relevant to the pathology of the human disease is uncertain. My own laboratory has reported evidence which suggests that deficiency or functional inefficiency of the C4 or C2 proteins of the classical pathway of complement are important predisposing causes of susceptibility [1]. Consequently, treating SLE with ciclosporin is probably not going to be the optimum therapy. Very carefully controlled trials are evidently going to be necessary to determine the answer.

Next, a few words about toxicity: this is clearly something that needs thought, and obviously the renal toxicity is what makes us most anxious. And what are the hopes for the future? Firstly, new variants of the drug may be less toxic. There is also the question that people may vary in susceptibility to this toxic effect. I believe that R. A. Sells and F. H. Bach have found substantial differences in toxicity of ciclosporin in different strains of mice. This direction of research is extremely important, and the results will be of great interest to us all. In addition, we should all be searching for limited-duration form of treatment. In this context, it seems that biliary cirrhosis may not be suitable for treatment with ciclosporin because of the long-term treatment required. The anomalous expression of Class II antigens during autoimmune diseases is known to occur on tissues which normally do not express these antigens. It might be of great importance to monitor the effect of ciclosporin on Class II antigen expression during long-term treatment with the drug.

Finally, the finding that prolactin and ciclosporin compete for the same receptor on the cell surface seems of great interest. It gives rise to many ideas. For example, there may be prolactin receptors on lymphocytes, which might explain the old observation that, normally, breast epithelial cells do not express Class II antigen but do so after lactation; also, competition of prolactin and ciclosporin for the same receptor might have something to do with the hair growth that occurs in some patients. One of the reports of toxic effects also included gynaecomastia, which again would seem to be related. This leads to questions about the effects of prolactin and pituitary hormones in general and their antagonists on the immune response, and whether these could be used to manipulate the immune response to the benefit of our patients.

Reference

1. Fielder AHL, Walport MJ, Batchelor JR, Rynes RI, Black CM, Dodi IA, Hughes GRV (1983) Family study of the major histocompatibility complex in patients with systemic lupus erythematosus: importance of null alleles of C4A and C4B in determining disease susceptibility. Br Med J 286:425–428

Subject Index

MIX
Papier aus verantwortungsvollen Quellen
Paper from responsible sources
FSC® C105338

If you have any concerns about our products,
you can contact us on
ProductSafety@springernature.com

In case Publisher is established outside the EU,
the EU authorized representative is:
Springer Nature Customer Service Center GmbH
Europaplatz 3, 69115 Heidelberg, Germany

Printed by Libri Plureos GmbH
in Hamburg, Germany